Paediatric Urology

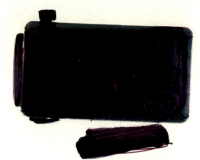

To Margaret and to Dorothy

Paediatric Urology
Second Edition

Edited by

D. Innes Williams
Director, British Postgraduate Medical Federation (University of London), London

J.H. Johnston
Urological Surgeon, Alder Hey Childrens Hospital, Liverpool

Butterworth Scientific

London   Boston   Sydney   Wellington   Durban   Toronto

First published 1968
Second edition 1982

© Butterworth & Co (Publishers) Ltd, 1982

British Library Cataloguing in Publication Data

Paediatric urology.–2nd ed.
  1. Pediatric urology 2. Genito-urinary organs–Diseases
  I. Williams, David Innes   II. Johnston, J.H.
  618.92′6   RJ466

  ISBN 0–407–35152–3

Phototypeset in 10/11 Baskerville by Scribe Design, Gillingham, Kent
Printed and bound by Mackays of Chatham Ltd

Preface to the Second Edition

This book was first published in 1968 under the editorship of D. Innes Williams and, although the rapidity of change in medical science is sometimes exaggerated, a new edition is clearly overdue. The scope of paediatric urology was defined in the 1960s and the groundwork of knowledge of the disorders to be treated was established, but the 1970s have seen a considerable increase in our understanding of the physiological aspects of urinary tract malformation and a much greater appreciation of the contributions that can be made to urology by other disciplines in medicine and science. The more diverse authorship of chapters in this new edition reflects our growing dependence upon the cooperative interests of our colleagues in nephrology, radiology, endocrinology, oncology and pathology, a reliance that has gone further in paediatric than in adult urology.

In clinical practice such collaborative work can only be fully achieved within a large hospital or a unit devoted to children. Both editors have been fortunate to work in such an environment and believe that the highest standards of paediatric urology can only be reached in such circumstances.

However, even in countries with advanced health care systems large numbers of children with urological disorders must be treated outside paediatric hospitals and this book is directed to all surgeons who undertake such work. Many will no doubt be urologists in training or in practice, whose chief concern is with adult disease; their continued interest in paediatrics is essential to the provision of appropriate care for the many children living long distances from specialized centres, but they also have a particular role to play in ensuring that the advances made in the more widely researched and better funded field of adult urology are applied to children's disorders. Equally, paediatric surgeons have a contribution to make to the treatment of urological disease and it is to be hoped that our book will be of value to them in training. For specialists outside surgery we aim at a reciprocal exchange of information. The urological surgeon needs to know something of oncology and similarly the oncologist must understand the problems and the possibilities of surgical treatment. This text is therefore intended for a wider audience than surgeons alone.

We are grateful to the various contributors to this volume for their cooperation in its production. Also we express our sincere thanks to the large number of junior staff and visitors in our respective departments who over many years have been involved in the management of patients, have helped in the assessment of results and, by their searching questions, have often stimulated reflection and research.

D. Innes Williams
J.H. Johnston

Contributors

Rosemarie A. Baillod, MB BS
First Assistant, Department of Nephrology and
Transplantation, Institute of Child Health,
London

T.M. Barratt, FRCP
Professor of Paediatric Nephrology, Institute of
Child Health, London;
Consultant Paediatric Nephrologist, Hospital
for Sick Children, Great Ormond Street and St.
Peter's Hospitals Group, London

Michael J. Dillon, MB, FRCP, DCH
Consultant Physician and Paediatric
Nephrologist, Hospital for Sick Children, Great
Ormond Street, London

Herbert B. Eckstein, MA, MD, MChir, FRCS
Consultant Paediatric Surgeon, Hospital for
Sick Children, Great Ormond Street, London
and Queen Mary's Hospital, Carshalton

Oswald N. Fernando, MB BS, DA, FRCS,
FRCS(Ed)
Consultant Surgeon, Department of Nephrology
and Transplantation, The Royal Free Hospital,
London

Isky Gordon, FRCR
Consultant Radiologist, Hospital for Sick
Children, Great Ormond Street, London

David B. Grant, MD, FRCP, DCH
Consultant Paediatric Endocrinologist, Hospital
for Sick Children, Great Ormond Street,
London

Frank Harris, MD, MMed, MB ChB, FRCP
Professor of Child Health, University of
Liverpool
Honorary Consultant Paediatrician, Alder Hey
Children's Hospital, Liverpool

Neville Harrison, MB BS, FRCS, LRCP,
DObstRCOG
Consultant Urologist, Royal Sussex County
Hospital, Brighton, Sussex

J.H. Johnston, MB, FRCS, FRCSI, FACS
Urological Surgeon, Alder Hey Children's
Hospital, Liverpool
Lecturer in Paediatric Urology, University of
Liverpool

John Martin, MB BS, FRCP, MRCS, DObstRCOG,
DCH
Consultant Paediatrician, Royal Liverpool
Children's Hospital and Alder Hey Children's
Hospital, Liverpool
Clinical Lecturer, Department of Child Health,
University of Liverpool

I.C.S. Norman, DM, FRCP
Professor of Child Health, University of
Southampton
Consultant Paediatrician, Southampton
General Hospital

P.G. Ransley, MA, MB BChir, FRCS
Consultant Urological Surgeon, Hospital for
Sick Children, Great Ormond Street and
St. Peter's Hospitals Group, London
Senior Lecturer in Paediatric Urology, Institute
of Child Health, University of London

Susan P.A. Rigden, MRCP
Lecturer in Paediatric Nephrology, Guy's
Hospital, London

R.A. Risdon, MD, FRCPath
Reader in Morbid Anatomy, The London
Hospital Medical College

Jean M. Smellie, DM, FRCP, DCH
Senior Lecturer in Paediatrics and Consultant
Paediatrician, University College Hospital,
London

D. Innes Williams, MD, MChir, FRCS
Director, British Postgraduate Medical
Federation, London

J.D. Williams, MD, BSc, MRCPath
Professor of Medical Microbiology, The London
Hospital Medical College

W. Keith Yeates, MD, MS, FR_S
Consultant Urologist, Newcastle University
Hospitals

Contents

1 Renal Function

T.M. Barratt

Introduction

The primary goal of the urologist is the preservation of renal function. With children there is an additional obligation to ensure optimum conditions for growth of the immature kidney. In this chapter basic aspects of renal physiology are not described because several accounts are readily available (Barratt, 1976). Instead the physiological development of the kidney, problems of assessment of renal function, metabolic aspects of young children and some fluid and electrolyte disturbances are reviewed.

Development of the kidney

Morphological aspects

Embryology

The pronephros develops in the human embryo during the third gestational week. Little is known of its function and it is rapidly superseded by the mesonephros which persists up to the 12th gestational week. The metanephros, which is the definitive kidney, is formed by the interaction of the ureteric bud arising from the lower end of the mesonephric duct with the nephrogenic blastema lying caudal to the mesonephros. The growing tip of the ureteric bud divides, undergoing 16 generations of branching, and secretes a substance that induces nephron formation in the blastema. Within the metanephros nephron development is centrifugal, the nephrogenic zone being in the outer cortex. The formation of new nephrons is essentially complete by the 36th week of gestation so that the full-term infant enters extrauterine life with his complete array of one million nephrons in each kidney (Potter and Thierstein, 1943; McCrory, 1972).

Postnatal growth

The combined weight of the kidneys at birth is approximately 25 g and this rises to 300 g in the adult. On the basis of DNA content Widdowson, Crobb and Milner (1972) concluded that the kidney of the full-term infant contains about 17 per cent of the adult number of cells. Net DNA synthesis ceases at 6 months of age and subsequent growth of the kidney is due to an increase in cell size rather than cell number. However, working on the rat kidney, Sands, Dobbing and Greatrix (1979) cast doubt on the neat division of phases of growth into hyperplasia characterized by an increase in cell number and hypertrophy in which there is an increase in cell size alone.

Microdissection studies show that the mean glomerular diameter in the middle cortical level of the neonatal kidney is 0.12 mm compared with an adult figure of 0.28 mm, whereas the proximal tubular length is only 1.73 mm in the neonate compared with 19.4 mm in the adult. The anatomical data suggest relative glomerular preponderance in the infant, and much of the increase in bulk of the kidney during early life is

1

due to growth of the proximal tubules, particularly in the most recently formed cortical nephrons (Fetterman *et al.*, 1965).

Renal function *in utero*

From the ninth week of gestation the metanephros secretes urine consisting essentially of an ultrafiltrate of plasma. In mid term there is still little tubular reabsorption of glomerular filtrate and the urinary flow rate is high (Alexander and Nixon, 1961); towards term salt and water reabsorption increases so that the urinary flow rate falls. The only known function of the fetal kidney is the maintenance of amniotic fluid volume: bilateral renal agenesis results in oligohydramnios with consequent intrauterine compression deformities and pulmonary hypoplasia but otherwise little disturbance of homeostasis because the placenta functions as an efficient kidney *in utero*.

Physiology of the infant kidney

Renal blood flow

Blood flow to the infant kidney is low compared to the adult organ, with a preferential distribution to the juxtamedullary area (Spitzer, 1978). During the first year of life there is a fourfold increase in the proportion of the cardiac output going to the kidneys, and the same phenomenon is evident whether renal blood flow is related to kidney weight or body surface area. Indirect estimation of renal plasma flow from the clearance of para-aminohippurate (PAH) is inaccurate, however, since the extraction of PAH is low, probably due to the higher fraction of renal blood flow perfusing medullary tissue. In the newborn puppy the ratio of blood flow in the superficial cortical nephrons to that in the juxtamedullary nephrons is 2:1, rising to 10:1 in the mature animal (Olbing *et al.*, 1973). Renal vascular resistance is high in the newborn and in the piglet it falls 10-fold during the first month of life (Gruskin, Edelmann and Yuan, 1970). Much of the rapid rise in renal blood flow in early life is due to the opening up of the vasculature in the superficial cortex.

Glomerular filtration

Inulin clearance, which is a measure of glomerular filtration rate (GFR), is low in relation to

Table 1.1 Glomerular filtration rate (ml/min per 1.73m^2 surface area) measured by inulin clearance in healthy individuals of different ages (data from Barratt and Chantler, 1975)

Age	GFR mean	GFR range ± 2 sd
Premature	47	29–65
2–8 days	38	26–60
4–28 days	48	28–68
35–95 days	58	30–86
1–5.9 months	77	41–103
6–11.9 months	103	49–157
12–19 months	127	63–191
2–12 years	127	89–165
Adult male	131	88–174
Adult female	117	87–147

body surface area or kidney weight during infancy (*Table 1.1*), principally due to the vascular factors described above. Permselectivity studies with polydisperse dextrans indicate restricted filtration of macromolecules by the neonatal glomerulus (Arturson, Groth and Grotte, 1971).

Proximal tubular function

The anatomical evidence of proximal tubular immaturity is reflected in decreased tubular reabsorption of endogenous amino acids, a low bicarbonate threshold and a low tubular maximum secretory capacity for PAH which is related to GFR. Data on the tubular maximum reabsorptive capacity for glucose are inconclusive. The excretion of low molecular weight protein, which is characteristic of renal tubular disease, is not a feature of the infant kidney, presumably because of a low filtered load resulting from the reduced permeability of the neonatal glomerulus to macromolecules (Barratt and Crawford, 1970).

Salt and water excretion

The infant kidney is less able than the adult organ to excrete a sodium load. For example, the fractional excretion of filtered sodium (sodium clearance/GFR) in an adult dog rises to 17 per cent following an infusion of isotonic saline 100 ml/kg body weight, but in a puppy only reaches 5 per cent (Goldsmith *et al.*, 1975). This phenomenon may be related to the diminished perfusion of the superficial nephrons which, with their short loops of Henle, are best adapted to the excretion of a sodium load.

During water diuresis the infant excretes a greater fraction of filtered water than the adult, suggesting that a larger proportion of the filtered sodium is reabsorbed by the distal nephron. The greater dependence on distal sodium reabsorption in the neonate is reflected in much higher plasma renin activity and aldosterone concentration (Dillon and Ryness, 1975) and in the more severe clinical expression of defects of mineralocorticoid biosynthesis such as congenital adrenal hyperplasia.

In response to water deprivation or exogenous ADH newborn infants concentrate their urine to only 600–700 mosmol/ℓ, whereas adults generally achieve 1200 mosmol/ℓ. This is largely due to low rates of urea excretion in neonates because the urinary concentrations of nonurea solutes are similar and the discrepancy is minimized by urea supplements or a high protein diet (Edelmann, Barnett and Tropkou, 1960).

Urinary excretion of acid

Infants tend to have a slightly lower plasma pH and bicarbonate concentration than adults. Although the bicarbonate threshold is also low in infants, data on the tubular maximum capacity to reabsorb bicarbonate are inconclusive because of the effects of concomitant volume expansion inherent in these studies. Immediately after birth there is a diminished urinary pH response to acidaemia, but by one week of age urinary pH values are as low as those of adults. Nevertheless net rates of acid excretion are low in babies because of low rates of excretion of phosphate and ammonia, which are the principal hydrogen ion acceptors. The infant excretes hydrogen ions in health at a rate close to maximum and has little reserve to cope with an acidotic stress.

Assessment of renal function

General considerations

Assessment of renal function in children with urological disorders necessitates care and familiarity with the methods, the precision and the sources of error of the techniques employed (Barratt, 1974a). Sick infants tolerate investigation poorly and methods that require repeated venepunctures, intravenous infusions or bladder catheterizations are rarely applicable in clinical practice. Problems arise with accurate timed urine collections because of losses and incomplete bladder emptying, and it is always prudent to check that creatinine excretion rates (urinary creatinine concentration times urinary flow rate) are of the expected order.

urinary creatinine concentration (mmol/kg body weight per day) = 0.132 + 0.004 × age (years) ± 0.026 (sd)

Allowance for body size

When evaluating renal function it is clear that some consideration must be given to the size of the individual as a whole. The problem of how to do so has not been satisfactorily resolved. It is customary to relate many physiological observations to body surface area, with a notional normal adult value of $1.73\,\text{m}^2$. On this basis most aspects of renal function appear immature, reaching 'adult' levels by the age of 2 years. However, the practice has insubstantial theoretical foundations. McCance and Widdowson (1952) proposed instead that it would be more logical to relate GFR to total body water, the domain over which the kidney exercises its excretory and regulatory function. A case can also be made for using extracellular fluid volume.

A similar problem arises in the estimation of surface area itself. The formula of Dubois and Dubois (1916) is commonly used, but it is based on meagre data in small infants.

surface area (cm^2) = weight $(\text{kg})^{0.425}$ × height $(\text{cm})^{0.725}$ × 71.84

The logarithmic transformation, which is convenient for pocket calculators, is

surface area (m^2) = antilog (0.425 log weight + 0.725 log height − 2.144)

An analysis of the estimation of surface area in infants was given by Haycock, Schwartz and Wisotsky (1978).

Glomerular function

There is no single test that gives an overall assessment of renal function, reflecting perhaps the bulk of functioning renal parenchyma. The GFR approaches this, but filtration equilibrium is achieved within the glomerular capillaries with reserve filtration area and therefore substantial damage to the glomerular capillary bed must occur before the GFR falls.

From the physiological point of view the glomeruli are ultrafilters and thus there are two functional expressions of damage, namely blockage, which is reflected in a fall in GFR, and leakage, which is manifested by the appearance in the urine of blood and protein. Assessment of leakage is described in Chapter 8. There are five tests commonly employed to assess GFR and they are ranked here in order of simplicity and inverse order of precision.

Plasma urea concentration

Urea production varies at least fourfold on conventional diets (see below). Urea clearance is less than GFR, due to back-diffusion, by an amount depending on the rate of urine flow. Thus metabolic factors are predominant in determining the plasma urea concentration. Although plasma urea concentration is deeply imbedded in the professional consciousness as a test of renal function, it is best discarded except as a measure of the degree of uraemia.

Plasma creatinine concentration

The plasma creatinine concentration is determined by the balance between creatinine production and creatinine clearance (excretion/plasma concentration). Creatinine production is a function of body weight (see above) and thus of the cube of height while creatinine clearance is related to body surface area and thus to the square of height. Hence plasma creatinine concentration rises with age (*Table 1.2*) and GFR can be predicted from the child's height and plasma creatinine concentration (Counahan *et al.*, 1976).

GFR/surface area (ml/min per $1.73\,\mathrm{m^2}$ surface area) = 38 height (cm)/plasma creatinine concentration ($\mu\mathrm{mol}/\ell$)

Measurement of plasma creatinine concentration in the laboratory has some technical problems, principally the detection of noncreatinine chromogens by the alkaline picrate reagent

Table 1.2 True plasma creatinine concentration ($\mu\mathrm{mol}/\ell$) measured by autoanalyser (data from Schwartz, Haycock and Spitzer, 1976)

| Age | Plasma creatinine concentration | | | |
| | Female | | Male | |
	mean	sd	mean	sd
1	31	4.4	36	8.8
2	40	6.2	38	10.6
3	37	7.0	40	9.7
4	41	10.6	40	9.7
5	40	9.7	44	9.7
6	42	9.7	46	10.6
7	47	10.6	48	12.3
8	47	9.7	50	12.3
9	48	9.7	52	14.1
10	48	11.4	54	19.4
11	53	11.4	55	12.3
12	52	11.4	57	14.1
13	55	12.3	60	18.5
14	57	11.4	63	21.1
15	59	19.4	67	19.4
16	57	13.2	65	22.0
17	62	17.6	70	15.8
18–20	63	16.7	81	15.0

used. Biochemistry laboratories serving paediatric urology departments should be encouraged to devote sufficient resources to providing a rapid, specific and reproducible service for plasma creatinine determination.

Creatinine clearance

This overestimates GFR as there is some tubular secretion of creatinine. It may be counterbalanced fortuitously by the tendency to overestimate plasma creatinine concentration due to noncreatinine chromogens. In some units a 24-hour urine collection is taken to minimize bladder emptying errors and to smooth out diurnal variation, but obviously the risks of urine losses are great and there are some advantages in short-term urine collections under diuretic conditions instead. Counahan *et al.* (1976) found that GFR could be predicted as accurately from the plasma creatinine concentration as from the 24-hour creatinine clearance, and there is therefore little to be gained from the additional burden of urine collection. However, there are circumstances in which the creatinine clearance rate is valuable, such as in divided renal function studies when the kidneys are drained separately, as an internal reference clearance for the assessment of for example phosphate or albumin excretion, and as an estimate of GFR where there is either muscle wasting with decreased creatinine production or oedema when single-shot techniques are inappropriate.

GFR estimates without urine collection

The difficulty inherent in accurate timed urine collections, particularly in children, has prompted research for other methods. Two are in current use, that is single-shot slope clearances and constant infusion techniques.

If a substance is rapidly mixed within its volume of distribution (V_D) and only cleared from the body by glomerular filtration, the GFR can be estimated from the rate of fall of plasma concentration after a single intravenous injection. Accurate measurement of low concentrations of the substance in plasma is essential and methods using radio-labelled compounds are generally the most suitable; ^{51}Cr-edetic acid (^{51}Cr-EDTA) and ^{99m}Tc-diethylene-triaminepentacetic acid (^{99m}Tc-DTPA) have proved useful. Several mathematical analyses are possible and the simplest requires only two blood samples 2 and 4 hours after the intravenous injection (Chantler and Barratt, 1972). The half-time ($t_{1/2}$) of the exponential disappearance is determined by plotting the plasma concentrations on a semilogarithmic scale, and an estimate of the volume of distribution is obtained by dividing the administered dose by the extrapolated zero-time plasma concentration. The GFR can then be calculated.

$$GFR = V_D \; \frac{0.693}{t_{1/2}}$$

This method has the merit of being very reproducible in the same individual, with a coefficient of variation of replicate GFR estimates that is 5 per cent. It is thus well suited to the detection of minor degrees of deterioration of renal function in urological patients.

If a substance cleared only by glomerular filtration is administered by constant intravenous infusion then in the equilibrium state the rate of infusion equals the rate of excretion. It can then be substituted in the clearance formula so that GFR can be calculated from the rate of infusion and the plasma concentration. The problem is that equilibrium may take a long time to achieve.

Inulin clearance

This remains the definitive method for determination of GFR against which all other techniques should be assessed. It requires constant intravenous infusion and accurately timed short periods of urine collection often necessitating catheterization, and the analytical methods are not easy.

Individual kidney GFR

In urological practice the need for an assessment of individual kidney function often arises. In these circumstances the relative function of the two kidneys is sufficient information, overall GFR being assessed in one of the ways described above. Clearly if urine from the two kidneys is draining separately then the divided creatinine clearance is a suitable measurement and opportunities to obtain such information should not be missed. Apart from this, methods of obtaining separate collections by ureteric catheterization or external occlusion are not convenient and radioisotopic means using 'area of interest' gamma camera analysis are most appropriate (*see* Chapter 2). In general such techniques depend on measurement of the rate of arrival of the radioisotope in the renal area and so depend on renal plasma flow rather than GFR.

Proximal tubular function

Renal glycosuria indicates a defect of proximal tubular function. Hypophosphataemia is suggestive as well, although it can also result from hyperparathyroidism or dietary phosphate depletion. A generalized aminoaciduria is characteristic, but perhaps the simplest screening test is detection in the urine of low molecular weight proteins such as beta$_2$-microglobulin or lysozyme (Barratt and Crawford, 1970) which are normally filtered by the glomerulus and reabsorbed by a pinocytic mechanism in the proximal tubule.

Urinary concentrating capacity

The capacity to concentrate the urine is an aspect of renal function very sensitive to urological disorders since it depends upon the integrity of the countercurrent system in the medulla. Obstructive uropathy in particular causes a major defect of urinary concentration. In most children over the age of 2 years deprived of fluid overnight the osmolality of the first urine specimen passed in the morning is over 900 mosmol/ℓ and a single such observation excludes a defect of urinary concentration. Formal and more prolonged water deprivation tests should be monitored closely so that the child does not lose more than 2–3 per cent of body weight. Under such circumstances normal children achieve a urinary osmolality of 1127 ± 128 (sd)mosmol/ℓ (Edelmann *et al.*, 1967a).

Failure to respond adequately to water deprivation can be due to pituitary or renal causes and the problem can be dissected further by observing the response to antidiuretic hormone (ADH). A synthetic analogue of ADH, D-deamino (8-D-arginine)vasopressin (DDAVP) is now generally used. It can be given by intranasal instillation of 10 µg in infants and 20 µg in older children (Aronson and Svenningsen, 1974), but if the response is inadequate there may be doubt as to whether the dose was properly administered. Thus intramuscular injection of 0.04 µg/kg body weight is preferable in critical cases. Urinary osmolality should rise above 750 mosmol/ℓ. In infants fluid intake should be restricted to match urine output and insensible losses in order to avoid the possibility of water intoxication.

Urinary acidification

The healthy kidney responds to metabolic acidosis by producing urine of pH less than 5.3 at any age with the exception of premature infants. A urinary pH less than 5.3 with a normal or only slightly reduced plasma bicarbonate concentration indicates an essentially normal acidification mechanism and certainly excludes distal renal tubular acidosis (*see* Chapter 29). Such an acidity is often found in the overnight urine specimen and obviates the need for further testing. Otherwise, ammonium chloride 75 mEq(4 g)/m^2 body surface area can be used as a moderate acid load, and the urinary pH should then fall below 5.3 (Edelmann *et al.*, 1967b). Urinary infection, particularly with Proteus, may interfere with urinary pH observations due to urea splitting and ammonia production.

Metabolic aspects of young children

Growth

The growing infant gains some 30 g in weight daily and of this approximately 25 g is water. About 1 g protein/kg body weight per day is incorporated into growing tissues and bone, along with sodium, potassium, calcium, phosphorus and other elements. In this respect growth relieves the kidney of an excretory load. McCance (1959) described growth as 'the third kidney' and reported protection from the effects of uraemia, hyperkalaemia and hyperphosphataemia by anabolism in the nephrectomized puppy (providing calorie intake was sufficient). The interaction of growth, calorie intake amd uraemia is further considered in Chapter 4.

Nutrition

A consideration of paramount importance in the metabolism of young children with renal disease is the difference in composition of human breast milk and cows' milk formulas (*Table 1.3*), even

Table 1.3   Representative dietary intakes and excretory loads expressed per kilogram body weight per day of infants on cows' milk and breast milk diets (data from Barratt, 1974b)

	Cows' milk	Breast milk
Water (ml)	150	100
Calories	100	100
Protein (g)	5	2
Sodium (mEq)	4	1
Potassium (mEq)	5	2
Phosphorus (mg)	150	23
Renal solute load (mosmol)	33	13
Hydrogen ion load (mEq)	6	1

though nowadays most of the artificial milks have protein and solute concentrations closer to those of human breast milk. The protein intake is more than twice as great from a cows' milk formula. Surplus protein not incorporated into growing tissues is broken down into urea, each gram of protein producing 0.3 g (5 mmol) of urea. With 1 g protein/kg per day being assimilated by growth then urea production on a protein intake of 2 g/kg per day is approximately 5 mmol/kg per day, whereas from a protein intake of 5 g/kg per day urea production is 20 mmol/kg per day. The implications for infants with chronic renal insufficiency are obvious.

The principal urinary solutes are urea, sodium, potassium and chloride and the solute load presented for excretion is determined by dietary intake and not by renal function. It can be estimated roughly in milliosmoles as **four** times the dietary protein intake in grams plus the dietary intake of sodium, potassium and chloride each expressed as milliequivalents (Ziegler and Fomon, 1971), and is thus 33 mosmol/kg per day in a baby fed cows' milk compared with 13 mosmol/kg per day in a breast-fed baby. With a conventional fluid intake urine volume is of the order of 100 ml/kg per day. Urinary osmolality in a breast-fed baby is thus about 130 mosmol/ℓ and in a baby fed cows' milk about 330 mosmol/ℓ. An infant who has lost the ability to concentrate the urine above 300 mosmol/ℓ, which is a defect commonly observed with urological disorders, is therefore in negative water balance on an intake of cows' milk of 150 ml/kg per day. He does not have effective thirst control and with impaired capacity to control urinary osmolality he has lost both limbs of the osmolar homeostatic mechanism. For such an infant cows' milk is like sea water for a shipwrecked sailor.

Body fluids and electrolytes

Water

Total body water (TBW) is 780 ml/kg in the full-term infant, falling to 600 ml/kg in the adult (Friis-Hansen, 1961). Extracellular fluid (ECF) is difficult to measure accurately or even to define with precision; it is generally taken to be the volume of distribution of a small solute whose intracellular concentration is negligible. The bromide space is easy to measure and amounts to 46 per cent of TBW in infants and 40 per cent in adults, but probably overestimates ECF by about 20 per cent (Barratt and Walser, 1969). Intracellular water (ICW) is taken as the difference between TBW and ECF.

The water intake of a baby is usually about 150 ml/kg per day. Of this about 25 ml/kg per day is incorporated into growing tissues and another 25 ml/kg per day is accounted for by insensible losses. Thus urine volume is about 100 ml/kg per day. Water balance is maintained by a homeostatic mechanism of which the afferent limb is ECF osmolality and the efferent limb is ADH which permits reabsorption of water from the collecting duct along the osmotic gradient established by the countercurrent system, thus reducing urine flow.

Sodium

The distribution of water between the intracellular and extracellular phases is determined by osmotic forces. Sodium and its attendant anion are the principal determinants of ECF osmolality. Therefore in states of salt and water depletion it is mainly ECF that is diminished, resulting in circulatory collapse, whereas with pure water depletion it is ICW that is decreased and the organ principally affected is the brain because of the volume constraints imposed by the skull. Conversely with pure water excess ICW is expanded, causing the syndrome of water intoxication, whereas salt and water excess increases ECF and leads to hypertension and oedema.

The concentration of sodium in ECF is determined by the relative amounts of sodium and water: a normal plasma sodium concentration is quite compatible with severe saline depletion or overload if there are equivalent changes in TBW. On the other hand hyponatraemia can imply water excess with normal body sodium levels (dilutional), sodium depletion with normal body water levels (depletional) or usually a mixture of the two. The distinction usually hinges upon a clinical assessment of ECF volume, particularly blood pressure. In equivocal cases a raised plasma renin activity is a helpful pointer to a state of sodium depletion.

Sodium excretion is determined ultimately by sodium intake and the need to maintain sodium balance. In states of sodium depletion urinary sodium can be reduced below 0.1 mEq/kg per day, except perhaps in premature infants. The afferent limb of the sodium homeostatic mechanism is responsive to ECF volume. The efferent limbs are the renin-angiotensin-aldosterone system, which controls distal tubular sodium absorption in exchange for potassium, and an as yet unidentified hormonal system (natriuretic hormone), which controls proximal tubular sodium reabsorption.

Potassium

Potassium is the principal intracellular cation. External potassium balance is under the control of the kidney and is regulated by aldosterone. If potassium excretion is impaired, as in renal failure, extracellular potassium concentration rises leading to dysfunction of cardiac muscle. With renal or gastrointestinal potassium losses ECF potassium concentration is initially maintained at the expense of intracellular potassium, which leaves the cell in exchange for hydrogen ions resulting in intracellular acidosis and extracellular alkalosis.

Hydrogen ions

Metabolism of a normal diet generates hydrogen ions in excess of bicarbonate, principally from breakdown of organic phosphates and sulphates. These hydrogen ions are excreted in the urine as titratable acidity and ammonium and amount to 1 mEq/kg per day in the breast-fed baby and as much as 6 mEq/kg per day in the infant fed cows' milk. Failure to excrete hydrogen ions results in a metabolic acidosis with a fall in plasma bicarbonate concentration. The change in ECF pH is minimized by compensatory hyperventilation (Kussmaul respiration) with hypocapnia.

Principles of parenteral fluid therapy

Parenteral fluid therapy is only indicated if the oral route is inadequate.

Correction of hypovolaemia

In states of circulatory collapse due to volume depletion 20 ml/kg body weight of blood, plasma or isotonic saline should be given rapidly.

Deficit replacement

If dehydration is perceptible then the water deficit is probably about 50 ml/kg, if moderate around 100 ml/kg, and if severe approximately 150 ml/kg. Probable deficits in infants with moderately severe dehydration are shown in *Table 1.4*. Deficits should be replaced over 4–6 hours, and more slowly in hypertonic states. Acidosis can be corrected simultaneously; a useful solution for isotonic dehydration with acidosis is sodium bicarbonate 4 mmol added to each 100 ml burette of 1/5N dextrose saline to give a final sodium concentration of 70 mEq/ℓ.

Maintenance requirements

The intravenous requirements for maintenance of fluid balance in infants are 120 ml/kg per day and approximately 2 mEq/kg per day of both sodium and potassium. About half this amount is required in the first few days of life and immediately after surgical operations. However, children with urological disorders frequently have defects of urinary concentration and sodium conservation so that they may not have the usual antidiuretic and antinatriuretic response to surgery. The practice of maintaining infants 'dry' in the postoperative period may not be appropriate for them.

Replacement of abnormal losses

Children with major defects of urinary concentration require a fluid intake up to 200 ml/kg per day. They may not tolerate preoperative restriction of oral fluids and may therefore need intravenous fluids during this period.

Excessive urinary sodium losses can, if not replaced, lead to salt and water depletion with secondary deterioration of renal function. This may occur dramatically after relief of urinary tract obstruction. In these circumstances the urinary sodium excretion usually rises in the postoperative period to about 2.5 mEq/kg per day (Ghazali and Barratt, 1974). Occasionally there is massive salt loss.

Nutrition

If it seems likely that there will be any delay in restitution of oral intake, early consideration should be given to the provision of amino acids, calories and vitamins parenterally (Harries, 1971).

References

Alexander, D.P. and Nixon, D.A. (1961) The foetal kidney. *British Medical Bulletin*, **17**, 112

Table 1.4 Probable deficits of water and electrolytes in moderately severe dehydration in infants (data from Dell, 1973)

Type of dehydration	Plasma sodium (mEq/ℓ)	Probable deficit (ml/kg)	(mEq/kg)
Hypertonic	>150	120–170	2–5
Isotonic	130–150	100–150	7–11
Hypotonic	<130	40–80	10–14

Aronson, A.S. and Svenningsen, N.W. (1974) DDAVP test for estimation of renal concentrating capacity in infants and children. *Archives of Disease in Childhood*, **49**, 654

Arturson, G., Groth, T. and Grotte, G. (1971) Human glomerular porosity and filtration pressure: dextran clearance analysed by theoretical models. *Clinical Science*, **40**, 137

Barratt, T.M. (1974a) Assessment of renal function in children. *In* Modern Trends in Paediatrics, 4th edn (edited by Apley, J.). Butterworths, London. p. 181

Barratt, T.M. (1974b) The nephrological background to urology. *In* Encyclopaedia of Urology, Vol. 15 (edited by Williams, D.I.). Springer, Heidelberg. Suppl. p. 1

Barratt, T.M. (1976) Fundamentals of renal physiology. *In* Scientific Foundations of Urology (edited by Williams, D.I. and Chisholm, G.D.). Heinemann, London. p. 19

Barratt, T.M. and Chantler, C. (1975) Clinical assessment of renal function. *In* Pediatric Nephrology (edited by Rubin, M.I. and Barratt, T.M.). Williams and Wilkins, Baltimore. p. 55

Barratt, T.M. and Crawford, R. (1970) Lysozyme excretion as a measure of renal tubular damage in children. *Clinical Science*, **39**, 457

Barratt, T.M. and Walser, M. (1969) Extracellular volume in individual tissues and whole animals: the distribution of radiosulfate and radiobromide. *Journal of Clinical Investigation*, **48**, 56

Chantler, C. and Barratt, T.M. (1972) Estimation of glomerular filtration rate from the plasma clearance of 51-chromium edetic acid. *Archives of Disease in Childhood*, **47**, 613

Counahan, R., Chantler, C., Ghazali, S., Kirkwood, B., Rose, F. and Barratt, T.M. (1976) Estimation of glomerular filtration rate from plasma creatinine concentration in children. *Archives of Disease in Childhood*, **51**, 875

Dell, R.B. (1973) Pathophysiology of dehydration. *In* The Body Fluids in Pediatrics (edited by Winters, R.W.). Little, Brown, Boston. p. 134

Dillon, M.J. and Ryness, J.M. (1975) Plasma renin activity and aldosterone concentration in children. *British Medical Journal*, iv, 316

Dubois, D. and Dubois, E.F. (1916) Clinical calorimetry: a formula to estimate the approximate surface area if height and weight be known. *Archives of Internal Medicine*, **17**, 863

Edelmann, C.M., Barnett, H.L. and Tropkou, V. (1960) Renal concentrating mechanism in newborn infants: effect of dietary protein and water content, role of urea and responsiveness to antidiuretic hormone. *Journal of Clinical Investigation*, **39**, 1062

Edelmann, C.M., Barnett, H.L., Stark, H., Boichis, H. and Rodriguez-Soriano, J. (1967a) A standardised test of renal concentrating capacity in infants and children. *American Journal of Diseases in Childhood*, **114**, 639

Edelmann, C.M., Boichis, H., Rodriguez-Soriano, J. and Stark, H. (1967b) The renal response of children to acute ammonium chloride acidosis. *Pediatric Research*, **1**, 452

Fetterman, G.H., Shuplock, N.A., Philipp, F.J. and Gregg, H.S. (1965) The growth and maturation of human glomeruli and proximal convolutions from term to adulthood: studies by microdissection. *Pediatrics*, **35**, 601

Friis-Hansen, B. (1961) Body water compartments in children: changes during growth and related changes in body composition. *Pediatrics*, **28**, 169

Ghazali, S. and Barratt, T.M. (1974) Sodium excretion after relief of urinary tract obstruction. *British Journal of Urology*, **46**, 373

Goldsmith, D.I., Drukker, A., Blaufox, M.D., Spitzer, A. and Edelmann, C.M. (1975) Response of the neonatal canine kidney to acute saline expansion. *In* Radionuclides in Nephrology (edited by Zum Winkel, K., Blaufox, M.D. and Funck-Brentano, J.L.). Thieme, Stuttgart. p. 45

Gruskin, A.B., Edelmann, C.M. and Yuan, S. (1970) Maturational changes in renal blood flow in piglets. *Pediatric Research*, **4**, 7

Harries, J.T. (1971) Intravenous feeding in infants. *Archives of Disease in Childhood*, **46**, 855

Haycock, G.B., Schwartz, G.J. and Wisotsky, D.H. (1978) Geometric method for measuring body surface area: a height and weight formula validated in infants, children and adults. *Journal of Pediatrics*, **93**, 62

McCance, R.A. (1959) The maintenance of chemical stability in the newly born: chemical exchange. *Archives of Disease in Childhood*, **34**, 361

McCance, R.A. and Widdowson, E.M. (1952) The correct physiological basis by which to compare infant and adult renal function. *Lancet*, ii, 860

McCrory, W.W. (1972) Developmental Nephrology. Harvard University Press, Cambridge

Olbing, H., Blaufox, M.D., Aschinberg, L.C., Silkalns, G.I., Bernstein, J., Spitzer, A. and Edelmann, C.M. (1973) Post-natal changes in blood flow distribution in puppies. *Journal of Clinical Investigation*, **52**, 2885

Potter, E.L. and Thierstein, S.T. (1943) Glomerular development in the kidney as an index of fetal maturity. *Journal of Pediatrics*, **22**, 695

Sands, J., Dobbing, J. and Greatrix, C.A. (1979) Cell number and cell size: organ growth and development and the control of catch-up growth in rats. *Lancet*, ii, 503

Schwartz, G.J., Haycock, G.B. and Spitzer, A. (1976) Plasma creatinine and urea concentration in children. Normal values for age and sex. *Journal of Pediatrics*, **88**, 830

Spitzer, A. (1978) Renal physiology and functional development. *In* Pediatric Kidney Disease (edited by Edelmann, C.M.). Little, Brown, Boston. p. 25

Widdowson, E.M., Crabb, D.E. and Milner, R.D.G. (1972) Cellular development of some human organs before birth. *Archives of Disease in Childhood*, **47**, 652

Ziegler, E.E. and Fomon, S.J. (1971) Fluid intake, solute load and water balance in infancy. *Journal of Pediatrics*, **78**, 561

2 Renal Diagnostic Imaging

Isky Gordon

Diagnostic imaging of the upper urinary tract has changed considerably over the last 10 years. In radiology fast film/screen combinations have been introduced allowing a significant reduction in radiation dose for all abdominal radiography. Simultaneously the development of other methods of imaging has made great progress. Recent advances in ultrasound can give an accurate delineation of structures in the neonatal abdomen and even in the fetus. The introduction of ^{99m}Tc radioisotopic studies allows a pathophysiological assessment of renal function. Computed tomography (CT) scanning is the newest modality of imaging available; new CT scanners will take less than 2 seconds per cut.

With these new techniques available in many hospitals there has been a reappraisal of renal imaging with the emphasis on an integrated approach which is necessary because of the different information provided by each modality. Ultrasound, radiology and CT scanning all give excellent anatomical detail while pathophysiological information is more accurately obtained with radioisotopes. There is thus the possibility of providing specific answers to clinical problems if the appropriate investigation or sequence of investigations is carried out.

Radiology

Radiology has been the backbone of imaging for the urologist over many decades. The intravenous urogram (IVU) is still an investigation invaluable to all urologists, but as other imaging techniques are developed the specific place of intravenous urography has become more clearly defined in particular clinical settings. Other simple radiographic techniques remain essential to the initial assessment and also to the follow-up of urological patients. For example radiographs of the hand and the knee are a sensitive index of renal osteodystrophy, and chest X-ray is the routine screening examination for patients suspected of having a Wilms' tumour or being followed up both during and after treatment of one.

IVU preparation and technique

A hungry dehydrated paediatric patient is an unhappy uncooperative child. Moreover in any paediatric urology clinic there are always a certain number of patients in chronic renal failure and so neither food nor liquid should be withheld. Rather, the parents should be encouraged to limit fluid intake and to give the child a *light* meal 2–3 hours before the examination. No specific bowel preparation is attempted. Sedation is very rarely required since a parent or guardian stays with the patient throughout the examination.

Using the less concentrated contrast media such as Hypaque 45 per cent or Conray 280 a maximum dose of 4 ml/kg can be administered intravenously, but 2 ml/kg usually suffices. Control radiographs are essential. After receiving intravenous contrast medium the patient is given a drink. A coned view of the renal areas is obtained within 2–4 minutes of completion of

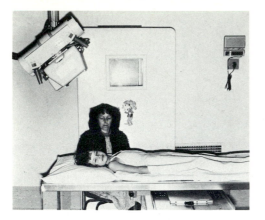

Figure 2.1. X-ray tube angled for the renal window view.

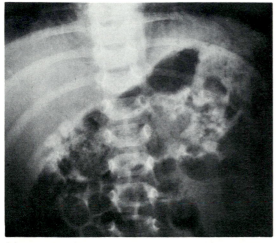

(a)

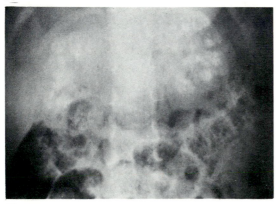

(b)

Figure 2.2. (*a*) This 2-year-old girl was known to have distal renal tubular acidosis. This is the coned control radiograph before the IVU. (*b*) The renal window view following the injection of contrast medium shows both kidneys to better advantage and the generalized nephrocalcinosis is clearly seen.

the injection. If this fails to show the renal outlines completely, a 'renal window' view is obtained between 7–10 minutes. For this the X-ray tube is angled at 35 degrees to the child's feet and centred on the xiphisternum (*Figure 2.1*) and the film is moved towards the feet by an appropriate distance. Such a radiograph enables the left kidney to be visualized through the gas-filled stomach and the right kidney through the liver. The small bowel and large bowel gas shadows are projected over the bony pelvis (*Figure 2.2*). This view frequently removes the necessity for tomography (Lucas, 1979).

If the course of the ureters is specifically relevant, a full-length film including the bladder is obtained at 5–7 minutes after the intravenous injection (*Figure 2.3*).

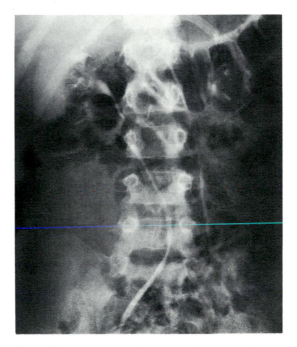

Figure 2.3. Retroperitoneal sarcoma. This 7-year-old girl presented with weakness on walking. Examination revealed fullness of the right side of the abdomen. The 7-minute full-length film reveals the displaced right ureter and demonstrates the normal left ureter as well.

A 'limited' or 'single-shot' IVU is adequate when certain follow-up patients are seen. Its disadvantage is that the renal outlines may not be visualized and therefore the appearance or progression of a renal scar cannot be followed adequately. However, the technique is very useful in those patients whose kidneys and upper collecting systems are normal at the outset, for example children with meningomyelocele or bladder pathology.

Antegrade pyelogram

Although a requirement for this investigation is relatively uncommon there is a clear-cut clinical indication. When there is dilatation of the upper collecting system but no lower ureter is seen on either the IVU or ultrasound then the level of the obstruction remains in doubt. Antegrade pyelographic injection is carried out under general anaesthesia immediately prior to formal surgical repair of the hydronephrosis. The patient is placed prone and under fluoroscopic control after intravenous injection of contrast medium a needle is inserted into the dilated calyx draining the lower pole. The major contraindication is a solitary kidney, since there is always some risk of haemorrhage.

Retrograde pyelogram

The indications for this procedure have decreased remarkably with the introduction of other imaging modalities. Nevertheless, retrograde pyelography is still indicated when adequate visualization of the upper collecting system has not been obtained. This is most frequently seen in children presenting in severe chronic renal failure without distended upper collecting systems. Rarely, malignancy or other pathology may be suspected in the nondistended renal pelvis or ureter of a good functioning kidney and when no other investigation has removed the clinical suspicion a retrograde pyelogram is decisive.

Catheter studies

Following surgical drainage, wherever an indwelling catheter is left *in situ* postoperatively a contrast examination can be carried out to ensure adequate emptying. This is useful when upper tract drainage has been performed at the time of urethral valve surgery (*Figure 2.4*).

Arteriography

This invasive investigation carries a significant morbidity rate due to damage to the intima of

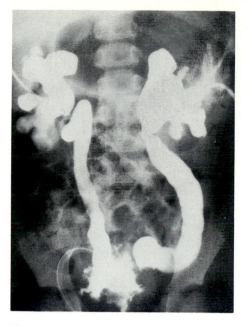

Figure 2.4. Urethral valves with bilateral ureterovesical junction obstruction. This 6-year-old boy presented in renal failure on peritoneal dialysis with the diagnosis of probable urethral valves. Despite continuous bladder catheter drainage the boy did not improve. Following bilateral nephrostomies this bilateral nephrostogram study was undertaken which shows secondary ureterovesical junction obstruction bilaterally.

the femoral artery, and some risk of fatality. Under the age of 10 years a general anaesthetic is required. Morbidity seems to be related to the age of the child, the period the catheter is in the artery and the skill of the radiologist. In general the smallest catheter capable of giving diagnostic images is used. A free-flush aortic injection is first carried out followed by selective renal arterial catheterization (Kirks, Firz and Harwood-Nash, 1976).

Arteriography is indicated chiefly in cases of suspected tumour and in trauma. When renal masses are found bilaterally and shown on ultrasound to be solid, or a mass lesion is discovered in a horseshoe kidney, in crossed fused renal ectopia, or in a solitary kidney, arteriography is required to delineate the exact arterial supply so that a partial nephrectomy can be considered (*Figure 2.5*). Selective arteriography does not, however, provide a reliable pathological diagnosis since a Wilms' tumour can show up as a relatively avascular mass

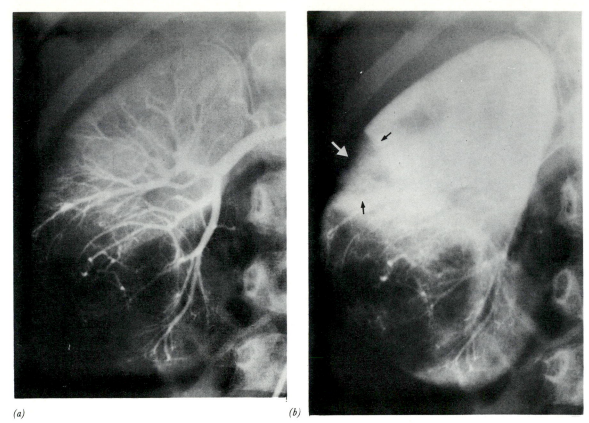

(a) *(b)*

Figure 2.5. Bilateral sequential Wilms' tumour. This 5-year-old girl had a left nephrectomy 18 months prior to this admission for a Wilms' tumour. She now presented in acute renal failure with haematuria and anuria with an expanded lower pole of the right kidney on the IVU, which on ultrasound appeared solid. The diagnosis of a sequential Wilms' tumour was made. (*a*) The early phase of this right selective renal arteriogram demonstrates the presence of an intrarenal mass in the lower pole displacing the arteries. (*b*) The late phase shows that this area is relatively avascular with only one or two abnormal vessels present. A second avascular area is seen in the peripheral aspect of the middle portion of the kidney which is avascular on the earlier phase (arrowed). This avascular area is supplied by the upper pole renal artery. Partial nephrectomy was ruled out and the patient was treated with cytotoxics. Exploration 1 year later revealed a scar in the middle portion of the right kidney and a renal mass was enucleated from the lower pole.

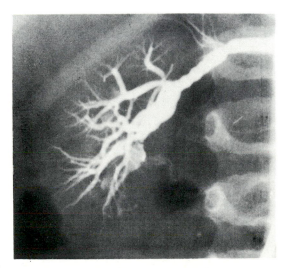

Figure 2.6. Fibromuscular hyperplasia. This child was found to have hypertension. The IVU was normal. This selective right renal arteriogram shows irregular areas of narrowing in the main renal artery as well as short narrow segments in the intrarenal vessels.

without malignant circulation and the possibility of a hamartomatous lesion cannot be excluded (Damascelli *et al.*, 1980; Andresen, Madsen and Steenskov, 1981).

When haematuria follows blunt trauma and does not settle with conservative management, or when the kidney is pyelographically nonfunctioning and the situation is not clarified by ultrasound, an arteriogram helps to plan surgery.

Other indications include hypertension (*Figure 2.6*) and suspected polyarteritis nodosa.

Radioisotopic studies

Images obtained by gamma camera after the injection of radiopharmaceuticals containing gamma emitting nuclides have revolutionized renal and skeletal diagnostic investigation during the last decade. Those radiopharmaceuticals effectively concentrated by the kidneys are agents labelled with ^{99m}Tc which emits single gamma rays of 140 keV and has a half-life of 6 hours. This radioisotope is eluted as pertechnetate from readily available molybdenum generators. Kits are available so that ^{99m}Tc labelling of different compounds can be undertaken in the hospital pharmaceutical laboratory. Sterility throughout the radiolabelling process is essential.

Dose of radioisotopes

A standard graph of body surface area versus fraction of adult dose is the basis of the calculation (*Table 2.1*). The surface area is calculated from the child's weight so that the fractional adult dose can be read directly from the graph.

Dynamic renal scan

^{99m}Tc-diethylenetriaminepentaceticacid (^{99m}Tc-DTPA) is filtered by the glomeruli of the kidney

and is neither reabsorbed nor excreted by the tubules. Injected intravenously as a bolus it gives accurate information on renal perfusion and glomerular filtration rate (GFR), and the collecting systems are also visualized. Its short half-life allows sequential scans at 48-hour intervals to assess perfusion and/or filtration when indicated, for instance following renal transplantation. No patient preparation is required.

The child is placed supine on a 1 cm foam mattress covering the camera face. Sedation is seldom required since the child is accompanied by a parent or a nurse, but a half-body vacuum immobilizer is useful with wriggly 2–4 year olds. A rapid intravenous bolus injection is made and the tubing flushed with saline; following the injection the study is recorded for 30 minutes.

When a computer is part of the system, recording should be continuous throughout the period. If only videotape is available then the first 7 minutes should be recorded with further information added at 10, 15 and 20 minutes. The films obtained show the following:

1. Blood pool images of the kidneys from 0–30 seconds
2. A renal image at 1 minute for 300 000 counts, noting the time
3. With the preset time of (2) images at 5, 10, 15 and 20 minutes. If possible, the bladder should be included (*Figure 2.7*).

The data available from the scan can be anatomical or physiological. The first anatomical information concerns the inferior vena cava. If the radioisotope is injected into a foot vein, which is our practice in a child with an abdominal mass or in acute renal failure, the patency and position of the inferior vena cava are seen routinely on the blood pool image (*Figure 2.10b*).

The image at 1 minute with normal renal function or later with diminished function outlines the functioning renal parenchyma. Normal calyces are not visualized and the renal pelvis is imaged at 4–5 minutes after the intravenous

Table 2.1   Radioisotope doses

	Adult dose (mCi)	Minimum dose (mCi)
^{99m}Tc-diethylenetriaminepentacetic acid (DTPA)	2.0	0.5
^{99m}Tc-dimercaptosuccinic acid (DMSA)	3.0	0.4
^{99m}Tc-methylene diphosphonate (MDP) (bone scan) 1 year plus	10.0	1.0
less than 1 year	7.5	1.0
^{99m}Tc-colloid (bone marrow)	3.0	0.5

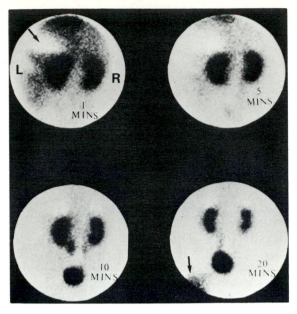

Figure 2.7. This 18-month-old girl with hypertension had a normal ^{99m}Tc-DTPA scan. The 1-minute image reveals the functioning renal parenchyma. The photon-deficient area above the left kidney (arrowed) probably represents a full stomach. The 5-minute image shows the radioisotope moving from the renal parenchyma into the collecting system. The 10-minute and 20-minute images show the progressive decrease in activity in the kidneys and the collecting systems with the radioisotope accumulating progressively in the bladder. The radioisotope below and to the left of the bladder on the 20-minute image lies in the nappy (arrowed).

injection. Often radioisotope is seen in the bladder on the 5-minute or 10-minute image, especially in neonates and infants with normal renal function. In the presence of dilated collecting systems delayed images are essential.

The ^{99m}Tc-DTPA scan is a measure of renal perfusion and GFR at the time it is carried out. All biochemical tests are a reflection of renal function over the 6–12 hours prior to the blood being obtained. The total dose of ^{99m}Tc-DTPA is usually contained in less than 1 ml of fluid and the solute load is therefore negligible even for neonates.

To assess perfusion and/or differential function, regions of interest (ROIs) over each renal area are marked and time-activity curves are generated. Background subtraction is also carried out. Only when a computer is available can the renal parenchyma be marked as an ROI separate from the ROI of the renal pelvis. When two ROIs can be obtained for each kidney, deconvolutional analysis can be performed so

that retention function can be determined (Diffey, Hall and Corfield, 1977; Britton, 1978). The objectives of this data analysis are to assess:

Renal time-activity curves (the renogram)

With background subtraction these curves show a characteristic shape. Phase one is the rapidly rising part usually lasting 30 seconds and is followed by phase two which shows a slower rise and lasts for up to 5 minutes ending in a peak. Phase three follows the peak; this is the phase of decreasing activity in the normal kidney. Phase one reflects renal perfusion and is a sensitive index for monitoring transplanted kidneysn (Hilson *et al.*, 1978). Phase two reflects glomerular filtration and phase three the emptying rate of the collecting system. Phase three can only be interpreted when the renogram up to the peak has been normal, that is there has been a peak.

Individual renal function

The parameters that can be determined quantitatively are the uptake and excretory functions of each kidney. Individual kidney GFR can be calculated if a 20-minute blood sample is obtained and detailed analysis applied to the renal curves (Piepsz *et al.*, 1978). Renal transit times can also be calculated from deconvolutional analysis. Obstructive uropathy has been distinguished by this method from obstructive nephropathy in an attempt to define which patients require surgery for obstruction (Whitfield *et al.*, 1978) but this work has not been validated in paediatric practice. Differential renal function can be calculted during phase two of the renogram, namely between 1.5–3 minutes after bolus injection. Background subtraction is also carried out over the same period (Pors Nielsen, Lehd Moller and Trap-Jensen, 1977; Tamminen, Ruhimaki and Tahti, 1978).

GFR

Using the same technique as with ^{51}Cr-edetic acid, an accurate GFR can be calculated using ^{99m}Tc-DTPA. The amount of ^{99m}Tc-DTPA injected must be accurately calculated and blood samples are obtained at 2 and 4 hours.

Dilatation of the collecting system

In an attempt to exclude obstruction in the

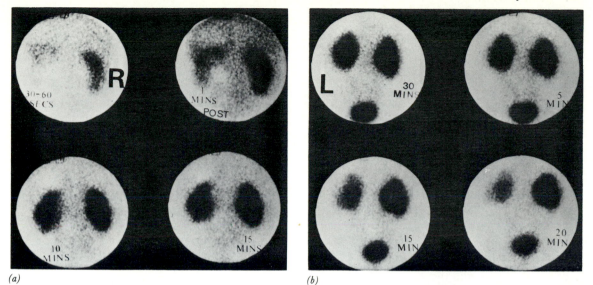

(a)   *(b)*

Figure 2.8. A ^{99m}Tc-DTPA scan with frusemide in pelviureteric junction obstruction. This 6-year-old boy was investigated for recurrent right-sided abdominal pain. He had a left pyeloplasty for a left pelviureteric junction obstruction 2 years prior to this examination. (*a*) The image between 30–60 seconds reveals the right kidney to be better perfused than the left. The 1-minute image shows that the right kidney accumulates the radioisotope more promptly than the left and the functioning renal parenchyma on the right is larger than on the left. Radioisotope can be seen in the collecting systems on both sides at 10 and 15 minutes with a progressive accumulation in the renal pelves. (*b*) The 30-minute image was obtained immediately prior to the injection of frusemide 20 mg intravenously. The images 5, 15 and 20 minutes after frusemide reveal significant washout of the radioisotope from the left kidney but no change in the right renal pelvis. A significant obstruction at the right pelviureteric junction was found at surgery.

presence of dilatation we routinely use intravenous frusemide 20–40 mg when the collecting systems have filled with radioisotope. A delayed image (250 K) of the renal areas, including as much of the bladder as possible, is obtained; the frusemide is then injected and images are obtained 5, 10 and 20 minutes afterwards (O'Reilly *et al.*, 1978). When there is dilatation of the collecting systems without obstruction the diuresis washes the radioisotope out of the renal tract. When an obstruction is present then frusemide has little or no effect (*Figures 2.8 and 2.9*).

Vesicoureteric reflux

Useful results are obtained from images taken during micturition at 3 hours after ^{99m}Tc-DTPA. In some institutions this is becoming the routine follow-up investigation in certain groups of patients, for example those with proven vesicoureteric reflux who are treated conservatively. The cooperation of the child is crucial.

Indications for dynamic scans

There is no other noninvasive method that can

accurately monitor various parameters of individual kidney function. If an obstruction has been diagnosed, preoperative and postoperative scans assess the effect of surgery. When renal damage has occurred, for example in reflux nephropathy or renal venous thrombosis, sequential scans assess individual renal function. In the case of urinary diversion the dynamic scan with frusemide allows more accurate assessment of both individual kidney function and the drainage from the kidneys.

It must be remembered that since the dynamic scan is dependent on renal function poor results are obtained in severe renal failure. ^{123}I-Hippuran is more useful in this situation but there is a level beyond which dynamic renal scans are of no use, usually when the serum creatinine level is above 500 μmol/ℓ.

Static renal scan

In the presence of poor renal function a high dose IVU frequently fails to provide the necessary information even with the use of tomography. This high dose IVU is not only unpleasant but also subjects the patient to a prolonged

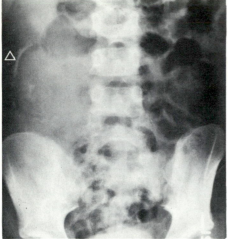

(a)

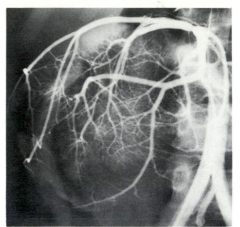

(e)

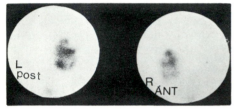

(b)

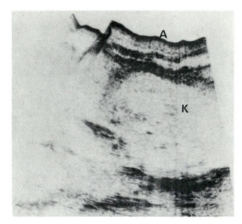

(c)

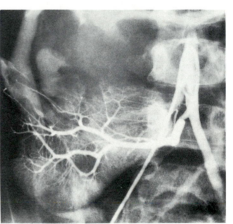

(f)

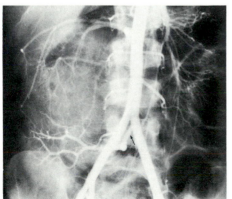

(d)

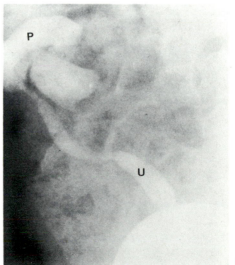

(g)

examination with a relatively high radiation dose. It is in this setting that ^{99m}Tc-dimercaptosuccinic acid (^{99m}Tc-DMSA) plays an important role. Other indications for its use include the small kidney as well as deteriorating renal function in the absence of dilated collecting systems (Bingham and Maisey, 1978). Accurate documentation and follow-up of renal scarring have been reported, showing that the ^{99m}Tc-DMSA scan is more accurate than the IVU (Merrick, Uttley and Wild, 1980). It may provide a sensitive index of segmental renal ischaemia in hypertension and is also useful in the presence of an intrarenal mass (*Figure 2.11*).

If relevant, for intravenous injection of ^{99m}Tc-DMSA a foot vein may be used so that the inferior vena cava is outlined. Scans of the abdomen are carried out approximately 2 hours later and posterior and oblique views are routine. With a horseshoe or pelvic kidney an anterior image is essential. Following intravenous injection approximately 50 per cent of the administered dose is localized in the kidneys by 1 hour and there is a very high cortical to medullary ratio. In the presence of obstruction, however, a ^{99m}Tc-DMSA scan may give false results because of excessive radioisotope in the dilated collecting system.

This investigation can provide information regarding both renal anatomy and renal function. Functioning renal parenchyma takes up the radioisotope. Renal function must be very poor for no renal image to be obtained and so focal or general loss of renal substance can be identified. Bowel gas is never a problem (*Figure 2.9b*).

Differential renal function can be assessed if the data are recorded from the posterior image. Data from the individual kidneys can then be used to calculate function in the same way as described for ^{99m}Tc-DTPA scans.

Bone scans

For a long time radioisotopic bone scans have been known to be more sensitive than radiographs in detecting metastases. However, in children—where neuroblastoma is often concerned—there may be diffuse marrow infiltration and in such circumstances controversy has arisen as to the value of the radioisotopic bone scan compared to a skeletal survey. If only the highest quality bone-scan images are accepted and close attention is given to the appearances of the metaphyses relative to the patient's skeletal maturity then the accuracy of bone scans increases significantly. At present all patients with neuroblastoma undergo a radiographic skeletal survey, a radioisotopic bone scan and also a radioisotopic bone marrow scan.

For the bone scan ^{99m}Tc-methylene diphosphonate (^{99m}Tc-MDP) is injected intravenously as a bolus. When indicated a foot injection can outline the inferior vena cava (*Figure 2.17*). Scans of the entire body including the extremities are obtained at 2 hours. The need for sedation is assessed at the time of the intravenous injection and if necessary diazepam is given intramuscularly 20 minutes before scanning.

For the bone marrow scan ^{99m}Tc-colloid is injected intravenously and the skeleton scanned 2 hours later.

Neuroblastoma is the only intra-abdominal mass that may take up ^{99m}Tc-MDP when there is no calcification in the tumour. When a 'hot' area is seen in the abdomen on a bone scan a confident diagnosis of neuroblastoma can thus be made (*Figure 2.10*).

An abnormal skeleton can be focally or generally affected. The metaphyses may simply show an increase in radioactivity which, if symmetrical, can lead the unwary to consider the bone scan normal. Focal hot areas may also be seen.

The ^{99m}Tc-colloid bone marrow scan can demonstrate patchy uptake of the radioisotope with a normal ^{99m}Tc-MDP bone scan. The author has seen a normal bone scan in the presence of an abnormal skeletal survey and

Figure 2.9. Xanthogranulomatous pyelonephritis in crossed fused renal ectopia, investigated by a sequence of imaging techniques. A retarded 7-year-old girl presented with diarrhoea and vomiting, and a right-sided intra-abdominal mass was felt. (*a*) This 10-minute IVU reveals distorted calyces in a rather low-lying kidney. The calyces are rather laterally located. (*b*) The ^{99m}Tc-DMSA scan reveals nonhomogeneous distribution of the radioisotope in the right kidney. The kidney lies abnormally low, close to the bladder and no left kidney is seen. (*c*) This is a longitudinal prone view of the right kidney on ultrasound demonstrating tissues of different echogenicity within the kidney (K). A = anterior abdominal wall. (*d*) Free-flush aortic injection reveals a right renal artery arising at L1–L2 and supplying the upper two-thirds of the renal substance. The second renal artery supplying the lower pole arises from the left common iliac artery (arrowed). (*e*) Selective right renal arterial injection reveals rather patchy perfusion of the right kidney but no definite pathological vessels. (*f*) This shows a relatively normal lower pole to the renal substance on selective angiography. The angiogram confirmed that this was a crossed fused renal ectopia. (*g*) The micturating cystogram reveals reflux into the right ureter and demonstrates the abnormal calyces and pelvis. An open biopsy confirmed the presence of xanthogranulomatous pyelonephritis in this crossed fused ectopia.

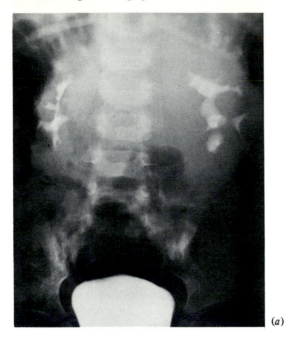

(a)

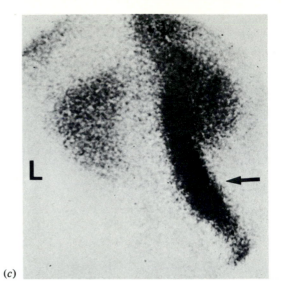

(c)

Figure 2.10. Neuroblastoma. This 18-month-old boy presented with abdominal swelling, diarrhoea for 4 days and general malaise. (*a*) The IVU shows a central abdominal mass compressing the left kidney and rotating the right kidney. (*b*) The radioisotopic bone scan shows the inferior vena cava displaced to the right by the mass at the time of injection (arrowed). (*c*) The scan of the lumbar spine at 2 hours shows homogeneous distribution of the radioisotope in the spine. Both kidneys are seen and above the left one there is an area of radioactivity due to the presence of tumour (arrowed). Biopsy proved this abdominal mass to be a neuroblastoma.

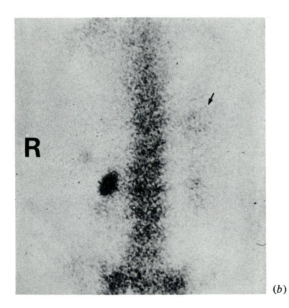

(b)

therefore feels these examinations are complementary and not mutually exclusive.

Ultrasound

Recent advances in ultrasound have resulted in high quality images with a resolution of 2–3 mm. No specific paediatric ultrasound unit is required although appropriate transducers to

examine neonates and infants are necessary. Sedation is rarely required and no patient preparation is needed so that this examination is easily performed, causes minimal discomfort, is truly noninvasive and involves no radiation. Because of its wide use in pregnancy the urologist can now be faced with an intrauterine diagnosis of an abdominal mass or hydronephrosis in the fetus.

Patients are scanned in the prone and supine positions both transversely and longitudinally. Certain areas are difficult to scan, including the upper pole of the left kidney which may be masked by the ribs posteriorly and the gastric air bubble anteriorly. Normal ureters are difficult to see above the pelvis, especially where they cross the transverse processes of the vertebrae.

Renal cortex

Since ultrasound looks at the kidney from every angle a small renal scar, which could be missed on the IVU, can be detected. The overall renal size can be measured and the two kidneys compared. If no kidney is seen on the left, this does not exclude the possibility of a small kidney overlying the 12th rib. On the right the absence of a kidney on ultrasound is more significant and is less likely to be due to a hypoplastic kidney.

Intra-abdominal mass

In this situation ultrasound should be the first investigation following the clinical examination. The origin of the mass, whether intrarenal or extrarenal, is revealed (*Figure 2.11*) and the opposite kidney, the inferior vena cava (*Figure 2.12*), the liver and other posterior abdominal wall structures can all be studied. The echographic appearance of the mass shows whether it is solid, and thus neoplastic, or cystic. When

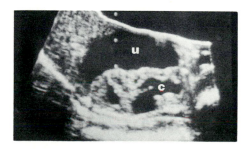

Figure 2.11. Posterior urethral valves with urinoma. In this 2 kg baby the diagnosis of hydronephrosis was made during the mother's antenatal ultrasound examination. Following birth posterior urethral valves were found. This longitudinal scan reveals the dilated calyces (c) and also shows the large leak of urine into the retroperitoneal tissues (urinoma) causing a transonic area (u).

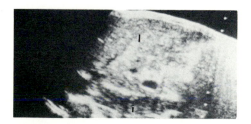

Figure 2.12. Wilms' tumour stage III. This longitudinal supine ultrasound examination reveals the normal texture of the liver (ℓ). The inferior vena cava is somewhat dilated and has echoes coming from within it. This child had a left Wilms' tumour with tumour extending into the renal vein and the inferior vena cava.

bilateral intra-abdominal masses on ultrasound suggest cystic disease, other members of the family should be examined in an attempt to determine which of the various groups of cystic disease of the kidneys is involved.

Calcification

Calcium is dense and casts an acoustic shadow on ultrasound giving a rather characteristic appearance. Significant calculi can therefore be detected by ultrasound but very faint calcification in a mass may be difficult to recognize (*Figure 2.13*).

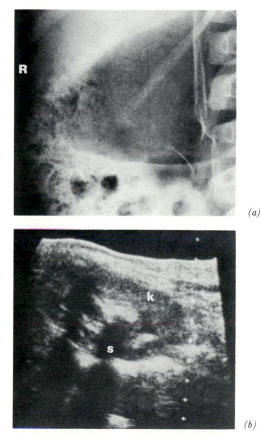

(a)

(b)

Figure 2.13. Nonopaque calculi. This 5-year-old girl presented in acute renal failure in coma. (*a*) The coned oblique view of the right renal area fails to demonstrate any abnormality in the region of the kidneys. (*b*) This longitudinal prone ultrasound scan of the right kidney reveals dense echoes within the kidney (k) casting acoustic shadows (s) which is a characteristic appearance of renal calculi. This child was found to have 2,6 dihydroxyadenine stones.

Collecting systems

The upper two thirds of the normal ureter is not visualized but a dilated ureter is readily seen. Ultrasound can assess the extent of the dilatation of the collecting system and so indicate the level of obstruction. Since ultrasound is independent of function a hydronephrotic nonfunctioning kidney or kidney element, such as the upper moiety of a duplex system, can be detected. When the renal pelvis is distended but no ureter is visualized a pelviureteric obstruction

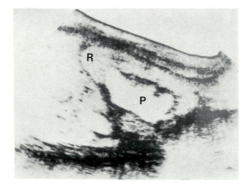

Figure 2.14. A longitudinal prone ultrasound scan of the left kidney reveals good functioning renal parenchyma (R) with dilatation of the calyces and the pelvis (P). No dilated ureter could be seen, strongly suggesting the site of obstruction to be the pelviureteric junction.

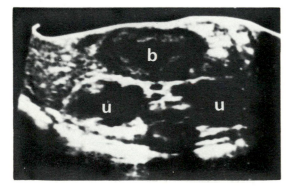

Figure 2.15. Prune belly. This is a transverse supine ultrasound image through the pelvis demonstrating the slightly thick-walled bladder (b) and the two dilated ureters behind the bladder (u).

can be diagnosed (*Figure 2.14*). The base of the bladder is always scanned, not only to determine the width of the ureters in their lower course (*Figure 2.15*) but also to look for ureteroceles in the bladder lumen.

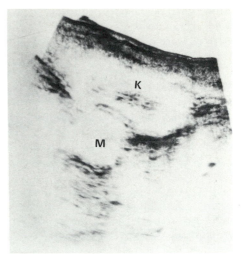

Figure 2.16. This 8-year-old girl had signs of early puberty for which she was investigated. The IVU was unequivocally normal. This longitudinal scan of the left kidney in the prone position shows a mass (M) situated anterior to the kidney (K) not causing any dilatation of the renal pelvis. The kidney itself is normal. At laparotomy a 6 cm tumour was removed from the renal hilum.

In the postoperative period a patient with pyrexia but no localizing signs should have an abdominal ultrasound examination looking for an accumulation of pus as well as observing the liver and the spleen. Another group of patients in whom ultrasound is useful are those with a hormonal imbalance suggesting excessive amounts of adrenal hormones. Ultrasound may well demonstrate one large gland or else show two normal glands and a tumour (*Figure 2.16*). The IVU remains an essential investigation in these patients.

CT scanning

The new generation of CT scanners have a cycle time of less than 20 seconds, and shortly machines with one not exceeding 2 seconds will be available. This is an important advance, permitting paediatric abdominal scans to be undertaken. The image obtained is an anatomical cross-section approximately 13 mm thick; longitudinal or angled images are not possible.

The scan is simply an anatomical representation of the area and different tissue densities are easily recognized. Excessive gas in the bowel and active peristalsis both cause significant degradation of the image. In part this can be overcome by antispasmodics such as hyoscine butylbromide.

Sedation is very important and general anaesthesia is used with infants and younger children. Intravenous contrast medium is given to outline both the parenchyma and the collecting systems when the unenhanced scan is equivocal or unhelpful. The entire examination lasts approximately 45 minutes.

Intra-abdominal mass

Examination for this condition is not routine and at the moment its major role is in helping the oncologist in the management of malignancy. Sequential scans are carried out in these patients to assess the size of the tumour mass in response to radiotherapy and/or chemotherapy.

Intrarenal mass

Rarely, both the IVU and ultrasound are equivocal, while a ^{99m}Tc-DMSA scan is noncontributory. In this situation the CT scan can be helpful.

Adrenal glands

Imaging of the adrenals is difficult. The IVU relies on a mass lesion of sufficient size to affect the position of the kidney. Ultrasound may run into difficulties when the gland overlies the rib. In such cases—especially in the obese patient— the CT scan is possibly the investigation of choice, but in the paediatric patient this remains a very difficult area.

The lungs in malignancy

The CT scan can pick up 2–3mm nodules in the chest and is more sensitive than lung tomography and lung fluoroscopy. Although it is the investigation of choice to determine how many metastases are present it is not available as a

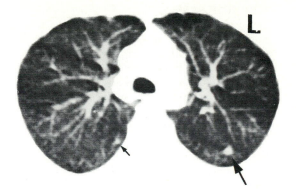

Figure 2.17. Wilms' tumour. The chest X-ray revealed one secondary in the left lung. This CT scan shows the secondary in the left lung and another smaller deposit in the right lung (both arrowed).

routine screening method (*Figure 2.17*). In Wilms' tumour when metastasis is seen on chest X-ray or tomography the role of CT chest scans is to ensure that there is only a solitary metastasis present.

The neonate

The immature kidney is susceptible to renal venous thrombosis and medullary necrosis and the potential for renal damage must not be worsened or precipitated by any imaging procedure. Intravenous contrast medium with sodium load and osmotic diuresis may be poorly tolerated by the neonatal kidney and acute renal failure may be aggravated. The IVU is therefore contraindicated in neonates who are ill or in renal failure. Moreover, during the first 48–72 hours after birth, failure to concentrate contrast medium in the presence of two normal kidneys has been noted. For these reasons it is inadvisable to use the IVU as the first-line investigation in the neonate.

The first examination should be by ultrasound. In renal failure this establishes the presence of the kidneys and also the state of the collecting systems. If a mass or bilateral masses are palpable the origin can be determined; solid bilateral masses may be due to renal venous thrombosis, medullary necrosis, infantile polycystic kidneys or nephroblastomatosis, while mesoblastic nephroma is unilateral. A cystic

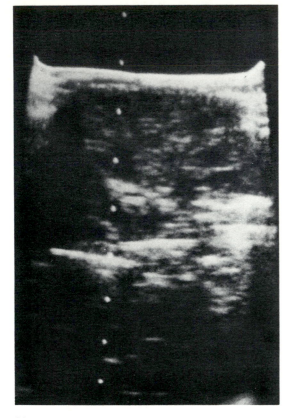

(a)

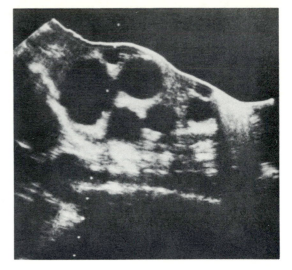

(b)

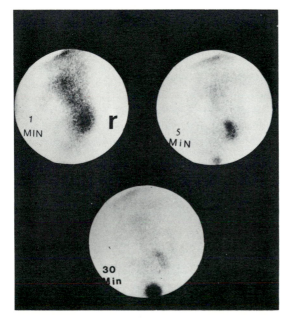

(c)

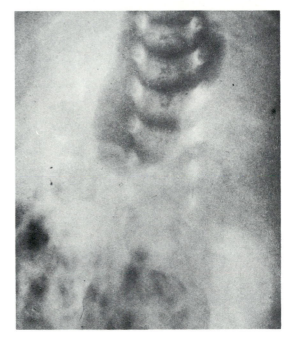

(d)

Figure 2.18. Multicystic kidney. This neonate was noted to
have an intra-abdominal mass at birth. (a) A right longitudinal prone ultrasound scan shows the normal right kidney.
(b) On the left are large circular echo-free areas and no
normal renal parenchyma is seen. (c) The ^{99m}Tc-DTPA
scan shows a normally functioning right kidney with
radioisotope in the bladder at 5 minutes but no activity on
the left side. The 30-minute image confirms the normal
drainage of the right kidney with no function on the left. (d)
The IVU at 1 week reveals a normal right kidney. This is the
renal window view showing the normal kidney to better
advantage. No contrast medium accumulated on the left. At
surgery a multicystic kidney was removed.

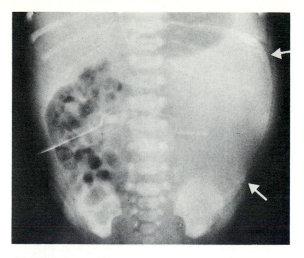

(a)

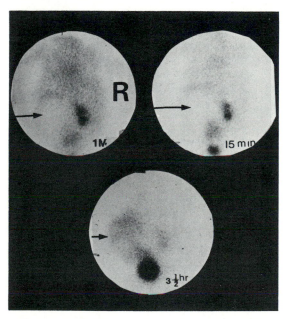

(b)

Figure 2.19. Pelviureteric obstruction in a neonate. The baby was noted to have a left abdominal mass at birth. (*a*) This shows the IVU on the first day of life 30 minutes after intravenous contrast medium was injected. No contrast medium is seen on the right and there is only a vague suggestion of a rim of contrast medium peripherally on the left (arrowed). (*b*) The 1-minute ^{99m}Tc-DTPA image shows the functioning right renal parenchyma. A large photon-deficient area is noted on the left (arrowed). It is again seen on the 15-minute image (arrowed). The 3½-hour image shows good drainage of the radioisotope from the right kidney with an accumulation in the previously noted photon-deficient area (arrowed) suggesting that the left kidney is obstructed. At surgery a left pelviureteric junction obstruction was found.

mass may be due to a multicystic kidney, a dilated renal pelvis in an obstructed system or, very rarely, adult polycystic disease in infancy.

The next investigation is either a micturating cystourethrogram (MCU) or a renal scan. The MCU may reveal reflux, thus outlining the upper collecting systems. The bladder, and in the male the urethra, should be outlined when an obstructive uropathy is suspected.

In renal failure a ^{99m}Tc-DTPA scan can be carried out to establish the extent of renal function. In the presence of an infection or metabolic acidosis a nonfunctioning kidney must not be equated with irreparable renal damage. Sequential scans should be used to aid management decisions. A ^{99m}Tc-DMSA scan should be carried out when there is a single enlarged kidney that is solid on ultrasound; this may aid in distinguishing between a mesoblastic nephroma and an acutely infected kidney.

The IVU is reserved to answer specific questions and should be carried out when the neonate is older than 72 hours, any infection present is under control and the metabolic state is stable. In polycystic disease it is essential to obtain a high quality IVU in the late neonatal period. In the infant with a multicystic kidney a ^{99m}Tc-DTPA scan should be obtained so that the function of the opposite kidney can be accurately assessed. When a neonate has a congenital anomaly, for example anorectal malformation or oesophageal malformation then an ultrasound examination in the neonatal period together with a one-shot IVU at 1 month of age suffices if both are normal.

Thus the first in the order of priority for imaging a neonate is an ultrasound examination. In renal failure or suspected obstructive uropathy an MCU should follow. Accurate assessment of renal function is obtained by radioisotopic scans. Intravenous urography is reserved for the older neonate and should always follow other imaging procedures.

Radiation dosimetry

It is not easy to equate the radiation doses to the patient from different examinations. During radiology and CT scanning that part of the body exposed receives the full dose of radiation while those parts not in the beam receive little or none.

Table 2.2   Dose in IVU (data from James, Wagner and Cooke, 1974)

Age (years)	Skin dose (mGy)	Mean whole-body dose (mGy)
1	2.0	0.3
5	3.0	0.4
10	5.0	0.6
15	7.5	0.7

Table 2.3   Dose of radionuclides (data from Bingham and Maisey, 1978)

	^{99m}Tc-DTPA ($\mu Gy/MBq$)	^{99m}Tc-DMSA ($\mu Gy/MBq$)
Kidney	11.4	168
Bladder	150	76
Whole body	4.3	4.3

In radiology doses are expressed as skin dose and mean whole-body dose (*Table 2.2*) while in CT scanning the dose is expressed in terms of energy imparted to the organ in the slice. Radioisotopes are given intravenously and thus the whole-body dose is a significant proportion of the radiation the patient receives while the target organ obviously receives a higher dose. With radionuclides the absorbed dose is dependent upon the dose of radioisotope administered and the function of the organ. For this reason absorbed radiation dose is expressed per unit of injected activity (*Table 2.3*).

Generally speaking ^{99m}Tc-DTPA gives a very low radiation dose to the kidneys and, with frequent bladder emptying, a low dose to the bladder. ^{99m}Tc-DMSA gives a higher renal dose but a lower bladder dose. Except for neonates, radioisotopes give a much lower dose than IVU. If tomography is used in the neonate the radiation is greater than with ^{99m}Tc-DTPA. The CT scan gives a higher radiation dose than the IVU.

With the introduction of SI units the following conversion factors operate. The absorbed dose is the rad or gray (Gy) where 10 mGy = 1 rad. The activity of radioisotopes is the curie (Ci) or becquerel (Bq) where 1 mCi = 37 MBq.

Doses in CT scanning were calculated by Wall, Green and Veerappan (1979) for a 75 kg man and given as energy imparted to the body (mJ) where 1J/kg = 1 Gy. Eight cuts of torso have a dose of 100 mJ (1.43 mGy) and a chest X-ray has a dose of 21 mJ (0.3 mGy).

References

Andresen, J., Madsen, B. and Steenskov, V. (1981) Radiological and clinical evaluation of twenty neuroblastomas. *Clinical Radiology*, **32**, 191

Bingham, J.B. and Maisey, M.N. (1978) An evaluation of the use of ^{99m}Tc-dimercaptosuccinic acid (DMSA) as a static renal imaging agent. *British Journal of Radiology*, **51**, 599

Britton, K. (1978). Radionuclides in renal imaging. *British Journal of Hospital Medicine*, **120**, 143

Damascelli, B., Gasparini, M., Barigozzi, P.L., Fossati-Bellani, F., Gabagnati, F., Prada, A. and Ceglia, E. (1980) Arteriography in childhood tumours. *Clinical Radiology*, **31**, 61

Diffey, B.L., Hall, F.M. and Corfield, J.R. (1977) The ^{99m}Tc-DTPA dynamic renal scan with deconvolutional analysis. *Journal of Nuclear Medicine*, **17**, 352

Hilson, A.J.W., Maisey, M., Brown, C.B., Ogg, C.S. and Bewick, M.S. (1978) Dynamic renal transplant imaging with Tc-99m DTPA (Sn) supplemented by a transplant perfusion index in the management of renal transplants. *Journal of Nuclear Medicine*, **19**, 994

James, A.E., Wagner, H.N. and Cooke, R.E. (1974) Paediatric Nuclear Medicine, 1st edn. Saunders, Philadelphia. p.47

Kirks, D.R., Firz, C.R. and Harwood-Nash, D.C. (1976) Paediatric abdominal angiography: a practical guide to catheter selection, flow rates and contrast doses. *Paediatric Radiology*, **5**, 19

Lucas, A. (1979) The window view of the renal area in infants and children. *Radiography*, **45**, 216

Merrick, M.V., Uttley, W.S. and Wild, S.R. (1980) The detection of pyelonephritic scarring in children by radioisotope imaging. *British Journal of Radiology*, **53**, 544

O'Reilly, P.H., Testa, H.J., Lawson, R.S., Farrar, D.J., Edwards, E.C. and Carroll, R.N.P. (1978) Diuresis renography in equivocal urinary tract obstruction. *British Journal of Urology*, **50**, 76

Piepsz, A., Denis, R., Ham, H.R., Dobbeleir, A., Schulman, C. and Erbsmann, F. (1978) A simple method for measuring separate glomerular filtration rate using a single injection of ^{99m}Tc DTPA and the scintillation camera. *Journal of Pediatrics*, **93**, 769

Pors Nielsen, S., Lehd Moller, M. and Trap-Jensen, J. (1977) ^{99m}Tc-DTPA scintillation camera renography: a new method for estimation of single kidney function. *Journal of Nuclear Medicine*, **18**, 112

Tamminen, T.E., Ruhimaki, E.J. and Tahti, E.E. (1978) A gamma camera method for quantitation of split renal function in children followed for vesicoureteric reflux. *Paediatric Radiology*, **7**, 78

Wall, B.F., Green, D.A.C. and Veerappan, R. (1979) The radiation dose to patients from EMI brain and body scanners. *British Journal of Radiology*, **52**, 189

Whitfield, H.N., Britton, K.E., Hendry, W.F., Nimmon, C.C. and Wickham, J.E.A. (1978) The distinction between obstructive uropathy and nephropathy by radioisotope transit times. *British Journal of Urology*, **50**, 433

3   Acute Renal Failure

T.M. Barratt and Susan P.A. Rigden

Introduction

The correct management of acute renal failure (ARF) in children demands close cooperation between nephrologist and urologist. Neither should embark on the care of such children without the services of the other because resuscitation, diagnosis, dialysis and definitive treatment are all interwoven in a rapidly evolving clinical situation often punctuated by medical or surgical surprises. The patterns of ARF in children are different from those in adults, with an overall better prognosis in the former and a greater proportion of cases with underlying urological abnormalities. There is, however, considerable variation in both the incidence and the aetiology of ARF in childhood from one geographical area to another and from one decade to the next (Barratt, 1971). Many forms of ARF are preventable so that the overall incidence in childhood is an accurate reflection of the general standards of child health and welfare in a community.

Pathogenesis

The secretion of urine depends on the integrity of the blood supply to the kidney, the normal functioning of the renal parenchyma and the patency of the urinary passages. There is thus merit in the time-honoured classification of ARF as prerenal, renal or postrenal. Nevertheless individual cases may be multifactorial and episodes of ARF may afflict kidneys that were previously healthy, or be superimposed on pre-existing renal disease (acute-on-chronic renal failure).

Prerenal factors

If renal perfusion pressure falls substantially, renal blood flow and glomerular filtration rate decline but tubular reabsorption of salt and water continues. There is oliguria with a urinary flow rate less than 0.5ml/kg per hour in infants, good quality urine of osmolality more than $300\,mosmol/\ell$, a urine/plasma urea concentration ratio greater than 5 and a urinary sodium concentration below $20\,mEq/\ell$. In such circumstances the urinary flow rate responds to diuretics, for instance frusemide 1–5 mg/kg intravenously, and returns to normal rapidly if renal perfusion pressure is restored. However, if renal hypoperfusion is prolonged the quality of the urine passed may decline and acute tubular necrosis (ATN) may supervene.

Central circulatory failure

The poor renal perfusion described above is a manifestation of circulatory failure which may be either central in origin with a poor cardiac output in spite of an adequate venous filling pressure, or peripheral with a low cardiac output because of hypovolaemia with a low filling pressure. When the distinction is not evident on clinical examination, measurement of the central venous pressure is helpful.

The low cardiac output and hypotension which may accompany cardiopulmonary bypass surgery is now the most common single cause of ARF necessitating dialysis at the Hospital for Sick Children, London (Barratt and Rigden, 1981). In such circumstances, providing volume replacement is adequate, a dopamine infusion is the most satisfactory form of circulatory support because it selectively increases renal blood flow.

Peripheral circulatory failure

On a global scale the hypovolaemia and contraction in extracellular fluid volume resulting from the salt and water depletion of gastrointestinal disease is probably the most important cause of ARF in childhood. Urinary salt wasting, which is common in children with urological disorders, may be responsible for acute-on-chronic renal failure. Plasma volume depletion due to protein loss may complicate burns or the nephrotic syndrome and cause prerenal uraemia. In all these circumstances correction of hypovolaemia is not only important in its own right but also prevents the development of ATN.

Renal factors

Acute tubular necrosis

ARF which is slowly reversible may complicate prolonged renal ischaemia or exposure to nephrotoxins and has been described as ATN. This terminology is not entirely satisfactory since necrosis is not always evident histologically. The major pathophysiological event appears to be in the renal circulation and the term vasomotor nephropathy is gaining currency (Oken, 1978). The common factor is decreased renal cortical perfusion possibly due to intranephron feedback inhibition resulting from increased sodium concentration in the tubular fluid at the level of the macula densa. There is evidence for the involvement of the renin-angiotensin system in this regulatory mechanism (Thurau, Boylan and Mason, 1979). Oliver, McDowell and Tracey (1951) showed by microdissection that there are two types of tubular lesion. With nephrotoxins such as mercuric chloride there is confluent and mainly proximal tubular necrosis with an intact basement membrane, whereas with ischaemia the tubular necrosis is patchy and more distal with focal ruptures of the basement membrane.

In children most cases of ischaemic ATN result from diarrhoeal dehydration, nephrotic hypovolaemia, burns, Gram-negative septicaemia, asphyxial delivery and cardiopulmonary bypass surgery. Nephrotoxic ATN may result from accidental ingestion of, for example, carbon tetrachloride or may be iatrogenic occurring as an adverse drug reaction especially to antibiotics such as cephaloridine and perhaps gentamicin. Some cases of ATN are multifactorial while in others no cause is apparent.

In adults the oliguric period averages 12 days while in children it is shorter and occasionally escapes notice. Some patients are never oliguric but pass urine of an insufficient quality to prevent uraemia. During the recovery period there may be a diuretic phase with inappropriate excretion of salt and water, although often this represents excretion of excess fluid retained during the oliguric phase. Ultimately recovery is complete.

ATN may be unilateral, for instance when complicating renal arterial clamping during urological surgery, and may also be responsible for oliguria following renal transplantation.

Acute cortical necrosis

Acute cortical necrosis implies death of the renal parenchyma but is not necessarily fatal since it can have a patchy distribution. It may follow prolonged severe renal hypoperfusion from any cause, although the most common circumstance is a severe episode of the haemolytic-uraemic syndrome (HUS).

Renal arterial occlusion

This is a rare lesion and an occasional complication of umbilical arterial catheterization during neonatal intensive care. ARF with hypertension results.

Renal venous thrombosis

The infant kidney is particularly prone to venous infarction, perhaps due to the high renal vascular resistance in early life (*see* Chapter 1). Most cases of renal venous thrombosis (RVT) occur in the first 3 months of life; the principal antecedents are perinatal anoxia (particularly in infants of diabetic mothers), hypernatraemic dehydration and cyanotic congenital heart disease (Arneil *et al.*, 1973). The thrombosis originates in small intrarenal veins and progresses centripetally; only rarely does it involve the inferior vena cava. Sometimes a similar pathological process affects the adrenal glands, resulting in an adrenal haematoma. There is often evidence of a generalized coagulation disorder with thrombocytopenia.

The clinical picture is of a firm enlarging kidney in a sick infant with oliguria and macroscopic haematuria. The nephrotic syndrome has only rarely been associated with RVT, and in such cases it is more probable that RVT is a consequence rather than the cause of the heavy proteinuria. Uraemia may be secondary to renal hypoperfusion or ATN and does not necessarily imply bilateral involvement. Even if both kidneys are involved, recovery of function is possible since the venous infarction can be patchy within the kidney. Most centres adopt a conservative approach to the management of RVT. Anticoagulants and fibrinolytic agents seem of little value, and urgent nephrectomy is inappropriate because it is difficult to predict the extent of recovery of function. Insofar as the thrombosis originates within the kidney thrombectomy is unlikely to be of value, and the risks involved in venography and surgery are high. The only situation in which surgery may be helpful is when the thrombosis appears to have originated in the inferior vena cava as suggested by leg oedema and cyanosis. Published data are inadequate to draw conclusions on this point.

Following venous infarction the affected kidney shrinks and may at this stage be difficult to distinguish from any other small irregularly contracted kidney. It may, however, be responsible for hypertension, and all cases of RVT need long-term follow-up with this in mind.

Medullary necrosis in infants can be regarded as a similar lesion in which venous infarction is confined to the medulla (Davies, Kennedy and Roberts, 1969), and the predisposing conditions are similar. An important consideration is that in sick infants radiological contrast media may cause the lesion, particularly in doses above 3 ml/kg body weight, for example during angiocardiography (Gruskin *et al.*, 1970). In the long term the condition results in calyceal clubbing similar to that of chronic pyelonephritis

except that there is no overlying cortical scar and vesicoureteric reflux is not present.

Haemolytic-uraemic syndrome

The combination of uraemia, haemolytic anaemia and thrombocytopenia occurring without overt cause is known as the idiopathic HUS (Lieberman, 1972). The disorder has a peak age incidence between 1–4 years, and is frequently preceded by a mild diarrhoeal illness. There are endemic areas such as Argentina and South Africa where the disease is common, appearing to afflict disproportionately the children of the upper socioeconomic classes. In nonendemic areas HUS often appears in microepidemics, suggesting an infectious agent although none has been regularly isolated.

The child presents with pallor, bruising, oliguria, oedema and hypertension. Investigations reveal anaemia with erythrocytic fragmentation, thrombocytopenia and uraemia. There is frequently evidence of intravascular coagulation with raised levels of circulating fibrin degradation products. The primary event appears to be endothelial damage with platelet activation particularly affecting the renal circulation, but the pathogenesis of the disorder is not understood.

Anticoagulant treatment with heparin and fibrinolytic therapy with streptokinase have both been advocated, although unsupported by controlled clinical trials. The most important aspect of treatment is careful management of the ARF itself, and more than 80 per cent of children recover completely without specific therapy. A few fail to recover any renal function and some others have residual proteinuria, hypertension and impaired renal function.

Pyelonephritis/septicaemia

Bacterial infection of the kidney is rarely sufficient on its own to cause ARF but may be an important contributory factor in obstructive uropathy. Septicaemia is frequently associated with ARF, partly on the basis of ATN and partly related to disseminated intravascular coagulation. Overwhelming infection in the neonate (particularly in males and principally with Gram-negative organisms) causes septicaemia, haematogenous pyelonephritis, disseminated intravascular coagulation, ARF and sometimes meningitis. Although the possibility of urological abnormality must not be over-looked in such infants, in fact the majority who present in this manner do not have an anatomical abnormality of the urinary tract.

Acute interstitial nephritis

This is a rare lesion sometimes occurring as a result of drug therapy such as with methicillin.

Acute glomerulonephritis

A few children with acute post-streptococcal nephritis are anuric at presentation. They generally recover completely, occasionally requiring short periods of dialysis. Crescentic nephritis (*see* Chapter 8) is a more sinister lesion. It can be a feature of several nephritides such as mesangiocapillary glomerulonephritis, Goodpasture's syndrome, Henoch-Schönlein purpura and polyarteritis nodosa. On the other hand there may be no recognized clinical association. The condition may improve on combined anticoagulant and immunosuppressant therapy.

ARF may complicate any variety of the nephrotic syndrome, in particular those with minimal changes in histology, due to the hypovolaemia associated with plasma protein depletion.

Postrenal factors

Congenital obstructive lesions

Urinary tract obstruction is usually congenital in origin and as such of long standing, but it may present as an acute emergency having been precipitated into ARF by urinary tract infection or saline depletion. The obstruction is usually infravesical and posterior urethral valves (*see* Chapter 21) are the most common lesion; nevertheless it may be in the upper urinary tract if there is a solitary functioning kidney.

Acquired obstructive lesions

Stones developing in a solitary kidney or bilaterally may present as ARF, and can have either an infective or a metabolic basis (*see* Chapter 29). Nonopaque stones are a particular challenge including stones in urate nephropathy in patients with leukaemia and other haematological malignancies, urate stones in the Lesch-Nyhan syndrome, xanthine stones, and dihydroxyadenine stones with adenosine-phosphoribosyl-transferase deficiency. Sulphadiazine crystalluria is now rare.

Other acquired obstructive lesions include neuropathic bladder and malignancy (particularly rhabdomyosarcoma) and other pelvic masses.

Pre-existing renal factors

Acute-on-chronic renal failure

If there is underlying chronic renal insufficiency, minor factors may precipitate acute-on-chronic renal failure. Such factors include salt depletion, urinary tract infection, urinary obstruction, hypertension and hypercalcaemia. Their importance is that they may confer an element of reversibility on what otherwise appears a hopeless situation.

An interesting variant of this theme is the effect of placental separation on the neonate with essentially functionless kidneys (*see* Chapter 1). Such babies are normal at birth (apart from the consequences of oligohydramnios) because the placenta functions as an efficient kidney, and in effect there is ARF from the moment of placental separation.

Acute presentation of chronic renal failure

An occasional case of chronic renal failure presents for the first time as advanced uraemia. Clues of chronicity may be given by poor growth and the presence of uraemic osteodystrophy. Almost any type of chronic nephropathy may show these characteristics, but in later childhood they are rather typical of juvenile nephronophthisis (medullary cystic disease).

Diagnosis

History

Clues to the underlying pathology of the renal failure may be found in the history. In males the character of the urine stream is of particular importance, although in infants a significant urethral obstruction may be present even with apparently normal micturition. A history of urinary tract infection is suggestive of a urological disorder. Diarrhoea and vomiting suggest saline depletion, but can also be a prelude to ATN, RVT or HUS, and can themselves be caused by pyelonephritis or uraemia. Exposure to drugs and other nephrotoxins should be reviewed. An upper respiratory infection suggests acute glomerulonephritis.

Examination

The physical examination is conducted with two principal considerations in mind, namely the severity of the uraemia and the underlying diagnosis. The state of consciousness is impaired in advanced uraemia and many children with this condition have convulsions. Respiratory drive may be poor in infants with overwhelming multisystem disorders of which ARF is only one facet, and assisted ventilation may be required. Hyperventilation (Kussmaul respiration) is a consequence of metabolic acidosis. Assessment of blood pressure and circulation provides a good guide to the state of hydration. Hypertension and peripheral or pulmonary oedema result from salt and water overload, whereas hypotension and diminished skin turgor indicate salt and water depletion.

Enlarged kidneys may represent hydronephrosis, cystic disease or venous infarction, but pyelonephritis or ATN may also cause some increase in renal size. A full bladder suggests infravesical obstruction.

Investigations

Blood and urine analysis

Plasma concentrations of electrolytes, urea, creatinine, calcium and phosphorus are estimated to indicate the severity of the biochemical disturbance. Blood-gas analysis reveals the degree of metabolic acidosis and the adequacy of ventilation. Haemoglobin determination and white blood cell and platelet counts provide useful information because anaemia with fragmented erythrocytes and thrombocytopenia is characteristic of HUS although it also occurs with septicaemia and RVT. A blood culture is almost always indicated.

Every drop of urine should be preserved for analysis. Routine tests for blood and protein should be supplemented by microscopy looking for red blood cells, casts, white blood cells, bacteria and crystals. The urine should be cultured, and evidence of a urinary tract infection is often a pointer to underlying urological disease. The osmolality and the urea and sodium concentrations should be measured to distinguish between prerenal and renal causes of oliguria.

Renal imaging

The diagnosis of urological abnormalities underlying ARF has been transformed in recent years by the advent of ultrasound, which in experienced hands can be reliably used to detect the presence of hydronephrosis. It is much easier to undertake the ultrasound study before a peritoneal catheter is inserted if time permits. If hydronephrosis is detected, the next investigation is a micturating cystourethrogram, leaving the child on catheter drainage if an infravesical obstruction such as urethral valves is demonstrated. A plain X-ray of the abdomen is needed to exclude opaque calculi, and may give some information on the renal outlines. Chest X-ray and X-ray of the wrist and hand for osteodystrophy should also be performed. In due course a ^{99m}Tc-diethylenetriaminepentacetic acid gamma-camera renal scan will provide information about renal perfusion and the relative function of the two kidneys.

With these techniques the intravenous urogram has a lesser role than formerly to play in diagnosis of the underlying cause of ARF. It is sometimes difficult to fit into the hectic schedule of resuscitation and diagnosis, but should not be omitted since it is often helpful in the precise anatomical definition of obstructive lesions. Similarly, there is still a place occasionally for cystoscopy and retrograde examination, for example in the diagnosis of nonopaque calculi.

Management

Resuscitation

The general principles of intensive care prevail, each system being reviewed in turn.

Ventilation

Of infants needing peritoneal dialysis 25 per cent also require assisted ventilation (Griffin, McElnea and Barratt, 1976). There may be inadequate ventilatory drive due to severe illness, convulsions or the consequences of anticonvulsant therapy. Pulmonary oedema accompanied by cyanosis is best managed by elective ventilation with positive end-expiratory pressure.

Circulatory collapse

Volume depletion with hypotension and no evidence of raised jugular venous pressure requires rapid volume expansion with plasma or normal saline 20 ml/kg body weight in the first instance. A good intravenous line is essential.

Hyperkalaemia

Circulatory collapse may be due to an arrhythmia complicating hyperkalaemia and these children should be connected to an ECG monitor. Hyperkalaemia is suggested by tall peaked T waves, and may in emergency be counteracted by intravenous administration of 10 per cent calcium gluconate 0.5 ml/kg. Oral or rectal calcium resonium 1 g/kg and correction of acidosis both tend to counteract hyperkalaemia. The use of glucose and insulin, while effective in driving potassium into the cells, is sometimes accompanied by troublesome hypoglycaemia

Convulsions

Children with ARF frequently convulse and there are many possible causes which should be considered, namely uraemia, hyponatraemia, hypernatraemia, hypocalcaemia, hypomagnesaemia and hypertension. Convulsions may also be part of the syndrome responsible for ARF, for example meningitis complicating septicaemia, or cerebral oedema. Convulsions during dialysis may be due to a rapid fall in plasma urea concentration leading to an osmotic gradient across the blood-brain barrier and fluid shifts into the brain, that is the dysequilibrium syndrome.

Many anticonvulsants tend to accumulate in renal failure. The most convenient is intravenous diazepam 0.25 mg/kg.

Hypertension and saline overload

A raised blood pressure almost invariably implies salt and water overload. If there is peripheral or pulmonary oedema as well, or if the jugular venous pressure is raised, then there is no doubt about the situation. Intake of salt and water should be minimized. Frusemide 5 mg/kg should be given intravenously and if the response is poor dialysis is probably indicated. When hypertension persists in spite of attempts at volume depletion, the blood pressure should be controlled with oral propranolol and hydrallazine 2 mg/kg per day of each, although beta-blockers should be avoided if there is pulmonary oedema or evidence of cardiac failure. If the control of hypertension seems an urgent matter, for example in encephalopathy, then parenteral hydrallazine 0.2 mg/kg intramuscularly or diazoxide 3 mg/kg intravenously can be used. In the presence of hypertension without other evidence of salt and water overload diazoxide is best avoided and a labetalol infusion is preferable (*see* Chapter 6).

Pulmonary oedema resulting from hypertension and volume overload is a deceptively dangerous situation and such patients require vigorous treatment and careful monitoring of blood gases. They may require assisted ventilation as described above.

Hypocalcaemia and tetany

Phosphate retention in ARF leads to reciprocal hypocalcaemia and tetany, but in infants convulsions are a more usual consequence of hypocalcaemia. Acidosis protects from tetany associated with hypocalcaemia, and thus rapid correction of acidosis by infusion of sodium bicarbonate may aggravate the problem. In infants ARF may also be complicated by convulsions due to hypomagnesaomia, while in older children and adults the plasma magnesium concentration tends to rise. The hyperphosphataemia can be controlled with aluminium hydroxide gel 0.5–1 ml/kg per day.

Metabolic acidosis

A severe uncompensated metabolic acidosis should be treated with intravenous sodium bicarbonate 2 mmol/kg (an 8.4 per cent solution contains 1 mmol/ml) provided that there is not volume overload and hypertension as outlined above. The sodium bicarbonate solution should be diluted, and it is often useful to ensure that the bulk of the sodium is given as bicarbonate rather than as chloride.

Sepsis

In many cases of ARF there is demonstrable or suspected sepsis, often with a Gram-negative organism in the urinary tract and blood stream. Gentamicin is the most useful antibiotic, but it should be remembered that it is excreted by the kidney and in concentrations above 10 μg/ml is ototoxic and nephrotoxic. A loading dose of 2 mg/kg should be given intravenously, and subsequently the blood level may be maintained by adding gentamicin to the dialysate in a concentration of 10 μg/ml.

Anaemia

Transfusion may be required if the haemoglobin concentration falls below 7 g/dl. It should never be embarked upon if there is still hypertension or any other feature of volume overload.

Conservative management

In the adult an intake of 0.25 g/kg body weight per day of protein of high biological value results in the minimum rate of urea production. The minimum protein intake in young children has not been established, and 1 g/kg body weight per day in infants over 3 months of age seems satisfactory. This is of course substantially less than the protein intake of an infant receiving a diet of cows' milk (5 g/kg body weight per day) or human breast milk (2 g/kg body weight per day), and it is often adequate merely to reduce the protein intake to the latter level.

The maximum benefit of such restricted protein diets may only be realized if an adequate calorie intake is achieved, that is at least 100 kcal/kg body weight per day and preferably more. This may be provided in the form of glucose polymer and lipid, although the carbohydrate concentration of the diet should not exceed 10 per cent or diarrhoea may ensue. However, often the problem in children with ARF is to ensure that calorie and minimum nitrogen requirements are met during the phase of acute illness. At this stage intravenous nutrition with Vamin, providing 1 g amino acids/kg per day, and calorie sources such as Intralipid or 10 per cent dextrose is very helpful.

Insensible water losses are related to surface area and hence on a weight basis are greater in the infant than in the adult. They are about 30 ml/kg body weight per day in the infant falling to 5 ml/kg body weight per day in the adult.

Dialysis

Indications

The decision to treat by dialysis is determined less by arbitrary criteria of blood chemistry than by an assessment of the probable course of the renal failure. Dialysis is indicated if the infant is hypercatabolic or if a prolonged period of oliguria is expected; if a quick return of renal function seems likely then conservative management may suffice and dialysis can be deferred. In practice, diuretic-resistant saline overload is perhaps the most important indication because correction of, for example, acidosis or anaemia is impossible under such circumstances without dialysis.

Haemodialysis versus peritoneal dialysis

Until recently there has been little question that peritoneal dialysis is preferable to haemodialysis in the management of children with ARF, although there has always been a small minority of patients in whom for technical reasons such as a burst abdomen peritoneal dialysis is impossible. The technical difficulties of infant haemodialysis have been access to the circulation, the large blood volume of the artificial kidney relative to that of the child, and hyperefficient dialysis causing the disequilibrium syndrome. An even greater problem, however, has been that the relative infrequency with which haemodialysis in small children is required has hindered the acquisition of the expertise necessary for the safe use of the artificial kidney by paediatric renal units.

The development of maintenance haemodialysis programmes in children has therefore opened the door to new technical solutions and some of the problems have now been overcome. Suitable paediatric arterial and venous shunts are available, and paediatric dialysers that require less than 10 per cent of the infant's blood volume for priming have been developed. It has been found important to relate the efficiency of the dialyser to the size of the child and urea clearances of 2–3 ml/kg body weight per minute are satisfactory. Nevertheless, even with these developments it is likely that most centres will rely on peritoneal dialysis in the immediate future for the treatment of ARF in children.

Setting up peritoneal dialysis

Under light sedation and local anaesthesia and with strict aseptic technique the peritoneal cavity is first filled with dialysate fluid (about 30 ml/kg body weight) through a small needle. This manoeuvre reduces the risk of perforation of a viscus. The peritoneal catheter itself should be moderately flexible, contain an internal stilette and have perforations that do not extend more than 3 cm from the tip. In infants it is often more convenient to insert the catheter in the left flank rather than in the customary subumbilical position, because it may be difficult to bury the perforations below the peritoneum in the latter site. There is also an increased risk of perforation of the bladder, which is an abdominal rather than a pelvic organ. A small skin incision is made and the catheter is inserted into the peritoneal cavity (it helps if the abdominal wall is made tense by the infant crying) and advanced towards the pelvis.

Some modifications of the standard adult equipment are required for infants, namely a burette to measure the input volume and a heating coil to minimize heat loss during dialysis. Ideally, the administration set should be manufactured as a single piece and not improvised from other intravenous equipment since junctions and three-way taps are potent sources of infection.

Dialysis regimen

Commercially available dialysate fluids may be used at all ages. A sodium concentration of 130 mEq/ℓ is usually optimum. The glucose concentration should not exceed 2 g/100 ml since higher concentrations cause such a rapid withdrawal along the osmotic gradient into the peritoneal cavity that hypovolaemic shock can ensue. Potassium should be added in a concentration of 4 mEq/ℓ if its serum level is not

elevated. Lactate is the usual metabolizable anion. However, the sick anoxic neonate may fail to convert it to bicarbonate and hence develop a lactic acidosis, and it is then necessary to prepare a dialysate containing bicarbonate instead.

A cycle volume of about 25–50 ml/kg body weight is usually satisfactory, but the amount tolerated varies in different children. Overdistension of the peritoneum is dangerous because it may cause respiratory embarrassment or, in the infant, apnoeic attacks. Under most circumstances it is convenient and adequate to use hourly cycles, that is allowing the fluid to run into the peritoneum for 10 minutes, to dwell for 20 minutes and to drain for 30 minutes. On this regimen with a dialysate glucose concentration of 1.4 g/100 ml the drainage usually exceeds the input by about 10 per cent. Assuming insensible losses of 20 ml/kg body weight per day this permits a fluid intake of about 120 ml/kg body weight per day plus the urine volume. Hypercatabolic states necessitate shorter cycles, which are best achieved by shortening the drainage phase since the efficiency of dialysis is related to the volume of fluid passing through the peritoneal cavity in unit time.

Accurate recording of the fluid balance estimated from dialysis input and return is important but susceptible to cumulative errors. The most useful observations are the child's weight and circulatory status, particularly blood pressure. Conversely when repeated weighing is difficult, for example in children on mechanical ventilators, or where other factors influence the cardiovascular signs of hydration, such as after cardiac surgery, control of fluid balance may become very difficult. In the latter circumstance monitoring of the central venous pressure is essential.

Complications

Certain difficulties may be encountered. Bleeding after insertion of the catheter is usually not as troublesome as it may at first appear, unless the infant has been given heparin. If bleeding does occur, it is helpful to add a small amount of heparin (200 iu/ℓ) to the dialysate to prevent blockage of the catheter. Bowel perforation is very unusual if the peritoneum is first filled with dialysate, but it may occur if the gut is grossly distended and is probably best managed by surgical exploration in young children. Difficulties in drainage of dialysate are infrequent in small children, probably because the omentum is not well developed and does not wrap around the catheter. Although infection is reasonably easy to eradicate in older children it is more serious in infants because septicaemia can disseminate from a peritoneal focus. At the first suggestion of peritonitis antibiotics should be added to the dialysate in a concentration that exceeds the minimum inhibitory concentration to the infecting organism while being less than the toxic blood level.

The dialysis regimen should be adjusted to permit a normal diet. Particular attention should be paid to the maintenance of nutrition during peritoneal dialysis. In infants a daily protein intake of at least 2 g/kg body weight and a calorie intake of 100 kcal/kg body weight should be provided as well as additional water-soluble vitamins. Protein depletion develops rapidly in small infants and plasma infusions may be required.

Integration with surgical management

The question of suitability of surgical intervention depends upon the urgency of operation. If there is an infected obstructed urinary tract then clearly surgical drainage is a matter of urgency. However, a minimum requirement before surgery is that there should be adequate control of volume status with correction of hyperkalaemia and acidosis. Usually catheter drainage buys sufficient time to permit these medical goals to be achieved.

Successful management of children with renal failure can only be achieved with the cooperation of several paediatric skills. A closely co-ordinated team of paediatric nephrologist, urologist, radiologist, nursing staff, pathologist and dietician all experienced in and equipped for the management of sick infants is essential, and any compromise of this arrangement will result in less than optimum results.

References

Arneil, G.C., McDonald, A.M., Murphy, A.V. and Sweet, E.M. (1973) Renal venous thrombosis. *Clinical Nephrology*, **1**, 119

Barratt, T.M. (1971) Renal failure in the first year of life. *British Medical Bulletin*, **27**, 115

Barratt, T.M. and Rigden, S.P.A. (1981) Management of the child after cardiac surgery: renal function and dialysis. *In* Proceedings of the First International Congress of Pediatric Cardiology (edited by Godman, M). In press

Davies, D.J., Kennedy, A. and Roberts, C. (1969) Renal medullary necrosis in infancy and childhood. *Journal of Pathology*, **99**, 125

Griffin, N.K., McElnea, J. and Barratt, T.M. (1976) Acute renal failure in early life. *Archives of Disease in Childhood*, **51**, 459

Gruskin, A.B., Oetliker, O.H., Wolfish, N.M., Gootman, N.L., Bernstein, J. and Edelmann, C.M. (1970) Effects of angiography on renal function in infants and piglets. *Journal of Pediatrics*, **26**, 41

Lieberman, E. (1972) Hemolytic-uremic syndrome. *Journal of Pediatrics*, **80**, 1

Oken, D.E. (1978) Pathogenetic mechanisms of acute renal failure. *In* Pediatric Kidney Disease (edited by Edelmann, C.M.). Little, Brown, Boston. p.189

Oliver, J., McDowell, M. and Tracey, A. (1951) The pathogenesis of acute renal failure with traumatic and toxic injury: renal ischaemia, nephrotoxic damage and the ischaemic insult. *Journal of Clinical Investigation*, **30**, 1305

Thurau, K., Boylan, J.W. and Mason, J. (1979) Pathophysiology of acute renal failure. *In* Renal Disease, 4th edn (edited by Black, D.A.K. and Jones, N.F.). Blackwell, Oxford. p.64

4 Chronic Renal Failure and Regular Dialysis

T.M. Barratt and Rosemarie A. Baillod

Introduction

Regular dialysis and renal transplantation have been established modes of treatment for chronic renal failure (CRF) for two decades, and have been systematically applied to children for one decade. The availability of these techniques leads to new considerations in the management of children with urological disorders, so that the paediatric urologist should be aware of current practice, and emphasizes as well the need for the close integration of paediatric nephrology and urology.

A substantial body of experience has accumulated which indicates that children fare as well as, if not better than, adults on renal replacement programmes (Chantler et al., 1979). Special consideration must nevertheless be given to these patients who not only are young in years but also may, as a consequence of their chronic illness, have grown poorly and not developed fully from the emotional, educational or social point of view. They cannot simply be regarded as small adults.

Epidemiology

Incidence

Comprehensive statistics on the incidence of CRF in childhood are not available. In Europe 351 children aged less than 15 entered renal failure programmes in 1978, but they accounted for only 2.9 per cent of all patients treated. With relation to the size of adult programmes the overall need for renal failure treatment in children is small (Brunner et al., 1979). In the most active countries the acceptance rate for treatment of children with CRF ranges from 1.0–2.4 per million total population per annum (Chantler et al., 1980). Of the children accepted for treatment up to and including 1978, 5 per cent were under 5 years, 26 per cent between 5–10 years and 69 per cent between 10–15 years (Chantler et al., 1980). There is not, however, adequate information on the number of children refused treatment on the grounds of other medical problems or age. In particular there are very few data on the mortality from CRF in those under 5 years old. This matter is now of some practical relevance because a few units have started to explore the possibilities of treatment of these young children (Hodson et al., 1978).

Aetiology

The underlying renal diseases in children accepted for treatment in Europe are given in Table 4.1. The distinction between pyelonephritis and renal dysplasia is somewhat insecure. In the Guy's Hospital programme 31 (41 per cent) of 75 children were classified as having pyelonephritis/reflux, congenital abnormalities or obstructive uropathy (Chantler et al., 1980). These are the children likely to have been under the care of a urologist at some stage, and their

Table 4.1   Primary renal disease in children entering renal failure programmes in Europe in 1978 (data from Chantler *et al.*, 1979)

Disease	Incidence (%)
Glomerulonephritis	34
Pyelonephritis	22
Cystic disease	8
Hereditary nephropathy	8
Renal hypoplasia/dysplasia	11
Renal vascular disease	2
Cortical/tubular necrosis	1
Other*	14

*Principally kidney tumours and haemolytic-uraemic syndrome

natural history might have been influenced by surgery. In addition, a reluctance to accept young children or those with urinary diversion may lead to an underestimate of the contribution of urological cases to the problem of CRF in childhood.

Decline of renal function

Assessment

In the presence of CRF renal function can, with sufficient precision for practical purposes, be inferred from the plasma creatinine concentration (*see* Chapter 1).

> glomerular filtration rate (ml/min per 1.73 m^2 surface area) = 38 height (cm)/plasma creatinine concentration (μmol/ℓ)

If the glomerular filtration rate (GFR) lies between 40–80 ml/min per 1.73 m^2 surface area, CRF is mild and asymptomatic; nevertheless the child should be routinely followed up to ensure that growth is adequate and to detect reversible factors, particularly hypertension, that adversely affect renal function. With a GFR between 20–40 ml/min per 1.73 m^2 surface area, CRF is moderately severe, growth failure is probable, there is a risk of development of osteodystrophy and the child's care should be supervised by a paediatric nephrologist. When the GFR is 10–20 ml/min per 1.73 m^2 surface area CRF is severe and may be symptomatic requiring careful dietary management; infants with this level of renal function require particularly careful management if optimum growth is to be achieved. When the GFR falls below 10 ml/min per 1.73 m^2 surface area (a plasma creatinine concentration more than 500 μmol/ℓ) the need for dialysis or transplantation is imminent.

Children with CRF due to glomerular disease deteriorate rapidly, particularly if they are hypertensive. On the other hand, the rate of progression of CRF in children with urological disorders is slow and survival for many years may be possible even with advanced renal failure, especially in infants. An estimate of the time at which renal replacement therapy may be required can be derived from projection of the plot of the GFR (derived from the reciprocal plasma creatinine concentration as described above) against age. It must nevertheless be emphasized that prediction of the outcome of CRF in infants is extremely difficult.

Reversible factors

In patients with CRF it is important to identify and correct reversible factors that cause further deterioration of renal function, namely salt depletion, urinary obstruction, urinary infection, hypertension, hypercalcaemia and drug nephrotoxicity. Of these salt depletion is the most commonly overlooked and urinary obstruction the most difficult confidently to exclude, especially in urological patients who have residual dilatation of the urinary tract in spite of previous surgery. Nevertheless, even when all the above factors have been excluded, with severe urological disorders there may be an inexorable decline of renal function often associated with proteinuria, suggesting that some aspect of the pathophysiology of renal failure may itself be damaging. Recent experimental evidence suggests that phosphate toxicity may be contributory (Haut *et al.*, 1980).

Pathophysiology of renal failure

Adaption to CRF

As GFR (and thus urea clearance) falls the plasma urea concentration rises until excretion again balances production, and in one sense the raised plasma urea concentration can be regarded as an adaptive response to the reduced GFR. In the equilibrium state the load of solute to be excreted is determined by dietary and metabolic factors rather than by renal function. Thus with a declining population of functioning nephrons there is an increased solute load per nephron, the behaviour of the kidney as a whole resembling that of a healthy kidney undergoing a solute diuresis resulting in a diminished flexibility of response to changes in extracellular fluid (ECF) volume and composition. This is the 'intact nephron' hypothesis (Platt, 1952).

Increased excretion per nephron is often only achieved at the expense of undesirable side effects. For example hypertension is the consequence of the chronic ECF overexpansion necessary to drive sodium excretion, and hyperparathyroid bone disease is the price to be paid for the maintenance of phosphate homeostasis. This is the 'trade-off' hypothesis (Bricker, 1972).

Uraemia

Uraemic toxins

The accumulation of urea and other products of protein catabolism in the body fluids is responsible for some of the symptoms of CRF collectively described as uraemia, namely ill health, lassitude, anorexia, nausea, vomiting and anaemia. It is not clear to what extent urea itself is responsible, or to what extent a raised plasma urea concentration is merely a marker of the retention of other nitrogenous substances. Bergström and Fürst (1978) listed 33 organic compounds that accumulate during uraemia such as the guanidine compounds including creatinine, and the low molecular weight peptides whose normal degradation pathway is glomerular filtration and reabsorption with catabolism in the proximal tubule. These are the so-called middle molecules which are resistant to dialysis (Scribner *et al.*, 1972); however, there are stringent criteria that must be met before any substance can be accepted as a uraemic toxin.

Nitrogen metabolism

Urea production is determined by net protein breakdown, which is the algebraic sum of protein anabolism and catabolism in the tissues.

Some urea nitrogen is recycled in the gut by bacterial action and the remainder is excreted by the kidney (Walser, 1980). Thus uraemia is exacerbated by increased dietary protein intake, decreased gastrointestinal recycling (for instance with tetracycline), increased tissue protein catabolism (such as with infections) and decreased anabolism. Protection from uraemia by anabolism is particularly important in children, who should be accumulating protein in growing tissues, but growth is often poor with renal failure. A major factor is calorie deprivation which is often a consequence of the anorexia associated with uraemia. However, there appear to be other factors in the uraemic state which are detrimental to protein anabolism (Jones, El-Bishti and Chantler, 1980).

Salt

In CRF the flexibility of sodium excretion is reduced. If the dietary sodium intake approaches the ceiling of sodium excretion then sodium balance can only be achieved by chronic ECF overexpansion resulting in hypertension and ultimately in peripheral and pulmonary oedema. Hypertension in CRF is almost always due to salt and water overload, although in a few instances it is renin-driven and resistant to saline depletion.

On the other hand if the dietary intake approaches the obligatory rate of sodium excretion, a deficit of body sodium ensues with contraction of the ECF volume and further impairment of renal function. Such salt-wasting states are typical of CRF due to renal dysplasia, pyelonephritis and obstructive nephropathy. They may be easily overlooked because the plasma sodium concentration is usually normal, and in the equilibrium state urinary sodium excretion must balance dietary intake. The diagnosis hinges on the physical signs of chronic ECF depletion, particularly postural hypotension, and on the results of a therapeutic trial of sodium supplementation.

Bone

The combination of osteomalacia/rickets, osteitis fibrosa and osteosclerosis associated with CRF is known as uraemic osteodystrophy (Avioli and Teitelbaum, 1978). The term 'renal rickets' is unsatisfactory, including as it does other forms of hypophosphataemic rickets associated with renal tubular disorders.

Vitamin D metabolism

It is now established that vitamin D_3 (cholecalciferol) after absorption from the gut is hydroxylated in the 25 position in the liver and then transported to the kidney. There it is further hydroxylated in the 1 position, forming 1,25-dihydroxycholecalciferol which is the active metabolite of vitamin D and promotes the absorption of calcium from the intestinal lumen (Haussler and McCain, 1977). With severe renal damage there is an acquired resistance to the action of vitamin D, impaired gastrointestinal absorption of calcium, and osteomalacia or (in the child) rickets.

Phosphate retention and hyperparathyroidism

With declining GFR the tendency to phosphate retention results in parathormone secretion which restores phosphate balance. However, the resultant secondary hyperparathyroidism leads to bony erosions (osteitis fibrosa) and osteosclerosis (Slatopolsky *et al.*, 1971). If unchecked, hyperphosphataemia causes metastatic calcification and accelerates the decline of renal function.

Growth

Retarded statural growth is characteristic of nearly all children with CRF. The most severely affected are those with a long history of CRF, in particular when this dates from the first year of life (Betts and Magrath, 1974), and thus children with urological disorders are especially at risk. Skeletal maturation is retarded as well and puberty may be delayed, particularly in boys.

A number of factors that interfere with growth in children with CRF have been identified. These include energy deprivation, uraemic osteodystrophy, metabolic acidosis, chronic salt or water depletion and anaemia (Holliday, 1978). The most important factor appears to be a poor energy intake due to anorexia, notably in

Table 4.2   Medical management of children with chronic renal failure

Problem	Assessment	Area of action
Renal function	Plasma creatinine	Review reversible factors: obstruction, urinary tract infection, salt depletion, high blood pressure, hypercalcaemia
Uraemia	Plasma urea, diet	Dietary protein and calorie intake
Salt depletion	Examination, blood pressure	Dietary sodium intake, sodium supplements
Water balance	Plasma sodium	Fluid intake
Hypertension	Blood pressure	Sodium intake, diuretics, antihypertensives
Acidosis	Plasma bicarbonate	Sodium bicarbonate supplements
Hyperkalaemia	Plasma potassium	Dietary potassium intake, calcium resonium
Hyperphosphataemia	Plasma phosphorus	Dietary phosphorus intake, Aludrox
Osteodystrophy	X-rays of wrist, hand and knee; plasma, calcium, phosphorus and alkaline phosphatase	Dietary calcium intake, control of hyperphosphataemia, vitamin D, dihydrotachysterol or 1-alpha-hydroxycholecalciferol therapy
Anaemia	Haemoglobin and red blood cell indices, serum iron and folate	Supplements of iron and folate
Infection	Urine culture	Antibiotics
Other drugs	Prescription sheet	Modification of drug dosage
Growth	Height, bone age	Review all the above, especially calorie intake
Education	School report	Communication
Social situation	Social worker's report	Communication
Psychological problems	Discussion	More discussion
Future plans		

infants who have developed unsatisfactory feeding habits because of the need to maintain a high fluid intake to make up for defects of urinary concentration. However, although energy deprivation in uraemic children prevents growth, energy supplementation does not necessarily result in normal growth rates. No characteristic endocrine deficiency has been found in uraemic children and hormone therapy has not so far been proven to be of value.

Practical aspects of management

Regular medical assessment

Children with CRF of moderate severity (GFR less than 40 ml/min per 1.73 m² surface area) should be seen at least every 3 months in an appropriate medical clinic and reviewed along the lines of the problem list in *Table 4.2*. Their diet should be monitored and their social and intellectual progress assessed. Height and weight should be measured and recorded on growth charts and blood pressure should be taken. Plasma electrolytes, urea, creatinine, calcium and phosphorus concentrations should be determined. X-rays of the hand, the wrist and the knee are required every 6 months–1 year for the detection and assessment of uraemic osteodystrophy, particularly in the early years. An overview of the whole family's life must be obtained, and it is a great help to have the cooperation of a dietician and a social worker in the clinic.

Diet

An adequate energy intake is essential to maintain protein anabolism and body growth. In babies an intake of 100 kcal/kg body weight per day is appropriate. In older children the intake should be at least as high as the recommended dietary allowance of a child of the same height and age (Department of Health and Social Security, 1969). Such a goal is easier to state than to achieve, particularly if fluid intake has to be restricted. Glucose polymers are a useful and inoffensive source of extra calories.

The dietary protein intake should be reduced if the plasma urea concentration is above 30 mmol/ℓ or if there are symptoms such as nausea and vomiting which might be attributable to uraemia. Extreme dietary protein restriction as practised in earlier years can result in malnutrition, and it is unwise to reduce the protein intake so that it provides less than 4 per cent of the total calories (about 1 g/kg body weight per day). For infants the most important consideration is that the protein intake of a breast-fed baby is only about 2 g/kg body weight per day whereas unmodified cows' milk formulas provide as much as 5 g/kg body weight per day. Often, therefore, the only dietary adjustment necessary is a change from a cows' milk formula to one with a protein content similar to that of breast milk.

Breast milk has other advantages. The sodium, potassium and phosphorus levels are low so that the osmolar load presented for excretion is reduced and thus there is a lesser problem of water balance in infants with a major defect of urinary concentration, such as is frequently found with obstructive uropathy or renal dysplasia. However, babies with CRF are often also salt-wasters, and in addition tend to lose bicarbonate, in which case supplemental sodium bicarbonate 2–4 mmol/kg body weight per day may be appropriate.

Hypertension

Blood pressure should be carefully monitored and controlled because hypertension is perhaps the major treatable factor responsible for late deterioration of renal function. In the first instance the dietary sodium intake should be reduced and if this is insufficient then sodium excretion should be promoted with a diuretic such as frusemide. For first-line antihypertensive treatment the combination of a beta-blocker such as propranolol or atenolol with a vasodilator such as hydrallazine or prazosin is appropriate. With proper appreciation of the role of salt and water overload, and with the modern range of antihypertensive drugs, refractory hypertension is now rare.

Osteodystrophy

Control of uraemic osteodystrophy is one of the most important and difficult aspects of the management of children with CRF. The phosphorus intake should be reduced by dietary phosphorus restriction and the use of phosphate-binding gels such as Aludrox so that the plasma phosphorus concentration is maintained at around the mean level found in healthy children of the same age. Vitamin D intake should be monitored, and in the presence of radiological evidence of osteodystrophy vitamin D therapy should be intensified. Supplements can be given in the form of large doses of vitamin D_3, dihydro-tachysterol, or one of the compounds already hydroxylated at the 1 position, namely 1-alpha-hydroxycholecalciferol or 1,25-dihydroxy-cholecalciferol. It is not yet established whether any of the three compounds are more effective than vitamin D_3 itself, except that they have a shorter biological half-life and therefore toxic episodes of hypercalcaemia resolve more rapidly.

Psychosocial factors

As in any chronic illness psychosocial factors loom large in the management of children with CRF. The vicious circle of depression, anorexia, growth failure, social withdrawal and further depression is a real risk. In cases where renal disease is present at birth an inappropriately dismal prognosis may be given to the parents, who then may prematurely mourn the loss of their child. Difficulties with feeding often lead to tensions, particularly as these children often appear to dislike solid food. As the growth deficit becomes apparent, reactions to the child are often determined by his physical size rather than by his chronological age and he tends to be infantilized; it is essential to ensure that the educational arrangements are appropriate to his age and maturity. Later, anxieties about the future grow and are increased by the interest of the media in kidney machines and transplants and the often-discussed possibility that there may be insufficient facilities for dialysis and transplantation.

Planning for the future

By the time the plasma creatinine concentration reaches 500 μmol/ℓ arrangements for the future should be under consideration. In general, developed countries should have adequate facilities for the treatment of all children with end-stage renal failure over the age of 5 years provided that they have no other major medical problems. The concept of selection of patients for treatment is becoming outmoded and instead management should be adjusted to the needs and resources of the family. Nevertheless both dialysis and transplantation demand discipline, and experience strongly indicates that lack of cooperation at all levels by patients and their families after transplantation, or in particular during haemodialysis, is a very serious medical hazard. Assessment of the parents' motivation is therefore a most important preliminary, since without continued emotional support for the child renal failure treatment becomes a burden for all and not least for the child himself.

Renal replacement programmes

Integration of dialysis and transplantation

Renal transplantation and regular dialysis must not be seen as competitive techniques for the management of end-stage renal failure but rather as different aspects of an integrated programme. One form of treatment leads to the other and back again, and good dialysis techniques must be developed to support a transplantation programme and provide alternative treatment if the transplant fails.

In view of the rigorously sustained discipline necessary for dialysis and of its long-term expense, successful transplantation is the goal. However, some patients prove to be untransplantable, for example due to recurrence of primary disease or just because they are poor recipients, and long-term dialysis is on occasion inescapable.

Transplantation is not a guaranteed treatment because of the risk of biological and technical mishaps, but sometimes the drive to transplant early without careful planning is due to the failure of dialysis.

Peritoneal dialysis or haemodialysis?

Until recently nearly all centres involved in long-term regular dialysis relied upon haemodialysis, reserving peritoneal dialysis for acute cases only. In the last few years, however, technical developments have led to a resurgence of interest in chronic peritoneal dialysis. A permanent indwelling Silastic catheter with a Dacron cuff which acts as an anchor and seals off the catheter tunnel is a painless prosthesis and can be used indefinitely; it has substantially reduced the problem of bacterial infection (Tenckhoff and Schecter, 1968). Intermittent peritoneal dialysis three to five times weekly can be undertaken in the home where biochemical control is adequate although blood pressure control is sometimes poor. The treatment is well tolerated and growth can be achieved.

Continous ambulatory peritoneal dialysis is a new development of considerable promise (Popovich *et al.*, 1978). According to the size and tolerance of the patient $1-2\ell$ of dialysate is introduced into the peritoneal cavity where it remains for 5–8 hours until drained out; the collapsible peritoneal dialysate bag is left attached and hidden within the patient's clothing. The principle is to make maximum use of the peritoneal membrane, and biochemical control is better than with intermittent peritoneal dialysis. In children continuous ambulatory peritoneal dialysis is a much simpler technique than regular haemodialysis, but it remains to be seen what the relative long-term clinical advantages of the two methods prove to be.

Regular haemodialysis

Principles

Although haemodialysis is a complex treatment demanding special skills, it can be mastered by a parent for treatment of the child in the home. In principle the blood is taken outside the body to be cleaned and physiologically balanced within an artificial kidney. Efficient reliable blood access and control of blood volume outside the body are vital to the procedure. The monitoring equipment is designed to protect the blood while outside the body from problems such as spillage,

abnormal chemistry, abnormal temperature and introduction of air and bacteria, and also to control the extracorporeal blood volume. Contemporary haemodialysis is a highly efficient method of changing blood biochemistry and as such is potentially dangerous, particularly in small individuals who are subject to rapid alterations in the volume and composition of their body fluid compartments. Short frequent dialysis allowing more even control of biochemistry should be the long-term aim of treatment.

Blood vascular access

Patients dependent on renal replacement therapy only survive as long as their blood vessels remain patent. Concern that blood vascular access is the Achilles' heel of renal failure has been present throughout the development of treatment programmes, and experience is essential in its management. Every approach to a blood vessel at any stage of the patient's life must be carefully assessed as to potential loss of the vessel or segments of its length, including intravenous infusion of irritant drugs, cutdown for intravenous infusions, and failed blood vascular access operations or ill conceived access sites with wasting of distal sites. Without reliable blood vascular access haemodialysis is impossible, inefficient or dangerous; the child becomes distraught and anxious and there is disruption of the family and a need for hospitalization.

Two methods of blood vascular access are in current use. These are the external Silastic Teflon arteriovenous shunt (Quinton, Dillard and Scribner, 1960) and the internal arteriovenous fistula (Brescia *et al.*, 1966).

External shunts

The great advantage of the external shunt is its immediate availability for use after insertion and the painless procedure of attachment to the dialysis equipment. However, external shunts have a limited life either because the vein becomes thickened due to the high pressure arterial blood, leading to a reduction in flow and to clotting, or because infection develops in relation to the Silastic Teflon material. Shunt clotting may also result from dislodgment of clots during the dialysis procedure, low blood pressure and accidental kinking of the tubing. If the flow can be re-established then heparinization is essential for 24 hours or longer until a good flow is established. Long-term anticoagulation is sometimes required. Failure to re-establish the flow requires revision of the shunt. Early active treatment of all shunt infections is vital.

Usually external shunts are inserted in the leg vessels. Cannulation of small peripheral arteries can be extremely difficult and infants under 10 kg may need to have thigh or upper arm vessels cannulated with special small paediatric vessel tips and Silastic tubing, whereas veins in general are easily dilated at all ages and can be cannulated with adult size vessel tips. There are in addition many special types of external shunts, for example Buselmeier *et al.* (1971) described a shunt specially designed for children. One of the authors has found straight Silastic tubing with a Dacron cuff as made for permanent peritoneal catheters very satisfactory: the straight line of tubing within the vessel facilitates declotting and the Dacron cuff ensures fixation and sealing of the tunnel and helps prevent infection. With this equipment the arterial section has an average life expectancy of 4 years and the venous section of 12–24 months.

Internal fistulas

In view of the anxiety related to external shunt clotting, infection, failure and the need for revision, the primary choice for all adult centres and most paediatric ones is the internal fistula. When well developed this is free from these problems and can last indefinitely.

Fistulas are generally created in the arm. There are a number of techniques, including the use of venous autograft and nonhuman prosthetic material. Usually two needles are required, one to take out the blood and the other to return it, but safe equipment is now available to allow good dialysis through a single needle. Nevertheless internal fistulas can take 4 weeks–4 months to develop the adequately dilated veins essential for their use. In addition attachment to dialysis equipment requires the skill to insert large diameter needles or cannulas each time dialysis takes place. The insertion of needles is always associated with some discomfort, and even after successful cannulation fistula dialysis can be uncomfortable due to the vein collapsing on to the needle.

Careful assessment and expertise are necessary to select the appropriate blood vascular access for any particular patient. It is very difficult to create a satisfactorily functioning internal fistula in a child under 15 kg.

Technical problems

The patient's weight is the main pointer in assessing technical problems (Baillod, 1978). As a rough guide the blood volume can be taken as 100 ml/kg body weight and the patient feels faint or distressed or loses consciousness if the extracorporeal volume exceeds 10 per cent of the blood volume, that is 100 ml in a 10 kg child and 200 ml in a 20 kg child. The equipment should therefore be chosen to give an extracorporeal volume of less than 70 ml in a 10 kg child and less than 130 ml in a 20 kg child.

Weight gain between dialyses should not exceed 10 per cent, because removal of more than this volume results in circulatory collapse during dialysis. The less weight gained between dialyses, the smoother the procedure becomes. Conversely if the patient does not cooperate and drinks or eats excessively, dialysis is more traumatic and has to be more frequent.

About 12–18 hours of dialysis per week is required depending on size, biochemical control and technical difficulties. If fistula access requiring needle insertion is used, dialysis is generally undertaken during three sessions each week. With an external shunt more frequent and shorter sessions, for instance 3 hours for five sessions per week, are more suitable for small children and allow a freer diet.

Small children under 18 kg are the most difficult to dialyse (Kjellstrand *et al.*, 1971). Skill is required and the dialysis programme must be adjusted to each individual's needs. Patients can usually only be dialysed in the recumbent position. Weight loss during dialysis must be very accurately monitored. Hypotension may occur, often causing abdominal pain rather than faintness. In larger patients (up to 25 kg) the initial dialyses can be as hazardous as in small children, but long-term treatment should be asymptomatic. Between 25–35 kg treatment is much smoother and these patients are usually able to get out of bed during dialysis.

Medical problems

Convulsions are unusual in well controlled dialysis unless there is an epileptic focus. If they do occur, it is towards the end of dialysis and routine intravenous diazepam may be helpful.

Hypertension can nearly always be controlled by proper assessment and maintenance of the true dry weight. A patient's weight can be quite steady for many months until an intercurrent illness such as a viral infection leads to loss of appetite and flesh weight. To continue to maintain the previous dry weight is in effect to retain salt and water, exacerbating hypertension and running the risk of pulmonary oedema. Antihypertensive drugs are only rarely required in well dialysed patients.

The anaemia of CRF is due in part to erythropoietin deficiency and tends to be more severe in children than in adults on dialysis. Basic requirements for haemoglobin synthesis such as iron, folate and vitamin B_{12} must be supplied. Blood loss from dialysis, nose bleeds or excessive blood sampling must be checked. Blood transfusions should be used cautiously since iron overload can occur, but rigorous avoidance of blood transfusion as previously practised is no longer necessary with better screening of blood products for hepatitis B antigen and the surprising observation that prior transfusion prolongs graft survival. Bilateral nephrectomy tends to aggravate anaemia to levels at which the patient is invariably symptomatic.

Disabling bone disease occurs in 14 per cent of children on long-term dialysis (Chantler *et al.*, 1979). Control of hyperphosphataemia by diet and phosphate-binding gels together with vitamin D and calcium supplements is appropriate. There is a surprising variation in the severity of osteodystrophy in different centres which has recently been shown to be due to variations in the aluminium content of the water supplies (Wing *et al.*, 1980). Severe osteodystrophy is sometimes associated with a neurological disorder known as dialysis dementia which fortunately has not been reported in children.

Dialysis organization

Regular dialysis in hospital appears to place less responsibility on the family than home dialysis but in fact the disruption of education and family life is very severe and travel may involve inordinate time and expense. The average time on dialysis before the first renal transplant ranges from 1–2.5 years in active European countries (Chantler *et al.*, 1980).

Although good medical care can in fact be provided with home dialysis if the parents are well motivated, the child thrives at the expense of parental energy and family life. Support services for home dialysis have to be superior to those provided for adults because often treatment cannot be delayed for 24 hours. A round-the-clock technical service is therefore necessary.

Results of treatment

Survival

Of the 1877 children accepted in Europe for treatment before 31 December 1978, 1330 (71 per cent) were still alive on that date. Of these 628 (47 per cent) were receiving hospital dialysis, 142 (17 per cent; 57 in the UK) home dialysis and 25 (2 per cent) peritoneal dialysis, and 575 (43 per cent) had a functioning transplant (Chantler *et al.*, 1979). Five-year patient survival of children on home dialysis was 84.6 per cent which is superior to that of adults and also to that of children on hospital dialysis (67.4 per cent) or following a live donor (75.6 per

Table 4.3 Patient survival according to age groups and different modes of treatment of children on the register of the European Dialysis and Transplant Association (data from Chantler *et al.*, 1980)

Treatment	Age (years)	Survival 1 year (%)	2 years (%)	5 years (%)
Hospital haemodialysis	0–14	87.6	79.9	65.7
	0–4	84.0	75.3	
	5–9	85.8	76.8	
	10–14	88.5	81.2	67.4
Home haemodialysis	0–14	95.0	92.0	84.6
Live donor grant	0–14	90.1	85.4	75.6
Cadaver graft	0–14	86.4	81.6	70.6

cent) or a cadaver (70.6 per cent) graft (*Table 4.3*). Of 340 children whose initial treatment was at least 8 years previously 142 (48 per cent) were known to be alive in 1979 (Chantler *et al.*, 1980).

Rehabilitation

On average, children established on home dialysis have only 8 per cent of their dialysis sessions in hospital (Wass *et al.*, 1977). Just 50 per cent of children on hospital haemodialysis attend school regularly (Chantler *et al.*, 1979) while on home dialysis regular education is usually achieved with school attendance records of 65 per cent (Wass *et al.*, 1977). Patient selection accounts for some of the differences between survival and rehabilitation statistics for children on hospital and home dialysis.

Growth

Growth is poor in prepubertal children on regular dialysis but improves at puberty (Wass *et al.*, 1977). After renal transplantation in prepubertal children growth is significantly better (Chantler *et al.*, 1979). The problem of growth on dialysis is exacerbated by the small size of many of these children on entering renal failure programmes.

Psychosocial adaptation

A detailed prospective study of children on home dialysis was undertaken by Wass *et al.* (1977). At the start of home dialysis 14 (56 per cent) of 25 children were considered to be emotionally disturbed. One year later 11 of these were coping satisfactorily but two others developed psychological difficulties so that at the end of the year only five (20 per cent) were considered disturbed. It is worrying, though, that at the beginning of the study five (20 per cent) of the families were disturbed and by the end of the year 12 (48 per cent) of them had problems. This was mainly a result of the parents' emotional stress and tiredness and the secondary effects on family relationships of having a child on dialysis in the home.

The provision of services for children with renal failure

There has been much debate on the problem of the optimum organization for the provision of services for children with renal failure. Fortunately the root of the problem is the low incidence of end-stage renal failure in children compared to adults. Thus services have been developed largely with the needs of the adult population in mind and the concentration of

affected children necessary for the development of adequate expertise has been difficult to achieve, often involving families in major travelling problems. Hence 839 children were being treated in as many as 240 centres in Europe in 1978; 218 (26 per cent) were in centres treating less than three children and only 353 (42 per cent) in centres treating 10 children or more (Chantler *et al.*, 1979). Only 14 centres were responsible for 10 or more children on dialysis. Many children are treated without the involvement of a paediatrician and are not in a children's ward. The European Dialysis and Transplant Association has defined a specialist paediatric centre as one that treats more than three children annually and has the resources of a paediatrician, a hospital school, a psychiatrist, a dietician and a children's ward. Less than 40 per cent of children are treated in such units in Europe and sadly the proportion has not risen since 1973. The matter is of more than doctrinaire importance, for both patient and cadaver graft survival are better and growth on dialysis is superior in children treated in specialized centres (Chantler *et al.*, 1979).

References

Avioli, L.V. and Teitelbaum, S.L. (1978) Renal osteodystrophy. *In* Pediatric Kidney Disease (edited by Edelmann, C.M.). Little, Brown, Boston. p.366

Baillod, R.A. (1978) Practical Aspects of Paediatric Dialysis. *In* Dialysis Review (edited by Davidson, A.M.). Pitman, London. p.248

Bergström, J. and Fürst, P. (1978) Uremic toxins. *Kidney International*, **13**, Suppl.9

Betts, P.R. and Magrath, G. (1974) Growth patterns and dietary intake of children with chronic renal insufficiency. *British Medical Journal*, ii 189

Brescia, M.J., Cimino, J.E., Appel K. and Hurwich, R.J. (1966) Chronic hemodialysis using venepuncture and a surgically created arteriovenous fistula. *New England Journal of Medicine*, **275**, 1089

Bricker, N.S. (1972) On the pathogenesis of the uremic state: an exposition of the "trade-off" hypothesis. *New England Journal of Medicine*, **286**, 1093

Brunner, F.P., Brynger, H., Chantler, C. Donckerwolcke, R.A., Hathway, R.A., Jacobs, C., Selwood, N. and Wing, A.J. (1980) Combined report on regular dialysis and transplantation in Europe, 1979. *Proceedings of European Dialysis and Transplant Association*, **16**, 4

Buselmeier, T.J., Santiago, E.A., Simmons, R.C., Najarian, J.S. and Kjellstrand, C.M. (1971) Arteriovenous shunts for pediatric hemodialysis. *Surgery*, **70**, 638

Chantler, C., Donckerwolcke, R.A., Brunner, F.P., Brynger, H., Hathway, R.A., Jacobs, C., Selwood, N.H. and Wing, A.J. (1979) Combined report on regular dialysis and transplantation of children in Europe, 1978. *Proceedings of the European Dialysis and Transplant Association*, **16**, 76

Chantler, C., Carter, J.E., Bewick, M., Counahan, R., Cameron, J.S., Ogg, C.S., Williams, D.G. and Winder, E. (1980) 10 years' experience with regular haemodialysis and renal transplantation. *Archives of Disease in Childhood*, **55**, 435

Department of Health and Social Security (1969) Recommended intakes of nutrients for the United Kingdom, *Reports of Public Health and Medical Subjects*, **120**

Haussler, M.R. and McCain, T.A. (1977) Basic clinical concepts related to vitamin D metabolism and action. *New England Journal of Medicine*, **297**, 979, 1041

Haut, L.L., Alfrey, A.C., Guggenheim, S., Buddington, B. and Schrier, N. (1980) Renal toxicity of phosphate in rats. *Kidney International*, **17**, 722

Hodson, E.M., Najarian, J.S., Kjellstrand, C.M., Simmons, R.L. and Mauer, S.M. (1978) Renal transplantation in children aged 1 to 5 years. *Pediatrics*, **61**, 458

Holliday, M.A. (1978) Growth retardation in children with renal disease. *In* Pediatric Kidney Disease (edited by Edelmann, C.M.). Little, Brown, Boston. p.331

Jones, R.W.A., El Bishti, M.M. and Chantler, C. (1980) The promotion of anabolism in children with chronic renal failure. *In* Topics in Paediatrics, 2: Nutrition (edited by Wharton, B.). Pitman, London. p.900

Kjellstrand, C.M., Shideman, J.R., Santiago, E.A., Mauer, M., Simmons, R.C. and Buselmeier, T.J. (1971) Technical advances in hemodialysis of very small pediatric patients. *Proceedings of Dialysis and Transplant Forum*, **1**, 124

Platt, R. (1952) Structural and functional adaptation in renal failure. *British Medical Journal*, i, 1313, 1372

Popovich, R.P., Moncrief, J.W., Nolph, K.D., Ghods, A.J.,

Twardowski, Z.J. and Pyle, W.K. (1978) Continuous ambulatory peritoneal dialysis. *Annals of Internal Medicine*, **88**, 449

Quinton, W., Dillard, D. and Scribner, B.H. (1960) Cannulation of blood vessels for prolonged hemodialysis. *Transactions of the American Society for Artificial Internal Organs*, **6**, 104

Scribner, B.H., Farrell, P.C., Milutinovic, J., and Babb, A.L. (1972) Evolution of the middle molecule hypothesis. *Proceedings of the 5th International Congress of Nephrology*, **3**, 190

Slatopolsky, E., Caglar, S., Pennell, J.P., Taggart D.D., Canterbury, J.M., Reiss, E. and Bricker, N.S. (1971) On the pathogenesis of hyperparathyroidism in chronic experimental renal insufficiency in the dog. *Journal of Clinical Investigation*, **50**, 492

Tenckhoff, H. and Schecter, A. (1968) A bacteriologically safe peritoneal access device. *Transactions of the American Society for Artificial Internal Organs*, **18**, 436

Walser, M. (1980) Determinants of ureagenesis, with particular reference to renal failure. *Kidney International*, **17**, 709

Wass, V.J., Barratt, T.M., Howarth, R.V., Marshall, W.A., Chantler, C., Ogg, C.S., Cameron, J.S., Baillod, R.A. and Moorhead, J.F. (1977) Home haemodialysis in children: report of the London Children's Home Dialysis Group. *Lancet*, i, 242

Wing, A.J., Brunner, F.P., Brynger, H., Chantler, C., Donckerwolcke, R.A., Gurland, H.J., Jacobs, C., Kramer, P. and Selwood, N.H. (1980) Dialysis dementia in Europe. *Lancet*, ii, 190

5 Renal Transplantation in Children

Oswald N. Fernando

Introduction

The management of renal failure in children and infants has been a therapeutic challenge and its solution is now well beyond the experimental stage. This condition presents unique problems of technique and of medical and surgical management of the patients. Careful selection and expertise can provide rehabilitation and a remarkably improved quality of life (Laplante *et al.*, 1970; Fine *et al.*, 1971; Najarian *et al.*, 1971; Weil *et al.*, 1976). Although transplantation has certainly proved to be more acceptable than prolonged dialysis, various problems still need elucidation.

Selection of cases

Incidence of renal failure

The incidence of end-stage renal failure in children has been variously put at two to three per million of population. Of these, one per million receives treatment (*Lancet*, 1978). Selection of the paediatric patient for renal failure treatment must be based on the long-term outlook of the initial pathology, the stage at which the disease is found and also various psychosocial considerations since the treatment has major implications for the family and for society as well as for the child. Considerable ethical and moral problems are brought into focus in deciding whether neonates and young children should receive therapy for renal failure, including transplantation. However, serious consideration needs to be given before appropriate therapy is denied.

Causes of renal failure

Glomerulonephritis accounts for almost half the children presenting in renal failure, and pyelonephritis for about 20 per cent (Scharer, Chantler and Donckerwolcke, 1978). Congenital obstructive uropathies, congenital hypoplasia, polycystic disease, Alport's syndrome, haemolytic-uraemic syndrome, cystinosis (Malekzadeh *et al.*, 1978), lupus erythematosus and hereditary nephropathy are rarer causes of end-stage renal failure. It must be noted that the number of children with chronic renal failure increases with age, and that drug-induced nephropathy is commoner in older children.

Recipient selection

Patients are accepted for renal failure therapy primarily as part of a comprehensive dialysis-transplantation programme. It is an essential aspect of management that treatment is carried out in specialist centres where facilities for children exist.

Following appropriate vascular access surgery, dialysis is commenced when the glomerular filtration rate has reached approximately 5 ml/min or when symptoms demand it. The criterion for a suitable recipient is the onset of irreversible renal failure (Fine, 1975). Infancy is a relative contraindication and the value of renal transplantation in neonates and infants needs to be established (Mauer *et al.*, 1975; Hodson *et al.*, 1978; Kwun *et al.*, 1978). Severe and even moderate mental retardation is a contraindication to transplantation. The presence of generalized systemic infection obviates transplantation, but this condition can be treated in the hope of eradicating it. Liver disease and malignancy are relative contraindications, although if a child with malignancy proves to be free from recurrence after 1 year then transplantation can be undertaken (Ehrlich, Goldman and Kaufman, 1974).

There are reservations regarding the suitability of patients with membranous proliferative glomerulonephritis, amyloidosis, cystinosis, diabetes, gout, oxalosis, Fabry's disease and Goodpasture's syndrome. However, patients with these conditions have received successful transplants. Recurrence of the original disease process in a graft contraindicates retransplantation. Patients with obstructive uropathy have been considered poor candidates for transplantation, but with suitable preparation such treatment can be successful. It is especially important that residual infection in the urinary tract is completely eradicated.

Donor selection and nephrectomy

It is generally agreed that live donor renal transplantation produces better results in children than cadaveric donor transplantation (Simmons *et al.*, 1976). There has been some reluctance on the part of surgeons to transplant paediatric kidneys into children or adults. Nevertheless, experimental evidence and clinical experience have clearly shown that kidneys from neonates and children can be transplanted quite successfully and that satisfactory glomerular filtration rates are attained rapidly (Kootstra *et al.*, 1974; Silber, 1976; Boczko, Tellis and Veith, 1978).

In managing the individual case, enquiries are first made as to the possibility of a live donor. Motivated adult family members are HLA-tested to select as nearly identical a tissue match as possible. Following selection, a mixed lymphocytic culture test and a direct crossmatch are carried out. The donor is given a thorough physical examination and a complete biochemical and haematological investigation is performed. Intravenous urography and aortography are carried out to assess the state of the donor renal tract. It is of great importance to keep the safety of the donor in mind, and all aspects of preoperative, intraoperative and postoperative care are geared towards this end.

Pretreatment of the live donor with azathioprine and prednisolone has been found to be useful. Intravenous fluids are administered prior to surgery to ensure an adequate intraoperative diuresis. Under normal circumstances an incision is made above the 11th rib and the kidney is approached extraperitoneally. The lower end of the incision is carried down far enough to have adequate ureteric exposure and the ureter is dissected along with a considerable amount of periureteric tissue. The renal vascular pedicle is dissected so as to obtain the maximum length of renal artery and renal vein. Care is taken not to stretch the artery and the vein and thereby compromise the circulation to the kidney. If the dissection of the kidney causes intrarenal arterial spasm it may be necessary to cease dissection momentarily or to inject papaverine sulphate into the periarterial tissues. After nephrectomy the kidney is immediately perfused with cold Collins solution and is transferred to the recipient (Collins, Bravo-Shugarman and Terasaki, 1969).

Cadaveric donor nephrectomy is carried out by a transabdominal approach and caval and aortic patches are obtained to facilitate vascular anastomoses.

Programme of management

Preparation of the recipient

Although it may be possible to proceed to live donor transplantation without haemodialysis, cadaveric transplantation calls for continuing haemodialysis or peritoneal dialysis and the patient should be available at all times in case a suitable donor presents. The patient is assessed thoroughly as for any major surgical procedure. General examination must necessarily include investigation for cardiac and respiratory problems. Hypertension needs to be controlled either by drugs or by bilateral nephrectomy. Peptic ulceration must be looked for and appropriate medication given or surgery undertaken. Bone problems due to secondary hyperparathyroidism often need elucidation prior to transplantation. Blood transfusion should be carried out if indicated and there are reports that transfusion may in fact result in longer graft survival (Festenstein *et al.*, 1976; Opelz and Terasaki, 1976).

Special attention is given to the genitourinary tract and major reconstructive surgery may be necessary prior to transplantation (Tunner *et al.*, 1971; Shenasky, 1976). Voiding patterns, frequency, enuresis and the quality of urethral flow are carefully assessed. It must be noted that a long period of dialysis may reduce the capacity of the bladder before transplantation. Excretory urography is often unsatisfactory and therefore voiding cystourethrography, cystoscopy and retrograde pyelography may have to be carried out. Cystometrograms are obtained to assess bladder capacity and the ability to produce a detrusor contraction is examined. Massive reflux, large polycystic kidneys or grossly infected kidneys may call for bilateral nephroureterectomy. Urethral valves or bladder neck problems need correction. Patients who are still passing urine and have infected, flaccid or neuropathic bladders that are considered nonsalvageable require ileal urinary diversion prior to transplant surgery (Kelly, Merkel and Markland, 1966; Firlit and Merkel, 1977).

Technique of transplantation

The technique of renal transplantation in the child is basically similar to that in the adult (Gonzalez *et al.*, 1970; Merkel, *et al.*, 1974; Shenasky, Madden and Smith, 1975). The kidney is placed in the right or left iliac fossa, the renal artery is anastomosed to the proximal end of the divided internal iliac artery and the renal vein is joined to the side of the external iliac vein. However, the vascular anastomotic technique requires modification in the small child, especially if an adult kidney is used. If the kidney is placed in the iliac fossa, anastomosis to the internal iliac artery and external iliac vein causes acute angulation of the blood vessels with resulting ischaemia. In the small child it is therefore necessary to site the anastomoses on the aorta and the inferior vena cava, either at the points of bifurcation or slightly higher (*Figure 5.1*). It is quite feasible to transplant an

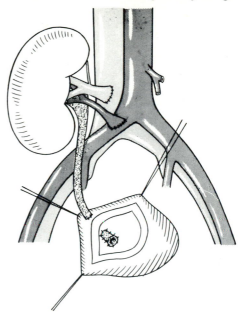

Figure 5.1. Technique of anastomoses and ureteric implantation.

adult kidney into a child, although it is preferable to use paediatric kidneys for paediatric recipients. When placing an adult kidney in a small child it is extremely important that an adequate circulating blood volume is maintained to ensure proper renal perfusion. Following release of the clamps, intentional hypervolaemia is necessary because the kidney diverts a considerable proportion of the patient's cardiac output and any hypovolaemia may precipitate acute tubular necrosis in the immediate postoperative period.

The ureter is anastomosed to the bladder by forming a short submucous tunnel and fashioning a nipple. Technical problems may arise in view of the small size of the bladder, particularly if the child has been on dialysis for a prolonged period of time. Hydrostatic distension of the bladder prior to transplantation often helps the location and placement of the ureter (Shenasky, Madden and Smith, 1975).

Immunosuppressive therapy

The standard immunosuppressive therapy for renal transplantation consists of azathioprine and a corticosteroid (either prednisolone or prednisone), commencing with an initial dosage of

2–4 mg/kg body weight per day. This is gradually reduced to a maintenance dosage of 1–2 mg/kg body weight per day of azathioprine and 0.5 mg/kg body weight per day of prednisolone. Children appear to tolerate azathioprine much better than adults, but the steroids seem to cause retardation of growth and maturation. It is therefore necessary to change to an alternate-day steroid regimen (Bell *et al.*, 1972; Potter *et al.*, 1975). Several series have confirmed that on alternate-day steroid therapy children grow adequately while continuing to have good renal function, although there is no growth spurt and no 'catch-up' growth (McEnery *et al.*, 1973; Reimold, 1973).

The patient is maintained on daily steroid therapy until renal function is quite stable. This may take 3–6 months, and in some cases longer. During conversion to the alternate-day schedule, accurate monitoring of renal function is necessary. One of two schemes can be used. First, the alternate-day prednisolone dose can be reduced by 0.5 mg every week until eventually the patient is maintained on 12–15 mg only on the alternate day. This process may take several months, and if at any time the programme of withdrawal of steroids aggravates rejection then it is necessary to return to a daily schedule and to cover the crisis with methyl prednisolone. In some centres it has been the practice to give prednisolone in double the daily dose on alternate days and to omit it on the others. The total dose is then gradually reduced.

Antilymphocytic and antithymocytic globulins have not proved to be as useful as was predicted in their immunosuppressive effects and therefore are not used routinely. Cyclophosphamide is often added, but one has to be very careful about severe bone marrow depression and hepatotoxic effects. In young children this drug is especially dangerous in view of its side effects related to gonadal depression and loss of hair. Irradiation is useful for rejection crises. The role of splenectomy, thymectomy and thoracic-duct drainage is highly questionable and only a few centres still use these modes of treatment. Newer immunosuppressive agents such as cyclosporin A and niridazole are being tried, but their efficacy is not yet proven.

Postoperative management

Paediatric renal allograft recipients require diligent postoperative care. Fluid and electrolyte balances need very careful monitoring, and over the first few days daily weight and hourly urine output measurements are important in assessing renal function. Bladder catheter drainage is maintained for approximately 1 week, and a normal diet is given as soon as possible.

Serial scanning using diethylenetriaminepentacetic acid (DTPA) or dimercaptosuccinic acid (DMSA) allows a quick assessment of vascular patency and helps discriminate between rejection and other complications. Intravenous urography, arteriography and biopsy are often of use in distinguishing rejection from obstructive phenomena. Constant clinical awareness of the many problems that may arise is most important in the postoperative period.

Rejection

This is still the main complication following renal transplantation. Hyperacute rejection occurs immediately following revascularization in the presence of preformed antibodies. Acute rejection can occur at any time in the early period following transplantation. Fever, hypertension, oliguria, weight gain and a rise in the blood urea and serum creatinine levels suggest the diagnosis. Biopsy often confirms the clinical findings, but should be used with discretion.

Acute rejection is treated by increasing the doses of immunosuppressive drugs. Methyl prednisolone is a potent steroid and is given as three pulse doses of 500–1000 mg/day. Other centres rely on increasing the steroids to the levels given on the day of operation and tailing them off as function improves.

Chronic rejection is a more insidious problem, with a gradual obliteration of the intrarenal vasculature. Treatment is often nonproductive and graft failure results.

Complications

Surgical

Surgical complications are related to the vascular and ureteric anastomoses and to sepsis (Fine *et al.*, 1973). Although serious haemorrhage is rare, if it occurs surgical intervention is needed rapidly. Administration of heparin in the immediate postoperative period for purposes of haemodialysis may provoke active bleeding.

Thrombosis of the renal artery or vein has disastrous consequences, with infarction and total loss of the functioning kidney. Urgent diagnosis and intervention may, however, salvage a kidney even though it may go through a period of acute tubular necrosis. Acute angulation and obstruction of the renal artery can be prevented by careful planning of the anastomotic site.

Urological

The incidence of urological complications in several series has been reported as 10–15 per cent (Edelbrock *et al.*, 1971). The mortality and morbidity rates of this particular aspect are exceedingly high. It therefore calls for meticulous attention to detail during the operative procedure and also in the technique of kidney harvesting. The preservation of the ureteric blood supply at the time of harvesting prevents most urological complications. Urinary leakage is a common early complication (McLoughlin, 1977). It may occur from the cystotomy, from the ureter as a result of necrosis or from the ureterovesical junction. A ureteric leak may be related to ischaemia as a result of a poor blood supply or of rejection. Subsequently, stenosis and hydronephrosis with consequent deterioration of function may occur, either acutely as a

result of oedema or more insidiously because of a cicatrizing process at the lower end of the ureter. Sterile reflux is not associated with any major consequences but infected reflux can result in septicaemia in the patient undergoing heavy immunosuppression with consequent loss of renal function.

Surgical correction must always be undertaken when there are urinary complications (Firlit, 1977). If an adequate length of ureter is available it may be possible to reimplant it into the bladder. Alternatively a Boari flap may be created, but the bladder may be particularly small and not amenable to this technique. Pyelovesicostomy has been carried out, and also pyeloureterostomy using the patient's own ureter. Low pressure uninfected reflux in the former instance does not appear to be significant and does not affect renal function. A rat-tail nephrostomy provides useful splintage in these ureters during the healing process.

Medical

Medical complications of transplantation are primarily related to the effect of immunosuppressive therapy and are summarized in *Table 5.1*. A few complications are peculiar to children (Martin, 1970; Potter *et al.*, 1970; Fine *et al.*, 1971; Lilly *et al.*, 1971). Hypertension is a

Table 5.1   Medical complications of transplantation

General	Increased susceptibility to infection	Protozoal Fungal (nocardial, cryptococcal) Bacterial (especially Gram-negative) Viral Pneumocystis
	Increased susceptibility to neoplasia especially reticuloses	
Effects due to steroids	Gastrointestinal tract	Peptic ulceration, colonic and small bowel perforation
	Musculoskeletal	Osteoporosis, avascular necrosis of hips, myopathy
	Cardiac	Hypertension
	Endocrine	Impaired growth, diabetes, secondary hyperparathyroidism
	Metabolic hyperlipidaemia Skin and face Eyes Psychiatric	Cushingoid facies, acne Cataracts
Effects due to azathioprine	Bone marrow depression Hepatic dysfunction Pancreatitis	

common complication (Malekzadeh *et al.*, 1975); it may be related to the steroid therapy, but can be associated with acute or chronic rejection and may also be secondary to renal arterial stenosis. In the early stages of hypertension drug therapy may produce adequate control, while for uncontrollable hypertension removal of the patient's own kidneys may be necessary. Renal arterial stenosis eventually causes a loss of function and needs surgical correction. Hepatic dysfunction has been reported (Malekzadeh *et al.*, 1972) and may be related to azathioprine toxicity, viral hepatitis or cytomegalovirus infection (Fine *et al.*, 1970, 1972). There have been a significant number of posterior subcapsular cataracts in children following transplantation (Fine *et al.*, 1975) and this has borne a direct relationship to the dosage of prednisolone. All patients therefore need assiduous ophthalmic supervision during the first few years, especially during high steroid dosage.

Linear growth is affected in children in renal failure (Grushkin and Fine, 1973; Hoda, Hasinoff and Arbus, 1975). If transplantation is carried out prior to fusion of the femoral and proximal tibial epiphyses (that is at a bone age of less than 12) growth potential is preserved. However, there is no catch-up growth, although generally boys seem to grow better than girls. Patients who have had high steroid dosage certainly show restricted growth. Alternate-day steroid therapy offers transplantation patients a better chance of optimum growth, but the adequacy of immunosuppression cannot be predicted.

Various psychosocial studies on the child and his family have shown that there is a considerable stress situation during dialysis and transplantation (Korsch *et al.*, 1973). These psychological upsets are related to obesity, cosmetic defects, problems with growth, activity restriction and anxiety regarding the status of the kidney. In some instances the aberration regarding cosmetic effect was so severe that patients deliberately withheld steroids and aggravated rejection crises even to the point of loss of the kidney.

Long-term results and retransplantation

The best results in terms of survival are obtained by home haemodialysis but successful transplantation produces near-complete rehabilitation of the child. Following transplantation, the overall patient survival rate in Europe after 3 years is 77 per cent for recipients of live donor kidneys and 74 per cent for recipients of cadaveric grafts. Fine *et al.* (1978) reported a 5-year survival rate of 78 per cent in 69 children with a live donor graft. Several other series have confirmed similar survival figures for transplantation. Failure to grow at a uniform rate remains a significant deterrent to complete rehabilitation, and this is related to the age at which the patient receives the graft. The quality of life after successful transplantation is excellent. It must, however, be noted that transplants undergo rejection and this can be traumatic physically and psychologically for the child and his family. The decision whether to retransplant must of course be made in each case individually according to the readiness with which the family will accept dialysis after a period of freedom from it (Fine *et al.*, 1973).

A multidisciplinary approach to the management of the child is important. Help from neurologists, urologists, occupational therapists, physiotherapists, child psychiatrists and social workers is essential while maintaining open discussions with the family and the child himself (*Lancet*, 1978; *British Medical Journal*, 1979).

In spite of all the technical and management problems involved it is in this area that the greatest potential lies for rehabilitation and a markedly improved quality of life.

References

Bell, M.J., Martin, L.W., Gonzales, L.L., McEnery, P.T. and West, C.D. (1972) Alternate day single dose Prednisolone therapy–a method of reducing steroid toxicity. *Journal of Pediatric Surgery*, **7**, 223

Boczko, S., Tellis, V. and Veith, F.J. (1978) Transplantation of children's kidneys into adult recipients. *Surgery, Gynaecology and Obstetrics*, **146**, 387

British Medical Journal (1979) Dialysis and transplantation in young children. Editorial, iv, 1033

Collins, G.M., Bravo-Shugarman, M. and Terasaki, P.I. (1969) Kidney preservation for transplantation. *Lancet*, ii, 1219

Edelbrock, H.H., Riddell, H., Mickelson, J.C., Grushkin, C.M., Lieberman, E. and Fine, R.N. (1971) Urologic aspects of renal transplantation in children. *Journal of Urology*, **106**, 934

Ehrlich, R.M., Goldman, R. and Kaufman, J.J. (1974) Surgery of bilateral Wilms tumour: the role of renal transplantation. *Urology*, **111**, 277

Festenstein, H., Sachs, J.A., Paris, A.M.I., Pegrum, G.D. and Moorhead, J.F. (1976) Influence of HLA matching and blood transfusion on outcome of 502 London transplant group renal graft recipients. *Lancet*, i, 157

Fine, R.N. (1975) Renal transplantation in children. *Advances in Nephrology*, **5**, 201

Fine, R.N., Grushkin, C.M., Anand, S., Lieberman, E. and Wright, H.T. (1970) Cytomegalovirus in children post renal transplantation. *American Journal of Diseases of Children*, **120**, 197

Fine, R.N., Edelbrock, H.H., Brennan, L.P., Grushkin, C.M., Korsch, B.M., Riddell, H., Stiles, Q. and Lieberman, E. (1971) Cadaveric transplantation in children. *Lancet*, i, 1087

Fine, R.N., Grushkin, C.M. Malekzadeh, M. and Wright, H.T. (1972) Cytomegalovirus syndrome following renal transplantation. *Archives of Surgery*, **105**, 564

Fine, R.N., Korsch, B.M., Brennan, L.B., Edelbrock, H.H., Stiles, Q.R., Riddel, H.I., Weitzman, J.J., Mickelson, J.C., Tucker, B.L., Grushkin, C.M. (1973) Renal transplantation in young children. *American Journal of Surgery*, **125**, 559

Fine, R.N., Korsch, B.M., Riddel, H., Stiles, Q.R., Edelbrock, H.H., Brennan, L.B., Heuser, E. and Grushkin, C.M. (1973) Second renal transplants in children. *Surgery*, **73**, 1

Fine, R.N., Offner, G., Wilson, W.A., Mickey, M.R., Pennisi, A.J. and Malekzadeh, M.H. (1975) Posterior sub capsular cataracts - post transplantation in children. *Annals of Surgery*, **182**, 585

Fine, R.N., Malekzadeh, M.H., Pennisi, A.J., Ettenger, R.B., Uittenbogaart, C.H., Negrete, V.F. and Korsch, B.M. (1978) Long term results of renal transplantation in children. *Pediatrics*, **61**, 641

Firlit, C.F. (1977) Unique urinary diversions of transplantation. *Journal of Urology*, **118**, 1043

Firlit, C.F. and Merkel, F.K. (1977) The application of ileal conduits in pediatric renal transplantation. *Journal of Urology*, **118**, 647

Gonzalez, L.L., Martin, L., West, C.D., Spitzer, R. and McEnery, P. (1970) Renal homotransplantation in children. *Archives of Survery*, **101**, 232

Grushkin, C.M. and Fine, R.N. (1973) Growth in children following renal transplantation. *American Journal of Diseases of Children*, **125**, 514

Hoda, Q., Hasinoff, D.J. and Arbus, G.S. (1975) Growth following renal transplantation in children and adolescents. *Clinical Nephrology*, **3**, 6

Hodson, E.M., Najarian, J.S., Kjellstrand, C.M. Simmons, R.L. and Mauer, S.M. (1978) Renal transplantation in children aged 1–5 years. *Pediatrics*, **61**, 458

Kelly, W.D., Merkel, F.K. and Markland, C. (1966) Ileal urinary diversion in conjunction with renal homotransplantation. *Lancet*, i, 222

Kootstra, G., Est, J.C., Dryburgh, P., Krom, R.A.F., Putnam, C.W. and Weil, R. (1974) Pediatric cadaver kidneys for transplantation. *Surgery*, **83**, 333

Korsch, B.M., Megrette, V.F., Gardner, J.E., Weinstock, C.L., Mercer, A.S., Grushkin, C.M. and Fine, R.N. (1973) Kidney transplantation in children: psychosocial follow up study on child and family. *Journal of Pediatrics*, **83**, 399

Kwun, Y.A., Butt, K.M.H., Kim, K.H., Kountz, S.L. and Moel, D.I. (1978) Successful renal transplantation in a 3 month old infant. *Journal of Pediatrics*, **92**, 426

Lancet (1978) Dialysis and transplantation in young children. Editorial, i, 26

Laplante, M.P., Kaufman, J.J., Goldman, R., Gonick, H.C., Martin, D.C. and Goodwin, W.E. (1970) Kidney transplantation in children. *Pediatrics*, **46**, 665

Lilly, J.R., Giles, G., Hurwitz, R., Schroter, C., Takagi, H., Gray, S., Penn, I., Halgrimson, C.G. and Starzl, T.E. (1971) Renal homotransplantation in pediatric patients. *Pediatrics*, **47**, 548

McEnery, P.T., Gonzalez, L.L., Martin, L.W. and West, C.D. (1973) Growth and development of children with renal transplants–use of alternate day steroid therapy. *Journal of Pediatrics*, **83**, 806

McLoughlin, M.G. (1977) The ureter in pediatric renal allotransplantation. *Journal of Urology*, **118**, 1041

Malekzadeh, M.H., Grushkin, C.M., Wright, H.T. and Fine, R.N. (1972) Hepatic dysfunction after renal transplantation in children. *Journal of Pediatrics*, **81**, 279

Malekzadeh, M.H., Brennan, P.L., Payne, V.C. and Fine, R.N. (1975) Hypertension after renal transplantation in children. *Journal of Pediatrics*, **86**, 370

Malekzadeh, M.H., Pennisi, A.J., Phillips, L., Ettenger, R.B., Uittenbogaart, C.H. and Fine, R.N. (1978) Growth and endocrine function in children with cystinosis following renal transplantation. *Transactions of the American Society for Artificial Internal Organs*, **24**, 278

Martin, L.W. (1970) Clinical problems encountered in renal homotransplantation in children. *Journal of Pediatric Surgery*, **5**, 207

Mauer, S.M., Kjellstrand, C.M., Buselmeier, T.J., Simmons, R.L. and Najarian, J.S. (1975) Renal transplantation in the very young child. *Proceedings of the European Dialysis and Transplant Association*, **11**, 247

Merkel, F.K., Ing, T.S., Ahmadian, Y., Lewy, P., Ambruster, K., Oyama, J., Suleiman, J.S., Belman, A.B. and King, L.R. (1974) Transplantation in and of the young. *Pediatric Urology*, **111**, 679

Najarian, J.S., Simmons, R.L., Tallent, M.B., Kjellstrand, C.M., Buselmeier, T.J., Vernier, R.L. and Michael, A.F. (1971) Renal transplantation in infants and children. *Annals of Surgery*, **174**, 583

Opelz, C., Terasaki, P.I. (1976) Prolongation effect of blood transfusions on kidney graft survival. *Transplantation*, **22**, 380

Potter, D., Belzer, F.O., Rames, L., Holliday, M.A., Kountz, S.L. and Najarian, J.S. (1970) The treatment of chronic uraemia in childhood–transplantation. *Pediatrics*, **45**, 432

Potter, D.E., Holliday, M.A., Wilson, C.J., Salvatierra, D. and Belzer, F.O. (1975) Alternate day steroids in children after renal transplantation. *Transplantation Proceedings*, **11**, 79

Reimold, E.W. (1973) Intermittent Prednisolone therapy in children and adolescents after renal transplantation. *Pediatrics*, **52**, 235

Scharer, K., Chantler, C. and Donckerwolcke, R.A. (1978) Replacement of renal function by dialysis. *Paediatric Dialysis*, **444**, 461

Shenasky, J.H. (1976) Renal transplantation in patients with urological abnormalities. *Journal of Urology*, **115**, 490

Shenasky, J.H., Madden, J.J. and Smith, R.B. (1975) Retroperitoneal renal transplantation in young children. *Urology*, **5**, 773

Silber, S.J. (1976) Growth of baby kidneys transplanted into adults. *Archives of Surgery*, **111**, 75

Simmons, R.L., Kjellstrand, C.M., Condie, R.M., Busel-
    meier, T.J., Thompson, E.J., Yunis, E.J., Mauer, S.M.
    and Najarian, J.S. (1976) Parent to child and child to
    parent kidney transplants. *Lancet,* i, 321
Tunner, W.S., Whitsell, J.C., Rubin, A.L., Stenzel, K.H.,
    David, D.S., Riggio, R.R., Schwartz, G.H. and Marshal,

V.F. (1971) Renal transplantation in children with cor-
    rected abnormalities of the lower urinary tract. *Pediatric
    Urology,* **106**, 133
Weil, R.W., Putnam, C.W., Porter, K.A. and Starzl, T.E.
    (1976) Transplantation in children. *Surgical Clinics of North
    America,* **56**, 567

6 Hypertension

Michael J. Dillon

It is becoming increasingly apparent that hypertension is not a disorder seen in just the adult population. Hypertension can and does occur in children, and if it is severe and untreated then it carries high morbidity and mortality rates (Still and Cottom, 1967). Unfortunately a lack of awareness of its existence all too frequently leads to serious delays in diagnosis which would never occur in adult practice where measurement of blood pressure is routine. Recently there has been an upsurge of interest in blood pressure measurement and hypertension in children. This appears to be due in part to the facts that adult essential hypertension is now thought to originate in childhood (Zinner *et al.*, 1974) and hypertension in children does not appear to be as rare as was formerly believed (Loggie, 1977). However the published data are difficult to interpret for several reasons including the lack of uniformity in the methodology of blood pressure measurement and the varying definitions used to identify young hypertensives.

Methods of blood pressure measurement

The most convenient means of measuring blood pressure in childhood remains the mercury sphygmomanometer. Nevertheless, with this method various sources of error are recognized, the most important being the cuff size. The standard recommendation is that the cuff should cover two thirds of the length of the upper arm but this is only appropriate if the upper arm is considered to start at the tip of the shoulder and extend to the elbow. A cuff that is too small produces an erroneously high blood pressure recording and can occasionally fail to occlude the underlying artery at all (Moss, 1978). For example Long, Dunlop and Holland (1971) found a difference of approximately 10 mmHg for the systolic and 7 mmHg for the diastolic values when using a cuff of 7.5 cm width instead of 12.4 cm. A useful rule of thumb is to use the largest cuff that still allows the vascular sounds to be heard easily with a stethoscope at the antecubital fossa (Steinfeld *et al.*, 1978).

It is now generally accepted that the fourth Korotkoff sound, corresponding to the point of muffling as the cuff is deflated, is the best estimate of the diastolic pressure (Blumenthal *et al.*, 1977). However, in some individuals (and especially in young children) no sounds are audible, while in others they are detectable continuously down to zero with no recognizable muffle on auscultation.

Several instruments have been developed in an attempt to overcome this type of difficulty. Instruments utilizing ultrasound based on the Doppler principle have been available for some time and in spite of doubts about the accuracy of the diastolic estimate (Whyte *et al.*, 1975) they have been shown to record reliably both systolic and diastolic pressures (Savage, Dillon and Taylor, 1979). Alternatively there are devices that record low frequency vibrations in arterial walls, that is infrasound. These are just as accurate for systolic pressure measurement but less so for diastolic (Savage, Dillon and Taylor, 1979).

Further indirect methods of recording blood pressure when the Korotkoff sounds cannot be heard, especially in infants, include palpation of the radial or brachial arteries and the so-called flush method. The former gives a gross estimation of systolic blood pressure which is usually 5–10 mmHg less than that obtained on auscultation. The flush method is cumbersome and only provides a mean blood pressure measurement.

Normal blood pressure and the definition of hypertension

Blood pressure varies directly with age and hence it is important to compare values in children with the normal range for age before interpretation is attempted. Normal ranges of childhood blood pressure have been published (Londe, 1966; Blumenthal *et al.*, 1977; André *et*

al., 1978; Leumann, 1979) but are hardly comparable in view of the variability in both the conditions of sampling and the techniques used for measurement. The ranges quoted in the *Report of the Task Force on Blood Pressure Control in Children* (Blumenthal *et al.*, 1977) are representative (*Figure 6.1.*) although they are pooled data from several different studies.

In view of these findings it is clearly inappropriate to consider a blood pressure of 140/90 mmHg as the upper limit of normal throughout childhood since a considerable number of hypertensive children with blood pressures less than this would remain undetected. This raises the difficult question of the definition of hypertension in childhood. Rather than absolute values, levels repeatedly exceeding a given percentile—for example the 90th (Londe *et al.*, 1971), the 95th (Blumenthal *et al.*, 1977) or the 97.5th (André *et al.*, 1978)—or exceeding two standard deviations above the mean (Rance *et al.*, 1974) are now becoming accepted limits. As a result a few apparently normal children are by definition considered to be hypertensive. In clinical practice there is no problem when the

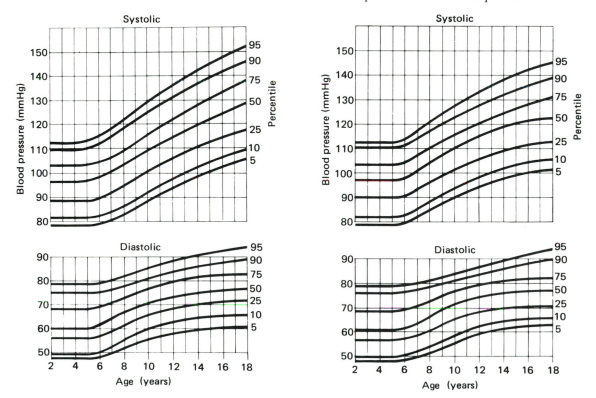

Figure 6.1. Percentiles of blood pressure measurement in boys (left) and girls (right) from the *Report of the Task Force on Blood Pressure Control in Children* (Blumenthal *et al.*, 1977).

hypertension is severe, and difficulties only arise in the borderline situation when blood pressure only just exceeds what is considered to be the normal range for age.

The incidence of hypertension

The exact incidence of hypertension in children and adolescents is not yet known but various authors have claimed that 1–11 per cent of children have a raised blood pressure (Loggie, 1977). However, many of these data were obtained from single examinations of the children in question, rather than from a series of recordings in the same subjects. If the blood pressure is measured on several separate occasions the incidence of hypertension decreases and in schoolchildren it has been found to lie between 1–3 per cent (Leumann, 1979).

The importance of blood pressure measurement

Severe sustained hypertension in childhood carries a high risk of morbidity and mortality if untreated (Still and Cottom, 1967). In 80–90 per cent of cases it is secondary to some underlying and often remediable, cause (Londe, 1978) and therefore there is a considerable advantage to be gained by its detection. The benefits of recognizing mild to moderate degrees of hypertension are not so clear cut. Nevertheless, since it is known that hypertension is a major factor in the genesis of arterial disease in adults (Kannel and Dawber, 1974) and that essential hypertension appears to have its origins in childhood (Londe *et al.*, 1971), there appears to be some value in identifying those at risk. From studies demonstrating familial aggregation of blood pressure it seems that hypertensive adults beget hypertensive children. Identification of these children may allow modification of early environmental factors which might counteract hypertensive familial traits or enable early treatment to be undertaken before serious sequelae ensue.

Causes of hypertension

When considering the causes of hypertension it is valuable to differentiate between transient and sustained increases in blood pressure. There are many conditions that may be associated with acute and usually short-lived increases in blood pressure in children. Within this category renal disease predominates and hypertension is frequently seen in acute glomerulonephritis, the haemolytic-uraemic syndrome, Henoch-Schönlein nephritis, acute renal failure from any cause and following renal transplantation as a feature of rejection or graft arterial stenosis. Hypertension is also seen after urological surgery (Berens, Linde and Goodwin, 1966) and may be due to disturbance of renal perfusion after the kidney has been handled or damaged. In addition transient hypertension can be seen with burns, poliomyelitis, the Guillain-Barré syndrome, familial dysautonomia and raised intracranial pressure, and on the administration of corticosteroids, the contraceptive pill and sympathomimetic medications (Londe, 1978). These are not dealt with here, although it is important to emphasize that some of the affected patients may go on to develop sustained hypertension at a later stage.

When considering sustained hypertension, the severity of the hypertension and the age group under consideration are important factors. Severe symptomatic hypertension is likely to be secondary to renal disease in the majority of cases (Londe, 1978). Mild hypertension detected incidentally as part of a routine clinical examination has a much greater chance of being primary or essential in nature (Londe, 1978). The main causes of sustained hypertension in children are given in *Table 6.1*.

Table 6.1 Causes of sustained hypertension in childhood

Coarctation of the aorta	
Chronic renal failure	
Renin-dependent hypertension	Renovascular disease
	Renal parenchymal disease
	Renal tumours
Catecholamine-excess hypertension	Neuroblastoma
	Phaeochromocytoma
Corticosteroid-excess hypertension	Iatrogenic
	Congenital adrenal hyperplasia
	Conn's and Cushing's syndromes
Essential hypertension	

Coarctation of the aorta

This constitutes the second most important cause of hypertension after renal disease and is seen in 10 per cent of paediatric patients with secondary hypertension (Leumann, 1979). The cause of hypertension in thoracic coarctation is complex and still not fully understood. Mechanical obstruction is the simplest explanation and the role of the renin-angiotensin system is controversial. Diagnosis is based on the finding of upper limb hypertension associated with delayed femoral pulses and a significant blood pressure difference between the arms and the legs. Detailed investigation and treatment come within the province of the cardiologist and the cardiovascular surgeon and are not dealt with here. Coarctation of the abdominal aorta may be associated with renal arterial narrowing and in this situation the hypertension is usually renin-dependent (*see* Chapter 7).

Chronic renal failure

Chronic renal failure from any cause may be associated with hypertension, which is usually due to sodium and water overload. The renin-angiotensin system is not thought to play a major role in this type of hypertension and treatment is orientated towards saline removal by dietary salt restriction, diuretics and dialysis. In spite of this there is some evidence of an abnormal relationship between circulating renin and exchangeable sodium in these patients (Davies *et al.*, 1973) and inappropriate renin release could play an additive role. In some patients the hypertension is refractory to saline depletion and these individuals have extremely high levels of plasma renin (Weidmann and Maxwell, 1975). Under these circumstances bilateral nephrectomy may be required to control the hypertension and drugs that block angiotensin II production by converting enzyme inhibition may also have a therapeutic role (Brunner *et al.*, 1978).

Hypertension associated with activation of the renin-angiotensin system

Conditions in which hypertension is associated with activation of the renin-angiotensin system include renal ischaemia due to various forms of renovascular disease, many varieties of parenchymal renal disease (but especially pyelonephritic scarring), renin-secreting tumours and malignant hypertension of any cause (Dillon, 1974). Secondary hyperaldosteronism with hypokalaemia tends to occur in the majority of these situations.

Physiology of the renin-angiotensin system

Renin is a proteolytic enzyme secreted by the juxtaglomerular cells of the afferent arterioles in response to a variety of stimuli. The most important of these is a decrease in renal arterial perfusion pressure, while changes in the sodium concentration of renal tubular fluid, sympathetic nervous activity, and plasma levels of potassium, antidiuretic hormone and prostaglandins also play a part. In addition there is evidence for negative feedback inhibition secondary to levels of angiotensin II in the circulation.

Renin acts on an alpha$_2$ globulin (renin substrate) synthesized by the liver, forming the relatively inactive decapeptide angiotensin I (*Figure 6.2*). Further hydrolysis by converting

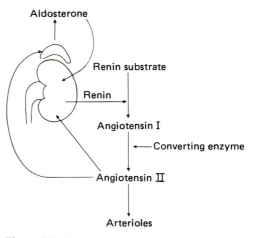

Figure 6.2. Simplified diagrammatic representation of the renin-angiotensin system. (From Dillon, 1974.)

enzyme in the lung, the plasma, the kidney and the vascular endothelium yields the most potent pressor substance known, namely the octapeptide angiotensin II. This is broken down by angiotensinases to smaller peptides of five to seven residues with much less biological activity. A specific role has been attributed to only one of these, a heptapeptide known as des,asp-angiotensin II (angiotensin III), which is far less active than angiotensin II as a pressor substance but equipotent as a stimulator of aldosterone production.

Angiotensin II acts on specific receptors in the arteriolar walls causing vasoconstriction. It also acts centrally on the area postrema of the medulla oblongata producing a central pressor effect. In the adrenal cortex it is the main determinant, perhaps with angiotensin III, of secretion by the zona glomerulosa of aldosterone which induces sodium and water reabsorption in the distal tubules. Aldosterone secretion is also stimulated by increased plasma potassium levels, ACTH secretion and sodium depletion.

Within the kidney angiotensin II appears to have contrasting actions dependent on its concentration. In small quantities it causes sodium and water retention and in larger amounts sodium and water excretion. These differing actions can be explained in terms of angiotensin II having on the one hand local homeostatic intrarenal actions, perhaps as part of a glomerulotubular feedback system, and on the other hand renal effects caused by an increase in systemic blood pressure. For a review of this complex subject see Oparil and Haber (1974), Peart (1975), Davis and Freeman (1976) and New and Levine (1978).

In infancy and childhood the renin-angiotensin system appears to be particularly active. The reason for this activity remains unclear although it may be related to greater dependence on this system's integrity for the maintenance of sodium balance and blood pressure control.

There are now many published reports demonstrating an inverse relationship between age and measurable components of the renin-angiotensin system including plasma renin activity (PRA) and plasma aldosterone concentration (Dillon and Ryness, 1975). In healthy children these plasma levels are almost entirely dependent on age and only marginally attributable to differences in other variables such as sodium intake. This inverse relationship extends into the neonatal period with particularly increased PRA and plasma aldosterone concentration in cord blood samples from vaginally delivered neonates (Dillon *et al.*, 1976).

The mechanism by which increased activity of the renin-angiotensin system is maintained in the young is still speculative. One possibility is that the young infant with relatively immature proximal renal tubular function is much more dependent than the older child or adult on distal tubular sodium reabsorptive mechanisms under renin-angiotensin control to maintain his sodium balance (Dillon, 1974). In practical terms it is essential to relate any values of peripheral venous renin or aldosterone to the normal range for age before attempting to interpret them.

Pathology of the renin-angiotensin system

The ischaemic kidney secretes renin and through the vasopressor effects of angiotensin II causes hypertension. There is some controversy as to whether the measurement of peripheral PRA has a diagnostic role in providing evidence of stimulation of the renin-angiotensin system in childhood hypertension (Robson, 1978; Leumann, 1979). However, it has been shown that in children with significant hypertension secondary to renovascular disease or pyelonephritic scarring the PRA is raised above the normal range for age in the majority of cases (*Figure 6.3*; Dillon and Ryness, 1975; Savage *et al.*, 1978). On the other hand, it is well known that hypertensive children can have an increased PRA without underlying renal disease

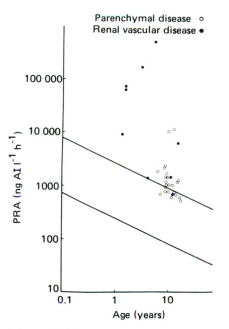

Figure 6.3. Plasma renin activity levels in hypertensive children with scarred kidneys and renovascular disease. The lines indicate the upper and lower limits of the normal range. (From Dillon, 1981.)

(Robson, 1978) while the converse rarely occurs. A very low PRA in a hypertensive child may be the clue to an underlying mineralocorticoid-excess state (New and Levine, 1978).

Measurement of peripheral PRA may also have a useful role in predicting which children with pyelonephritic scarring will subsequently develop hypertension. Since approximately 10 per cent of children with renal scarring become hypertensive (Wallace, Rothwell and Williams, 1978) it is of some importance to identify those at risk of this complication. If overproduction of renin is the cause of hypertension in this situation then early measurement of PRA may have predictive value. In a recent study by Savage *et al.* (1978) eight out of 100 normotensive children with renal scarring had peripheral PRA values above the normal range for age. It remains to be seen whether these are the ones who go on to develop hypertension at a later stage.

Renal venous renin measurements

Determination of bilateral renal venous renin levels has been established as an important diagnostic procedure to identify surgically curable forms of renal hypertension in adults (Stockigt *et al.*, 1972) and this technique has now been applied successfully to the investigation of hypertensive children (Godard, 1977; Dillon, Shah and Barratt, 1978; Robson, 1978). Gerdts *et al.* (1979) recently established a reference range for renal venous PRA ratios in normotensive children free from renal disease. This study supported a ratio of 1.5 as an accept-

able upper limit of normality for the interpretation of renal venous PRA ratios in the investigation of children with suspected renal hypertension.

In hypertensive children in whom renal venous renin measurements have been taken, the ratio of 1.5 has been shown to be a good predictor of surgical success in patients with renal lesions amenable to surgical treatment. In fact 100 per cent surgical success can be obtained in terms of subsequent blood pressure control when a renal venous renin ratio above 1.5 is used as an indication for operation (*Figure 6.4*; Dillon, Shah and Barratt, 1978). However, some reports have doubted the value of this method of investigating childhood hypertension because of an unacceptably high incidence of false-negative main venous ratios (Godard, 1977). It may be possible to eliminate this problem by the use of segmental renal venous sampling to identify local sources of renin release (Schambelan *et al.*, 1974). A similar technique can be applied to hypertensive post-transplantation patients in an attempt to identify whether the graft or the original kidneys are contributing to the hypertension (Dillon, Shah and Barratt, 1978).

Pharmacological blockade of angiotensin II and converting enzyme

Pharmacological means of blocking the action or production of angiotensin II have been developed which may have diagnostic and therapeutic roles. Saralasin (1-sar-8-ala-angiotensin

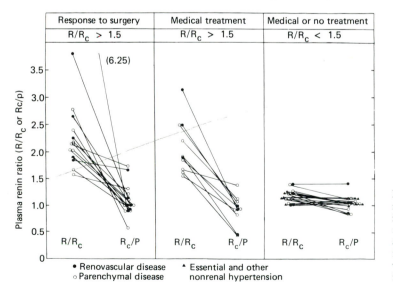

Figure 6.4. Renal venous plasma renin ratios in hypertensive children divided into groups according to the ratio and the response to treatment. (From Dillon, Shah and Barratt, 1978.) R = PRA in renal vein from diseased kidney; R_c = PRA in renal vein from contralateral kidney; P = PRA in caudal inferior vena cava.

II) is a competitive angiotensin II inhibitor that has been found to be a valuable tool for detecting an angiotensinogenic component in certain types of hypertension (Streeten *et al.*, 1975). A significant decrease in blood pressure coupled with an increase in PRA on infusion of saralasin intravenously under controlled conditions is the criterion by which the response is judged (Baer *et al.*, 1977). In children this test can be helpful in demonstrating the involvement of the renin-angiotensin system in various types of hypertension, although interpretation can be difficult (Favre *et al.*, 1979).

The oral converting enzyme inhibitor Captopril (S.Q.14225) initially looked promising as another diagnostic test for hyper-reninaemic hypertension, but has proved to be disappointing in this context. It now appears that this drug is capable of nonspecifically lowering the blood pressure in a variety of conditions. In spite of this it is clearly an agent with enormous therapeutic potential (Brunner *et al.*, 1978).

Plasma renin-aldosterone profiles and urinary steroid analysis

See Corticosteroid-excess hypertension.

Renovascular disease

This is discussed in detail in Chapter 7. However, it is worth emphasizing that renal arterial stenosis can be familial and can be associated with idiopathic hypercalcaemia, Marfan's syndrome, rubella and, most importantly, neurofibromatosis.

In terms of diagnostic imaging, intravenous urography and renal arteriography are of proven value, and dynamic renal scanning with ^{99m}Tc-diethylenetriaminepentacetic acid may also have a useful role (*see* Chapter 2). Peripheral plasma renin measurements, perhaps coupled with a saralasin test, can identify a renin-dependent hypertensive state. Divided renal venous renin determinations can then localize the site or sites of renin release and allow prediction of surgical success if revascularization surgery or nephrectomy is planned (*see* Pathology of the renin-angiotensin system).

Renal parenchymal disease

Although there are many types of disease affecting the renal parenchyma, the commonest and

most important in terms of causing hypertension is pyelonephritic scarring. This type of coarse renal scarring causes two thirds of all severe hypertension in childhood (Still and Cottom, 1967) and is associated almost exclusively with vesicoureteric reflux and urinary tract infection in early life (Smellie and Normand, 1975). *See* Chapters 2, 10 and 15 for more detailed discussion on this subject.

Hypertension is usually a late sequel (Heale, 1977), rarely developing in the first 5 years of life and in some cases first detected in the malignant phase in late childhood. It has been shown that approximately 10 per cent of children with renal scarring become hypertensive (Holland, Kotchen and Bhathena, 1975; Wallace, Rothwell and Williams, 1978) and in view of the relationship between hypertension and late deterioration of renal function (Heale, 1977) this is clearly an important and worrying complication.

The genesis of hypertension in these cases is not clear, although the renin-angiotensin system probably plays an important part (Holland, Kotchen and Bhathena, 1975; Siegler, 1976; Savage *et al.*, 1978). Not only is peripheral PRA increased in the majority of children with pyelonephritic scarring and hypertension (Savage *et al.*, 1978), but also divided renal venous renin measurements can, as in renovascular disease, localize sources of renin release within the kidney or kidneys (Dillon, Shah and Barratt, 1978). However, a word of caution is required when surgical management of the hypertension by nephrectomy or partial nephrectomy is being considered. Although in unilateral disease with a normal contralateral kidney and lateralization of renin release to the affected side nephrectomy is likely to cure the hypertension (Dillon, Shah and Barratt, 1978) in bilateral disease in which disparity of function is less marked and renal venous renin ratios are equivocal medical treatment is to be preferred.

Other causes of parenchymal disease that can be associated with hypertension include chronic glomerulonephritis, the haemolytic-uraemic syndrome, dysplastic and hypoplastic kidneys and polycystic renal disease (Gill *et al.*, 1976). Hypertension can also occur after irradiation of the kidney (Vidt, 1977) and this must be an important consideration when planning treatment for renal or other abdominal malignant disease. The so-called Ask-Upmark kidney or segmental hypoplasia is considered by some to be caused by an arterial occlusion very early in development and hence to be an example of renovascular disease (Royer *et al.*, 1971) and by others to represent a polar pyelonephritic scar (Bernstein, 1978). In practical terms the origin matters very little, and for all intents and purposes this kidney can be handled in the same way as one with pyelonephritic scarring.

Finally the kidney following renal venous thrombosis may, after shrinkage, cause hypertension many years after the original event (Arneil *et al.*, 1973; *see* Chapter 7).

Renal tumours

This infrequent cause of hypertension can be associated with nephroblastoma (Ganguly *et al.*, 1973), rare renin-producing tumours of the juxtaglomerular cells called haemangiopericytomas (Robertson *et al.*, 1967) and renal hamartomas (Hirose *et al.*, 1974).

In Wilms' tumour hypertension may be due to distortion of the renal vasculature resulting in ischaemic hyper-reninaemia, but evidence is becoming available which implicates excessive renin production by the tumour itself (Ganguly *et al.*, 1973).

Since the first haemangiopericytoma was described by Robertson *et al.* (1967) 12 or more other patients affected have been reported, approximately half of them children (Leumann, 1979). The tumours are always small and difficult to locate even with selective renal arteriography. Peripheral plasma renin is increased and divided renal venous renin measurements allow identification of the site of the lesion within the affected kidney. Nephrectomy results in cure and so far no evidence of malignancy has been reported. *See* Chapter 32 for more detailed discussion of renal neoplasms.

Catecholamine-excess hypertension

Catecholamine-excess hypertension is caused by a functioning neural crest tumour. This can take the form of a phaeochromocytoma, a neuroblastoma or a ganglioneuroma. Phaeochromocytomas can arise in the adrenal medulla or at any site in the sympathetic chain. In children they account for 2 per cent of the causes of secondary hypertension (Leumann, 1979). Boys are affected twice as often as girls and approximately two thirds of childhood phaeochromocytomas

reported in the literature occurred in the adrenal medulla (Stackpole, Melicow and Uson, 1963). The most frequent extra-adrenal sites include the region of the adrenals (with no direct involvement of them), the aortic bifurcation and the renal hilum (Stackpole, Melicow and Uson, 1963). Although phaeochromocytomas are usually sporadic they are occasionally familial and are associated with Von Recklinghausen's disease, Von Hippel-Lindau's disease, and Sipple's syndrone, that is medullary carcinoma of the thyroid, multiple mucosal neuromas, phaeochromocytoma and hyperparathyroidism. Hypertension was sustained in 88 per cent of paediatric cases reviewed by Stackpole, Melicow and Uson (1963) and the clinical symptoms observed were headaches in 75 per cent, sweating in 67 per cent, nausea and vomiting in 48 per cent, visual disturbances in 37 per cent, abdominal pain in 32 per cent, polydipsia and polyuria in 31 per cent, convulsions in 22 per cent and acrocyanosis in 22 per cent.

The diagnosis of phaeochromocytoma is established by demonstrating increased urinary excretion of catecholamines or their metabolites. The commonest screening test is the measurement of urinary vanillylmandelic acid (Hakulinen, 1971) although a normal level does not exclude the diagnosis (Lieberman, 1978). Specific measurements of urinary and plasma noradrenaline and adrenaline may be helpful in this situation (Moss, Greenbaum and Sever, 1980). The phentolamine test and therapeutic trial of phenoxybenzamine have their place in diagnosis but both can give misleading results.

Localization of the tumour may be difficult, especially if multiple sites are involved. Ultrasound, arteriography (after alpha-adrenergic blockade), computed tomography and vena caval catecholamine sampling are all useful (Loggie, 1971; Leumann, 1979).

Treatment is surgical but must only be undertaken after full alpha-adrenergic blockade has been achieved with oral phenoxybenzamine 1–4 mg/kg per day. Usually beta-blockers are required in addition to counteract the tachycardia produced and also in some circumstances to block the effects of excess adrenaline production. Resistance to oral alpha-blockers has been reported (Robinson *et al.*, 1977) and in this circumstance the use of alpha-methyltyrosine, which inhibits the conversion of tyrosine to dopa, has been advocated (Robinson *et al.*, 1977). During surgical removal of the tumour short-acting parenteral alpha-blockers must be available to cope with the sudden increase in blood pressure that may occur if the tumour is handled. Phentolamine is well established in this context but labetalol (Cumming and Davies, 1979) is proving to be a particularly valuable agent. It is also critically important to treat the hypotension that follows removal of the tumour rapidly with blood volume expansion.

The long-term outlook is good in the majority of cases and the incidence of malignancy is low and of the order of 5–10 per cent (Leumann, 1979). For an account of neuroblastoma *see* Chapter 33.

Corticosteroid-excess hypertension

This is a relatively rare cause of hypertension in childhood. Apart from extraneously administered corticosteroids, it can result from certain forms of congenital adrenal hyperplasia, Conn's syndrome, Cushing's syndrome and so-called apparent mineralocorticoid-excess states. The hypertensive forms of congenital adrenal hyperplasia are 11-beta-hydroxylase deficiency and 17-alpha-hydroxylase deficiency (New and Levine, 1978). In the former there is virilization and accumulation of deoxycorticosterone and deoxycortisol. PRA is suppressed and the hypertension is thought to be due to excess deoxycorticosterone. In 17-alpha-hydroxylase deficiency the majority of patients have a female phenotype and the hypertension is also considered to be due to excess deoxycorticosterone secretion. *See* Chapter 48 for further details and available treatment.

Cushing's syndrome is commonly associated with hypertension and 21 of 26 cases reported by Loridan and Senior (1969) had increased blood pressure. The hypertension is thought to be due to the mineralocorticoid effect of excess cortisol. However, an increase in renin substrate and hence angiotensin II may play a part. The cause in childhood is most commonly an adrenal carcinoma or adenoma (New and Levine, 1978). *See* Chapter 33 for details of treatment.

Conn's syndrome or primary hyperaldosteronism is extremely rare in childhood. It can be caused by an aldosterone-producing tumour but is more commonly due to bilateral adrenal hyperplasia (New and Levine, 1978). Peripheral PRA is suppressed and plasma aldosterone increased. Surgery is the treatment of choice for tumours while long-term spironolactone may be necessary for hyperplasia (Conn, 1974). Dexamethasone-suppressible hyperaldosteronism is a rare familial form (New and Levine, 1978) in which remission of the hypertension comes about with glucocorticoid therapy.

Apparent mineralocorticoid-excess states have recently been recognized and comprise hypertension, hypokalaemic alkalosis and decreased PRA and plasma aldosterone concentration (New and Levine, 1978). This type of hypertension responds to spironolactone and triamterine and is made worse by administered ACTH. It is thought that these children may have modified metabolism of adrenal steroids giving rise to a relative increase in some unusual cortisol metabolites with the ability to cause hypertension (Shackleton *et al.*, 1980).

Essential hypertension

A diagnosis of essential hypertension can only be made after the exclusion of all known causes of hypertension. The prevalence of essential hypertension is extremely difficult to ascertain but seems to be less than 3 per cent in schoolchildren. It is perhaps slightly higher in black males (Leumann, 1979).

Clinical features of hypertension

Symptoms of hypertension in childhood vary considerably and all too often are totally lacking. There appear to be some differences in the presenting features according to the age of the child. During infancy congestive cardiac failure, respiratory distress, failure to thrive, vomiting, irritability and convulsions are the commonest features whereas in older children headache, nausea, vomiting, polydipsia, polyuria, visual symptoms, tiredness, irritability, cardiac failure, facial weakness, epistaxis and growth retardation are seen most frequently (Gill *et al.*, 1976; Dillon, 1978; Leumann, 1979). Unfortunately, children can present with features of malignant hypertension including loss of consciousness, fits and hemiplegia with only minimal preceding symptomatology (Dillon, 1979). Palpitations, sweating and pallor may suggest an underlying phaeochromocytoma but these symptoms can also occur at times with renovascular causes of hypertension.

Physical examination may reveal signs of cardiomegaly or evidence of hypertensive retinopathy. There may also be specific signs associated with the underlying cause of the hypertension, for example delayed pulses and blood pressure differences between the upper and lower limbs in coarctation of the aorta, a bruit in the abdomen or flank in renovascular disease (a rare occurrence), café au lait patches in neurofibromatosis with renal arterial stenosis, abdominal masses in nephroblastoma and neuroblastoma, and cushingoid features or evidence of virilization in disturbances of adrenocortical function.

Of these signs and symptoms it is worth specially emphasizing the importance of three features. Headache is the commonest presenting symptom (Leumann, 1979) and may precede the detection of the hypertension by months or even years. Failing vision or even blindness may be secondary to retinopathy, cortical damage or infarction of the optic nerves (Dillon, 1978; Hulse, Taylor and Dillon, 1979). The last is an extremely serious complication since it can lead to permanent visual loss. Finally, lower motor neurone facial weakness is a presenting feature in a significant number of hypertensive children (Hulse, Taylor and Dillon, 1979) and the blood pressure should always be measured in a child presenting with this symptom.

Investigations

There is now a wide range of investigative procedures that can be utilized in the evaluation of children with hypertension (*Table 6.2*). Some of these are routine tests easily undertaken in most hospitals while others are more refined methods only available in specialized units.

Simple tests can provide valuable information that may either establish the diagnosis or allow rational decisions to be made about which specific tests are appropriate. However, critical interpretation of the results is important since hypertension can cause secondary effects that may be diagnostically misleading. For example renal failure and proteinuria may be due to the hypertension and need not imply the presence of primary renal disease.

The severity and duration of hypertension can often be gauged by ECG changes or radiologically by the heart size. Intravenous urography may reveal evidence of renal asymmetry or scarring and a late nephrogram followed by a prolonged dense pyelogram may show unilateral renal arterial stenosis or renal displacement in

Table 6.2   Investigation of children with sustained hypertension

	Routine tests	Special tests
Blood	Full blood picture	Peripheral plasma renin
	Electrolytes, urea, creatinine	Peripheral plasma aldosterone
	Calcium	Peripheral plasma catecholamines
		Glomerular filtration rate with ^{51}Cr-EDTA
Urine	Microscopy and culture	Urinary steroid excretion
	Protein estimation	Urinary catecholamines
	Vanillylmandelic acid	
Imaging	Chest X-ray	Abdominal ultrasound
	Skull X-ray	Renal scintillography
	Intravenous urography	Aortography, renal and adrenal arteriography
	Micturating cystourethrography	Angiocardiography
		Adrenal venography
		Brain and abdominal computed tomography
Other	Electrocardiography	Main and segmental renal venous renin estimations
	Bone marrow	Catecholamine estimations in the inferior vena cava and adrenal veins
		Adrenal venous steroid estimations
		Rogitine test
		Saralasin test
		Echocardiography
		Cardiac catheterization
		Dexamethasone suppression test

the presence of a suprarenal mass (*see* Chapter 2). This investigation should be undertaken only when the blood pressure is controlled in view of the solute load provided by the contrast medium. Micturating cystography can add further information about the presence or absence of vesicoureteric reflux or an obstructive uropathy such as urethral valves. These techniques are of proven value (Chrispin and Scatliff, 1973; Robson, 1978), but it is worth remembering that abdominal ultrasound and both dynamic (^{99m}Tc-diethylenetriaminepentacetic acid) and static (^{99m}Tc-dimercaptosuccinic acid) renal scanning also have useful roles. Ultrasound can provide valuable information about renal shape, size and texture quite apart from its ability to detect extrarenal lesions (Koenigsberg, Freeman and Blaufox, 1978; Robson, 1978). It also has the advantage of being noninvasive and does not carry the risk of a solute load in the presence of hypertension. Static renal imaging provides an alternative means of demonstrating renal anatomy whereas dynamic imaging reflects renal perfusion and can be useful in demonstrating circumstances in which this is compromised, for example renal arterial disease (Koenigsberg, Freeman and Blaufox, 1978). However, the technique has not superseded renal arteriography as the investigation of choice when attempting to demonstrate anomalies of the renal vasculature.

Measures of the activity of the renin-angiotensin system and the utilization of means of selectively blocking its action have already been dealt with. Similarly details of the investigation of corticosteroid-excess and catecholamine-excess states have been described in detail.

Finally, since many children with accelerated hypertension have neurological complications the availability of a brain scanner is of considerable value.

Treatment

The treatment of hypertension is a very controversial subject in both adults and children (Dillon, 1978, 1979; Lieberman, 1978; Siegel and Mulrow, 1978; Sinaiko and Mirkin, 1978). It can be considered under the following headings:

1. Treatment of the acute hypertensive emergency
2. Medical treatment of moderate to severe chronic hypertension
3. Surgical treatment of moderate to severe chronic hypertension
4. Treatment of mild hypertension.

The acute hypertensive emergency

Emergency management is indicated when the level of blood pressure is a threat to life or the normal function of vital organs. Drugs with rapid actions are necessary but require careful handling to prevent the development of sudden hypotension (*Table 6.3*; Hulse, Taylor and Dillon, 1979; Ledingham and Rajagopalan, 1979).

Table 6.3   Drug treatment of the acute hypertensive emergency (see text for details of administration)

Drug	Dose	Action	Comment
Labetalol	1–3 mg/kg per h IV (total 0.5–5.0 mg/kg)	Alpha-blocker and beta-blocker	Drug of choice; use alone; stop infusate when blood pressure is controlled; effective 4–6 hours
Sodium nitroprusside	0.5–8.0 μg/kg per min IV	Direct vasodilator	Very short duration of action; only effective while being infused
Diazoxide	2–10 mg/kg IV bolus	Direct vasodilator	Can cause hyperglycaemia, hypotension and salt and water retention
Hydrallazine	0.1–0.2 mg/kg IV or IM	Direct vasodilator	Can cause tachycardia, headache and flushing
Minoxidil	0.1–0.2 mg/kg PO	Direct vasodilator	Rapidly effective even though orally administered
Frusemide	1–2 mg/kg IV	Diuretic	Avoid unless saline overload is obvious
Phentolamine	0.1–0.2 mg/kg IV	Alpha-blocker	Hypertensive crisis of phaeochromocytomas

Intravenous hydrallazine and reserpine were at one time considered to be the drugs of choice in this situation (Etteldorf, Smith and Johnson, 1956). These were superseded by intravenous diazoxide (McLaine and Drummond, 1971) which remains a very valuable tool in the management of severe hypertension. However, the risk of sudden hypotension after a bolus injection of this agent has necessitated the introduction of drugs that on incremental infusion can very finely control the blood pressure during this critical early phase of management. Sodium nitroprusside (Luderer *et al.*, 1977) and labetalol (Cumming and Davies, 1979) are ideal in these circumstances, and the latter is becoming the first-line drug of choice for the hypertensive emergency. The new oral hypotensive minoxidil (Pennisi *et al.*, 1977) also has a place in the management of patients who fail to respond adequately to standard therapy and it appears to be almost as effective as the above parenteral preparations.

Many children have salt depletion on presentation with severe hypertension and the administration of diuretics with other hypotensive agents may result in severe volume depletion and a precipitous drop in blood pressure. Unless saline overload is an obvious threat to life it is probably safer to reserve diuretics until the hypertensive state is stabilized. Serious neurological sequelae can be associated with a rapid reduction in blood pressure (Hulse, Taylor and Dillon, 1979; Ledingham and Rajagopalan, 1979). Failure of autoregulatory mechanisms can cause inadequate perfusion of the brain, the spinal cord and the optic nerves with resulting ischaemic damage (Hulse, Taylor and Dillon, 1979; Ledingham and Rajagopalan, 1979). Maintaining the blood pressure during acute treatment at a level where autoregulation

Table 6.4   Drug treatment of moderate to severe chronic hypertension (see text for details of administration)

Drug	Oral dose initial (per kg/day)	maximum (per kg/day)		Comment
Propranolol	1–2 mg	15 mg	Beta-blocker	Drug of choice; contraindicated in asthma and cardiac failure
Hydrallazine	1–2 mg	8 mg	Direct vasodilator	Drug of choice; occasionally causes reversible lupus syndrome; reflex tachycardia is avoided by use of a beta-blocker as well
Chlorothiazide	10 mg	40 mg	Diuretic	Useful for mild hypertension; may need potassium supplementation
Frusemide	0.5–1.0 mg	15 mg	Diuretic	Often necessary with vasodilator drugs and in renal failure; potassium supplementation necessary
Prazosin	0.05–0.1 mg	0.4 mg	Direct vasodilator and alpha-blocker	Well tolerated; introduce carefully since hypotension can occur with a large initial dose
Minoxidil	0.1–0.2 mg	1–2 mg	Direct vasodilator	Extremely effective in refractory hypertension; side effects hirsutism and saline retention
Captopril	0.3 mg	5 mg	Converting enzyme inhibitor	Recently released for clinical use; remarkably effective in renin-dependent hypertension
Methyldopa	5 mg	40 mg	Central alpha-adrenergic stimulator	Main problem is sedation and depression
Bethanidine	0.4 mg	10 mg	Postganglionic adrenergic blocker	Marked postural hypotension
Diazoxide	5 mg	25 mg	Direct vasodilator	Saline retention, hyperglycaemia and hirsutism
Clonidine	5 μg	30 μg	Central alpha-adrenergic stimulator	Depression; reflex hypertension on withdrawal
Phenoxybenzamine	1 mg	4 mg	Alpha-sympathetic blocker	Useful for oral control of blood pressure in phaeochromocytoma before surgery; often needs a beta-blocker because of reflex tachycardia
Spironolactone	1 mg	3 mg	Competitive aldosterone antagonist	Potassium retention and gynaecomastia

can still function may prevent these complications. This usually means that the blood pressure must be reduced a little more slowly than hitherto recommended and kept somewhat above the normal range for age by intravenous saline or plasma if necessary (Hulse, Taylor and Dillon, 1979).

Medical treatment of moderate to severe chronic hypertension

Management depends on the underlying cause of hypertension. A wide variety of drugs is available (*Table 6.4*) but at present the most effective treatment seems to be a combination of a peripheral vasodilator, for example hydrallazine, and a beta-blocker such as propranolol (Dillon, 1978; Siegel and Mulrow, 1978). A diuretic may also be required to offset the salt and water retention that occurs with the use of peripheral vasodilators. Alternative agents that are available include prazosin (Sinaiko and Mirkin, 1978) and minoxidil (Pennisi *et al.*, 1977). Although advocated by some, methyldopa, clonidine and bethanidine are not ideal for routine use in childhood. The new converting enzyme inhibitor, captopril, is certainly beginning to prove valuable in the treatment of renin-dependent hypertension resistant to other agents (Brunner *et al.*, 1978). In catecholamine-excess states oral phenoxybenzamine coupled with a beta-blocker such as propranolol is indicated as a prelude to surgery. In Conn's syndrome due to adrenal hyperplasia spironolactone is indicated and in other mineralocorticoid-excess states hydrocortisone, dexamethasone or triamterine may be appropriate (*see* relevant preceding sections).

Surgical treatment of moderate to severe chronic hypertension

This may consist of resection of a narrowed aortic segment in coarctation; removal of an adrenal or renal tumour, revascularization or nephrectomy in renovascular disease; and nephrectomy or partial nephrectomy in certain types of renal parenchymal disease. Decisions concerning which kidney to remove or revascularize are made in part on detailed radiological studies coupled with renal venous renin measurements (*see* relevant section above and Chapters 7 and 32).

Treatment of mild hypertension

This is in many ways the most difficult area. It is important to balance the risks of prolonged drug treatment against those of leaving mild hypertension untreated. The dilemma is still unresolved since the natural history of childhood hypertension remains ill defined. However, from the adult literature there is good evidence that patients with borderline hypertension tend to develop more severe hypertension and suffer excess mortality and morbidity related to this (Julius, 1978). There is at present no reason to conclude that children behave differently. Decisions about treatment depend on the height of the blood pressure, its constancy, what is considered to be the underlying cause, and the presence or absence of various risk factors such as obesity and a hypertensive family history (Julius, 1978). If a child is symptomatic or there is evidence of cardiomegaly or left ventricular hypertrophy on chest X-ray or ECG then treatment is probably indicated.

Simple measures may be tried first, such as weight reduction and salt restriction. However, drugs may be necessary. Initially they may take the form of a thiazide diuretic alone, with the addition later on of a more powerful hypotensive such as propranolol if indicated.

References

André, J.L., Deschamps, J.P., Valantin, G. and Gueguen, R. (1978) Pression artérielle chez l'enfant et l'adolescent: valeurs normales et définition de l'hypertension. *Nouvelle Presse Medicale*, **7**, 2576

Arneil, G.C., MacDonald, A.M., Murphy, A.V. and Sweet, E.M. (1973) Renal venous thrombosis. *Clinical Nephrology*, **1**, 119

Baer, L., Parra-Carrillo, J., Radichevich, I. and Williams, G.S. (1977) Detection of renovascular hypertension with angiotensin II blockade. *Annals of Internal Medicine*, **86**, 257

Berens, S.C., Linde, L.M. and Goodwin, W.E. (1966) Transitory hypertension following urologic surgery in children. *Pediatrics*, **38**, 194

Bernstein, J. (1978) Renal hypoplasia and dysplasia. *In* Pediatric Kidney Disease (edited by Edelmann, C.E.). Little, Brown, Boston. p.541

Blumenthal, S., Epps, R.P., Heavenrich, R., Lauer, R.M., Lieberman, E., Mirkin, B., Mitchell, S.C., Naito, V.B., O'Hare, D., McFate Smith, T., Tarazi, R.C. and Upson, D. (1977) Report of the task force on blood pressure control in children. *Pediatrics*, **58**, Suppl. p.797

Brunner, H.R., Gavras, H., Turini, G.A., Waeber, B., Chappuis, P. and McKinstry, D.N. (1978) Long term treatment of hypertension in man by an orally active angiotensin-converting enzyme inhibitor. *Clinical Science and Molecular Medicine*, **55**, Suppl. 4, p.293

Chrispin, A.R. and Scatlif, J.H. (1973) Systemic hypertension in childhood. *Pediatric Radiology*, **1**, 75

Conn, J.W. (1974) Primary aldosteronism and primary reninism. *Hospital Practice*, **9**, 131

Cumming, A.M.M. and Davies, D.L. (1979) Intravenous labetalol in hypertensive emergency. *Lancet*, i, 929

Davies, D.L., Beevers, D.G., Briggs, J.D., Medina, A.M., Robertson, J.I.S., Schalekamp, M.A., Brown, J.J., Lever, A.F., Morton, J.J. and Tree, M. (1973) Abnormal relation between exchangeable sodium and the renin-angiotensin system in malignant hypertension and in hypertension with chronic renal failure. *Lancet*, i, 683

Davis, J.O. and Freeman, R.M. (1976) Mechanisms regulating renal disease. *Physiological Reviews*, **56**, 1

Dillon, M.J. (1981) Application of study of the renin-angiotensin system to paediatric urology. *In* Hypertension in Children and Adolescents (edited by Giovanni, G., New, M.I. and Gorini, S.). Raven, New York. p. 137

Dillon, M.J. (1974) Renin and hypertension in childhood. *Archives of Disease in Childhood*, **49**, 831

Dillon, M.J. (1978) Hypertension in childhood. *Update*, **17**, 1409

Dillon, M.J. (1979) Recent advances in evaluation and management of childhood hypertension. *European Journal of Pediatrics*, **132**, 133

Dillon, M.J. and Ryness, J.M. (1975) Plasma renin activity and aldosterone concentration in children. *British Medical Journal*, iv, 316

Dillon, M.J., Gillin, M.E.A., Ryness, J.M. and De Swiet, M. (1976) Plasma renin activity and aldosterone concentration in the human newborn. *Archives of Disease in Childhood*, **51**, 537

Dillon, M.J., Shah, V. and Barratt, T.M. (1978) Renal vein renin measurements in children with hypertension. *British Medical Journal*, ii, 168

Etteldorf, J.N., Smith, P.D. and Johnson, C. (1956) The effect of reserpine and its combination with hydrallazine on blood pressure and renal hemodynamics during the hypertensive phase of acute nephritis in children. *Journal of Pediatrics*, **48**, 129

Favre, L., Boerth, R.C., Braren, V., Dean, R.H. and Hollifield, J.W. (1979) Angiotensin II blockade by Saralasin in the evaluation of hypertension in children. *Kidney International*, **15**, Suppl.9, p.75

Ganguly, A., Gribble, J., Tyne, B., Kempson, R.L. and Luetscher, J.A. (1973) Renin secreting Wilms' tumour with severe hypertension: report of a case and brief review of renin-secreting tumors. *Annals of Internal Medicine*, **79**, 835

Gerdts, K.-G., Shah, V., Savage, J.M. and Dillon, M.J. (1979) Renal vein renin measurements in normotensive children. *Journal of Pediatrics*, **95**, 953

Gill, D.G., Mendes da Costa, B., Cameron, J.S., Joseph, M.C., Ogg, C.S. and Chantler, C. (1976) Analysis of 100 children with severe and persistent hypertension. *Archives of Disease in Childhood*, **51**, 951

Godard, C. (1977) Predictive value of renal-vein renin measurements in children with various forms of renal hypertension: an international study. *Helvetica Paediatrica Acta*, **32**, 49

Hakulinen, A. (1971) Urinary excretion of vanillylmandelic acid of children in normal and certain pathological conditions. *Acta Paediatrica Scandinavica*, **212**, Suppl. 1

Heale, W.F. (1977) Hypertension and reflux nephropathy. *Australian Paediatric Journal*, **13**, 56

Hirose, M., Arakawa, K., Kikuchi, M., Kawasaki, T., Omotu, T., Kato, H. and Nagayana, T. (1974) Primary reninism with renal hamartomatous alteration. *Journal of the American Medical Association*, **230**, 1288

Holland, N.H., Kotchen, T. and Bhathena, D. (1975) Hypertension in children with chronic pyelonephritis. *Kidney International*, **8**, Suppl. 5, p.243

Hulse, J.A., Taylor, D.S.I. and Dillon, M.J. (1979) Blindness and paraplegia in severe childhood hypertension. *Lancet*, ii, 553

Julius, S. (1978) Clinical and physiological significance of borderline hypertension in youth. *Pediatric Clinics of North America*, **25**, 35

Kannel, W.B. and Dawber, T.R. (1974) Hypertension as an ingredient of a cardiovascular risk profile. *British Journal of Hospital Medicine*, **11**, 508

Koenigsberg, M., Freeman, L.M. and Blaufox, M.D. (1978) Radionucleide and ultrasound evaluation of renal morphology and function. *In* Pediatric Kidney Disease (edited by Edelmann, C.M.). Little, Brown, Boston. p.236

Ledingham, J.G.G. and Rajagopalan, B. (1979) Cerebral complications in the treatment of accelerated hypertension. *Quarterly Journal of Medicine*, **48**, 25

Leumann, E.P. (1979) Blood pressure and hypertension in childhood and adolescence. *Ergebnesse der Inneren Medizin und Kinderheilkunde*, **43**, 109

Lieberman, E. (1978) Hypertension in childhood and adolescence. Ciba Clinical Symposia, Vol.30, No.3. Summit, New Jersey

Loggie, J.M.H. (1971) Systemic hypertension in children and adolescents: causes and treatment. *Pediatric Clinics of North America*, **18**, 1273

Loggie, J.M.H. (1977) Prevalence of hypertension and distribution of causes. *In* Juvenile Hypertension (edited by New, M.I. and Levine, L.S.). Raven, New York. p.1

Londe, S. (1966). Blood pressure in children as determined under office conditions. *Clinical Pediatrics*, **5**, 71

Londe, S. (1978) Causes of hypertension in the young. *Pediatric Clinics of North America*, **25**, 55

Londe, S., Bourgoignie, J.J., Robson, A.M. and Goldring, D. (1971) Hypertension in apparently normal children. *Journal of Pediatrics*, **78**, 569

Long, M., Dunlop, J.R. and Holland, W.W. (1971) Blood pressure recording in children. *Archives of Disease in Childhood*, **46**, 636

Loridan, L. and Senior, B. (1969) Cushing's syndrome in infancy. *Journal of Pediatrics*, **75**, 349

Luderer, J.R., Hayes, A.H., Dubynsky, O. and Berlin, C.M. (1977) Long term administration of sodium nitroprusside in childhood. *Journal of Pediatrics*, **91**, 490

McLaine, P.N. and Drummond, K.N. (1971) Intravenous diazoxide for severe hypertension in childhood. *Journal of Pediatrics*, **79**, 829

Moss, A.J. (1978) Indirect methods of blood pressure measurement. *Pediatric Clinics of North America*, **25**, 3

Moss, S., Greenbaum, R. and Sever, P.S. (1980) Preoperative localization of a phaeochromocytoma using plasma noradrenaline concentrations in multiple site samples. *Journal of the Royal Society of Medicine*, **73**, 139

New, M.I. and Levine, L.S. (1978) Adrenocortical hypertension. *Pediatric Clinics of North America*, **25**, 67

Oparil, S. and Haber, E. (1974) The renin-angiotensin system. *New England Journal of Medicine*, **291**, 389, 446

Peart, W.S. (1975) Renin-angiotensin system. *New England Journal of Medicine*, **292**, 302

Pennisi, A.J., Takahashi, M., Bernstein, B.H., Singsen, B.H., Vittenbogaart, C., Ettenger, R.B., Malekzadeh, M.H., Hanson, V. and Fine, R.N. (1977) Minoxidil therapy in children with severe hypertension. *Journal of Pediatrics*, **90**, 813

Rance, C.P., Arbus, G.S., Balfe, J.W. and Kooh, S.W. (1974) Persistent systemic hypertension in infants and children. *Pediatric Clinics of North America*, **21**, 801

Robertson, P.W., Klidjian, A., Harding, L.K., Walters, G., Lee, M.R. and Robb-Smith, A.H.T. (1967) Hypertension due to a renin-secreting tumour. *American Journal of Medicine*, **43**, 963

Robinson, R.G., De Quattro, V., Grushkin, C.M. and Lieberman, E. (1977) Childhood pheochromocytoma: treatment with alpha methyl tyrosine for resistant hypertension. *Journal of Pediatrics*, **91**, 143

Robson, A.M. (1978) Special diagnostic studies for the detection of renal and renovascular forms of hypertension. *Pediatric Clinics of North America*, **25**, 83

Royer, P., Broyer, M., Habib, R. and Nouaillie, Y. (1971) L'hypoplasie segmentaire du rein chez d'enfant. *In* Actualites Nephrologiques de l'Hôpital Necker. Flammarion, Paris. p.151

Savage, J.M., Dillon, M.J., Shah, V., Barratt, T.M. and Williams, D.I. (1978) Renin and blood pressure in children with renal scarring and vesicoureteric reflux. *Lancet*, ii, 441

Savage, J.M., Dillon, M.J. and Taylor, J.F.N. (1979) Clinical evaluation and comparison of the Infrasonde, Arteriosonde, and mercury sphygmomanometer in measurement of blood pressure in children. *Archives of Disease in Childhood*, **54**, 184

Schambelan, M., Glickman, M., Stockigt, J.R. and Biglieri, E.G. (1974) Selective renal-vein renin sampling in hypertensive patients with segmental renal lesions. *New England Journal of Medicine*, **290**, 1153

Shackleton, C.H.L., Honour, J.W., Dillon, M.J., Chantler, C. and Jones, R.W.A. (1980) Hypertension in a four-year-old child: gas chromatographic and mass spectrometric evidence for deficient hepatic metabolism of steroids. *Journal of Clinical Endocrinology and Metabolism*, **50**, 786

Siegel, N.J. and Mulrow, P.J. (1978) The management of hypertension. *In* Pediatric Kidney Disease (edited by Edelmann, C.M.). Little, Brown, Boston. p.457

Siegler, R.L. (1976) Renin-dependent hypertension in children with reflux nephropathy. *Urology*, **7**, 474

Sinaiko, A.R. and Mirkin, B.L. (1978) Clinical pharmacology of antihypertensive drugs in children. *Pediatric Clinics of North America*, **25**, 137

Smellie, J.M. and Normand, I.C.S. (1975) Bacteriuria, reflux and renal scarring. *Archives of Disease in Childhood*, **50**, 581

Stackpole, R.H., Melicow, M.M. and Uson, A.C. (1963) Phaeochromocytoma in children: report of 9 cases and review of the first 100 published cases with follow-up studies. *Journal of Pediatrics*, **63**, 315

Steinfeld, L., Dimich, I., Reder, R., Cohen, M. and Alexander, H. (1978) Sphygmomanometry in the pediatric patient. *Journal of Pediatrics*, **92**, 934

Still, J.L. and Cottom, D. (1967) Severe hypertension in childhood. *Archives of Disease in Childhood*, **42**, 34

Stockigt, J.R., Noakes, C.A., Collins, R.D., Schambelan, M. and Biglieri, E.G. (1972) Renal vein renin in various forms of renal hypertension. *Lancet*, i, 1194

Streeten, D.H.P., Anderson, G.H., Freiberg, J.M. and Dalakos, T.G. (1975) Use of an angiotensin II antagonist (Saralasin) in the recognition of "angiotensinogenic" hypertension. *New England Journal of Medicine*, **292**, 657

Vidt, D.G. (1977) Hypertension induced by irradiation to the kidney. *Archives of Internal Medicine*, **137**, 840

Wallace, D.M.A., Rothwell, D.L. and Williams, D.I. (1978) The long-term follow-up of surgically treated vesicoureteric reflux. *British Journal of Urology*, **50**, 479

Weidmann, P. and Maxwell, M.H. (1975) The renin-angiotensin-aldosterone system in terminal renal failure. *Kidney International*, **8**, Suppl. 5, p.219

Whyte, R.K., Elseed, A.M., Fraser, C.B., Shinebourne, E.A. and De Swiet, M. (1975) Assessment of Doppler ultrasound to measure systolic and diastolic blood pressures in infants and young children. *Archives of Disease in Childhood*, **50**, 542

Zinner, S.H., Martin, L.F., Sacks, F., Rosner, B. and Kass, E.H. (1974) A longitudinal study of blood pressure in childhood. *American Journal of Epidemiology*, **100**, 437

7 Renal arterial disease

J.H. Johnston

Intrinsic renal arterial obstruction

Obstructive disease involving the renal arteries in children occurs in several forms but the main manifestation and usually the presenting clinical feature of each is hypertension. Since the various conditions are uncommon, and since the opportunity to carry out a complete morphological and histological study of each is rare, a precise pathological classification is difficult. However, in the present state of knowledge the following lesions can be recognized.

Coarctation

Coarctation is a congenital annular stenosis involving usually the proximal part of one or both renal arteries. The condition is hereditary in some instances (Kaufman and Fay, 1974). In the 8-year-old child described by Guntheroth, Howry and Ansell (1963) identical lesions were present in the splenic and left femoral arteries as well as in the renal artery.

Fibromuscular mural dysplasia

Mural dysplasia is the commonest cause of intrinsic renal arterial obstruction during childhood and is an important cause of hypertension in that age group. Its aetiology is unknown but the occurrence of the disease in three siblings has been described (Halpern, Sanford and Viamont, 1965) suggesting that hereditary factors are involved. From arteriographic studies Aurell (1979) pointed out that the condition can be acquired. Mural dysplasias are commoner in the female and are peculiar to the renal arteries. In about one third of cases the lesion is bilateral. As a rule a normally sited renal artery and kidney are affected although an aberrant vessel may be diseased on its own or in addition (Hunt et al., 1962). Mural dysplasia has also been described in the artery supplying a pelvic kidney in a child with hypertension (Wylie, Perloff and Wellington, 1962).

Fibromuscular mural dysplasia occurs in several forms. Lesions involving the tunica media are commonest. Hamburger et al. (1968) described three forms of medial disease but emphasized that the autonomy of each is not fully established. In subadventitial perimuscular fibrosis there is a ring of connective tissue occupying more than half of the media; the internal and external elastic laminas and the intimal and adventitial coats are normal or minimally affected. With fibromuscular medial hyperplasia, which is the commonest form of mural dysplasia, zones of proliferation of the musculature alternate with zones in which the muscle is thin, elastic fibres are few and microaneurysms may occur. The condition may be localized to the main renal artery, usually involving the distal two thirds, or may extend into its branches; infrequently the disease is restricted to a primary branch or to a segmental intrarenal vessel (Niall and Murphy, 1965). In diffuse fibrosis of the media the muscle fibres are replaced by collagen.

Adventitial and intimal forms of mural dys-plasia are rare. In each there is diffuse fibrous thickening of the relevant arterial tunic. The adventitia may show infiltration by lymphocytes and plasma cells, especially around the vasa vasorum. Intimal hyperplasia of the renal arteries, in some cases with aortic involvement in addition, has been reported in infants with hypertension (Formby and Emery, 1969).

Neurofibromatosis

It has long been known that a child with neurofibromatosis is liable to hypertension because of the coexistence of phaeochromocytoma or aortic coarctation. More recently it has become recognized that hypertension with neurofibromatosis may be due to specific renal arterial

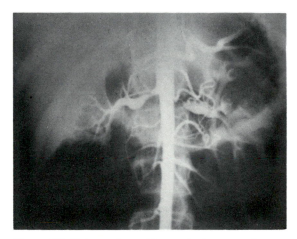

Figure 7.1. Right renal arterial stenosis. Aortogram in a 5-year-old girl with neurofibromatosis and malignant hypertension. Revascularization of the right kidney failed but hypertension was subsequently cured by nephrectomy. She also suffered occlusion of the right internal carotid artery at its bifurcation.

lesions. Grad and Rance (1972) and Tilford and Kelsch (1973) reported examples in young children. As a rule there are other obvious clinical manifestations of neurofibromatosis such as sub-cutaneous tumours and café au lait spots which indicate the diagnosis. The pathology of the arterial lesions depends upon the size of the vessels affected (Reubi, 1945). In arterioles intimal thickening predominates. In somewhat larger vessels there is muscular and elastic disorganization of the media, often with microaneurysms, and the lesions may resemble

those seen in polyarteritis nodosa. In the main arterial trunks cellular nodules occur in the adventitia and the vasa vasorum.

Diagnosis

The definitive diagnosis of occlusive renal arterial disease is made by selective renal angiography. The radiological appearances vary with different lesions. Arterial coarctation shows as an annular constriction close to the origin of the artery. With fibromuscular hyperplasia of the media there are alternating zones of arterial narrowing and dilatation producing a characteristic beaded appearance. Other forms of dysplasia generally lead to smooth concentric stenoses of varying lengths. With all types of arterial narrowing post-stenotic dilatation of the vessel is common. Collateral vessels to the kidney from the lumbar, iliac and ureteric arteries are often well developed and they may produce a notched appearance of the pelvis and ureter on pyelography.

Surgical treatment

The investigation of the child with hypertension and the indications for surgical intervention are discussed in Chapter 6.

Surgery for occlusive disease of the renal artery causing hypertension may be directed to excision of the ischaemic renal parenchyma or to revascularization of the same by reconstructive arterial surgery or intraluminal dilatation. Nephrectomy is indicated in cases of unilateral disease when the distribution of the arterial pathology prohibits reconstruction or the kidney is severely atrophic and unable to make any useful contribution to overall renal function. Partial nephrectomy may be possible if the disease is restricted to a primary or segmental branch.

Various reconstructive procedures can be employed depending upon the site and the extent of the arterial involvement. With annular coarctation resection of the affected segment and reanastomosis may be possible. Alternatively the vessel may be widened by the insertion of a patch graft of vein or Dacron. For more extensive arterial disease the gap following excision of the narrowed portion may be bridged by a graft of internal saphenous vein or internal iliac artery. In children Kaufman and Fay (1974) prefer autologous tissue to synthetic prostheses because of the uncertain fate of the latter in the long term. As an alternative to resection of the diseased artery the obstructed segment may be short-circuited by a bypass graft between the aorta and the renal artery distal to the obstruction. Kaufman and Fay (1974) employ autotransplantation of the kidney to the internal or external iliac vessels if an *in situ* repair is difficult or the aorta is affected by progressive disease. The ureter is left intact and its function remains normal despite its circuitous course to the bladder. Arterioplasties are performed under intraoperative mannitol and heparin cover and without renal cooling. Interrupted sutures are employed in order to allow the vascular anastomoses to grow proportionately to the vessels involved.

Percutaneous transluminal dilatation of the renal artery under radiological control has been shown to be effective in relieving hypertension caused by mural fibroplasia (Millan and Madias, 1979).

Extrinsic renal arterial obstruction

Hypertension due to external compression of the renal artery may occur as a result of local developmental abnormalities. Cases have been reported in which the artery was crossed and partly obstructed by musculotendinous fibres from the crus of the diaphragm (Kincaid, 1966) or the psoas muscle (D'Abreu and Strickland, 1962) or by nerve fibres from the lumbar sympathetic chain (Sutton *et al.*, 1963). Hypertension may rarely result from displacement of the kidney stretching the renal artery or from arterial compression by a post-traumatic haematoma or a tumour mass. Sinaiko *et al.* (1973) reported the case of an 8-year-old boy in whom the aorta and the renal arteries were involved in and partly obstructed by a form of retroperitoneal fibrosis.

Middle aortic syndrome

The middle aortic syndrome is probably a form of Takayasu's disease which as originally described was localized to the aortic arch. In this disorder a nonspecific stenosing arteritis possibly due to an autoimmune reaction associated with tuberculous infection involves the subdiaphragmatic aorta and the origins of its major branches. The syndrome occurs mainly in young women, although it has been encountered in children, and most cases have been from the Far East. The acute phase is characterized by a variety of nonspecific features such as fever, anaemia, pleural effusion, polyarthralgia, pericarditis and haemoptysis. Later, ischaemic effects are evident in the alimentary tract, with intestinal angina, and in the kidneys, with hypertension. The possibility of surgical relief of the hypertension by vascular reconstruction procedures depends upon the extent of the disease. If the iliac vessels are uninvolved, renal autotransplantation to the iliac fossa may be effective.

Renal arterial aneurysm

Aneurysm of the renal artery presenting in childhood is usually of saccular form and typically occurs at a point of vascular bifurcation in the renal hilum. It is presumed that the lesion is due to the existence of a congenital localized deficiency in the arterial wall similar to that causing berry aneurysm of the circle of Willis, and intracranial and renal arterial aneurysms may coexist. The condition is often bilateral. The youngest case recorded was in a boy aged 4 months (Rahill *et al.*, 1974).

Complications are common. Rupture of the aneurysm may cause severe retroperitoneal haemorrhage or thrombosis may occlude the renal artery causing infarction of the kidney. Hypertension often develops when the aneurysm compresses the renal artery or one of its major branches. A bruit is audible over the kidney. Radiography commonly shows a ring-shaped opacity due to calcification of the sac wall. Pyelography may reveal pelvicalyceal distortion or there may be diffuse or localized parenchymal atrophy resulting from ischaemia. The aneurysm is demonstrated by angiography.

Treatment depends upon the local pathology. It may be possible to resect the aneurysm alone or along with its vessel of origin and preserve at least part of the kidney. Often, however, the main renal artery is extensively involved or the kidney is severely atrophic so that nephrectomy is unavoidable.

Arteriovenous fistula

Renal arteriovenous fistulas are of various types and have various causes. A congenital fistula may be single or may take the form of a cirsoid angiomatous malformation with multiple intercommunicating vessels. Acquired intraparenchymal fistulas may follow penetrating, or less often blunt, injuries or may occur as a result of such surgical procedures as nephrolithotomy, partial nephrectomy and percutaneous renal biopsy. A fistula may develop between the stumps of the renal artery and vein after nephrectomy, especially if a transfixing mass ligature is employed and the renal bed is infected.

A history of previous injury or operation may be relevant in diagnosis. The patient may present with high output cardiac failure and cardiomegaly. Haematuria is common. On occasions there is diastolic hypertension possibly caused by localized parenchymal ischaemia. A large arteriovenous communication such as may occur following nephrectomy causes systolic hypertension, a low diastolic pressure and a collapsing pulse. In most of these cases a bruit is audible over the fistula.

Intravenous urography commonly shows a space-occupying lesion distorting the pelvicalyceal system, and 'cobblestone' filling defects may exist as a result of compression by dilated vessels. The definitive diagnosis is made by selective renal arteriography which may demonstrate an angiomatous malformation, rapid filling of the renal vein and prompt visualization of the inferior vena cava. The renal artery and renal vein proximal to the fistula are dilated.

An arteriovenous fistula following renal biopsy often closes spontaneously so that early intervention is usually unnecessary (Hirschman, Klein and Blumberg, 1971). In persistent cases the communication may be obliterated by arterial embolization with autologous blood clot (Bookstein and Goldstein, 1973). For larger fistulas, either congenital or acquired, excision of the fistulous mass or ligation of feeding vessels may be effective. If such procedures are not feasible, partial or total nephrectomy is generally needed.

Renal arterial thrombosis

Thrombosis of the renal artery can occur following closed trauma or as a result of pre-existing arterial disease or aneurysm. In an initially normal artery, thrombosis causing hypertension is a recognized complication of umbilical arterial catheterization employed in the management of critically ill newborn babies. Plumer, Mendoza and Kaplan (1975) reported seven cases, three of which were treated by nephrectomy, with survival in two. In the six cases of Adelman *et al.* (1976) renal arterial narrowing due to mural thrombi was demonstrable on angiography. The infants were managed by hypotensive drugs and all became normotensive, four of them no longer needing medication. Cases of acute neonatal thrombosis of the renal artery of unknown causation were recorded by Woodard, Patterson and Brinfield (1967) and by Cook, Marshall and Todd (1966). The presenting features were haematuria and cardiac failure due to hypertension. Intravenous urography demonstrated renal nonfunction. In each patient nephrectomy was performed successfully.

Renal arterial embolism

Embolism of the renal artery has occurred in infancy from thrombosis arising in an aneurysmal dilatation of a patent ductus arteriosus (Zuelzer, Kurnetz and Fallon, 1951). Early ligation of a patent ductus, which is now accepted therapy, avoids the complication.

References

Adelman, R., Goetzman, B., Vogel, J., Wennberg, R. and Merten, D. (1976) Neonatal renovascular hypertension: a non-surgical approach. Presented at the Western Society for Pediatric Research, Carmel, California

Aurell, M. (1979) Fibromuscular dysplasia of the renal arteries. *British Medical Journal*, i, 1180

Bookstein, J.J. and Goldstein, H.M. (1973) Successful management of post-biopsy arteriovenous fistula with selective arterial embolization. *Radiology*, **190**, 535

Cook, G.T., Marshall, V.F. and Todd, E. (1966) Malignant renovascular hypertension in a newborn. *Journal of Urology*, **96**, 863

D'Abreu, F. and Strickland, B. (1962) Developmental renal artery stenosis. *Lancet*, ii, 517

Formby, D. and Emery, J.L. (1969) Intimal hyperplasia of the aorta and renal vessels in an infant with hypertension. *Journal of Pathology*, **98**, 205

Grad, E. and Rance, C.P. (1972) Bilateral renal artery stenosis in association with neurofibromatosis: report of two cases. *Journal of Pediatrics*, **80**, 804

Guntheroth, W.G., Howry, C.L. and Ansell, J.S. (1963) Renal hypertension: a review. *Pediatrics*, **31**, 767

Halpern, M.M. Sanford, H.S. and Viamont, M. (1965) Renal artery abnormalities in three hypertensive sisters. *Journal of the American Medical Association*, **194**, 512

Hamburger, J., Richet, G., Crosnier, J., Brentano, J.L.F., Antoine, B., Ducrot, H., Mery, J.P. and de Montera, H. (1968) Pathologic changes in the renal vessels. *In* Nephrology. Saunders, Philadelphia, London, Toronto. p.1201

Hirschman, A., Klein, M.J. and Blumberg, A.G. (1971) Spontaneous disappearance of iatrogenic renal arteriovenous fistula. *Journal of Urology*, **105**, 4

Hunt, J.C., Harrison, E.G., Kincaid, O.W., Bernatz, P.E. and Davis, G.D. (1962) Idiopathic fibrous and fibromuscular stenoses of the renal arteries associated with hypertension. *Proceedings of Staff Meetings of the Mayo Clinic*, **37**, 181

Kaufman, J.J. and Fay, R. (1974) Renal hypertension in children. *In* Reviews in Paediatric Urology (edited by Johnston, J.H. and Goodwin, W.E.). Excerpta Medica, Amsterdam. p.201

Kincaid, O.W. (1966) Renal angiography. Year Book Medical Publishers, Chicago

Millan, V.G. and Madias, N.E. (1979) Percutaneous translumenal angioplasty for severe renovascular hypertension due to renal artery medial fibroplasia. *Lancet*, i, 993

Niall, J.F. and Murphy, L. (1965) Segmental renal artery stenosis with hypertension in childhood. *Medical Journal of Australia*, **2**, 372

Plumer, L.B., Mendoza, S.A. and Kaplan, G.W. (1975) Hypertension in infancy. The case for aggressive management. *Journal of Urology*, **113**, 555

Rahill, W.J., Molteni, A., Hawking, K.M., Koo, J.H. and Menon, V.A. (1974) Hypertension and narrowing of the renal artery in infancy. *Journal of Pediatrics*, **84**, 39

Reubi, F. (1945) Neurofibromatose et lesions vasculaires. *Schweize Medizinische Wochenschrift*, **75**, 463

Sinaiko, A., Najarian, J., Michael, A.F. and Mirkin, B.L. (1973) Renal autotransplantation in the treatment of bilateral renal artery stenosis: relief of hypertension in an 8 year old boy. *Journal of Pediatrics*, **83**, 409

Sutton, D., Brunton, F.J., Foot, E.C. and Guthrie, J. (1963) Fibromuscular, fibrous and non-atheromatous renal artery stenosis and hypertension. *Clinical Radiology*, **14**, 381

Tilford, D.L. and Kelsch, R.C. (1973) Renal artery stenosis in childhood neurofibromatosis. *American Journal of Diseases of Children*, **126**, 665

Woodard, J.R., Patterson, J.H. and Brinfield, D. (1967) Renal artery thrombosis in newborn infants. *American Journal of Diseases of Children*, **114**, 191

Wylie, E.J., Perloff, D. and Wellington, J.S. (1962) Fibromuscular hyperplasia of the renal arteries. *Annals of Surgery*, **156**, 592

Zuelzer, W.W., Kurnetz, R. and Fallon, R. (1951) Circulatory diseases of infancy and childhood: occlusion of the renal artery. *American Journal of Diseases of Children*, **81**, 21

8 Glomerular Disease and Haematuria

T.M. Barratt

Classification of glomerulonephritis

The term glomerulonephritis encompasses a number of disorders, many of which appear to be mediated by immunological processes, affecting the glomeruli. The bewildering rapidity with which fashions in nomenclature change indicates that a satisfactory system of classification for the glomerulonephritides has not yet evolved. Three levels of description can be discriminated (Cameron, 1979). First there is the clinical manifestation, that is the syndrome of the glomerular disorder, for example the 'nephrotic syndrome'; this level of classification has historical priority (Bright, 1836) and by many criteria remains the most valid. Secondly the advent of percutaneous renal biopsy has permitted morphological classification and introduced new terminology such as 'focal glomerulonephritis'. Finally there is a level of description based on pathogenesis, for example 'immune-complex disease', which might be preferred were it not for the ignorance that surrounds the mechanisms of most glomerular diseases.

Experience has shown that there is poor correlation between these three descriptive levels. Thus immune-complex disease, even with the same antigen, may result in a wide range of histological appearances each of which in turn may have various clinical manifestations. There have been some reasonably constant clinico-pathological associations, but unfortunately this has led to a tendency to extend to one level a descriptive term more suitable for another. It is, for instance, inappropriate to use the morphological term focal glomerulonephritis to describe the clinical syndrome of recurrent haematuria. Other examples of similar associations leading to imprecise nomenclature are 'minimal-change nephrotic syndrome' (steroid-responsive nephrotic syndrome) and 'crescentic nephritis' (rapidly progressive glomerulonephritis).

Pathogenesis of glomerulonephritis

Two principal lines of evidence point to immunological mechanisms in the pathogenesis of glomerulonephritis (Peters, 1981). First, immunoglobulins and complement components can often be demonstrated in the glomeruli by immunofluorescence techniques, sometimes with associated depression of serum complement. Secondly, there are a number of experimental animal models of nephritis which depend upon manipulation of the immunological system. From the conceptual point of view the simplest mechanism is autoimmunity, the production of antibody to kidney tissue, but it is very rare in childhood and most glomerulonephritis appears to result from the deposition or formation *in situ* in the glomeruli of immune complexes containing both antigen and antibody.

Immune-complex nephritis

Reaction of antigen with antibody results in the formation of immune complexes which are rapidly removed from the circulation by the reticuloendothelial system. Under certain conditions, particularly when there is antigen excess, smaller complexes are formed which remain in solution in the circulation to be deposited in the glomeruli and elsewhere in the tissues, eliciting an inflammatory response with recruitment of the complement, polymorphic and coagulation systems. The antibody and the antigen (if known) can usually be demonstrated in the kidney by immunofluorescence, generally as granular deposits on the epithelial side of the basement membrane. In this system the antibody does not have a special affinity for the kidney, which becomes involved as an innocent bystander of the immunological reaction. Numerous methods are now available for the detection of circulating immune complexes, but it is far from certain whether those detected in the serum are in fact responsible for the glomerulonephritis (Levinsky, 1981).

The antigens involved may be exogenous or endogenous. Exogenous antigens include bacterial (for example streptococcal), viral (such as hepatitis B) and protozoal (for instance malarial) types, and can also be derived from drugs or parenteral administration of foreign proteins (for example serum sickness). Endogenous antigens may be shielded autoantigens such as double-stranded deoxyribonucleic acid (in systemic lupus erythematosus) or thyroglobulin, or carcinoma-associated neoantigens. Nevertheless, in the majority of cases the antigen is not known. The characteristics of the immune response to antigen are a major factor in the genesis of immune-complex disease, and it has been proposed that the persistence of circulating immune complexes in some individuals exposed to relatively widely distributed antigens may be viewed as a form of immunodeficiency (Soothill and Steward, 1971).

Other mechanisms

Autoimmune disease with circulating antibody to glomerular basement membrane is the mechanism involved in some patients with crescentic nephritis, and may be associated with lung haemorrhage (Goodpasture's syndrome). There is a characteristic immunofluorescence pattern with linear deposition of immunoglobulin in the basement membrane.

In many forms of glomerular disease, for example steroid-responsive nephrotic syndrome, evidence of immunological involvement is only circumstantial. In others, notably hereditary nephritis (Alport's syndrome), there is no evidence at all of involvement of immunological mechanisms.

Manifestations of glomerular injury

The filtration process

The initial step in the formation of urine is the production of an ultrafiltrate of plasma by the glomeruli. This is a passive process, being driven by the balance between capillary hydrostatic and oncotic pressures, and is regulated by the renal plasma flow and the glomerular surface area available for filtration (Brenner *et al.*, 1977). The kidney is a very vascular organ and the renal blood flow accounts for one quarter of the cardiac output; the blood flow through each adult glomerulus is approximately 1 ml/24 h.

The ultrafiltrate of plasma from within the capillary lumen traverses the endothelial cell, the basement membrane and the interdigitating foot processes of the epithelial cells to reach the space of Bowman's capsule and enter the lumen of the proximal tubule from which selective active reabsorption takes place. The glomerular filtration rate in the adult is approximately 120 ml/min, or 180 ℓ/24 h, and thus a volume of fluid equivalent to the total body water leaves the glomeruli every 4–6 hours.

The glomerular filtrate is free of red blood cells, and proteins of molecular weights above 40 000 are largely excluded from it. The actual site of the filtration barrier is believed to be at the slit pores of the epithelial cells, where a high density of fixed anionic radicals leads to a selectively greater exclusion of circulating polyanions such as albumin (Brenner, 1978).

The chief manifestations of glomerular disease arise in two ways: first abnormal leakiness of the glomeruli resulting in the appearance in the urine of red blood cells (haematuria) or excessive amounts of protein (proteinuria), and secondly blockage of the glomeruli leading to a reduction of glomerular filtration rate and ultimately renal failure. Although it is the degree of blockage that is the principal determinant of the outcome, it is usually the phenomena attributable to glomerular leakage which first draw attention to the disorder. The presence of haematuria commonly prompts referral of the child to a urologist in the first instance, and therefore in this chapter the greatest emphasis is placed on those varieties of glomerular disease that may present with haematuria alone.

Haematuria

Even small amounts of blood added to urine cause obvious macroscopic haematuria. The most convenient screening test is carried out with Hemastix, which are strips impregnated with a buffered mixture of organic peroxide and orthotolidine. The peroxidase-like activity of haemoglobin and myoglobin and some of their degradation products catalyses the oxidation of orthotolidine to a blue derivative.

The presence of haematuria should be confirmed by microscopic examination of a fresh uncentrifuged urine specimen. As well as distinguishing haematuria from haemoglobinuria or myoglobinuria, microscropy may reveal the presence of red blood cell or granular casts, which immediately point to a parenchymal source of bleeding.

In the past considerable attention has been paid to the measurement of red blood cell excretion rates, but the marked temporal variation makes such precision of little value.

Proteinuria

Proteinuria may result from increased glomerular permeability (so-called glomerular proteinuria) or decreased tubular reabsorption of low molecular weight proteins normally present in the glomerular filtrate (so-called tubular proteinuria). The use of boiling or salicylsulphonic acid for the detection of protein has been superseded by Albustix. These are paper strips impregnated with tetrabromophenol blue buffered in citrate at pH 3.5. Urinary protein, particularly albumin, binds with the dye and causes a colour change by displacement of the transformation range of the indicator. Proteinuria present in the upright position but not in the recumbent one is not pathological.

Screening tests depend upon the protein concentration and are thus affected by the urine flow rate; quantitative protein excretion rates are more precise. Although haematuria may affect nonspecific measurements of protein excretion, a simple and reliable assessment of glomerular permeability can be gained from the immunochemically determined albumin/creatinine concentration ratio (Barratt, 1974). Significant albuminuria accompanying haematuria strongly suggests parenchymal origin of the blood.

Further description of the abnormality of glomerular permeability in states of heavy proteinuria is provided by consideration of the relative clearances of proteins of different molecular size (differential protein clearances or selectivity of proteinuria). When the clearance of a larger protein is substantially less than that of a smaller one, the proteinuria is said to be highly selective. The ratio of the clearance of IgG (molecular weight 166 000) to that of albumin (molecular weight 70 000) is a convenient estimate of selectivity and may be used to characterize the nephrotic syndrome. If the ratio is less than 10 per cent then minimal histological changes and a response to steroids are virtually certain, whereas if it is greater than 20 per cent then steroid resistance is more probable.

Morphology of glomerulonephritis : renal biopsy

Methods

The widespread application of percutaneous renal biopsy for the investigation of glomerular disease in childhood has led to a very refined understanding of renal histopathology. Considerable technical skill and experience are necessary in the interpretation of renal biopsies and they should not be undertaken except in specialized centres with full access to all histological techniques and a sufficient throughput of material, for example 25 cases annually.

Light-microscopic examination of renal biopsy material necessitates special fixation and very skilled cutting of $2\,\mu m$ thin sections. A wide range of stains are helpful, the periodic acid Schiff stain being the most useful for routine purposes. Snap-frozen material is required for immunofluorescence studies, which are essential in the investigation of haematuria. Special techniques are required for the processing of tissue for electron microscopy, which is also mandatory for the investigation of haematuria, particularly if there is a familial element. To ensure that there are glomeruli in all three specimens it is helpful if the pathologist examines the biopsy core immediately and divides it under the dissecting microscope.

Normal appearance

The normal glomerulus consists of a tuft of capillaries invaginated into the blind end of the proximal tubule which forms Bowman's capsule. The capillaries are fed by an afferent and drained by an efferent arteriole; they are lined by endothelial cells and supported by mesangial cells and matrix. Mesangial cells differ from endothelial cells in that they do not come into contact with the capillary lumen. Together the two types of cells are called endocapillary cells because both lie within the basement membrane which is continuous with the equivalent structure in the proximal tubule. Outside the basement membrane lie the epithelial cells and the cells of Bowman's capsule, and jointly these are called extracapillary. In health the capillary loops are patent, the mesangial matrix is sparse and the basement membrane is a thin even structure. Epithelial cells are more prominent in childhood than in the mature glomerulus.

Terminology

The borders of normality are difficult to define and there is often disagreement, especially over the distinction between normal glomeruli and mild proliferative lesions. In order to err on the side of conservatism the trend is now to admit minor variations of doubtful pathological significance into a category formally designated as minimal histological abnormality on light microscopy or, more briefly, minimal change.

An increase in the number of cells in the capillary tuft is known as proliferation and the term is qualified by the type of cell involved, for example 'mesangial proliferative' which is virtually synonymous with 'endocapillary proliferative'. Extracapillary proliferation usually results in the formation of epithelial cell crescents, and this condition is known as crescentic nephritis. If polymorphonuclear leukocytes are present, the term exudative proliferation is sometimes applied. When all the glomeruli are involved the process is termed diffuse, but if some are abnormal and others normal it is described as focal. In this manner terms such as focal endocapillary proliferative glomerulonephritis are built up.

Sclerosis of a glomerulus may be global, that is involving the whole structure, or segmental. Focal segmental glomerulosclerosis is a lesion quite frequently observed in children with a steroid-resistant nephrotic syndrome, whereas focal global glomerulosclerosis is not necessarily an abnormal finding in young children.

Thickening of the basement membrane is implied by the term membranous, and if there are no proliferative features the condition is known as membranous nephropathy. If there is proliferation as well, the appropriate term is membranoproliferative glomerulonephritis; confusingly, for rather unsatisfactory reasons this last condition is also known as mesangiocapillary glomerulonephritis.

Practical procedure

Percutaneous renal biopsy is now an established procedure for the investigation of glomerular disease and has a low, while not negligible, complication rate. Before embarking on a biopsy the presence of two functioning kidneys must be confirmed by intravenous urography, the results of coagulation studies and the platelet count must be normal, and hypertension and uraemia must be controlled. Blood should be cross-matched and informed parental consent obtained.

Most investigators use either the Franklin modification of the Vim Silverman needle or the disposable Tru-Cut. Local anaesthesia with sedation is suitable for most children except very young and nervous ones. It matters less which form of sedation is used than that the whole procedure is conducted in an atmosphere of confident calm, and it is very helpful to have an assistant whose sole function is to hold the child's hand and talk him through the biopsy.

The safety and the success of the procedure

are much improved if the kidney is localized by fluoroscopy following intravenous injection of contrast medium. The child lies prone on the X-ray table and the lower pole of the kidney is identified during the nephrogram phase. Local anaesthesia is given and the depth of the kidney determined with an exploratory needle. The biopsy needle is advanced just beneath the renal capsule and its position checked by fluoroscopy (the tip of the needle moves synchronously with the renal shadow during respiratory excursions). It is safest if the child does not breathe while the biopsy is being taken. Only one kidney should be sampled at a session, and not more than four attempts should be permitted.

Following biopsy the child should remain in bed for 24 hours with regular observation of his pulse and blood pressure. The commonest complication is bleeding, either retroperitoneal or into the urinary tract. Retroperitoneal bleeding has been shown by routine postbiopsy computed tomography to occur frequently, but is rarely massive; it may, however, become secondarily infected or precipitate an exacerbation of systemic lupus erythematosus. Urinary bleeding is also common and occasionally massive, resulting in troublesome clot colic and requiring transfusion. If bleeding is prolonged there may be a traumatic arteriovenous fistula, which can be plugged by embolization under arteriographic control. Sometimes the bleeding can be arrested with epsilonaminocaproic acid. Very rarely nephrectomy is required. In the nephrotic child cellulitis can easily spread from the skin incision and may be disquietingly severe. Additionally, the risks of general anaesthesia are increased in the prone oedematous child. Although with care and experience the risks of renal biopsy can be substantially reduced, they remain a serious consideration to be balanced against the value of the information likely to be obtained.

Syndromes of glomerulonephritis

The acute nephritic syndrome

The acute nephritic syndrome is characterized by the sudden onset of haematuria, proteinuria, oliguria, oedema, hypertension and uraemia; it is the syndrome described by Ellis (1942) as type I nephritis. Salt and water retention is responsible for the hypertension and if marked may result in pulmonary oedema or encephalopathy. The oliguria may be severe and amount to acute renal failure. Classically the syndrome is described as following an infection with a nephritogenic strain of beta-haemolytic streptococcus in the throat or skin. In these circumstances there is a rise in the antistreptolysin-O titre and depression of C3. Renal histology shows initially an acute exudative proliferative glomerulonephritis with prominent humps on the epithelial side of the basement membrane, and later a simple mesangial proliferative picture. Although there may be occasional bouts of haematuria for some months in the convalescent phase, follow-up studies show complete recovery of renal function.

The same clinical picture may be found in a number of other renal diseases, in several of which the prognosis is not as good as in acute post-streptococcal glomerulonephritis (*Table 8.1*).

With the improvement in the general health of children in the community and with the widespread use of penicillin there has been a marked decline in the incidence of streptococcal infections, and the acute nephritic syndrome is now much less common than it used to be. However, the corollary is that the proportion of

Table 8.1 Varieties of the acute nephritic syndrome

Post-streptococcal*
Following other acute bacterial infections*:
  staphylococcus, pneumococcus, syphilis (congenital)
Subacute bacterial endocarditis
Shunt nephritis (bacterial colonization of ventriculoatrial shunts)*
Following viral infections: mumps, Epstein-Barr (infectious mononucleosis), hepatitis B (Australia-antigenaemia)
Malaria
Mesangiocapillary (membranoproliferative) glomerulonephritis*†
Crescentic nephritis
Antiglomerular-basement-membrane-antibody nephritis (with lung haemorrhage this is Goodpasture's syndrome)†
Henoch-Schönlein purpura†
Polyarteritis†
Systemic lupus erythematosus*
Radiation nephritis
Idiopathic

---

*Plasma C3 may be reduced
†May be complicated by crescentic nephritis

cases that are not post-streptococcal is greater, and the individual case needs therefore to be treated with greater circumspection. In particular there is a need to identify as early as possible cases of crescentic nephritis, because these may be amenable to treatment by immunosuppression, anticoagulation or plasmapheresis provided anuria has not set in; otherwise they carry a grim prognosis for renal function (rapidly progressive glomerulonephritis). A renal biopsy should be undertaken in children with the acute nephritic syndrome if renal function continues to deteriorate or if there are atypical features, especially if the plasma C3 concentration is normal.

The nephrotic syndrome

The term nephrotic syndrome applies to any condition in which there is heavy albuminuria and hypoalbuminaemia and hence oedema (Ellis's type II nephritis). The fall in plasma albumin concentration results in a decrease in plasma oncotic pressure, disturbance of the Starling equilibrium and a seepage of extracellular fluid from the intravascular to the interstitial compartment. There is thus a reduction in the plasma volume resulting in hypovolaemia with relative polycythaemia; sodium reabsorption is enhanced, which aggravates the oedema. The hypovolaemia may result in peripheral circulatory failure and shock, and predisposes to thrombosis including renal venous thrombosis (Barratt, 1979a).

The nephrotic syndrome may be secondary to the glomerulonephritis of an overt systemic disorder, such as Henoch-Schönlein purpura or systemic lupus erythematosus, or may be primary without extrarenal manifestations other than those attributable to proteinuria. The primary nephrotic syndrome may be associated

with one of several different histological patterns (*Table 8.2*), but in general two major groups can be discerned according to the response to corticosteroid therapy.

In the majority of nephrotic children there is a highly selective proteinuria (see above) responsive to corticosteroid therapy, and no histological abnormality (that is minimal change) of the glomeruli is apparent on light microscopy. This syndrome is variously called idiopathic nephrotic syndrome and steroid-responsive nephrotic syndrome. The last term is the most useful since it makes no assumptions about histology or pathogenesis. Steroid response and minimal change histology correlate so well that routine renal biopsy is not necessary in this group.

Steroid-responsive nephrotic syndrome is more common in boys with a peak age at onset of 3 years; macroscopic haematuria does not occur and the plasma C3 concentration is normal. Hypertension is not a feature, and if renal failure is present then it is attributable to the poor renal perfusion resulting from hypovolaemia. There is an associaton with atopy and other clues suggest an immunopathogenesis, although the mechanisms involved are unclear (Barratt, 1979b). One third of affected children have only a single episode, one third have an occasional relapse and one third relapse frequently, often suffering from corticosteroid toxicity (particularly growth retardation). Relapses ultimately cease, however, and renal failure does not ensue.

A more stable remission can be induced with alkylating agents, particularly cyclophosphamide and chlorambucil, but their disquieting potential for toxicity prompts caution in their usage. Among other problems the administration of either drug to boys before puberty may result in testicular atrophy and azoospermia, although the evidence to date suggests that this

Table 8.2 Pathology and steroid response in the childhood nephrotic syndrome (modified from Churg, Habib and White, 1970)

Histological category		Total	Steroid-resistant
Minimal change		98	5
Focal glomerulosclerosis		12	10
Proliferative glomerulonephritis	Mesangioproliferative	4	1
	Crescentic	4	4
	Membranoproliferative	6	5
Membranous		2	2
Advanced chronic glomerulonephritis		1	1

is rare with the 8-week course of cyclophospha-mide usually given for the nephrotic syndrome (Barratt, 1979a). Longer courses of cyclophos-phamide may also result in haemorrhagic cysti-tis which is occasionally followed by bladder fibrosis and possibly neoplasia.

It is apparent from *Table 8.2* that children with a steroid-resistant nephrotic syndrome are a heterogeneous group. Factors suggesting ster-oid resistance in a nephrotic child are an age at onset of less than 3 months or over 10 years (particularly if female), macroscopic haematur-ia or a past history of acute nephritic syndrome, hypocomplementaemia and poorly selective proteinuria. The prognosis is similarly heter-ogeneous. Children with minimal change, mesangial proliferative or membranous lesions tend to improve, whereas one third of those with mesangiocapillary (membranoproliferative) glomerulonephritis or focal glomerulosclerosis develop renal failure within 5 years of diagnosis (Cameron, 1979), and patients with crescentic nephritis deteriorate rapidly. Steroid-resistant nephrotic syndrome with minimal histological changes responds to cyclophosphamide, and crescentic nephritis possibly responds to com-bined immunosuppression and anticoagulation; otherwise no specific therapy is available for these glomerular disorders. However, control of hypertension is essential.

Isolated haematuria

Haematuria naturally suggests the possibility of a urological disorder, in particular tumour, hyd-ronephrosis or stone. It warrants a careful cli-nical examination, an intravenous urogram and a renal ultrasound examination, irrespective of other evidence such as casts or albuminuria suggestive of a glomerular disorder. Neverthe-less, several forms of glomerular disease may have haematuria as their sole clinical manifesta-tion. Isolated bouts of haematuria may occur for many months after an episode of acute post-streptococcal glomerulonephritis or Henoch-Schönlein purpura, so that an accurate history is essential. While considering medical causes of haematuria, sickle-cell disease or trait and coagulation disorders or thrombocytopenia must not be forgotten.

Isolated haematuria is a feature of the early stages of familial glomerulonephritis, especially the variety associated with nerve deafness (Alport's syndrome). Typically there is persis-tent microscopic haematuria with macroscopic exacerbations; initially the deafness may involve high frequencies only and thus escape notice. The disorder is inherited as an autosomal reces-sive condition with marked sex modification : males are much more severely affected. The family history may only be revealed by a careful enquiry about distant relatives. The diagnosis can be confirmed by electron microscopy of the biopsy specimen, which shows a characteristic splitting of the basement membrane. It is distur-bingly easy to overlook the possibility of Alport's syndrome among the population of children with haematuria and yet the diagnosis is very important, not only for its genetic implications but also because the prognosis is much worse than in other forms of isolated haematuria, with renal failure often developing in the second or third decade of life.

Recurrent bouts of haematuria with com-pletely normal urine between attacks form a common syndrome in childhood; experience shows that the outcome is generally good, and the syndrome is known as benign recurrent haematuria. The episodes of haematuria are frequently provoked by strenuous exercise or an upper respiratory infection (without the 10-day delay characteristic of acute post-streptococcal glomerulonephritis), and may be accompanied by abdominal or loin pain. In about half the cases light microscopy of renal biopsy specimens shows focal proliferative glomerulonephritis, while in the remainder no abnormality can be discerned. In the majority of cases (but not in all of them) immunofluorescence shows the deposi-tion of IgA principally, and IgG and C3 as well, in the mesangium (Berger, Yaneva and Hing-lais, 1971); the condition is variously described as Berger's disease, IgA-deposit disease and IgA-IgG nephropathy. These patients tend to have raised plasma IgA concentrations as well. The condition in childhood is benign and does not require treatment; the main purpose in establishing a biopsy diagnosis is to prevent anxiety on the part of the patient or his doctors and forestall unnecessary urological investiga-tions.

Little is known about the IgA-negative chil-dren with recurrent haematuria. This group needs a careful repeat of the radiological inves-tigations 6 months to 1 year after presentation to make sure that nothing was overlooked the first time round.

Miscellaneous syndromes of urological interest

There are a few varieties of glomerular disease which the urologist may occasionally encounter and which thus require brief discussion.

Shunt nephritis

Infection of ventriculoatrial shunts in children with hydrocephalus results in a syndrome akin to subacute bacterial endocarditis. Haematuria, proteinuria and a mild degree of renal failure accompany fever, anaemia and hepatosplenomegaly. Bacteria of low grade pathogenicity such as *Staphylococcus epidermidis* are usually responsible. The condition responds to appropriate antibiotic therapy, but it is generally necessary to remove the shunt.

Drug-induced nephritis

Cystinuric patients treated with D-penicillamine occasionally develop the nephrotic syndrome as a consequence of drug toxicity.

Radiation nephritis

Radiation nephritis is characterized by the slow development of proteinuria, hypertension and renal failure, often associated with microscropic haematuria. With modern radiotherapeutic techniques it is now uncommon, although it is important to note that chemotherapeutic agents (particularly actinomycin D) may sensitize the kidney to radiation damage.

Nephritis associated with nephroblastoma

An interesting syndrome has recently been recognized which is characterized by male pseudohermaphroditism, glomerular disease and nephroblastoma (*British Medical Journal*, 1978). The nephritis may antedate clinical presentation of the tumour by several years. A partial syndrome may occur without the genital anomaly, especially in younger cases or those with bilateral tumour. Careful attention of the pathologist to glomerular morphology in the kidney surrounding the tumour may suggest the disorder which in the past has been confused with radiation nephritis. Removal of the tumour does not necessarily prevent the progression to renal failure.

Henoch-Schönlein nephritis

A purpuric papular rash accompanied by arthritis, abdominal pain and later nephritis characterizes Henoch-Schönlein disease. Apart from its importance as a cause of haematuria and renal failure, the urologist should be aware of the fact that it may occasionally present with a painful testicular swelling difficult to differentiate from torsion. Polyarteritis may also cause testicular pain associated with nephritis.

Glomerular lesions in end-stage urological disorders

Patients with severe renal damage associated with obstructive uropathy or vesicoureteric reflux appear to develop a nephropathy that inexorably deteriorates in spite of satisfactory correction of the urological abnormality. There is usually moderate proteinuria (not necessarily attributable to hypertension), and there are occasional reports of glomerular deposits of immunoglobulin demonstrated by immunofluorescence. Whether there are secondary immunological factors resulting in glomerulonephritis is not known and the matter warrants further investigation.

Practical approach to the child with haematuria

The principal investigation in the child with haematuria is the intravenous urogram, which is nowadays supplemented (but not replaced) by ultrasound examination. It should be performed in all children with haematuria without exception, even if there is clear-cut evidence of nephritis, and it should be repeated after 1 year if the haematuria persists and no cause is apparent.

If the intravenous urogram is normal then evidence for glomerular disease should be reviewed, in particular a past history or family history of nephritis, the presence of oedema or hypertension, the detection in the urine of casts or proteinuria, the plasma C3 concentration and the state of renal function reflected in the plasma creatinine concentration. A renal biopsy is needed if there is persistent proteinuria with the haematuria or if there is a positive family history.

Assuming that no clues have so far emerged, attention must be paid to the possibility of a lower urinary source of bleeding, especially if the haematuria occurs at the beginning or end of the urinary stream or if there are other micturition symptoms. The postmicturition bladder film of the intravenous urogram is sometimes worth reviewing, but children with haematuria whose symptomatology points to the lower urinary tract need definitive cystourethroscopy carefully performed so that repetition is not necessary. For the majority who do not have such symptoms routine cystoscopy is most unrewarding and is generally agreed to be unnecessary. Arteriography also has a poor yield as well as being invasive, and is not required unless there are other indications in addition to the haematuria.

The question that then remains is whether children with haematuria not so far diagnosed need renal biopsy for diagnosis. Practice varies among paediatric nephrologists on this point. There are some situations fraught with anxiety on the part of the child, his parents and his medical advisers in which a positive diagnosis (for example of IgA nephropathy) is a considerable help in the overall management of the case. On the other hand renal biopsy is an invasive procedure, does not always provide a definitive answer, and in this group of patients does not yield a diagnosis pointing to the need for a specific treatment or even one indicating a poor prognosis. Thus routine renal biopsy is not necessary in these patients, although it requires the confidence born of experience to appreciate that recurrent isolated haematuria without urological abnormality is a common and generally benign disorder of childhood, and to resist the pressures leading to overinvestigation.

References

Barratt, T.M. (1974) Assessment of renal function in children. *In* Modern Trends in Paediatrics, 4th edn (edited by Apley, J.). Butterworths, London. p.181

Barratt, T.M. (1979a) Nephrotic syndrome. *In* Paediatric Therapeutics (edited by Valman, H.B.). Blackwell, Oxford. p.81

Barratt, T.M. (1979b) The steroid-responsive nephrotic syndrome of childhood: pathogenesis and treatment. *Australian Paediatric Journal*, **15**, 17

Berger, J.G., Yaneva, I.H. and Hinglais, N. (1971) Immunohistochemistry of glomerulonephritis. *Advances in Nephrology*, **1**, 11

Brenner, B.M. (1978) Molecular basis of proteinuria of glomerular origin. *New England Journal of Medicine*, **298**, 826

Brenner, B.M., Bohrer, M.P., Baylis, C. and Deen, W.M. (1977) Determinants of glomerular permselectivity: insights derived from observations *in vivo*. *Kidney International*, **12**, 299

Bright, R. (1836) Cases and observations illustrative of renal disease accompanied by the secretion of albuminous urine. *Guy's Hospital Reports*, **1**, 338

British Medical Journal (1978) Two children with kidney disease. Clinico-pathological Conference, ii, 867

Cameron, J.S. (1979) The natural history of glomerulonephritis. *In* Renal Disease, 4th edn (edited by Black, D.A.K. and Jones, N.F.). Blackwell, Oxford. p.329

Churg, J., Habib, R. and White, R.H.R. (1970) Pathology of the nephrotic syndrome in children: a report for the International Study of Kidney Disease in Children. *Lancet*, i, 1299

Ellis, A. (1942) Natural history of Bright's disease: clinical, histological and experimental observations. *Lancet*, i, 34

Levinsky, R.J. (1981) Principles of detection of immune complexes. *In* Clinical Aspects of Immunology, 4th edn (edited by Gell, P.G.H., Coombs, R.R.A. and Lachmann, P.J.). Blackwell, Oxford. In press

Peters, D.K. (1981) The kidney in allergic disease. *In* Clinical Aspects of Immunology, 4th edn (edited by Gell, P.G.H., Coombs, R.R.A. and Lachmann, P.J.). Blackwell, Oxford. In press

Soothill, J.F. and Steward, M.W. (1971) The immunopathological significance of the heterogeneity of antibody affinity. *Clinical and Experimental Immunology*, **9**, 193

9 Urinary Tract Infection

J.D. Williams

Microbiology

Infection in the urinary tract can be defined in quantitative terms. Generally the presence of 10^5 or more organisms of a single bacterial species per millilitre means that the microorganisms are actively multiplying in the bladder urine. There are exceptions to this rule, for instance mixed infections with two or more species may occur in patients undergoing invasive urological procedures and organisms may be present at a total concentration of 10^5 organisms/ml. However, the growth of two or more organisms usually denotes that an unsatisfactory specimen of urine has been examined and in some circumstances less than 10^5 organisms/ml may indicate a significant infection particularly when *Proteus mirabilis* is involved.

The urine specimen

The value of microbiological examination of the urine depends primarily on the quality of the specimen examined. Misleading results may be obtained due to contaminating organisms washed into the urine from the skin and subsequently multiplying to exceed 10^5 organisms/ml. Spurious 'infections' of this type are very common, especially in children, and examination of several successive specimens of urine may be necessary to clarify the position. Cleansing of the genitalia should be carried out with soap and water only (if skin disinfectants gain access

to the urine this may reduce the bacterial count) and the urine collected in a sterile bottle. The urine should be stored at 4°C and examined as soon as possible after collection. Delays of more than 2 hours before examining unrefrigerated urine or of 24 hours for refrigerated specimens allow bacterial multiplication sufficient to distort the microbiological results.

Examination of the urine for formed elements

Microscopic examination of the urine is usually carried out as a guide to the presence of infection. White blood cells have been much studied and considerable efforts have been made to standardize methods that give an accurate assessment of their concentration in urine, although the presence of microscopic bacteriuria correlates more closely to the presence of urinary infection than does a raised white blood cell content. Haematuria is a common finding in urinary tract infection and a search for red blood cells is part of the microscopic examination of the urine.

Quantitative estimates of the formed elements in urine can be done using a haematological counting chamber. The urine should be freshly taken; if it has been standing, even for only a few minutes, it should be well mixed and a drop of the uncentrifuged specimen placed under the coverslip and examined under reduced illumination. When 10^5 or more bacteria are present the organisms can usually be clearly seen in the counting chamber, and the presence of visible bacteria correlates very closely with subsequent culture findings. The white blood cells may be counted and the number expressed as cells per cubic millimetre. Normally very few white blood cells are excreted in the urine, the limits of normal being approximately 200 000–400 000 per hour. A concentration of more than 10 white blood cells/mm^3 indicates a raised white blood cell excretion rate (Little, 1964). The limitations of white blood cell counting to detect infection are many, for example there may be an extraneous source of white blood cells in the skin, vagina or urethra, and several other forms of urinary pathology (such as stone) may be accompanied by white blood cells in the urine. Furthermore urinary tract infection may be present in the absence of white blood cells, particularly when the infection is asymptomatic. The use of the presence of red blood cells as a guide to the diagnosis of urinary tract infection is affected by similar factors which should be taken into consideration in the interpretation of the findings.

Urine culture

Urine culture requires the use of quantitative methods. Simple dilution techniques, such as the culture of 0.1 ml of a 1/100 dilution of the urine, are available and give the most accurate results. When collection and storage of specimens are of a high order of efficiency the difference between infected and noninfected urine is so marked that semiquantitative methods are commonly used. In these techniques small wire loops of standard size or strips of blotting paper are used to transfer an aliquot of urine to the culture plate which is then inoculated in a standard way (Leigh and Williams, 1964). These provide sufficiently accurate methods for most purposes.

In addition to standard bacteriological methods several tests are now available to enable cultures to be made immediately after collection of the urine. There are several varieties of dip slides which comprise a carrier for flat strips of culture media. The slides are dipped into the urine, allowed to drain and incubated. The results obtained allow some quantitative assessment of the number of bacteria present and correlate closely with those from standard bacteriological methods (Guttman and Naylor, 1967). Examination of the slides can be carried out by the clinician who has acquired some knowledge of microbiology and the interpretation of culture plates. Alternatively, the inoculated slides can be transported or posted to a laboratory for incubation, and this also enables antibiotic susceptibility tests to be carried out when necessary.

For the examination of large numbers of urine specimens simple chemical tests have been tried. Modification of the Greiss tests for nitrites in urine carried out after incubation with added nitrate (Sleigh, 1965) and the use of a reducible dye (triphenytetrazoliumchloride; Simmons and Williams, 1962) were the most widely used although they had the limitation that positive results required further examination by culture techniques. One unfulfilled expectation of chemical tests was the hope that they could provide a result within a few minutes while the patient was still in the clinic. This would greatly simplify the diagnosis of urinary tract infection, but so far no such facility is available (Kass, 1975).

Causative organisms

Most organisms present in the urine in urinary tract infection are aerobic bacteria and predominantly Gram-negative rods. Anaerobic bacteria, parvobacteria and viruses are very rarely implicated. The organisms isolated reflect the origins of the infecting species, which are derived from the aerobic microflora of the intestine and the perineum and include *Escherichia coli*, *P. mirabilis* and aerobic micrococci; less common are faecal streptococci of groups D and B. Infections that arise in association with invasive procedures on the urinary tract have a more varied bacterial flora, including Klebsiella species, *Pseudomonas aeruginosa* and Serratia, which depends upon and reflects the flora of the particular hospital environment. Organisms derived from the respiratory tract, for example *Haemophilus influenzae* and *Streptococcus pneumoniae*, also occur but are unusual. Microaerophilic corynebacteria may be found in cultures from the urethra and are sometimes seen in large numbers in the urine. The role of these organisms in symptomatic infections is a matter of current debate.

In girls the commonest organism isolated is *E.coli* which accounts for about 90 per cent of the isolated strains. *P. mirabilis*, micrococci, *Strep. faecalis* and other bacteria are found in the remaining cases. In boys, however, *P. mirabilis* has been reported to be more common than *E. coli*. Maskell, Hallett and Pead (1975) found 59 per cent of infection in boys under 12 years to be due to *P. mirabilis* compared to 29 per cent associated with the isolation of *E.coli* and other coliforms.

Pathogenesis

In discussing why and how urinary tract infections arise one must consider factors that may be present in the infecting organisms and in the host.

Pathogenic mechanisms in infecting organisms

E. coli is the most frequent urinary pathogen and is the organism that has been most studied in the search for mechanisms of pathogenicity. The two mechanisms that *E. coli* exhibits are invasiveness and the production of exotoxins. In the urinary tract most work has concentrated on the antigenic structure of the cell envelope and in particular the O and K antigens. The O antigens enable *E. coli* to be divided into about 150 serotypes. In infantile gastroenteritis certain O types have been implicated in invasive infection and a parallel was considered to exist between enteropathic strains causing diarrhoeal disease and uropathic strains causing urinary tract infection. Certainly some O serotypes of *E. coli* are commonly found in urinary tract infection, notably O1, O2, O4, O6, O18 and O75. These strains, however, are also most commonly isolated from stool flora and their frequent presence in urinary infection reflects their prevalence in the main source of infecting strains. These common O serotypes are also the most often encountered in abdominal sepsis. Animal experiments have failed to show any enhancement of virulence associated with O serotypes in experimental pyelonephritis.

The K antigens of *E. coli* play a role in the pathogenesis of urinary tract infection but this is related to the amount of K antigen present rather than to the specific serological type. Strains containing abundant K antigen are able to colonize the urinary tract and may be more invasive than K-negative strains because of their effects on phagocytosis and on complement activity. In urinary tract infection no parallel exists to the *E. coli* K88 strain which adheres tightly to the mucosa of the intestinal tract of pigs and gives rise to severe gastroenteritis.

Serological typing of *E. coli* strains is therefore of no value as a guide to their pathogenic potential. It is now mainly used as a helpful tool in differentiating persistent infection from reinfection in patients with recurrent episodes of urinary tract infection.

Proteus species present special pathogenic features related to the production of urease which leads to the formation of ammonia and the alkalinization of the urine. The latter produces two adverse effects. First precipitation of phosphates in the urine while still in the urinary passages can lead to formation of stone, which in addition to the adverse effects of the stone itself leads to difficulties in eradicating the infection. Secondly many antimicrobial agents, notably nitrofurantoin and most beta-lactam antibiotics, are less active at alkaline pHs and one may have to resort to aminoglycosides for treatment of Proteus infection. Other virulence factors associated with *P. mirabilis* are the occurrence of K antigens in the envelope of many strains and the presence of pili that enable attachment to the pelvic mucosa (Silverblatt and Ofek, 1975).

Of the various subdivisions of coagulase-negative cocci one type predominates in community-acquired urinary tract infection. These are strains of Micrococcus type III which are almost always novobiocin-resistant and thus simply recognized (Meers, Whyte and Sandys, 1975). The fact that this group of organisms shares some cell wall constituents with *Staphylococcus pyogenes* may relate to their virulence. No explanation has been found for their predilection for the urinary tract.

Other organisms that gain access to the urinary tract and produce infection are usually associated with instrumentation and other invasive procedures. In the normal urinary tract these organisms do not appear and the infections arise from impairment of host defences rather than any specific pathogenic potential in the urinary tract.

Host factors

Access of organisms to the bladder

Most studies on the access of organisms to the bladder from the perineum have been done on adult females (O'Grady *et al.*, 1970; Marsh, Murray and Panchamia, 1972) but the findings are probably applicable also to children. Spoiling of the perineal area by faeces and colonization of the skin, preputial sac or vulva are common in children. The relative shortness of the urethra in childhood may predispose to urinary tract infection. Nevertheless, it is only in a proportion of subjects colonized in this way that the organisms enter the bladder and only in a fraction of these that they manage to establish a foothold in the bladder urine. ·The balance between the virulence of the organisms and the normal host defences requires some distortion before infection supervenes. The predilection of *P. mirabilis* for boys has been related to some unspecified effect of prostatic secretions (Maskell, Hallett and Pead, 1975). In girls it is likely that the K antigens of *E. coli* are sufficient to initiate infection in some patients.

Immunological aspects

It is unlikely that circulating antibody has any effect in reducing the incidence of ascending urinary tract infection. In the experimental animal immunization with K antigen reduces the severity but not the frequency of infection and has no effect on kidney scarring (Radford *et al.*, 1974). Antibodies may also be present in the urine, especially when there is proteinuria. The IgG and IgM groups have little protective effect (Asscher, 1978) but local production of secretory IgA is probably of some importance. Children with recurrent urinary tract infection may show a fivefold increase in secretory IgA levels in the urine (Jodal *et al.*, 1970). Burdon (1976) has shown that most urinary IgA arises from the urethra and in normal circumstances this may have the effect of preventing the attachment of bacteria to the mucosa, colonization and ascending infection.

Identification of the site of infection

An infection situated in a kidney subject to an anatomical or physiological abnormality is more difficult to eradicate and more prone to relapse than one confined to the lower urinary tract. Bilateral ureteric catheterization with culture of the ureteric urine is the only accurate method by which one can determine whether the infection is proceeding from the upper part of the urinary tract. Although such a procedure may be justifiable as a clinical research measure it does not appear to be an essential investigation in the majority of cases of recurrent urinary tract infection. In relapsing infection it is sometimes helpful to know if the infection is localized in the kidney, and a variety of noninvasive procedures have been suggested to provide this information. Of these tests serum antibody levels against the infecting organism and the presence of antibody-coated bacteria in the urine are the ones that have been most widely studied.

Two types of circulating antibody have been detected in the serum of patients with urinary tract infection, namely an agglutinating antibody (Percival, Brumfitt and de Louvois, 1964; Brumfitt and Percival, 1965) and a haemagglutinin. Results obtained with the two techniques are not comparable. While the presence of high circulating antibody levels correlates with the presence of a renal infection there are many exceptions and antibody levels may be of little help in the individual patient. For example Turck (1978) found titres of haemagglutinating antibody greater than 512 in 10 of 39 patients with renal bacteriuria and only one of 40 patients with bladder bacteriuria. In a study of antibody levels in children over a long period Smellie *et al.* (1973) found some cases in which a raised titre might have been expected and none occurred and others in which a high titre was found but renal growth proceeded normally.

Several studies have shown an association between antibody-coated bacteria in the urine and the presence of a renal infection (Jones, Smith and Sanford, 1974; Thomas, Shelokov and Forland, 1974). Not all workers have achieved the close correlation found in the earlier studies, as the discussion following the paper by Fries *et al.* (1978) shows. Tests for antibody-coating of bacteria in the urine do not appear to be widely used at present, even though the techniques using fluorescent antihuman-globulin sera are easy to perform.

Fairley *et al.* (1967) suggested a method for localization which was less invasive than ureteric catheterization. The technique involves catheterization of the bladder which is then treated with washout and neomycin to reduce the bacterial count. The rate at which the bacteriuria recovers differentiates a renal infection (rapid recovery of bacteriuria) from bladder infection (slow recovery of bacteriuria). This test has received several modifications using forced diuresis and/or diuretics to increase the urine flow, and in experienced hands it can give helpful data in the few patients for whom such information is necessary.

Underlying urinary tract disease

The presence of structural and/or functional abnormality of the urinary tract does not necessarily lead to an increased incidence of ascending infection. However, once organisms have been introduced into an abnormal tract it is easier for them to become established and more difficult for them to be removed either by the normal defence mechanisms or by active treatment.

Asymptomatic infections and covert bacteriuria

The symptoms of urinary tract infection can be mild or indefinite even in adults. In children, where they may be even less clearly expressed, many infections remain undiagnosed and numerous studies have been done in an attempt to detect occult or covert cases of infection. The epidemiological work carried out by Kunin and his colleagues delineated the extent of the problem (Kunin, Zacha and Paquin, 1962; Kunin, Deutscher and Paquin, 1964; Kunin, 1970, 1972). Many large studies have been carried out in the UK and particularly in Dundee (Savage *et al.*, 1969), Manchester (Cohen and Eirew, 1973) and Cardiff and Oxford (McLachlan *et al.*, 1975). Most programmes mounted to detect bacteriuria have shown an incidence of just less than 1 per cent in preschool girls (rather less in boys) and 1–2 per cent in girls of school age. The detection rate of asymptomatic infection in boys of school age is much less. In infancy there is a higher occurrence in boys of both symptomatic and asymptomatic infection which has been reported to be in the region of 2 per cent (Reindke *et al.*, 1975).

Despite all the effort that has been expended over the years on screening programmes for detecting bacteriuria in children they have not become established as part of general paediatric care. It is worthwhile examining the reasons for this. The logistic problems in collecting and examining quickly large numbers of urine specimens from apparently healthy children are formidable and if some immediate culture technique is used, such as dip slides, the costs are high. The bacteriuria is commonly intermittent and therefore the number of bacteriuric children uncovered by a single specimen is small. Invasive investigations such as cystourethography and excretory urography are needed to identify those children especially at risk of continuing renal damage, but these techniques require scarce resources and can be unpleasant for the child and his parents. Furthermore some studies indicate that both in infancy (Reindke *et al.*, 1975) and in schoolchildren (Cohen and Eirew, 1973) urinary tract infections are often accompanied by symptoms that point to some abnormality in the child. In the absence of screening programmes bacteriological examination of the urine should be carried out whenever there is the slightest suspicion that a child's illness may be due to urinary tract infection.

References

Asscher, A.W. (1978) Immune response to urinary tract infections. *In* Modern Topics in Infection (edited by Williams, J.D.). Heinemann, London. p.83

Brumfitt, W. and Percival, A. (1965) Serum antibody response as an indication of renal involvement in patients with significant bacteriuria. *In* Progress in Pyelonephritis (edited by Kass, E.H.). Davis, Philadelphia. p.118

Burdon, D.W. (1976) Immunological reaction to urinary infection: the nature and function of secretory immunoglobulins. *In* Scientific Foundations of Urology, Vol.1 (edited by Williams, D.I. and Chisholm, G.D.). Heinemann, London. p.192

Cohen, G.J. and Eirew, R.C. (1973) The Manchester schools survey; the first 5,000. *In* Urinary Tract Infection (edited by Brumfitt, W. and Asscher, A.W.). Oxford University Press, London. p.16

Fairley, K.F., Bond, A.G., Brown, R.B. and Habersberger, P. (1967) Simple test to determine the site of urinary tract infection. *Lancet*, ii, 427

Fries, D., Jacques, L., Del Graissy, F., Delavelle, F. and Arvis, G. (1978) Immunofluorescence studies in the localisation of urinary tract infection. *In* Infections of the Urinary Tract (edited by Kass, E.H. and Brumfitt, W.). University of Chicago Press, Chicago. p.136

Guttman, D. and Naylor, G. (1967) Dip-slide aid to quantitative urine culture in general practice. *British Medical Journal*, iii, 343

Jodal, A., Hanson, L.A., Holmgren, J. and Kaijser, B. (1970) Studies of antibodies and immunoglobulin levels in urine from children with urinary tract infections caused by *E.coli. Acta Paediatrica Scandinavica*, **206**, Suppl. p.78

Jones, S.R., Smith, J.W. and Sanford, J.P. (1974) Localisation of urinary tract infection by detection of antibody-coated bacteria in urinary sediments. *New England Journal of Medicine*, **290**, 591

Kass, E.H. (1975) Epidemiological aspects of infections of the urinary tract. *In* Infections of the Urinary Tract (edited by Kass, E.H. and Brumfitt, W.). Chicago University Press, Chicago. p.1

Kunin, C.M. (1970) A ten year study of bacteriuria in school girls; a final report on the bacteriologic, urologic and epidemiologic findings. *Journal of Infectious Diseases*, **122**, 982

Kunin, C.M. (1972) Epidemiology and natural history of urinary tract infection in children. *In* Urinary Tract Infection and its Management (edited by Kaye, D.). Mosby, St Louis. p.156

Kunin, C.M., Zacha, E. and Paquin, A.J. (1962) Urinary tract infection in childhood. *New England Journal of Medicine*, **266**, 1285

Kunin, C.M., Deutscher, R. and Paquin, A.J. (1964) Urinary tract infection in schoolchildren; an epidemiological, clinical and laboratory study. *Medicine*, **43**, 81

Leigh, D.A. and Williams J.D. (1964) Method for the detection of significant bacteriuria in large groups of patients. *Journal of Clinical Pathology*, **17**, 498

Little, P.J. (1964) A comparison of the urinary white cell concentration with the white cell excretion rate. *British Journal of Urology*, **36**, 360

McLachlan, M.S.F., Meller, J.T., Verrier-Jones, R., Asscher, W.A., Fletcher, E.W.L., Mayon White, R.T., Legindham, J.G., Smith, J.C. and Johnston, H.H. (1975) The urinary tract in school girls with covert bacteriuria. *Archives of Disease in Childhood*, **50**, 253

Marsh, F.P., Murray, M. and Panchamia, P. (1972) The relationship between bacterial cultures of the vaginal introitus and urinary infection. *British Journal of Urology*, **44**, 368

Maskell, R., Hallett, R.J. and Pead, L. (1975) Urinary tract infection in boys aged 2 to 12 years. *In* Infections of the Urinary Tract (edited by Kass, E.H. and Brumfitt, W.). University of Chicago Press, Chicago. p.26

Meers, P.D., Whyte, W. and Sandys, G. (1975) Coagulase-negative staphylococci and micrococci in urinary tract infections. *Journal of Clinical Pathology*, **28**, 270

O'Grady, F.W., McSherry, M.A., Richards, B. and O'Farrell, S.M. (1970) Introital enterobacteria, urinary infection and the urethral syndrome. *Lancet*, ii, 1208

Percival, A., Brumfitt, W. and de Louvois, J. (1964) Serum antibody levels as an indication of clinically inapparent pyelonephritis. *Lancet*, ii, 1027

Radford, N.J., Chick, S., Ling, R., Coles, G.A. and Asscher, A.W. (1974) The effect of active immunisation on ascending pyelonephritis in the rat. *Journal of Pathology*, **112**, 169

Reindke, B., Daschner, F., Morgenroth, H., Belchradsky, B., Leuthner, G. and Marget, W. (1975) Value of screening for bacteriuria in infancy. *In* Infections of the Urinary Tract (edited by Kass, E.H. and Brumfitt, W.). Chicago University Press, Chicago. p.31

Savage, D.C.L., Wilson, M.J., Ross, E.M. and Fee, W.M. (1969) Asymptomatic bacteriuria in girl entrants to Dundee primary schools. *British Medical Journal*, iii, 75

Silverblatt, F.J. and Ofek, I. (1975) Effects of pili on susceptibility of *Proteus mirabilis* to phagocytosis and adherence to bladder cells. *In* Infections of the Urinary Tract (edited by Kass, E.H. and Brumfitt, W.). University of Chicago Press, Chicago. p.49

Simmons, N.A. and Williams, J.D. (1962) A simple test for significant bacteriuria. *Lancet*, i, 1377

Sleigh, D.A. (1965) Detection of bacteriuria by a modification of the nitrite test. *British Medical Journal*, i, 765

Smellie, J.M., Pursell, R., Prescod, N. and Brumfitt, W. (1973) Relationship between serum antibody titre and radiological findings in children with urinary tract infection. *In* Urinary Tract Infection (edited by Brumfitt, W. and Asscher, A.W.). Oxford University Press, London. p.31

Thomas, V., Shelokov, A. and Forland, M. (1974) Antibody-coated bacteria in the urine and the site of urinary tract infection. *New England Journal of Medicine*, **290**, 588

Turck, M. (1978) Importance of localization of urinary tract infection in women. *In* Infections of the Urinary Tract (edited by Kass, E.H. and Brumfitt, W.). University of Chicago Press, Chicago. p.114

10 Urinary Tract Infection: Clinical Aspects

Jean M. Smellie and I.C.S. Normand

Introduction

Urinary tract infection (UTI) may be defined as the persistent presence within the urinary tract of actively multiplying organisms. It occurs during childhood in some 5 per cent of girls and 2 per cent of boys, placing it among the commonest of childhood bacterial infections. The urinary pathogen is usually one of the patient's own bowel commensals and it is reasonable to assume that the development of a UTI indicates some form of breakdown of the intrinsic defences of the urinary tract against bacterial colonization by the bowel flora. It must therefore be regarded as a sign, which is often the only one, of urinary tract disorder.

In the majority of children such infection causes neither damage to the kidney nor impairment of future health. In a small number, however, it may be the first sign of serious underlying pathology such as obstructive uropathy or it may unmask a long-standing disease process such as the coarse renal scarring of chronic atrophic pyelonephritis or reflux nephropathy. Pyelonephritic renal scarring causes two thirds of serious hypertension in the young and like obstructive uropathy is a major cause of renal failure in children and young adults requiring dialysis or renal transplantation.

Reflux of urine from the bladder into the ureters can be demonstrated after eradication of bacteriuria in over a third of children who present with UTI. It is almost invariably found in those with renal scarring and in such children there is also good reason to believe that the morphology of the renal papillae can allow calycotubular backflow of urine (intrarenal reflux; Ransley and Risdon, 1978). In this way bacteria in bladder urine can be propelled into the substance of the kidney whenever the bladder pressure is sufficient to reverse urine flow in the renal papilla. It is becoming increasingly clear that renal scarring seldom occurs for the first time after childhood and indeed that the most serious and extensive scarring is likely to develop during the first 5 years of life in children with UTI who also have both vesicoureteric reflux (VUR) and intrarenal reflux (Rolleston, Maling and Hodson, 1974; Smellie and Normand, 1975).

If infective damage of the urinary tract is to be minimized, both infection and its associated problems must be recognized as early as possible and dealt with effectively. It must be stressed that throughout childhood the symptoms of UTI are an unreliable guide both to the state of the urinary tract and to the extent of renal involvement. One of the unfortunate characteristics of the infant and the young child is that at a time when the rapidly growing kidney appears to be most vulnerable to the effects of bacterial invasion the nonspecific symptoms of infection render the clinical diagnosis most difficult.

Aetiology

Escherichia coli is the commonest urinary pathogen and is responsible in pure growth for

80–90 per cent of first and a slightly lower proportion of recurrent infections. Other urinary invaders include *Klebsiella aerogenes*, *Streptococcus faecalis*, micrococci and enterococci, and *Proteus mirabilis*. These are all bowel commensals and the urinary pathogen is usually found simultaneously and with the same resistance pattern in the faecal and the periurethral floras of girls with recurrent infection. In boys, in whom Proteus infections are common, this organism may also be recovered simultaneously from the preputial sac. Proteus infection is particularly associated with stone formation.

The urinary tract is usually infected by organisms ascending the urethra (except in the newborn period when bacterial spread to the kidney may be haematogenous) and the short urethra in the female, especially if there is periurethral colonization, may partly explain the high incidence of UTI in girls. Invasion of the bladder is likely to be facilitated by local irritation.

Causes of breakdown in bladder defences

Urine flow may be obstructed mechanically as a result of malformation such as posterior urethral valves or functionally because of bladder neuropathy or detrusor-sphincter incoordination (Allen, 1977). Also, residual urine can collect either in large bladder diverticula or following the return of refluxed urine from the ureter to the bladder.

An increase in residual urine has been a common finding in females with recurrent infection (MacGregor and Wynne Williams, 1966; Shand *et al.*, 1970; Lindberg *et al.*, 1975) and bladder emptying may be incomplete in the child who voids only twice a day or whose gross chronic faecal overload displaces the bladder (Neumann, de Domenico and Nogrady, 1973). Normal micturition can also be inhibited by

Table 10.1   Radiological findings in children with symptomatic urinary infection aged 0–12 years

Finding		Percentage
No structural defect		50
Defects requiring surgery e.g. obstruction, stones, diverticula etc.		8
Vesicoureteric reflux { with renal scarring		12
{ no renal scarring		23
Renal scarring without vesicoureteric reflux		1
Malformations without either obstruction or reflux		6

Colonization and bacterial multiplication within bladder urine, itself a good culture medium, are normally prevented by the natural defence processes of which regular complete emptying of the bladder is the most important (O'Grady and Cattell, 1966; Hinman and Cox, 1967). Protection is also provided through the dilution by freshly formed urine of organisms entering the bladder; the resistance of the bladder mucosa to bacterial attachment; the desquamation, leukocytic activity and inflammatory response of the bladder mucosa and vesical wall (Orikasa and Hinman, 1977); and other local and general immunological responses (Hanson, 1973). Anything that interferes with these functions or causes urinary stasis may thus predispose to infection.

painful napkin dermatitis or by vulval inflammation of any cause. Nevertheless, only a small proportion of young children with dysuria are found to have infected urine.

Significance of abnormalities

Urinary tract abnormalities are found in about 50 per cent of children with UTI, with a slight male preponderance. Substantially higher rates that have been reported usually include diagnoses such as meatal stenosis and radiological bladder neck obstruction which are now generally discounted (*Table 10.1*).

Abnormalities requiring surgical correction

These are found in 8 per cent of children with UTI. They include such conditions as diverticula, stones and ureteroceles and it is those causing obstruction to urine flow that are the most serious because of the damaging effect of infection in the presence of obstruction and back-pressure.

Vesicoureteric reflux

This is the commonest abnormal finding on investigation of children with UTI. It occurs in 35–40 per cent of children with either symptomatic or covert bacteriurias discovered on screening. Because of its tendency to disappear spontaneously with time (Smellie, 1967) reflux is found in a higher proportion of infants with bacteriuria and a lower proportion of older schoolchildren (*Table 10.2*).

VUR is important in children with UTI not only because it can convey organisms from the bladder to the kidney but also because the residual urine formed by the return of refluxed urine encourages reinfection. For these reasons VUR is almost invariably found in children with chronic pyelonephritic renal scarring. However, due to its natural tendency to regress and disappear it is found in less than 50 per cent of adults with such scarring (Vermillion and Heale, 1973).

Although renal scarring is already established in approximately 30 per cent of children found to have VUR, the intravenous urogram (IVU) is essentially normal in half of the children with reflux when they are first investigated. In children over 5 years of age the appearances usually remain normal despite continuing moderate reflux and symptomless bacteriuria (Cardiff-Oxford Bacteriuria Study Group, 1978). Fresh scarring occasionally follows symptomatic infection if VUR is present (Smellie *et al.*, 1975).

Renal scarring

This is found in 12–25 per cent of children with UTI, whether this is symptomatic infection or

Table 10.2 Renal scarring of the chronic atrophic pyelonephritic type and vesicoureteric reflux in childhood urinary tract infection (data from Smellie and Normand, 1979)

Reference	Schoolgirls with bacteriuria found on screening	Renal scars (%)	Vesicoureteric reflux (%)
Kunin, Deutscher and Paquin (1964)	Total children	13.1	18.5
	Total white children	15.7	22.5
	White 5–9 years	13.9	33.0
	White 10–14 years	20.0	14.2
Savage *et al.* (1969)	5 years	15.0	40.0
Savage *et al.* (1973)	5–14 years	23.0	35.0
Asscher *et al.* (1973)	Total children	20.0	29.0
	5–7 years	12.0	29.2
	8–12 years	25.0	28.2
Newcastle Asymptomatic Bacteriuria Research Group (1975)		15.0	21.0
Lindberg *et al.* (1975)		10.0	20.7
Edwards *et al.* (1975)		17.0	25.0

Reference	Children with symptomatic urinary infection aged 0–12 years	Renal scars (%)	Vesicoureteric reflux (%)
Smellie *et al.* (1964)	Age 0–12 years	13.0	34.0
	Recurrent infection	26.0	40.0
Wein and Schoenberg (1972)	Girls	13.0	35.0
Winberg *et al.* (1974)	First infection	6.0	
Shannon (1972)	Age 0–1 year	8.0	49.0
Drew and Acton (1976)	Newborn	4.0	46.0

bacteriuria detected on screening. The incidence is higher in older children and those with a history of repeated infections than in infants and young children. It must be re-emphasized that in children this scarring is almost invariably accompanied by past or present VUR although the proportion of children with reflux showing renal scarring increases with age (Smellie and Normand, 1968).

Unlike VUR, which tends to regress spontaneously, renal scarring is permanent and its sequelae may develop whether the associated reflux continues, disappears or is corrected surgically. Thus bilateral chronic pyelonephritic scarring remains one of the main causes of renal failure requiring dialysis or renal transplantation. It accounted for 27 per cent of young adults undergoing these treatments in Europe by 1977 and 24 per cent in 1978 (*Proceedings of the European Dialysis and Transplant Association*, 1977, 1978). Hypertension is increasingly becoming recognized as a transient or permanent result of scarring of one or both kidneys, even years after surgery has terminated VUR (Wallace, Rothwell and Williams, 1978; Smellie and Normand, 1979). The continued follow-up of children with renal scarring is therefore assuming increasing importance whether or not reflux persists, so that hypertension can be recognized early and the necessary treatment instituted.

Anomalies

Defects such as duplex systems or solitary kidneys *without VUR or obstruction to flow* are found in approximately 7 per cent of children with UTI. The prognosis is good but the familial association of duplex systems with VUR and potential renal scarring is significant and should always be taken into consideration if siblings develop UTI (Atwell *et al.*, 1977).

Half the children with UTI have *no structural defect* of the urinary tract and their renal prognosis is excellent. A small group have recurrent symptomatic infection and suffer distressing symptoms and school absence. It appears that even schoolgirls with bacteriuria discovered on screening have a greater risk of recurrent UTI in early adult life (Gillenwater, Harrison and Kunin, 1979) so that this is by no means an unimportant group.

Recognition of infection

Urine collection

In order to establish the diagnosis, which depends upon demonstrating significant bacteriuria, urine samples of suitable quality must be collected and correctly processed as described in Chapter 9.

Time must be spent, particularly in infancy, upon the practical problem of urine collection since decisions about unpleasant and expensive investigations and prolonged treatment and follow-up are determined by the bacteriological findings.

Clean or midstream sample

There is no problem in the older child who can pass a midstream specimen to order after local cleansing with tap water. A dip slide held in the stream (a dipstream specimen) or dipped in the freshly passed urine sample obviates the problems of overgrowth by contaminant organisms if there is any likelihood of delay in handling the sample.

Bag specimen

In infants and children too young to cooperate a plastic collecting bag, for example a Hollister U-bag, may be applied to the cleansed perineum. (If any antiseptic solution is used, this must be removed by rinsing with water and drying). The infant or toddler is then held upright or made to adopt a position that allows voided urine to run into the dependent part of the bag out of contact with the perineal skin. As soon as voiding occurs the bag should be removed and the urine delivered into a sterile container after snipping the lower corner of the bag. In this way most of the contamination that has impaired the collecting bag's reputation can be eliminated. This method is best used in domiciliary and outpatient practice where the mother is available to supervise its use and has time to do so; it is notoriously unreliable when used on the ward in hospital. While a positive culture from bag urine in an infant requires confirmation by direct collection of bladder urine a negative result may be of great importance.

Suprapubic aspiration

The collection of urine by direct bladder puncture has been widely applied with minimal complications in young children. It is particularly useful in the newborn infant when a rapid unequivocal result is needed, in the very ill infant or young child as part of diagnostic bacteriological screening before starting antibacterial treatment, to confirm a positive culture obtained from bag urine, and when 'mixed' growths have been obtained from two or more voided samples.

In infants the procedure is only attempted if the bladder is palpable suprapubically or if a bag is dry after 1 hour in position on a normally hydrated infant. Urine should be obtained on insertion, not withdrawal, of the needle to avoid contamination of the needle tip by penetration of the bowel.

Catheter specimen

The disposable fine polythene catheters now available have overcome many of the earlier objections to catheterization. An urgent diagnostic sample may be obtained in this way in the infant who is ill or dehydrated or whose bladder is not palpable. This method should be avoided if urethral or bladder neck obstruction is suspected or balanitis is present, because of the risk of trauma or of introducing infection.

Criteria for diagnosis

Significant bacteriuria

The diagnosis of UTI can be made with certainty only on the demonstration of significant bladder bacteriuria. The usual criterion for this is a pure growth of 10^5 or more organisms per millilitre in girls or 10^4 or more organisms per millilitre in boys obtained on culture of a urine sample either freshly passed or chilled to 4°C immediately after voiding. These figures may be affected by, for example, diuresis if fluids are offered when a sample is difficult to obtain and pure growths of 10^3–10^5 organisms require repeat cultures. *Any* pure growth of organisms in bladder urine obtained by suprapubic aspiration or urethral catheterization is significant. In an acute symptomatic infection one sample is usually sufficient to give an unequivocal answer, but where the diagnosis is in doubt and the child is not ill the collection of at least two is desirable. A mixed growth of organisms generally indicates contamination and requires a repeat test, although very rarely two organisms may infect the obstructed urinary tract. Equivalent values have been determined for direct microscopy of the fresh uncentrifuged urine, dip-slide culture and the filter-paper screening technique (*see* Chapter 8).

Pyuria

Pyuria is a sign of inflammation within the urinary tract and is not alone diagnostic of UTI. In uncentrifuged fresh urine white blood cell counts of more than $10/mm^3$ in boys and more than $50/mm^3$ in girls are considered abnormal. Significant pyuria usually but not always accompanies symptomatic UTI and can be a useful adjunct to the clinical diagnosis in the febrile child who has received antibacterial treatment before collection of a diagnostic urine sample. No pyuria is found in half the schoolchildren with bacteriuria identified by screening. Very rarely children with apparently sterile pyuria are identified. In those with renal scarring this has sometimes been attributed to bacterial L-forms, while a search for fastidious or anaerobic organisms (Maskell, Pead and Allen, 1979) or even for the tubercle bacillus may be rewarded. When pyuria is associated with a mixed growth of organisms the source is usually the perineum or vagina.

Other

Microscopic and macroscopic haematuria may occur and have also been reported with viral cystitis. The finding of proteinuria is of no value in the diagnosis of UTI.

Presentation of urinary tract infection

The presentation and symptoms of UTI in infancy and childhood are variable and misleading and are influenced by the age and the sex of the child, the underlying cause and any preceding treatment. For this reason it cannot be too

Table 10.3   Main symptoms in 200 children (148 girls and 52 boys) with urinary infection presenting or born in hospital; 65 per cent had no symptoms related to the urinary tract (data from Smellie et al., 1964)

Principal symptoms on presentation	Age on diagnosis 0–1 month	1 month–2 years	2–5 years	5–12 years	Total
Excessive weight loss or slow weight gain, feeding problems	24	16	3	–	43
Jaundice	20	–	–	–	20
Screaming attacks, irritability, 'colic'	–	6	2	–	8
Offensive or cloudy urine	–	4	6	–	10
Diarrhoea	8	7	–	–	15
Vomiting	11	13	7	2	33
Fever (rigors)	5	17(2)	25(2)	33	80(4)
Convulsions	1	3	4	3	11
Haematuria	–	3	7	4	14
Frequency or dysuria	–	2	15	27	44
Enuresis	–	–	12	19	31
Abdominal pain	–	–	10	29	39
Loin pain	–	–	–	8	8
No. of children	45	45	44	66	200

strongly emphasized that the diagnosis will be repeatedly missed or delayed if urine cultures are not carried out in children with a wide variety of clinical symptoms. Completely symptomless bacteriuria is uncommon but may be discovered either on population screening or during or following antibacterial treatment or prophylaxis of UTI.

Symptoms in relation to age

The distribution of the main symptoms in relation to age in 200 children with UTI presenting or born in hospital is shown in *Table 10.3*. The most striking observations are that nearly half presented under the age of 2 and that in this youngest age group the classic symptoms usually associated with UTI in older children were absent. An early age of onset of UTI has been the widespread finding of paediatricians (Smellie et al., 1964; Stansfeld, 1966; Winberg et al., 1974) and of surveys in general practice (Mond, Grüneberg and Smellie, 1970; Cohen, 1972; Randolph, Morris and Gould, 1975). Reports of a high incidence at a later age come from surgical clinics where presentation depends upon referral and from some general practice studies when the symptoms of infants with UTI were perhaps not recognized.

THE NEWBORN PERIOD
UTI may be part of a general septicaemia or may occur by the more usual ascending route.

The symptoms are those of any infection at this age, with poor feeding, failure to thrive, poor colour and perhaps fever, vomiting or diarrhoea, sleepiness, lassitude and slow weight gain. Bacteraemia is usually present. Jaundice is common in neonatal coliform infections and the urine should always be cultured in the sick jaundiced infant. Even at this age symptomless bacteriuria may be found on screening (Abbott, 1972).

THE FIRST 2 YEARS
The presenting symptoms of UTI, namely slow weight gain, misery, fretfulness, diarrhoea, vomiting and febrile convulsions, are often mistaken for teething or feeding problems or disregarded altogether.

BETWEEN 2–5 YEARS
Nonspecific symptoms of general ill health, recurrent upper respiratory infection, constipation or fever continue to be common complaints. There may also be a delay in gaining normal control of micturition and occasionally there is haematuria. Dysuria and increased frequency are more often the result of local irritation and are rather a rare symptom of bacteriuria.

OVER THE AGE OF 5
The expected symptoms of fever, frequency, dysuria, haematuria and abdominal or loin pain do occur but, especially in girls, they may still be minimal or nonspecific. Here the differential diagnosis is from the acute abdomen, functional

enuresis (which may coexist) and musculo-skeletal pain related to posture, fashion footwear and exercise.

Sex variation of symptoms

During the newborn period boys with UTI equal or outnumber girls. The sexes are equally affected through infancy and in later childhood girls predominate by four times in symptomatic infection and by more than 10 times in bacter-iuria found on screening. The complaints in boys are more likely to be related to the urinary tract, and in infancy even boys presenting with fairly trivial or brief symptoms such as a feeding problem or a mild fever may be found to have infection of a grossly malformed urinary tract.

Symptoms in relation to the underlying cause

It is virtually impossible to predict from the presenting symptoms whether an underlying structural defect is present. Investigation of a classic attack of acute pyelonephritis may subsequently reveal no abnormality, while a renal stone or an unsuspected ureterocele may be discovered on investigating bacteriuria in an infant presenting with symptoms as diverse as constipation, low grade fever or a feeding problem. Haematuria may be found with acute

infection of either the bladder or the kidney. In boys there is an increasing chance of finding either a congenital or an acquired urinary tract abnormality when there are repeated infections.

It would clearly be helpful to be able to recognize VUR clinically and the authors have compared the presenting symptoms of UTI in 246 children with and 498 without reflux. In those with VUR there was a slightly higher incidence of fever, particularly if renal scarring was also present, and of bed-wetting over the age of 5. These differences were not statistically significant and there were no clinical features clearly distinguishing between children with and without VUR (*Table 10.4*). Among the children with reflux, however, the proportion with renal scarring who had a previous history of UTI (46 per cent) was significantly higher than that of those with no renal scarring (19 per cent; Smellie, Normand and Katz, 1981).

Symptoms in relation to preceding treatment

It is likely that undiagnosed bacteriuria may sometimes be eliminated when antibiotics are given for another concurrent infection, so that recent antibacterial treatment should be enquired about when searching for UTI. Indeed the diagnosis of UTI may sometimes be delayed for months or even years if the child also suffers

Table 10.4 Main presenting symptoms, previous history of proved recurrent infection and centile height on presentation in 744 children with and without vesicoureteric reflux

		Children without vesicoureteric reflux			Children with vesicoureteric reflux			Total
		X-ray normal (n=431)	X-ray abnormal (n=67)	Total (n=498)	Intravenous urogram normal (n=143)	X-ray abnormal (n=103; scars 76)	Total (n=246)	(n=744)
		(%)	(%)	(%)	(%)	(%)	(%)	(%)
Main presenting symptoms	fever	33	48	35	50	67	57	42
	abdominal or loin pain	28	36	29	38	30	35	31
	enuresis aged 5 or over	36	37	36	34	51	42	38
Past history	two or more proven urinary tract infections	25	33	26	19	40*	28	27
Height	10 centile or less	12	16	12	4	20	11	12
	90 centile or more	14	19	14	14	16	15	15

*46 per cent of patients with scarred kidneys had a past history of two or more proven urinary tract infections

from a recurring problem such as bronchitis requiring antibacterial treatment.

In addition it is known that untreated bacteriuria may be self-limiting and intermittent both in infancy (Abbott, 1972) and in schoolgirls (Cardiff-Oxford Bacteriuria Study Group, 1978). For these reasons it is rarely possible either to exclude a past history of UTI or to say retrospectively at what age a child first developed bacteriuria unless regular cultures were made in infancy and during any early disorder or illness.

Clinical history and examination

These should concentrate on the factors predisposing to infection, the presence of adequate physical growth and the exclusion of both obstructive or neuropathic lesions of the bladder and hypertension.

Initial treatment

The presence of more or less free urethral drainage distinguishes most infections of the urinary tract from closed bacterial infections elsewhere. Therapeutic success may require only a delicate tilt of the balance between the rate of urine formation, the frequency of micturition, the volume of residual urine and the bacterial multiplication rate in the bladder.

In the great majority of children with UTI a symptomatic and bacteriological response is obtained within 48 hours to any drug to which

the infecting organism is sensitive, although in practice 7–10 days antibacterial treatment is usually prescribed. However, the bladder usually remains susceptible to infection and over two thirds of children develop a further infection which is almost always a reinfection with a fresh bowel organism. This most often happens in the ensuing 6 months and the likelihood of recurrence represents a major problem in the management of children with UTI.

If the infection persists or is replaced by an organism resistant to the drug prescribed, or if there is a rapid recurrence due to the original infecting organism or serotype after treatment is discontinued (relapse) then obstruction, continuing stasis or calculus must be suspected. Infection may also persist or only clear slowly in children with severely impaired renal function.

Antibacterial treatment

The choice of drug is influenced by the expected sensitivities of urinary pathogens in the local environment. For instance, a higher proportion of urinary organisms are sensitive to the usual antibacterials if they are grown from domiciliary patients rather than hospital inpatients. The drug chosen may also depend on the effect any preceding antibacterial treatment has had upon the bowel flora and on the likely tissue and urinary concentrations of the drug.

Suggested drugs and dosages are given in *Table 10.5*. Penicillin and gentamicin are useful when septicaemia is suspected in the very sick child and infant but the latter should be discontinued as soon as possible because of the

Table 10.5   Drugs used for the treatment and prophylaxis of urinary infection in children

Drug	Dosage therapeutic mg/kg per day	prophylactic mg/kg per day
Sulphonamide	100	20–25
Co-trimoxazole		
(sulphamethoxazole)	(20)	(10–5)
(trimethoprim)	(4)	(2–1)
Trimethoprim	4	2–1
Ampicillin	50	–
Amoxycillin	20–25	–
Nitrofurantoin	4–5	1–2
Nalidixic acid	40–50	15–20
Gentamicin	2–3	
Cephaloridine	15–30	
Carfecillin	30–60	
Hexamine mandelate		250–500 mg three times daily with acidified urine

risk of nephrotoxicity. Modification of the dosage may be needed if renal function is impaired.

Urine should ideally be cultured at 48 hours and 7–10 days after the start of treatment, and at intervals of 2–3 months over the succeeding year whether or not the child has symptoms. Many recurrences during or after treatment are quite symptomless and are only recognized by routine follow-up urine culture.

In the very small proportion of children with persistent or relapsing infection in whom obstruction is suspected, repeated changes of antibacterial drug only encourage the growth of multiresistant organisms and investigation should be expedited rather than delayed because of this.

Other measures

The management of the acute infection does not stop with the prescription of antibacterial treatment. Fluid intake should be liberal and constipation corrected. When the urinary tract is free from infection the dosage can be reduced to prophylactic levels until investigations are complete.

Initial investigation

Purpose

Investigation is undertaken to assess renal function, to identify serious lesions which may require surgical relief, to diagnose VUR which may lead to renal scars and to detect any abnormality rendering the urinary tract susceptible to infection. Investigation also helps in designing an effective therapeutic programme appropriate to the individual child and in establishing the likely prognosis.

Methods and uses

Plasma creatinine concentration is the routine test of renal function. The maximum concentrating capacity of the kidneys is impaired for some weeks after renal infection but this is seldom tested except for research purposes. Tests to determine the site of infection based for example on *E. coli* antibody levels, the ESR and the C-reactive protein and antibody coating of bacteria have been studied although to date they have not proved sufficiently discriminatory in children for routine clinical use. Chemical and immunological methods have also been examined to find a noninvasive way of diagnosing VUR and these too have so far been disappointing.

The IVU provides information about renal size, shape and function and should be performed in *all* children with proven UTI. In over two thirds of children found to have bacteriuria UTI recurs with or without symptoms within 2 years so that it is more logical to identify those at risk *before* renal damage has occurred. Moreover, in view of the symptomatology in young children it is seldom possible to be confident that the presenting infection is in fact the first one.

In addition to renal features the ureteric calibre and peristalsis and the bladder capacity and its emptying facility can be assessed. The state of the bowels can be seen and a loaded colon identified, particularly when it is producing deformity of the bladder. Lower spinal defects and calcification within the renal tract may be seen on the preliminary plain film. An IVU identifies most of the patients at risk and needing follow-up or further investigation. If the kidneys remain normal to the age of 7, the parents can be largely reassured.

The initial IVU should be carried out immediately (after checking renal function) when obstruction or stone is suspected. Otherwise antibacterial dosage can be reduced to a prophylactic level and the IVU postponed for 2 weeks. Provided that the urine remains sterile, nothing will be lost and the effect of any renal enlargement during the acute phase upon the baseline for renal growth assessment is avoided.

Micturating cystourethrography (MCU) may be an unpleasant experience for a child and, even with an image-intensifier, necessarily exposes the gonads to some irradiation. Nevertheless it is at present the most accurate means of identifying VUR (*Tables 10.1 and 10.2*).

Until a more acceptable alternative is routinely available MCU should be done in all infants and children aged 5 or under with a proven UTI, and in those over 5 if there is a duplex, scarred or small kidney, or a dilated ureter or renal pelvis on the IVU. It is also useful after repeated infections to obtain information about bladder capacity, bladder emptying and residual urine, and to detect diverticula and other possible causes of recurrence. In some centres MCU is performed before infection has developed in newborn infants whose first-degree relatives have renal scarring or severe VUR.

It is undesirable to carry out MCU during an acute infection. An interval of at least 2 weeks free from bacteriuria, with low dosage antibacterial cover, is usually advised.

Follow-up

General principles of further management

The purpose of treatment is to *prevent* or limit renal damage and to *prevent* troublesome symptomatic reinfections. Management of children liable to suffer from these problems includes appropriate surgical correction of underlying defects, measures to avoid urinary stasis, long-term low dosage antibacterial prophylaxis to guard against reinfection of the susceptible urinary tract, and follow-up control.

Surgery

Children with obstruction, stone, diverticula and possibly gross VUR require surgical treatment with follow-up to confirm operative success and freedom from reinfection on urine culture. It is particularly important that infection should be prevented during any postoperative urinary stasis.

If the unobstructed refluxing urinary tract becomes infected, any reflux-stopping surgery should be delayed until the infection has been eliminated and the urinary tract kept free from infection by antibacterial prophylaxis for some weeks. For example in the Stanford experience (Govan *et al.*, 1975) fresh scars were identified postoperatively in a number of children undergoing ureteric reimplantation. In 45 per cent of these children there had been a symptomatic UTI within the 2 weeks preceding reimplantation (Friedland, 1979).

Measures to reduce stasis

Attention to detail is essential in the care of these children. A careful clinical history including both bowel and bladder emptying habits, social aspects and family history often identifies likely factors and indicates remedies so as to reduce unnecessary and unpleasant investigation.

When the abnormal susceptibility of the bladder to infection is due to a functional rather than a structural cause, modification of the child's habits may help to restore the normal bladder defences. Recommendations include the following:

1. *Regular complete voiding*. There may be problems of incomplete or infrequent voiding, for example in the toddler who has recently acquired voluntary bladder control and with no time to spare empties the bladder just partially but sufficiently for comfort, or in the schoolgirl who does not use the school toilets because they are unsavoury or inaccessible or who is reluctant to waste playtime in a queue. The latter can develop a considerable increase in bladder capacity and the overstretched detrusor later contracts incompletely. Most of these problems can be corrected by a word from the mother to the teacher or nursery supervisor and by a reminder at home. Voiding before leaving school, going out to play or watching television is a helpful recommendation. Double or triple micturition at bedtime ensures complete bladder emptying at least once a day.
2. *Drinks*. A regular drink with main meals and at mid-morning and mid-afternoon is advisable, with reminders of this routine before camping holidays and long journeys and in hot weather.
3. *Bowels*. Dietary regulation with bran and brown bread may be sufficient but long-standing constipation may require continuous laxatives given over several months.
4. *Local irritants*. Threadworms are often overlooked but may cause dysuria even when there is no UTI. Nylon pants, especially in strong colours, are best replaced with white cotton ones. If UTI follows swimming in heavily chlorinated water then local vaseline, zinc paste or barrier cream may protect the labia from irritation. Antiseptics or surface-tension lowering agents such as bubble-bath are best avoided when bathing.

Low dosage antibacterial prophylaxis

Purpose

Low dosage antibacterial prophylaxis is prescribed to prevent reinfection of the urinary tract, which is likely to remain susceptible even after the presenting infection has been eradicated. It is not intended to suppress partially treated bacteriuria. It is important that this is explained to the parent and to the child who is old enough to understand, otherwise there is a tendency for treatment to be stopped as soon as the symptoms disappear (Normand and Smellie, 1965).

Drugs

The ideal antibacterial drug for prophylactic use is effective against most urinary pathogens, well tolerated, free from side effects, absorbed high in the alimentary tract so that any effect on the lower bowel flora is minimized, excreted in a high concentration in the urine and of low cost. Co-trimoxazole, nitrofurantoin and trimethoprim are the drugs that at present most nearly fulfil these criteria. Short-acting sulphonamides are effective in outpatient practice but ampicillin, which promotes the emergence of a resistant bowel flora, is not a satisfactory prophylactic drug (*Table 10.5*). Prophylaxis should be given in the lowest dosage compatible with maintaining sterility of the bladder urine and over long periods the dosage can be reduced to the minimum that is effective, which is often appreciably less than that recommended. Failure of prophylaxis may result from the use of too high a dosage, thereby inducing bowel flora resistance. The practice of rotating drugs has no merit in children. Compliance can be improved by considering the timing of administration in relation to family routine and the child's preference for liquid or tablet preparations. The use of tablets should always be encouraged and dental care emphasized if elixirs are chosen.

Monitoring

Regular urine cultures should be made and the authors do this at 2 weeks, 1 month, 2 months and 3 months, and then 3-monthly, both during and for 1 year after low dosage prophylaxis. We do not discontinue prophylactic antibacterials for this purpose since 48 hours is quite long enough for reinfection to occur, negating the purpose of prophylaxis which is to maintain the urinary tract sterile so long as the bladder defences are impaired. A further urine culture is necessary if *any* growth is obtained or there is significant pyuria.

Efficacy

Low dosage prophylaxis is very effective in preventing recurrence of UTI when appropriate drugs and dosages are used. Reinfection *during* prophylaxis with co-trimoxazole combined with other measures already described was reduced to the order of one recurrence per 22 patient years in a group of infected children with or without VUR who had no outflow obstruction (Smellie *et al.*, 1976). Moreover, in the radiologically normal urinary tract there was a significant reduction in the reinfection rate *after* a period of prophylaxis (Smellie, Katz and Grüneberg, 1978). A possible explanation for this is that during the infection-free period afforded by prophylaxis bladder mucosal inflammation subsides and voiding and bowel habits can be corrected (the latter often requiring several months). Recurrences following a period of prophylaxis are more often symptomless than those after only a short course of treatment.

Duration

Reinfection is most likely to occur in the first 6 months after a symptomatic infection, with a progressively decreasing risk subsequently. In children without VUR or renal scarring the authors usually recommend prophylaxis for 6–12 months depending upon their previous history. If there is VUR, prophylaxis is continued for as long as this persists when there is no renal scarring and until the kidneys are fully grown when there is.

Side effects

No significant side effects have been reported in children maintained for long periods on the low dosages recommended of nitrofurantoin, co-trimoxazole or short-acting sulphonamides. Annual blood and platelet counts are usually carried out during long-term use of these drugs.

Recurrences after prophylaxis

These represent not a failure of antibiotic treatment but a failure to remedy the underlying cause of urinary tract susceptibility. They are often quite symptomless and provided that VUR or obstruction does not occur there is no immediate indication for antibacterial treatment. Follow-up should continue, with checking of bowel and voiding habits. If the recurrence is accompanied by symptoms then a short course of chemotherapy is required. A two-film IVU may be indicated after more than one symptomatic recurrence.

In the small group of children with normal X-rays who remain free from infection during prophylaxis but repeatedly have a symptomatic recurrence after it is stopped, the standard prophylactic dosage can be reduced every 3 months. Even a weekly dose of co-trimoxazole may be effective in preventing these recurrences.

Follow-up control

Bacteriology

Urine cultures should be continued until there has been a complete year of freedom from infection without antibacterial treatment. Dip slides, which can be posted, have proved a convenient method of ensuring regular bacteriological follow-up if the patient lives at a distance from the laboratory. Their use can be of considerable diagnostic value during febrile episodes in children liable to suffer from recurrent UTI.

Radiology

Normal renal growth assessed by the measurement of renal length on serial two-film IVUs and related to the child's growth in height (or if this is unavailable to the increase in vertebral lengths) provides a sensitive indication of normal renal development (Hodson, 1968; Eklöf and Ringertz, 1976). Observations of renal substance thickness, calyceal changes and renal outline can also identify early scarring.

Serial measurements are made in children with VUR or renal scarring, usually after 1 year in infancy and at intervals of 2–3 years thereafter or 6 months after a severe symptomatic presenting infection. A one-film IVU may be repeated if there are recurrent symptomatic infections and is essential following surgical procedures involving the vesicoureteric junction, including ureteric reimplantation, generally after an interval of 2 or 3 months.

While normal renal growth and function are the primary objectives in the management of children with UTI who have VUR, the progress of reflux can be monitored clinically in the older child by the presence and the volume of residual urine on a second micturition. When there is no appreciable residue then cystography can be repeated. Radionuclide and ultrasound techniques are likely to be used increasingly in follow-up (*see* Chapters 2 and 15).

If possible, both hospital admission and general anaesthesia should be avoided. All follow-ups should be arranged with minimal disruption of home and school life.

Further management in specific groups of children

Vesicoureteric reflux and renal scarring

If there is no lower tract obstruction or stone formation the only children with UTI likely to have or develop renal scarring or impaired renal growth are those with VUR.

Prevention of scarring

Renal scarring is usually already present when a child with UTI is first investigated and there are not many well documented reports of new scars developing in normal kidneys. It is now becoming clear that the majority of fresh scars originate when infected urine refluxes up to a kidney in which there are probably compound papillae allowing intrarenal reflux to occur, although this may not always be seen radiologically. Extensive scarring mostly develops in the early years of life (*Table 10.6*; Rolleston, Maling and Hodson, 1974; Smellie *et al.*, 1975). Scarring may be prevented or at least postponed by rapid recognition and immediately effective treatment of the first infection occurring in a child with

VUR. This should be followed by low dosage prophylaxis.

Urinary tract infection with vesicoureteric reflux

The indications for surgical correction of VUR are considered in Chapter 15. In the majority of children with UTI found to have VUR surgical intervention is unnecessary since reflux into ureters without marked dilatation stops spontaneously in time in over 80 per cent and renal growth proceeds normally if the urinary tract is kept free from infection (Edwards *et al.*, 1977). (A later recommendation of surgery may be made on social grounds for noncompliance.) Until the results of controlled trials of the long-term effect of treatment on renal growth are available the management of the child with UTI and more severe VUR requires individual consideration. Most reports of renal growth following surgical correction of VUR have failed to dissociate any possible mechanical benefits of stopping reflux from those of confining infection to the bladder.

The alternative to surgery is not simply to do nothing but involves a strictly supervised medical regimen to prevent further infection as already outlined with attention to compliance, regular urine culture and follow-up of renal growth. The authors continue low dosage prophylaxis in children with UTI who have VUR and unscarred kidneys until the reflux stops or the kidneys are fully grown (Smellie *et al.*, 1981). Short courses of treatment for recurrences of infection are not advisable because of the increased risk of renal scarring (Lenaghan *et al.*, 1976).

Infection with vesicoureteric reflux and renal scarring

If scarring is present, the authors continue prophylaxis until renal growth is complete in the mid to late teens (Smellie, 1979). It seems likely, as Ransley and Risdon (1978) suggest, that contraction of established renal scars may deform adjacent papillae rendering their collecting-duct orifices incompetent and making intrarenal reflux possible with a risk of further scarring, so that vigilance in preventing further infection is imperative. When renal function is impaired, antibacterial dosage may need mod-

ification and nephrotoxic drugs should be avoided. Regular blood pressure checks are important for the early detection of hypertension.

The progress of these children can be gauged by renal growth and function together with the development and extension of renal scarring, and if this is already present then by the blood pressure. Whether reflux continues or not is essentially a secondary issue.

Recurrent infection following surgery

Provided that there is no renal scarring or obstruction at the ureterovesical junction on a postoperative IVU, children with UTI following ureteric reimplantation should be treated as if they had normal urinary tracts. In the case of residual obstructive renal damage persisting after surgical relief of obstruction or removal of stones, continued follow-up with urine culture and renal functional assessment is advisable.

Symptomless bacteriuria

If there is no VUR, obstruction or renal scarring then there is no indication for treatment of symptomless bacteriuria but follow-up urine cultures should be made. All bacteriuria should be treated or prevented if VUR or renal scarring is present.

Prognosis

The long-term consequence of childhood UTI can be assessed in terms of renal growth and function, recurrent bacteriuria, hypertension, and the child's general health, growth and well-being.

Bacteriuria

In the majority of affected children UTI is a recurring problem and the outcome of treatment depends upon identifying and correcting the cause of the increased susceptibility of the urinary tract to infection. Provided that there is no obstruction to urine flow, recurrences can be almost completely prevented by long-term low dosage prophylaxis and such further infections as do occur can usually be traced to failure to comply with the antibacterial regimen.

The renal prognosis is excellent in all children who have a normal IVU and no VUR or obstruction, even if there is recurrent symptomatic or symptomless infection. This includes those in whom VUR has stopped spontaneously or on successful ureteric reimplantation and those with duplex or other renal anomalies but otherwise normal urinary tracts. In these circumstances parents and others caring for the child can be confidently reassured. A significantly higher incidence of recurrent infection is found in young adult women who had bacteriuria at school, although renal insufficiency does not develop (Gillenwater, Harrison and Kunin, 1979).

Infection with vesicoureteric reflux

The presence of VUR alters the situation. However, with long-term prophylactic regimens VUR stops spontaneously in time in over 80 per cent of children with undilated refluxing ureters and in 40 per cent of those with dilated ones, even if these drain scarred kidneys. Renal growth is also normal in over 90 per cent of children in whom recurrent infection is prevented even during continued VUR (Smellie, 1967; Edwards *et al.*, 1977).

Schoolgirls over 5 years old with covert bacteriuria and radiologically normal kidneys are unlikely to develop renal scarring notwithstanding the presence of continuing bacteriuria and despite the persistence of mild to moderate

VUR, although fresh scars may appear in previously scarred kidneys exposed to infection through refluxing ureters (Claësson and Lindberg, 1977; Cardiff-Oxford Bacteriuria Study Group, 1978). Symptomatic infection when VUR is present can be followed by fresh scarring of the previously normal kidney up to the age of 10 or 12, while extensive focal scarring has usually occurred by the age of 5 (*Table 10.6*). The incidence of such late scarring in children presenting with symptomatic UTI and having VUR who are maintained on continuous prophylactic regimens is less than 2 per cent (Normand and Smellie, 1979). Persistence of VUR in a greater proportion of ureters and a higher risk of fresh renal damage have been reported in children who received intermittent short courses of treatment for recurring infections rather than continuous prophylaxis against them (Lenaghan *et al.*, 1976).

Infection with renal scarring

In children with small irregularly scarred kidneys drained by dilated ureters the prognosis is least good: infection is most likely to recur, renal growth is most likely to be slow, VUR is least likely to stop, and hypertension is most likely to be a hazard. It is not yet known how much, if any, of such severe scarring is superimposed on congenital dysplastic elements or how much is acquired and potentially preventable. The long-term influence on renal growth and scarring which the surgical correction of VUR may have, compared with the prevention of infection until reflux stops naturally, should be elucidated by the results of controlled trials currently in progress.

Table 10.6   Fresh scars developing in previously normal kidneys (data from Smellie and Normand, 1979)

Reference	Number of children with normal kidneys developing fresh scars	Vesico-ureteric reflux	Infection	Age of scarring
Penn and Breidahl (1967)	9	9	9	2–8 years
Smellie and Normand (1968, 1975)	10	10	10	3 months–10 years
Bergström *et al.* (1972)	3		3	0–6 months
Rolleston, Maling and Hodson (1974)	3	3		10 days–3 years
Filly *et al.* (1974)	4	4	4	Under 10 years
Randolph, Morris and Gould (1975)	3	3	3	6 months–3½ years
Lenaghan *et al.* (1976)	24	24	24	
Shah, Robins and White (1978)	5	5	5	2–9 years
Heale and Ferguson (1979)	44	44	44	4–10 years

Provided that renal function is normal and blood pressure is normal or controlled when the child with renal scarring is first seen there is no deterioration in renal function as long as further symptomatic infections are prevented. It is becoming clear, however, that at least 10 per cent of children with focal renal scarring develop significant hypertension if observed for a sufficient length of time, independent of whether VUR has been corrected or not (Wallace, Rothwell and Williams, 1978; Smellie and Normand, 1979). Uncontrolled hypertension may cause further renal deterioration (Holland, 1979) and it may well be that the early onset of hypertension or a liability to pre-eclamptic toxaemia will emerge as the most common and important consequence of childhood UTI with renal scarring.

Screening

Screening for bacteriuria has been carried out in children to establish the prevalence of unrecognized bacteriuria. Because of the association of bacteriuria with renal scarring, screening programmes have also been undertaken in the hope that early identification of a precursor of renal damage might offer an opportunity for its prevention or limitation.

In schoolchildren the feasibility of such screening programmes has been established, particularly using dip slides, and prevalences of 0.04 per cent in boys and a consistent 1–2 per cent in girls have been found. A single screening is insufficient and when repeated annually the increment has brought the incidence in girls during their school years to about 5 per cent. Due to the low rate of symptomless bacteriuria in schoolboys most of the surveys carried out in schoolchildren have been confined to girls. They have shown that symptoms occur in many children found to have bacteriuria on screening, although these are not sufficiently troublesome to cause them to consult a doctor, and so the term covert bacteriuria has replaced that of true asymptomatic bacteriuria. If untreated, the bacteriuria may be intermittent and may disappear spontaneously, while antibacterial treatment may be followed by symptomatic infection. It has been suggested that chemotherapy may disturb a symbiotic host-parasite relationship since certain differences have been noted in the organisms causing covert bacteriuria. A wider range of bacterial strains of which more are rough and untypable and less are closely correlated with bowel flora, with less bacterial adhesion, is found in those with covert bacteriuria.

However, the incidence of abnormalities and urinary tract defects is similar to that found in symptomatic infection (*Table 10.2*). By the age of 5, 12–20 per cent of girls with covert bacteriuria have acquired renal scars which is a similar proportion to those with symptomatic UTI. Some of these patients have a past history of symptomatic infection (Savage *et al.*, 1969) virtually always associated with VUR, and so it seems that screening on school entry is too late to have a significant impact on the prevention of fresh scarring. In the Cardiff-Oxford study untreated girls with bacteriuria and normal kidneys did not develop fresh scars during 4 years observation. New scars did develop, though, in 27 per cent of girls with initially scarred kidneys; all had VUR and were exposed to recurrent or persistent bacteriuria.

In order to prevent scarring developing in normal kidneys bacteriuria must clearly be identified before the age of 5 and some preliminary studies have been carried out in preschool children. It is much more difficult and expensive to effect comprehensive screening in this age group and to be of value such screening must be repeated. Bacteriuria confirmed by suprapubic aspiration was found in 1 per cent of newborn babies on screening (Abbott, 1972). This was symptomless in the majority and in many it was self-limiting. There was no renal abnormality on the IVU, but eight of 14 infants with bacteriuria had VUR.

The alternative approaches for the early detection of significant bacteriuria are ongoing screening programmes in general practice with urine culture in any sick infant on presentation, and routine screening of all infants at intervals of 6–12 months. The cost-effectiveness of such schemes has not yet been established and in the meantime a higher index of suspicion in the primary care physician is essential if early diagnosis of UTI is to be made (Mond, Grüneberg and Smellie, 1970).

Conclusion

UTIs are common in childhood but seldom have serious immediate or long-term consequences. In the majority of children the kidneys are normal on presentation and if there is no obstruction to flow and no VUR they remain so. In these children recurrent symptomatic infections can largely be prevented without too much investigation or parental anxiety.

The vulnerable few in whom hypertension or renal failure may ensue are those with the secondary effects of obstruction or stone and those in whom there is potential renal damage when the refluxing urinary tract becomes infected.

References

Abbott, G.D. (1972) Neonatal bacteriuria: a prospective study in 1,460 infants. *British Medical Journal*, i, 267

Allen, T.D. (1977) The non-neurogenic neurogenic bladder. *Journal of Urology*, **117**, 232

Asscher, A.W., McLachlan, M.S.F., Verrier Jones, E.R., Meller, S.T., Sussman, M., Harrison, S., Johnston, H.H., Sleight, G. and Fletcher, E.W. (1973) Screening for asymptomatic urinary tract infection in schoolgirls, *Lancet*, ii, 1

Atwell, J.D., Cook, P.L., Strong, L. and Hyde, I. (1977) The interrelationship between vesico-ureteric reflux, trigonal abnormalities and a bifid pelvicalyceal system: a family study. *British Journal of Urology*, **49**, 97

Bergström, T., Larson, H., Lincoln, K. and Winberg, J. (1972) Studies of urinary infection in infancy and childhood. 1280 patients with neonatal infection. *Journal of Pediatrics*, **80**, 858

Cardiff-Oxford Bacteriuria Study Group (1978) Sequelae of covert bacteriuria in schoolgirls. *Lancet*, i, 889

Claësson, I. and Lindberg, U. (1977) Asymptomatic bacteriuria in schoolgirls, a follow-up study of the urinary tract in treated and untreated asymptomatic bacteriuria. *Radiology*, **124**, 179

Cohen, M. (1972) Urinary tract infections in children: females aged 2 through 14, first two infections. *Pediatrics*, **50**, 271

Drew, J.H. and Acton, C.M. (1976) Radiological findings in newborn infants with urinary infection. *Archives of Disease in Childhood*, **51**, 628

Edwards, B., White, R.H.R., Maxted, H., Deverill, I. and White, P.A. (1975) Screening methods for covert bacteriuria in schoolgirls. *British Medical Journal*, i, 463

Edwards, D., Normand, I.C.S., Prescod, N. and Smellie, J.M. (1977) Disappearance of vesicoureteric reflux during long-term prophylaxis of urinary tract infection in children. *British Medical Journal*, ii, 285

Eklöf, O. and Ringertz, H. (1976) Kidney size in children, a method of assessment. *Acta Radiologica*, **17**, 617

Filly, R., Friedland, G.W., Govan, D.E. and Fair, W.R. (1974) Development and progression of clubbing and scarring in children with recurrent urinary tract infections. *Radiology*, **113**, 145

Friedland, G.W. (1979) Post-reimplantation renal scarring. *In* Reflux Nephropathy (edited by Hodson, J. and Kincaid-Smith, P.). Masson, New York. p.323

Gillenwater, J.Y., Harrison, R.B. and Kunin, C.M. (1979) The natural history of bacteriuria in schoolgirls. *New England Journal of Medicine*, **301**, 396

Govan, D.E., Fair, W.R., Friedland, G.W. and Filly, R.A. (1975) Management of children with urinary tract infections: the Stanford experience. *Urology*, **6**, 273

Hanson, L.A. (1973) Host-parasite relationship in urinary tract infections. *Journal of Infectious Diseases*, **127**, 726

Heale, W.F. and Ferguson, R.S. (1979) The pathogenesis of renal scarring in children. *In* Infections of the Urinary Tract (edited by Kass, E.H. and Brumfitt, W.). University of Chicago Press. p.101

Hinman, F. and Cox, C.E. (1967) Residual urine volume in normal male subjects. *Journal of Urology*, **97**, 641

Hodson, C.J. (1968) Radiological diagnosis of renal involvement. *In* Urinary Tract Infection (edited by O'Grady, F. and Brumfitt, W.). Oxford University Press, London. p.108

Holland, N.H. (1979) Reflux nephropathy and hypertension. *In* Reflux Nephropathy (edited by Hodson, J. and Kincaid Smith, P.). Masson, New York. p.257

Kunin, C.M., Deutscher, R. and Paquin, A. (1964) Urinary infection in schoolchildren: an epidemiological, clinical and laboratory study. *Medicine (Baltimore)*, **43**, 91

Lenaghan, D., Whitaker, J.G., Jensen, F. and Stephens, F.D. (1976) The natural history of reflux and long term effects of reflux on the kidney. *Journal of Urology*, **115**, 728

Lindberg, U., Bjure, J., Haugstbedt, S. and Jodal, U. (1975) Asymptomatic bacteriuria in schoolgirls: relation between residual urine volume and recurrence. *Acta Paediatrica Scandinavica*, **64**, 437

MacGregor, M.E. and Wynne Williams, C.J.E. (1966) Relation of residual urine to persistent urinary infection in childhood. *Lancet*, i, 893

Maskell, R., Pead, L. and Allen, J. (1979) The puzzle of "urethral syndrome": a possible answer? *Lancet*, i, 1058

Mond, N.C., Grüneberg, R.N. and Smellie, J.M. (1970) Study of childhood urinary tract infection in general practice. *British Medical Journal*, i, 602

Neumann, P.Z., de Domenico, I.J. and Nogrady, M.B. (1973) Constipation and urinary tract infection. *Pediatrics*, **52**, 241

Newcastle Asymptomatic Bacteriuria Research Group (1975) Asymptomatic bacteriuria in schoolchildren in Newcastle-upon-Tyne. *Archives of Disease in Childhood*, **50**, 90

Normand, I.C.S. and Smellie, J.M. (1965) Prolonged maintenance chemotherapy in the management of urinary infection in childhood. *British Medical Journal*, i, 1023

Normand, I.C.S. and Smellie, J.M. (1979) Vesicoureteric reflux: the case for conservative management. *In* Reflux Nephropathy (edited by Hodson, J. and Kincaid Smith, P.). Masson, New York. p.281

O'Grady, F. and Cattell, W.R. (1966) Kinetics of urinary tract infection, I and II. *British Journal of Urology*, **38**, 149, 156

Orikasa, S. and Hinman, F. (1977) Reaction of the vesical wall to bacterial penetration. *Investigative Urology*, **15**, 185

Penn, I.A. and Breidahl, P.D. (1967) Ureteric reflux and renal damage. *Australia and New Zealand Journal of Surgery*, **37**, 163

Randolph, M.F., Morris, K.E. and Gould, E.B. (1975) The first urinary tract infection in the female infant. *Journal of Pediatrics*, **86**, 342

Ransley, P.G. and Risdon, R.A. (1978) Reflux and renal scarring. *British Journal of Radiology*, Suppl. p.14

Rolleston, G.L., Maling, T.M.J. and Hodson, C.J. (1974) Intrarenal reflux and the scarred kidney. *Archives of Disease in Childhood*, **49**, 531

Savage, D.C.L., Wilson, M.I., Ross, E.M. and Fee, W.M. (1969) Asymptomatic bacteriuria in girl entrants to Dundee Primary Schools. *British Medical Journal*, iii, 75

Savage, D.C.L., Wilson, M.I., McHardy, M., Dewar, D.A.E. and Fee, W.M. (1973) Covert bacteriuria of childhood. *Archives of Disease in Childhood*, **48**, 8

Shah, K.J., Robins, D.G. and White, R.H.R. (1978) Renal scarring and vesico-ureteric reflux. *Archives of Disease in Childhood*, **53**, 210

Shand, D.G., Nimmon, C.C., O'Grady, F. and Cattell, W.R. (1970) Relation between residual urine volume and response to treatment of urinary infection. *Lancet*, i, 1305

Shannon, F.T. (1972) Urinary tract infection in infancy. *New Zealand Medical Journal*, **75**, 282

Smellie, J.M. (1967) Medical aspects of urinary infection in children. *Journal of the Royal College of Physicians of London*, **1**, 189

Smellie, J.M. (1979) Management of urinary tract infection. *In* Paediatric Therapeutics (edited by Valman, H.B.). Blackwell, Oxford. p.60

Smellie, J.M. and Normand, I.C.S. (1968) Experience of follow-up of children with urinary tract infection. *In* Urinary Tract Infection, (edited by O'Grady, F.B. and Brumfitt, W.). Oxford University Press, London. p.123

Smellie, J.M. and Normand, I.C.S. (1975) Bacteriuria, reflux and renal scarring. *Archives of Disease in Childhood*, **50**, 581

Smellie, J.M. and Normand, I.C.S. (1979) Reflux nephropathy in childhood. *In* Reflux Nephropathy (edited by Hodson, J. and Kincaid Smith, P.). Masson, New York. p.14

Smellie, J.M., Hodson, C.J., Edwards, D. and Normand, I.C.S. (1964) Clinical and radiological features of urinary infection in childhood. *British Medical Journal*, ii, 1222

Smellie, J.M., Edwards, D., Hunter, N., Normand, I.C.S. and Prescod, N. (1975) Vesico-ureteric reflux and renal scarring. *Kidney International*, **8**, S65

Smellie, J.M., Grüneberg, R.N., Leakey, A. and Atkin, W.S. (1976) Long-term low-dose co-trimoxazole in prophylaxis of childhood urinary tract infection: clinical aspects. *British Medical Journal*, ii, 203

Smellie, J.M., Katz, G. and Grüneberg, R.N. (1978) Controlled trial of prophylactic treatment in childhood urinary tract infection. *Lancet*, ii, 175

Smellie, J.M., Normand, I.C.S. and Katz, G. (1981) A comparison of children with urinary tract infection with and without vesico-ureteric reflux. *Kidney International*, **20**

Smellie, J.M., Edwards, D., Normand, I.C.S. and Prescod, N. (1981) Effect of vesico-ureteric reflux on renal growth in children with urinary tract infection. *Archives of Disease in Childhood*, **56**, 593

Stansfeld, J.M. (1966) Clinical observations relating to incidence and aetiology of urinary tract infections in children. *British Medical Journal*, i, 631

Vermillion, C.D. and Heale, W.F. (1973) Position and configuration of the ureteral orifice and its relationship to renal scarring in adults. *Journal of Urology*, **109**, 579

Wallace, D.M.A., Rothwell, D.L. and Williams, D.I. (1978) The long-term follow-up of surgically treated vesicoureteric reflux. *British Journal of Urology*, **50**, 479

Wein, J. and Schöenberg, H.W. (1972) A review of 402 girls with recurrent urinary tract infection. *Journal of Urology*, **107**, 329

Winberg, J., Andersen, H.J., Bergström, T., Jacobsson, B., Larson, H. and Lincoln, K. (1974) Epidemiology of symptomatic urinary tract infection in childhood. *Acta Paediatrica Scandinavica*, Suppl. 252

11 Urinary Tract Infection: Localized Inflammatory Lesions

J.H. Johnston

Renal infections

Renal carbuncle

Formerly the majority of renal abscesses in children were the result of haematogenous inoculation of the parenchyma by staphylococci secondary to furunculosis or other lesions. In recent years, possibly due to more liberal use of effective antibiotics for cutaneous staphylococcal infections, the picture has changed. Most renal abscesses are now caused by Gram-negative organisms, especially *Escherichia coli*, and in the majority of instances they are not a consequence of bacteraemia. Staphylococcal abscesses are most commonly single and well circumscribed. With abscesses caused by coliform organisms the lesion has more resemblance to a segmental pyelonephritis (Costas, Rippey and van Blerk, 1972) and there are often less obvious inflammatory changes elsewhere in the kidney. Vesicoureteric reflux is a common association (Timmons and Perlmutter, 1976), suggesting that the renal condition is the result of ascending infection. Infrequently the abscess ruptures into the perinephric tissues.

The child presents with loin pain and fever. Flank tenderness may be present or an enlarged kidney may be palpable. Although there are often no pre-existing symptoms of urinary tract infection, significant coliform bacilluria is common. On intravenous urography the kidney is relatively immobile on respiration because of perinephritis; there is a bulge on the renal outline and an intrarenal space-occupying lesion which may be suggestive of a neoplasm (*Figure 11.1*). Arteriography may on occasions be unhelpful in distinguishing between a chronic abscess and a tumour since new vessels develop in the infective granulation tissue and dilate in response to injected adrenalin as does the neovasculature in a malignant lesion (Shenoy, Culver and Arani, 1977). Ultrasound may reveal a sonolucent mass or there may be internal echoes due to loculation of pus. The localization of administered ^{67}Ga-citrate in the inflammatory lesion can be detected by gamma-camera or rectilinear scanning.

During the acute phase a renal abscess, whether of staphylococcal or coliform causation, often resolves with intensive chemotherapy. Needle aspiration or drainage may be needed for an intrarenal or perirenal collection of pus but nephrectomy should rarely be required.

Xanthogranulomatous pyelonephritis

In this condition cholesterol-containing material is found within an inflammatory lesion in the kidney parenchyma. A yellow crystalline or amorphous substance is visible macroscopically. Histologically there are sheets of foam cells in inflammatory and fibrous tissue. In children the disorder is most commonly seen in cases of pyonephrosis secondary to infection calculi and Proteus bacilluria, but it may occur as a consequence of infection superimposed on a pelviureteric obstruction (Abbate and Meyers,

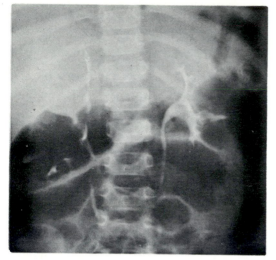

(a)

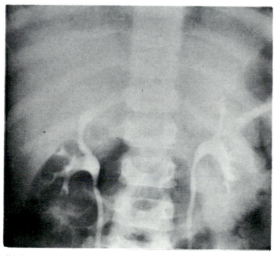

(b)

Figure 11.1. Renal carbuncle. (*a*) Intravenous urogram in a boy with a right renal swelling of gradual onset, low fever only, and sterile urine. There is a large mass in the upper pole of the right kidney with ill defined renal margins At exploration a large abscess was drained and the pus grew only anaerobic streptococci on culture. (*b*) Intravenous urogram 3 months later showing complete recovery.

1976). Urinary cytology may reveal foam cells in the sediment. Infrequently xanthogranulomatous pyelonephritis occurs without pre-existing urinary tract pathology (Ceccarelli, Wurster and Chandor, 1970) when it may simulate a neoplasm on intravenous urography. Treatment depends on the local pathology. As a rule the affected kidney parenchyma is incapable of recovering useful function and nephrectomy,

heminephrectomy or partial nephrectomy is generally needed.

Cystitis

Acute cystitis due to bacterial infection is a common occurrence in girls, causing symptoms of frequency and urgency of micturition, wetting and stinging on voiding. Constitutional symptoms and fever are rare in the absence of ascending infection resulting from vesicoureteric reflux. Since endoscopy is rarely performed during the acute attack the mucosal appearances can only be surmised. The condition responds rapidly to the appropriate antimicrobial therapy although recurrence or persistent asymptomatic bacilluria is a common sequel.

A variety of specific and nonspecific forms of acute and chronic cystitis have been described, sometimes with adjectival appellations owing more to the pictorial imagination of endoscopists than to a precise evaluation of the pathology involved.

Acute haemorrhagic cystitis

Haematuria can occur with severe degrees of acute bacterial cystitis caused by coliform and other organisms. In the absence of bacilluria viral infections have been incriminated. Adenovirus type 11 was reported by Mufson and Belshe (1976) to be causative of haemorrhagic cystitis in 51 per cent of cases in Japan and 23 per cent in Chicago. The condition is commoner in males. Rapid resolution is usual while recurrence is possible.

Eosinophilic cystitis

This rare form of cystitis can affect all ages and Kessler, Clark and Kaplan (1975) described a case in a 5-day-old infant. In children in the USA it is commoner in blacks than in caucasians. The symptomatology is that of severe bacterial cystitis and there is often haematuria, but although pyuria is present the urine is sterile. Urography frequently shows some degree of upper tract dilatation and there may be filling defects on the cystogram. Cystoscopy reveals raised yellow-red lesions 5–10 mm across, especially in the bladder dome. Histology of the mucosal elevations shows vascular engorgement, oedema, and eosinophilic and plasma-cell infiltration of the submucosa. The condition often lasts for weeks or months but there is a tendency for spontaneous improvement and ultimately complete resolution.

The aetiology is uncertain. An allergic mechanism is suggested by the occasional occurrence of eosinophilia. Perlmutter, Edlow and Kevy (1968) found an increased antibody titre to *Toxocara cani*, a parasite found in dogs and cats, and suggested that infestation by this organism may be responsible. Antihistamines and steroids have been employed for treatment, frequently without leading to any obvious hastening of symptomatic or pathological regression. It remains doubtful whether eosinophilic cystitis should be regarded as a disease entity since infiltration by eosinophils is found in a variety of infective and neoplastic bladder lesions.

Proliferative cystitis

With this condition, often loosely termed cystitis cystica, multiple solid or cystic nodules 2–3 mm in diameter are seen on the mucosa especially over the trigone and the posterior and lateral bladder walls. Histologically a variety of proliferative pathological changes may be found. There may be small epithelial-lined cysts (cystitis cystica), solid submucosal nests of epithelial cells (Von Brunn's nests), accumulations of mucus-secreting glands (cystitis glandularis) or, most commonly, lymphoid follicles (cystitis follicularis). Rarely the mucosal swellings are so pronounced that they produce filling defects on cystography and the radiological and endoscopic appearances may then simulate sarcoma botryoides (Varsano *et al.*, 1975). In the majority of cases in which proliferative cystitis is seen urinary tract infection exists and the mucosal changes, although ultimately reversible, generally indicate that chronic bacilluria is to be expected (Kaplan and King, 1970).

With cystitis follicularis Uehling and King (1973) found increased excretion of immunoglobulin A, suggesting that immunological factors may be involved. However, the exact relationship between proliferative cystitis and infection is uncertain. Sarma (1970) found cystitis

follicularis to be present commonly in patients with vesical carcinoma in the absence of bacilluria. The prognostic significance of cystitis glandularis as regards a predisposition to malignancy also remains undecided. Edwards, Hurm and Jaeschke (1972) described an adenocarcinoma developing in a patient with cystitis glandularis but Andersen and Hensen (1972) found that proliferative mucosal changes of all forms, often involving the renal pelvis and the urethra as well as the bladder, were present at each of 15 routine autopsies in adults.

Interstitial cystitis

Interstitial cystitis, which is characterized by a low capacity and ultimately fibrotic and contracted bladder that causes intolerable frequency of micturition, is mainly a disease of adult women. The pathogenesis is obscure. An auto-immune reaction has been suggested (Silk, 1970) as have psychogenic factors since the patients are often of a highly emotional nature. The mucosal ulceration described by Hunner (1914) is largely artefactual, resulting from distension of the contracted mucosa and submucosa during endoscopy. When the severity of the symptoms exceeds that of the demonstrable pathological changes the diagnosis of interstitial cystitis is often more a matter of opinion than of fact.

The author has never seen the condition in a child but Geist and Antolak (1970) claimed to have encountered 21 childhood cases presenting between the ages of 3–16 years which responded to treatment with hydrostatic bladder distension. Nevertheless, the symptomatology in their patients appeared to be no different from that of ordinary enuresis with daytime symptoms due to an uninhibited immature bladder. Farkas, Waisman and Goodwin (1977) described two cases of interstitial cystitis in adolescent girls with large bladder ulcer and fibrous replacement of the detrusor. They recommended that if conservative therapy with steroids and hydrostatic distension is ineffective then surgical excision of the diseased portion of the bladder and vesical enlargement by ileocystoplasty should be performed. However, the disease may subsequently extend to involve the ileal segment.

Nephrogenic adenoma

This rare form of metaplasia of the bladder mucosa is caused by nonspecific bacterial infection following the use of an indwelling catheter. It is most often seen in young males and Kalloor and Shaw (1973) described a case in a 16-year-old boy. Haematuria and dysuria occur, often some time after the removal of the catheter. Cystoscopy reveals raised red papillomatous lesions suggestive of a bladder tumour. Histology of the lesion demonstrates glandular spaces resembling renal tubules. The condition does not tend to regress spontaneously and diathermy fulguration of the papillary elevations is indicated. Malignant degeneration has been recorded (Molland *et al.*, 1976).

Phosphate-encrusted cystitis

Cystitis with phosphatic mucosal encrustations occurs mainly in elderly men but the author has encountered the condition in a 10-year-old boy with a urethral stricture. Residual bladder urine is infected by urea-splitting organisms such as Proteus or Pseudomonas which leads to alkalinization of the urine and calcium phosphate deposition on areas of mucosal ulceration or necrosis. Treatment requires relief of urinary obstruction and restoration of complete bladder emptying. Elimination of infection by chemotherapy, acidification of the urine by oral ammonium chloride and repeated bladder irrigation with 0.5 per cent acetic acid encourage the dissolution of phosphatic accumulations and prevent further encrustation. Detachment of adherent plaques by endoscopic manipulation may be necessary.

Malakoplakia

Malakoplakia occurs mainly in cases of urinary tract infection affecting adults, although it has been reported during childhood (Morrison, 1944). Flat brown-yellow plaques are found on the mucosal surface of the bladder and possibly elsewhere in the urinary tract in addition. The plaques contain small calcified spheres, that is Michaelis-Gutmann bodies. McClurg *et al.* (1973) showed by electron microscopy that intracellular bacteria exist in the mucosa. The condition is due to a deficiency in the mononuclear cells in the lesions of cyclic 3', 5' guanosine monophosphate. As a result the cells are unable to release lysosomal enzymes which impairs their ability to digest phagocytosed bacteria. Zornow *et al.* (1979) treated three cases successfully by the control of infection and the administration of bethanechol chloride to enhance bladder tone and emptying.

Chemical cystitis

A variety of chemical agents arriving at the bladder by introduction into the lumen, by excretion in the urine or in the blood stream may damage the vesical wall and produce differing degrees of pathological change.

Cyclophosphamide cystitis

Haemorrhagic cystitis in patients receiving cyclophosphamide occurs as a result of mucosal irritation by drug metabolites excreted in the urine. The onset of symptoms may be delayed for several weeks after the last dose of the drug has been given, especially if oral treatment has been employed: following intravenous therapy the sequence of events is more rapid. Symptoms of frequency and urgency precede the development of severe haematuria. Cystoscopy reveals vascular engorgement, oedema, telangiectases and mucosal haemorrhages and ulceration. In severe cases sloughing of the mucosa may occur and is followed by fibrous replacement of the musculature, mural calcification and bladder contracture. Carcinoma has occurred as a late complication in adults and fibrosarcoma of the bladder has been reported in a 12-year-old boy who had had 7 years of cyclophosphamide treatment for Hodgkin's disease (Rupprecht and Blessing, 1973).

Prevention of cystitis in patients receiving cyclophosphamide may be achieved by ensuring a high urine output to dilute the metabolites and by frequent voiding to shorten their contact time with the bladder mucosa. Bladder irrigation with 20 per cent acetylcysteine may be employed to neutralize the excretion products.

Treatment of the established condition often requires that the bladder is first irrigated to free it of clots. Endoscopic fulguration of bleeding points may be possible or bleeding may be controlled by hydrostatic compression employing an inflated balloon fitted to a urethral catheter. Various chemical corrosives have been applied locally in order to coagulate and destroy the damaged bladder mucosa and allow re-epithelialization of a normal mucous membrane. Silver nitrate as a 1 per cent solution may be instilled through a catheter to produce an eschar of silver chloride. However, anuria has been reported as a complication from obstruction of the ureteric orifices or from precipitation of the salt in the renal tubules if vesicoureteric reflux is present (Raghavaish and Soloway, 1977). Although intravesical 10 per cent formalin can be effective it carries the risks of bladder rupture (Scott, Marshall and Lyon, 1974) and of inducing ureteric reflux and causing fatal papillary or cortical necrosis (Kalish, Silber and Herwig, 1973) and so the ureters should be occluded by Fogarty catheters during its use (Bright *et al.*, 1977). Rao *et al.* (1978) reported a fatality resulting from systemic absorption of formaldehyde which led to acute tubular necrosis. Duckett, Peters and Donaldson (1973) advocated the use of phenol as follows. At open cystotomy 100 per cent phenol 30 ml and glycerine 30 ml are instilled into the bladder; after 1 minute the solution is washed out and replaced by absolute alcohol for a further 1 minute; finally the bladder is irrigated with saline. If local therapy fails, Pyeritz *et al.* (1978) found a continuous intravenous infusion of vasopressin to be effective.

THAM necrosis

Alkalinizing drugs such as tris-hydroxymethylaminomethane (THAM) and sodium bicarbonate have been used in the management of acidosis in the newborn. In high concentrations THAM has a direct cellular toxic effect and in hyperosmolar solution it can lead to vascular spasm and tissue destruction. Necrosis of the bladder may occur following its administration through an umbilical arterial catheter.

Ether cystitis

Lebowitz and Effmann (1978) reported two cases in which ether was injected into the inflating channel of a Foley catheter in order to rupture an obstructed balloon. Leakage of ether caused severe cystitis and in one case bladder contracture resulted which necessitated urinary diversion. The recommended method of managing a nondeflatable Foley balloon is to inject liquid paraffin along the occluded channel.

Methacillin cystitis

Methacillin, which is employed in the treatment of staphylococcal infections in infancy, may cause mucosal ulceration of the bladder and haematuria (Yow *et al.*, 1976).

Prostatitis and urethritis

Prostatic infections are rare during childhood. Staphylococcal abscess leading to retention of urine has been reported in the newborn (Mann, 1960) and was probably due to a blood-borne inoculation from umbilical sepsis. A periprostatic haematoma with secondary infection, possibly the result of rectal perforation by a thermometer, has been described as causing urinary obstruction in infancy (Williams and Martins, 1960). Chronic prostatitis with prostatic calculi is an occasional complication of neuropathic bladder with detrusor-sphincter dyssynergia in boys, particularly when the urine is infected with urea-splitting organisms (*Figure 11.2*). Micturating cystourethrography demonstrates reflux from the obstructed urethra into the prostatic ducts.

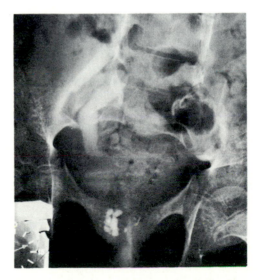

Figure 11.2. Prostatic calcification in a boy with neuropathic bladder.

Urethritis in girls may be caused by chemical irritation from the use of detergents to produce a bubble-bath. In children of either sex similar symptoms, often with urethral bleeding, may result from swimming in heavily chlorinated pools. In boys urethritis leading to pain on voiding and urethral haemorrhage is a relatively common condition in which the urine is sterile and the cystourethrogram is normal. Urethroscopy reveals inflammatory changes involving mainly the bulbar urethra (Williams and Mikhael, 1971). It is probable that the infection is of viral causation. Attacks may recur for months but urethral stricture has not occurred in the author's experience nor has it been reported in the literature. Similar symptoms of painful micturition and postvoiding bleeding in boys may be caused by a diverticular dilatation of the lacuna magna of the fossa navicularis of the glandular urethra and this lesion should be excluded by endoscopy and urethrography (Sommer and Stephens, 1980).

Condylomata acuminata are soft papillary growths that appear on moist cutaneous and mucocutaneous surfaces. The lesions, believed to be caused by a viral infection, are encountered mainly in adults but have been described in a 3-year-old boy when they involved the urethra and presented as condylomas projecting from the meatus (Copulsky, Whitehead and Orkin, 1975). Treatment requires excision and fulguration of the papillomas.

References

Abbate, A.D. and Meyers, J. (1976) Xanthogranulomatous pyelonephritis in childhood. *Journal of Urology*, **116**, 231

Andersen, J.A. and Hensen, B.F. (1972) The incidence of cell nests, cystitis cystica and cystitis glandularis in the lower urinary tract revealed by autopsies. *Journal of Urology*, **108**, 421

Bright, J.F., Tosi, S.E., Crichlow, R.W. and Selikowitz, S.M. (1977) Prevention of vesicoureteral reflux with Fogarty catheters during formalin therapy. *Journal of Urology*, **118**, 950

Ceccarelli, F.E., Wurster, J.C. and Chandor, S.B. (1970) Xanthogranulomatous pyelonephritis in an infant. *Journal of Urology*, **104**, 755

Copulsky, J., Whitehead, E.D. and Orkin, L.A. (1975) Condylomata acuminata in a three year old boy. *Urology*, **5**, 372

Costas, S., Rippey, J.J. and van Blerk, P.J.P. (1972) Segmental acute pyelonephritis. A precursor to renal carbuncle or abscess. *British Journal of Urology*, **44**, 399

Duckett, J.W., Peters, P.C. and Donaldson, M.H. (1973) Severe cyclophosphamide haemorrhagic cystitis controlled with phenol. *Journal of Pediatric Surgery*, **8**, 55

Edwards, P.D., Hurm, R.A. and Jaeschke, W.H. (1972) Conversion of cystitis glandularis to adenocarcinoma. *Journal of Urology*, **108**, 568

Farkas, A., Waisman, J. and Goodwin, W.E. (1977) Interstitial cystitis in adolescent girls. *Journal of Urology*, **118**, 837

Geist, R.W. and Antolak, S.J. (1970) Interstitial cystitis in children. *Journal of Urology*, **104**, 922

Hunner, G.L. (1914) A rare type of bladder ulcer in women. *Transactions of the Southern Surgical and Gynecological Association*, **27**, 247

Kalish, M., Silber, S.J. and Herwig, K.R. (1973) Papillary necrosis as a result of intravesical instillation of formalin. *Urology*, **2**, 315

Kalloor, G.J. and Shaw, R.E. (1973) Nephrogenic adenoma of the bladder. *British Journal of Urology*, **46**, 91

Kaplan, G.W. and King, L.R. (1970) Cystitis cystica in childhood. *Journal of Urology*, **103**, 657

Kessler, W.O., Clark, P.L. and Kaplan, G.W. (1975) Eosinophilic cystitis. *Urology*, **6**, 499

Lebowitz, R.L. and Effmann, E.L. (1978) Ether cystitis. *Urology*, **12**, 427

McClurg, F.V., D'Angostino, A.N., Marten, J.H. and Race, G.J. (1973) Ultrastructural demonstration of intracellular bacteria in 3 cases of malakoplakia of the bladder. *American Journal of Clinical Pathology*, **60**, 780

Mann, S. (1960) Prostatic abscess in the newborn. *Archives of Disease in Childhood*, **35**, 396

Molland, E.A., Trott, P.A., Pris, A.M.I. and Blandy, J.P. (1976) Nephrogenic adenoma: a form of adenomatous metaplasia of the bladder. *British Journal of Urology*, **48**, 453

Morrison, J.E. (1944) Malakoplakia of the bladder. *Journal of Pathology*, **56**, 67

Mufson, M.A. and Belshe, R.B. (1976) A review of adenoviruses in the etiology of acute haemorrhagic cystitis. *Journal of Urology*, **115**, 191

Perlmutter, A.D. Edlow, J.B. and Kevy, S.V. (1968) Toxocara antibodies in eosinophilic cystitis. *Journal of Pediatrics*, **73**, 340

Pyeritz, R.E., Droller, M.J., Bender, W.L. and Saral, R. (1978) An approach to the control of massive haemorrhage in cyclophosphamide-induced cystitis by intravenous vasopressin: a case report. *Journal of Urology*, **120**, 253

Raghavaish, N.V. and Soloway, M.S. (1977) Anuria following silver nitrate irrigation for intractable bladder haemorrhage. *Journal of Urology*, **118**, 681

Rao, M.S., Bafna, B.C., Chugh, K.S., Dutta, T.K., Singhal, P.C., Vaidyanathan, S., Bhat, V.H. and Gupta, C.L. (1978) Fatal complication of intravesical formalin during control of intractable haemorrhage from radiation cystitis. *Urology*, **11**, 588

Rupprecht, L. and Blessing, M.H. (1973) Fibrosarcoma of the bladder and seven years chemotherapy of Hodgkin's disease in childhood. *Deutsche Medizinische Wochenschrift*, **98**, 1663

Sarma, K.P. (1970) On the nature of cystitis follicularis. *Journal of Urology*, **104**, 709

Scott, M.P., Marshall, S. and Lyon, R.P. (1974) Bladder rupture following formalin therapy for haemorrhage secondary to cyclophosphamide therapy. *Urology*, **3**, 364

Shenoy, S.S., Culver, G.J. and Arani, D.T. (1977) Renal carbuncle. Simulation of tumor response to epinephrine. *Urology*, **10**, 601

Silk, M.R. (1970) Bladder antibodies in interstitial cystitis. *Journal of Urology*, **103**, 307

Sommer, J.T. and Stephens, F.D. (1980) Dorsal urethral diverticulum of the fossa navicularis: symptoms, diagnosis and treatment. *Journal of Urology*, **124**, 94

Timmons, J.W. and Perlmutter, A.D. (1976) Renal abscess: A changing concept. *Journal of Urology*, **115**, 299

Uehling, D.T. and King, L.R. (1973) Secretory immunoglobulin-A excretion in cystitis cystica. *Urology*, **1**, 305

Varsano, I., Savir, A., Grunebaum, M., Vogel, R. and Johnston, J.H. (1975) Inflammatory processes mimicking bladder tumors in children. *Journal of Pediatric Surgery*, **10**, 909

Williams, D.I. and Martins, A.G. (1960) Periprostatic haematoma and prostatic abscess in the neonatal period. *Archives of Disease in Childhood*, **35**, 177

Williams, D.I. and Mikhael, B.R. (1971) Urethritis in male children. *Proceedings of the Royal Society of Medicine*, **64**, 133

Yow, M.D., Taber, L.H., Barrett, F.F., Mintz, A.A., Blackenship, G.F., Clark, G.E. and Clark, D.I. (1976) A ten year assessment of methicillin-associated side effects. *Pediatrics*, **58**, 329

Zornow, D.H., Landes, R.R., Morganstern, S.L. and Fried, F.A. (1979) Malakoplakia of the bladder: efficacy of bethanechol chloride therapy. *Journal of Urology*, **122**, 703

12 Urinary Tract Infection: Tuberculosis and Other Specific Infections

J.H. Johnston

Tuberculosis

Genitourinary tuberculosis during childhood is now rare in most civilized countries, although examples are occasionally encountered in older children who have previously had miliary, pulmonary, glandular or osseous tuberculosis.

Pathology

Tuberculosis of the kidney is a blood-borne extension of an established tuberculous lesion elsewhere in the body. The bacilli lodge in the glomeruli and the first lesions are minute cortical tubercles. In this early phase both kidneys are affected but healing can occur in one while the condition progresses in the other. Organisms pass from the cortex through the tubules and a coalescence of tubercles forms in a renal papilla. Caseation is followed by ulceration into the related calyx (*Figure 12.1*). Several such papillary lesions may form simultaneously or consecutively. The cavities in the papillae tend to enlarge into the renal pyramids. Stenosis of the calyceal neck causes retention of caseous material which often undergoes calcification.

An open calyceal lesion leads to extension of the infection into the renal pelvis and the ureter. The primary changes are mucosal tubercles and later ulceration occurs and fibrosis of the muscular wall develops. Inflammatory strictures may form, particularly at the pelviureteric and ureterovesical junctions, and result in the formation of a closed tuberculous pyonephrosis or

pyoureteronephrosis. Bladder involvement is originally evident in the vicinity of the ipsilateral ureteric orifice and subsequently there is diffuse cystitis with ulceration. The ureteric orifice becomes rigidly open, allowing vesicoureteric reflux. At first the inflamed bladder is spastic but

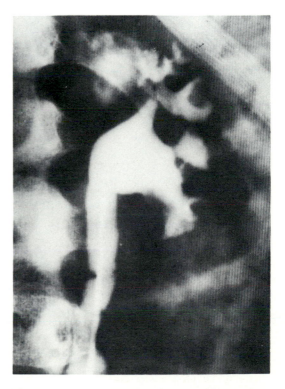

Figure 12.1. Renal tuberculosis. A retrograde pyelogram in a boy of 8 years showing an ulcerative lesion of the upper calyx of the left kidney associated with calcification and slight dilatation of the ureter.

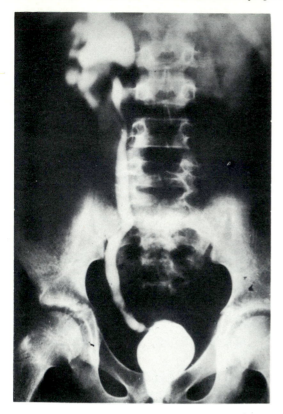

Figure 12.2. A tuberculous contracted bladder in a 13-year-old boy following left nephrectomy for advanced disease. The micturating cystogram shows a small capacity bladder with reflux into the right ureter, which because of the extreme contraction of the dome appears to enter high in the bladder. There is a dilated posterior urethra.

as the disease progresses it becomes fibrotic and irreversibly contracted. As a consequence, hydroureteronephrosis may develop in the contralateral uninfected ureter and kidney (*Figure 12.2*).

Tuberculosis of the male genital tract is virtually unknown during childhood unless there is advanced disease involving the urinary tract and other systems.

Clinical features

Symptoms develop following the ulceration of a papillary lesion into a calyx. Haematuria is common and is associated with diurnal and nocturnal frequency of micturition and with pain on voiding. Loin pain or ureteric colic may result from the passage of blood clot or caseous material. Loss of weight and colour with sweating and fever are the general manifestations. Although the tuberculin test is generally positive, the reaction is significant only in the young child who has not received BCG inoculation. The urine is acid in reaction, contains leukocytes and is sterile on routine culture. The erythrocyte sedimentation rate may be normal or moderately elevated.

Diagnosis

Chest and abdominal radiography are required to determine whether pulmonary disease exists or renal or mesenteric glandular calcification is present. On intravenous urography an early ulcerocavernous lesion shows as either an irregular enlargement of a calyx or a calyx communicating with a ragged cavity extending into the parenchyma. Cystoscopy may reveal a diminished bladder capacity and cystitis of varying degree and extent, possibly with submucosal tubercles. In advanced cases extensive mucosal ulceration and the rigidly open 'golf-hole' ureteric orifice are typical.

Confirmation of the diagnosis rests on the demonstration of *Mycobacterium tuberculosis* in the urine. Drugs such as tetracycline, chloromycetin, kanamycin and gentamicin should be stopped for at least 1 week before the urine is examined. Organisms are often excreted intermittently and in small numbers so that a minimum of three early morning specimens must be examined histologically and cultured. With improved culture techniques animal inoculation is not required routinely. The sensitivity of the organism to various antituberculous drugs must be determined.

Treatment

Chemotherapy

Two or more drugs to which the bacillus is sensitive should be used in combination in order to lessen the possibility of it becoming drug-resistant. Inpatient hospital treatment is no longer considered necessary and the patient can be treated at home, provided that satisfactory supervision is possible. Gow (1978) uses a combination of rifampicin 450 mg, isoniazid 300 mg and pyrazinamide 1 g daily. The drugs are taken orally at night just before retiring, for a period of 2 months. Then the pyrazinamide is discontinued and rifampicin 450 mg and isoniazid 600 mg are given three times a week for a further 2 months. If the response has been satisfactory, therapy can then be stopped. With young children the drug dosages must be reduced according to body weight.

Rifampicin is contraindicated in the presence of hepatic disease and hepatic function tests are needed at weekly intervals. Isoniazid may have toxic effects on the nervous system and peripheral neuritis or convulsions can occur. The neurotoxic action is due to competitive inhibition of pyridoxine metabolism and may be prevented by the administration of pyridoxine 25–50 mg daily.

Patients are reviewed clinically and by intravenous urography and culture of three early morning urine specimens at 3 months after the conclusion of chemotherapy and then twice more at 6-monthly intervals. If the results of the investigations are satisfactory, routine follow-up is discontinued after 15 months. However, when there is renal calcification indicating the presence of a focus to which drugs may not have had access, observation is required indefinitely.

Surgery

Urinary tuberculosis is curable by chemotherapy alone provided that there is no obstructive uropathy and the focus has an adequate blood supply. Surgery may be needed to maintain or provide free urine drainage or to remove accumulations of avascular caseous material which may harbour tubercle bacilli.

Obstructive lesions develop most commonly at the calyceal neck, at the pelviureteric junction and in the lower ureter. A closed-off calyx with a collection of caseous matter may be evident on pyelography as a focus of calcification or a segment of kidney devoid of a collecting system. As a rule the cavity can be emptied by aspiration through a wide bore needle under radiographic control so that open operation is avoided (Gow, 1978).

Stricture at the pelviureteric junction requires prompt intervention to avert the development of complete obstruction and thus early destruction

of the kidney. Pyeloureteroplasty by the Anderson-Hynes (Anderson, 1963) technique is applicable in most cases. Lower ureteric stenosis existing at the time of first presentation may respond to prednisolone in addition to the routine chemotherapy. If no improvement is apparent within 6 weeks then reimplantation of the ureter above the stricture into the bladder using a reflux-preventing technique is indicated.

Partial nephrectomy is required for a calcified lesion in a kidney pole that is increasing in size in spite of chemotherapy. Nephrectomy is indicated for a grossly diseased kidney that is non-functioning or which even if the infection is eradicated can make no useful contribution to overall renal function. Ureterectomy is needed in addition if the ureter is infected.

Fibrous contracture of the bladder causing severe frequency of micturition can be relieved by enterocystoplasty and this technique has largely eliminated the need for cutaneous or colonic urinary diversion (Abel and Gow, 1978).

Schistosomiasis (bilharziasis)

The parasites that cause schistosomiasis are various trematode worms. *Schistosoma haematobium* and less often *S. mansoni* are those responsible for urinary tract involvement. The disease is common in Middle Eastern countries and in tropical Africa.

Life cycle

The ova of the schistosomes are excreted from an infested human in the urine or faeces. When they reach fresh water, free-swimming ciliated miracidia are released and penetrate the skin of the intermediate host, namely a snail of the Bulinus or the Physopsis group. An asexual phase of development then occurs and mature tadpole-like cercariae leave the snail to swim in the water. Humans become infected by bathing in infested water, when the cercariae pierce the skin and enter the circulation. A sexual phase of development then occurs and mating of male and female cercariae occurs in the portal venous system. The fertilized female migrates to the pelvis where ovulation occurs in the mucosal venules of the lower urinary tract.

Pathology

Living bilharzial ova cause a chronic granulomatous inflammatory reaction in the bladder mucosa, the lower ureter, the posterior urethra and the scrotal organs or the vagina. Dead ova undergo calcification. In the bladder minute tubercles form near the ureteric orifices and later larger conglomerations produce polypoid mucosal lesions. In chronic disease atrophy of the mucosa occurs and calcified ova are then visible at cystoscopy to give the characteristic appearance of a 'sandy patch'. Mucosal ulceration may follow. Invasion of the vesical musculature causes fibrosis and bladder contraction. The ureterovesical valve is destroyed and vesicoureteric reflux follows. Secondary bacterial infection is common and calculi may form on nuclei of bilharzial debris. Finally bladder carcinoma (often of squamous type) may develop, frequently at a relatively early age: Brumskine, Dragan and Sanvee (1977) reported this complication in a 5-year-old boy.

Schistosomiasis of the ureter involves mainly the lower third. The mucosal changes are similar to those occurring in the bladder. Mural calcification and fibrous stenosis develop and are followed by hydroureteronephrosis.

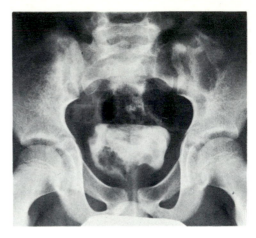

Figure 12.3. Bilharziasis of the bladder in a 9-year-old boy. The cystogram during intravenous urography shows multiple filling defects due to mucosal polyps.

Clinical features

Penetration of the skin by the cercariae may lead to the Kabure itch, a transient allergic reaction with fever and local itching and urticaria. The Katayama phase, which is a toxaemic state with generalized manifestations, is rare. Urinary tract symptoms begin 2–5 months after skin perforation with frequency of micturition, dysuria and terminal haematuria.

Diagnosis

The diagnosis of urinary schistosomiasis is made by histological demonstration of the typical terminal-spined ova in the urine. Cystoscopy reveals the characteristic mucosal changes. Intravenous urography may show 'egg-shell' calcification of the bladder or the lower parts of the ureters, and in the cystogram upper tract dilatation and filling defects due to mucosal polyps may be present (*Figure 12.3*). Eosinophilia occurs, especially in the early invasive stage of the disease. The complement fixation test and similar serological investigations are unreliable since false-negative and false-positive reactions are common (Gray, 1978).

Treatment

In the presence of active disease before the development of complications the parasite can be eliminated by chemotherapy. The drugs employed are potentially dangerous and care is required in their use in the presence of cardiac or hepatic disease or anaemia. During therapy the patient must be kept at rest. Various drugs may be employed (Honey, 1978). Lucanthone is administered by mouth twice daily as a 3-day course and in a total dose of 70 mg/kg; transient nausea and mental confusion may occur and although some 50 per cent of cases are cured by one course, a second may be needed. Niridazole is given orally twice daily in a dosage of 25 mg/kg per day for 7 days; convulsions are a possible complication especially in the presence of hepatic disease. Hycanthone has the advantage that it can be given by injection in a single dose of 2.5–3.5 mg/kg body weight; it is related to Lucanthone and may be similarly toxic especially if the patient is anaemic. Metrifonate is less toxic than the other drugs and is taken by mouth in a dosage of 7.5 mg/kg at 2-week intervals to a maximum of three doses.

Surgery may be needed for the removal of calculi, the relief of ureteric or bladder outlet obstruction, the enlargement of a contracted bladder or the treatment of carcinomatous change.

Moniliasis

Candida albicans is widely distributed in nature and is a common commensal in man, occurring particularly in the pharynx, the intestinal tract and the vagina. It is found in the faeces in 10–12 per cent of normal individuals. The fungus becomes pathogenic when the body defences are lowered by various means. For example antibiotic therapy destroys bacteria so that Candida has less competition for environmental growth factors, and debilitating diseases such as neoplasia, diabetes and haemopoietic disorders causing neutropenia reduce tissue resistance. Corticosteroids and immunosuppressive drugs depress cell-mediated immunity so that transplant recipients are at particular risk of monilial infection. The prolonged use of indwelling catheters provides a ready route of entry for the fungus into the urinary tract.

Urinary tract moniliasis occurs in several clinical forms. Systemic candidiasis is a septicaemic state that may involve the kidney secondarily or originate from it and causes acute monilial pyelonephritis with abscess formation. In primary renal candidiasis bezoars composed of masses of mycelia and spores may obstruct the renal pelvis or the ureter. With monilial cystitis, cystoscopy reveals thrush-like patches on the vesical mucosa and fungus balls may form in the bladder. Asymptomatic candiduria exists when there is colonization of the urinary tract without tissue invasion and occurs mainly in patients with indwelling catheters who are receiving antibiotics.

The diagnosis of urinary candidiasis is made by the identification of the fungus in an uncontaminated urine specimen. The serum precipitin test is positive when there is organ involvement while a negative result can indicate colonization without significant tissue invasion. Treatment depends upon the type and the severity of the infection. Asymptomatic candiduria generally requires no treatment other than the removal of the predisposing factors, although monilia may continue to be excreted for some weeks afterwards. Alkalinization of the urine discourages multiplication of the organism.

Various antifungal drugs are available. Nystatin can be used as a 10 per cent suspension for bladder irrigation in cases of monilial cystitis or for oral use for the elimination of alimentary tract fungus (the drug is not absorbed). Amphotericin B can also be employed as a 5 per cent solution for local lavage while for systemic disease it is given intravenously since there is little intestinal absorption; prolonged therapy is often necessary and this drug is very toxic. Immediate side effects include vomiting, phlebitis, fever and headache, and nephrotoxicity, hepatotoxicity and anaemia may be later sequelae. 5-Fluorocytosine has advantages over amphotericin B in that it is less toxic and can be given by mouth; however, some strains of Candida may be resistant to it. For severe systemic disease Michigan (1976) employs a combination of amphotericin B and 5-fluorocytosine provided that renal function is sufficiently good to allow use of the former and the fungus is shown to be sensitive to the latter. Surgery may be needed for the removal of an obstructive monilial bezoar.

Hydatid disease

A hydatid cyst is the larval stage of a tapeworm, namely *Taenia echinococcus*. In the primary host (dog, cat, fox or wolf) the worms inhabit the intestinal mucosa and ova are excreted in the faeces. The intermediate host (man, sheep or cattle) becomes infested by swallowing the ova. The cycle is completed when a contaminated carcass of an intermediate host is eaten by a primary host. Human hydatid disease is endemic in cattle-raising and sheep-raising areas, and children usually become infected by close contact with infested dogs.

Pathology

In the human alimentary tract the ova liberate embryos which penetrate the bowel wall to enter the portal venous system. Many embryos become arrested in the liver and this is the commonest site of hydatid disease. Others reach the lungs and from there they may be disseminated to any part of the body. The tissues of the host produce an inflammatory adventitious capsule around the embryo. The hydatid cyst itself has two layers: the outer is composed of an elastic lamina while the inner, the germinal membrane, produces brood capsules which may become detached to form daughter cysts inside the main one. The brood capsules contain scolices which are immature heads of *T. echinococcus* endowed with suckers and hooklets. Calcification of the cyst wall commonly occurs.

Hydatid involvement of the kidney is rare. Slim *et al.*(1971) reported 35 patients under the age of 15 years with hydatid disease in Lebanon and the kidney was affected in only one. The cyst forms in the kidney parenchyma but as it enlarges it often ruptures into the pelvis, discharging daughter cysts and scolices. Involvement of the rest of the urinary tract is usually extrinsic. For instance the ureter may be obstructed by a retroperitoneal cyst or intraperitoneal rupture of a hepatic cyst may cause implantation of daughter cysts in the rectovesical pouch where they may displace the bladder, interfere with micturition and cause bilateral upper tract dilatation (Keramidas *et al.*, 1980).

Clinical features and diagnosis

Renal hydatid causes flank pain. Haematuria may follow the perforation of a parenchymal cyst into the pelvis and it is then associated with ureteric colic and the passage of ruptured daughter cysts, resembling grape skins, in the urine. Rarely, urinary retention occurs from the accumulation of debris in the bladder. As a rule a loin swelling is palpable. Radiography may show renal enlargement and ring-shaped calcification. When the cyst is intact, intravenous urography shows distortion of the pelvicalyceal system and infiltration of contrast medium between the parasite and the adventitious capsule can produce a characteristic crescentic opacity. A ruptured cyst which allows entry of contrast medium from the pelvis gives a soap-bubble appearance because of its content of daughter cysts (Kirkland, 1966). Eosinophilia is inconstant and is present most often shortly after cyst rupture. The Casoni intradermal test and the Ghedini-Weinberg complement fixation test are of diagnostic value if positive, but false-negative reactions may occur.

Treatment

Surgery is required since there is no specific drug treatment available. The main intraoperative risk is rupture of the cyst which may cause anaphylactic shock and disseminate daughter cysts and scolices. Adrenalin and hydrocortisone should be immediately available and the wound must be protected by packing. When the cyst is exposed, and before enucleation is begun, its fluid contents are aspirated by needle and syringe and a scolicidal solution is injected. Meymerian *et al.* (1963) found 0.1 per cent hydrogen peroxide and 0.005 per cent cetrimide to be just as effective, and less damaging to body tissues, as the formerly customary formalin. Following a 5-minute interval to allow the scolicidal agent to take effect the cyst contents are evacuated by suction and the parasite is then removed through an incision in its adventitious capsule. Hydatid cyst confined to one or other kidney pole may be more readily treated by partial nephrectomy than by cyst enucleation. However, very often the disease is so advanced by the time the diagnosis is made that nephrectomy is unavoidable.

Actinomycosis

Actinomyces bovis is an anaerobic organism that is often found as a harmless saprophyte in the mouth or the intestinal tract. Tissue invasion may occur because of a lowering of general or local resistance or due to symbiosis between Actinomyces and other bacteria. A chronic suppurative inflammation results, with the formation of granulation tissue and the occurrence in the pus of aggregations of branching filaments which form the characteristic yellow 'sulphur' granules.

Actinomycosis is rare in childhood and involvement of the kidney is very exceptional: Kretschmer and Hibbs (1936) reviewed five cases. Renal infection may be apparently primary, when there is no recognizable portal of entry of the organism, or secondary, when the kidney is affected from a focus elsewhere either by direct extension or by metastatic spread through the blood stream.

Clinically renal actinomycosis causes a debilitating febrile illness with a painful loin mass. Perinephric abscess formation may be followed by the development of chronic discharging sinuses. There is usually no disturbance of micturition but the urine may contain leukocytes and erythrocytes and Actinomyces may be detected by microscopy or by culture under anaerobic or microaerophilic conditions. Pyelography reveals renal enlargement and pelvicalyceal distortion which may simulate a neoplasm or tuberculosis.

Treatment is by penicillin and 1–12 million units daily may be needed for several months before the infection is eradicated (Peabody and Seabury, 1960). Nephrectomy is generally needed when there is extensive kidney involvement.

References

Abel, B.J. and Gow, J.G. (1978) Results of caecocystoplasty for tuberculous bladder contracture. *British Journal of Urology*, **50**, 511

Anderson, J.C. (1963) Hydronephrosis. Heinemann, London

Brumskine, W., Dragan, P. and Sanvee, L. (1977) Transitional cell carcinoma and schistosomiasis in a 5 year old boy. *British Journal of Urology*, **49**, 540

Gow, J.G. (1978) Personal communication

Gray, D.R. (1978) Protozoal infections. *In* Scientific Foundations of Family Medicine (edited by Fry, J., Gambrill, E. and Smith, R. Heinemann, London. p.281

Honey, R.M. (1978) Urinary bilharziasis. *In* Scientific Foundations of Family Medicine (edited by Fry, J., Gambrill, E. and Smith, R.). Heinemann, London. p.531

Keramidas, D.C., Doulas, N. Anagnostou, D. and Voyatzis, N. (1980) Bilateral hydronephrosis and hydroureter due to hydatid cyst in the pouch of Douglas. *Journal of Pediatric Surgery*, **15**, 345

Kirkland, K. (1966) Urological aspects of hydatid disease. *British Journal of Urology*, **38**, 241

Kretschmer, H.L. and Hibbs, W.G. (1936) Actinomycosis of the kidney in infancy and childhood. *Journal of Urology*, **36**, 123

Meymerian, E., Luttermoser, G.W., Frayha, G.J., Schwabe, C.W. and Prescott, B. (1963) Host-parasite relationships in echinococcosis: laboratory evaluation of chemical scolicides and adjuncts to hydatid surgery. *Annals of Surgery*, **158**, 211

Michigan, S. (1976) Genitourinary fungal infections. *Journal of Urology*, **116**, 390

Peabody, J.W. and Seabury, J.H. (1960) Actinomycosis and nocardiosis. A review of basic differences in therapy. *American Journal of Medicine*, **28**, 99

Slim, M.S., Khayat, G., Nash, A.T. and Jidejian, Y.D. (1971) Hydatid disease in childhood. *Journal of Pediatric Surgery*, **6**, 440

13 Anomalies of the Kidney

D. Innes Williams

Congenital absence of the kidney

Bilateral renal agenesis is very rare and always fatal. Often the lower urinary tract is absent or at least minute, with no permeable urethra. Other severe abnormalities may occur in the same child, some of them due to oligohydramnios when the absence of fetal urine flow results in scanty amniotic fluid, the uterine wall presses upon the fetus and deformities result. One of the consequences is pulmonary hypoplasia, presumably caused by restricted chest movements *in utero*, and respiratory failure is commonly the cause of death soon after birth in bilateral renal agenesis. If the lungs are expanded, their lack of elasticity may cause a minor rupture and a spontaneous pneumothorax. Pressure upon the limbs is apt to produce talipes and other deformities. A characteristic facies (Potter, 1946) is a feature of many cases, but since similar facies are associated with other causes of oligohydramnios it is possible that this too is a pressure effect. Where respiratory function is adequate the absence of kidneys results in death from renal failure.

The rate of onset of symptoms depends upon the management of the child. When normal feeds are given to satisfy the infant's appetite oedema soon appears and the plasma creatinine level rises rapidly. If only minimal quantities of fluid and feeds are allowed, life can be prolonged for as much as a week. The severe concurrent anomalies of the urinary tract make renal implantation inappropriate. With bilateral multicystic kidney and complete urethral obstruction similar complications may occur.

Unilateral agenesis is relatively common and is associated with contralateral hypertrophy. Seipelt, Zoellner and Hilgenfeld (1970) suggested that this enlargement is due to increased size of the nephrons rather than increased number. The solitary kidney may itself be subject to congenital abnormalities and is perhaps more liable to disease. A degree of malrotation, ectopia or ureteric widening is often seen. Sometimes it is difficult to decide whether the dilatation results from obstruction or simply from the raised urine flow from the solitary organ. Unilateral agenesis more often affects the left side and a considerable proportion of cases are associated with other abnormalities, especially imperforate anus. The situation has been reviewed by Emmanuel, Nachman and Aronson (1974).

Unilateral agenesis is usually first suspected from the intravenous urogram, and absence must be distinguished from failure of function. Ultrasound scanning identifies most cases of nonopacified kidney although it occasionally misses a very small organ, particularly one on the left or displaced into the pelvis. Scans with ^{99m}Tc-dimercaptosuccinic acid show any functioning renal element. Cystoscopy and retrograde pyelography are old-fashioned but occasionally useful investigations: if there is no ureter there is no kidney. Nevertheless the cystoscopist must be aware that the ureteric orifice can sometimes be missed and that even when a clear-cut hemitrigone is seen a ureter may be present but ectopic.

Any treatment is directed towards the solitary kidney and any pathology observed in it.

Embryology of malrotated, fused and ectopic kidneys

When the ureteric bud is first seen the metanephrogenic tissue that gathers around it is in a position corresponding to the sacral region. It is clear, therefore, that to reach the normal adult position a change must occur which may reasonably be described as ascent. This process cannot, however, be regarded as an independent migration of the metanephros and nor is it likely that simple growth in length of the ureteric bud can push its clumsy cap upwards. The ascent is complicated by, and perhaps partly due to, changes in shape of the organ during development.

From the 6–10 mm stage the metanephros moves cranially along with the lower pole of the mesonephros. This movement essentially results from the straightening of the tail curvature which occurs at this stage, and no active effort is required of the kidney. The metanephros is next brought into contact with and diverted by the large umbilical arteries running forwards from the aorta to the abdominal wall (ultimately the common iliac arteries) so that the axis of the organ is shifted and the caudal pole brought up against the sacral vertebrae. Growth of the kidney is then rapid and, since the caudal pole is fixed, takes place chiefly at the cranial end; with the increase in length the renal pelvis soon reaches the level of the arteries and subsequently passes them. When the kidney measures 14 mm the cranial pole reaches the lower border of the first lumbar vertebra, which is its definitive position. After this elongated stage the kidney again becomes rounded and the caudal pole is drawn up away from the sacrum. At the 22 mm stage the kidney lies alongside the first three lumbar vertebrae and subsequent changes during fetal life are merely due to variation in size of the adjacent liver and suprarenal glands. During the first year of postnatal life the lower pole of the kidney frequently extends down to the iliac crest and the subsequent growth in length of the lumbar region results in an apparent upward movement, although the kidney itself is passive (Felix, 1912; Gruenwald, 1943).

In the very early stages the metanephrogenic cap lies chiefly lateral to the tip of the ureteric bud, but it is soon shifted so that the ureter lies in front. This relationship persists until the kidney has reached the lumbar region, when a rotation occurs which brings the renal pelvis into its usual medial or anteromedial position. During the ascent the metanephros makes use of a succession of mesonephric arteries in order to obtain its blood supply, the lower arteries degenerating after the upper ones have taken over.

The pelvic ectopic kidney may be regarded as the result of failure of this process of ascent; the ureter is short and springs from the anterior surface, and the blood supply is derived from the lower aorta or the common iliac arteries. The suprarenal glands have an entirely separate origin from the genital folds and are thus normal in position, although they do not of course show the normal moulding.

The fused kidney probably results from a defect at the 8–10 mm stage, when the two organs are pressed closely together between the two umbilical arteries. If fusion is complete then further ascent is impossible and the resulting 'cake' or 'disc' kidneys are pelvic in position. If fusion is incomplete, the rapid growth of the upper poles may continue in the normal way, leaving the lower poles joined by an isthmus of renal tissue lying behind the ureters. In these horseshoe kidneys ascent proceeds up to the point where the isthmus is brought into contact with the inferior mesenteric artery. On very rare occasions fusion of the upper poles above the vessels is observed.

In crossed ectopia, when both kidneys lie in the same loin more or less fused and the ureters enter the bladder in the normal position, the uncrossed kidney is often cranial to the other one and it has been postulated that fusion occurs when one metanephros ascends further than its fellow (Carleton, 1937). However, in other cases the two kidneys lie side by side and there are several anomalies on the side of the empty loin, for instance hemivertebra and congenital dislocation of the hip. The accompanying skeletal abnormalities were seen by Cook and Stephens (1977) as evidence of severe lateral curvature of the fetal lumbosacral spine, which they suggested could result in both ureteric buds meeting the same nephrogenic cord and thus inducing a crossed and fused organ.

Malrotation

It has been shown that in the normal fetal kidney the pelvis rotates from the anterior to the medial position late in development. Failure of this process leaving the pelvis facing anteriorly is a relatively common abnormality sometimes accompanying ectopia and/or fusion. Rarely the rotation goes too far, giving a posteriorly directed renal pelvis. The rotation element is not itself productive of symptoms or secondary pathology but the renal pelvis remains broad-based and dome-like with the ureter leaving from the top of the dome. There is thus no graded funnel from which peristaltic waves can easily propel a bolus of urine down the ureter. Therefore, not only does the renal pelvis of the malrotated kidney appear larger than normal in pyelograms because of its broad base but also a true hydronephrosis is likely to occur.

Ectopic kidney

The simple ectopic kidney is occasionally encountered in childhood, usually as an incidental finding during the investigation of abdominal pain, recurrent infection or enuresis. The kidney itself may be palpable as a mass within the abdomen lying in the iliac fossa. A thoracic ectopic kidney may be a surprise finding in a chest X-ray and curiously the kidney itself is often healthy. Although all anomalous kidneys are somewhat more liable to disease than normal ones, simple ectopia is very seldom responsible for symptoms (Kelalis, Malek and Segura, 1973; Donahoe and Hendren, 1980).

The fused pelvic kidney in which the whole mass lies in front of the sacrum may well give rise to diagnostic problems. The blood supply is variable but usually enters the anterior surface of the kidney. The two ureters are short and relatively wide (*Figure 13.1*) and complicating reflux is not uncommon.

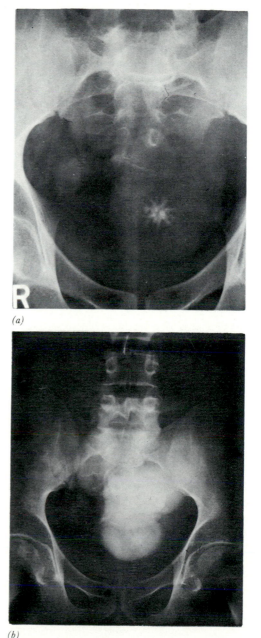

(a)

(b)

Figure 13.2. Solitary pelvic kidney with hydronephrosis and stone. *(a)* Straight X-ray. *(b)* Intravenous urogram.

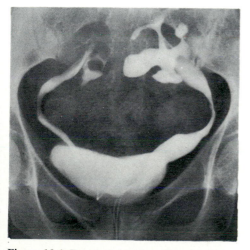

Figure 13.1. Fused pelvic kidney. Retrograde pyelogram showing deformed calyces and slightly dilated ureters.

The solitary pelvic kidney is the most likely of all this group of malformations to develop pathological complications. It usually takes the form of a flattened irregular disc a little to one side of the midline in the sacral area. The blood supply may be derived from the aorta or the iliac arteries. Major vessels most often lie in front of the disc, while a few short arteries may enter from behind. The renal pelvis is anteriorly directed but may break up immediately into calyces so that little extrarenal pelvis is present. The ureter can enter the bladder on either side and is relatively short and slightly dilated.

Hydronephrosis is a common complication of the solitary pelvic kidney, with huge excavated calyces and a narrowed pelviureteric junction. Complicating stones may be present (*Figure 13.2*). Episodes of exacerbation of obstruction present with rising plasma creatinine levels and a tense abdominal swelling which is often mistaken for a full bladder on clinical examination. Its real nature is recognized only after catheterization. This emergency situation may well have required nephrostomy drainage before the child is seen by the urologist and subsequent pyeloplasty can present many difficulties because of both the friability of the tissues following the initial drainage and the absence of a capacious renal pelvis. It may be necessary to perform a ureterocalycostomy rather than any standard operation. The early results are satisfactory but in the long run renal function may be inadequate. As with other anomalous hydronephrotic kidneys there is apt to be a late onset in the second or third decade of proteinuria, hypertension and renal failure.

Horseshoe kidney

Like other renal abnormalities horseshoe kidney may be found in children with no relevant complaint, particularly because it is commonly associated with other congenital abnormalities. The condition may well be revealed during the radiological investigation of cardiac anomalies. It is commoner in the male and interestingly is often a concomitant of Turner's syndrome.

All forms of renal pathology may occur in the horseshoe kidney on a unilateral or bilateral basis and the anomaly may create special problems in treatment, for example in nephroblastoma where the excision must cut through the isthmus. Hydronephrosis is the commonest complication of a horseshoe kidney as well as of other forms of malrotated kidney. It was formerly customary to identify the point where the ureter crosses the isthmus as the site of obstruction. In fact this is very infrequently observed. The hydronephrosis is seldom accompanied by a dilated upper ureter unless there are complicating obstructions due to the crossing of renal vessels in the hilum immediately overlying the ureter (*Figures 13.3 and 13.4*). In general the

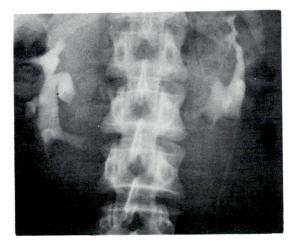

Figure 13.3. Horseshoe kidney. Intravenous urogram in an uncomplicated case.

correction of hydronephrosis demands pyeloplasty, which can be modified from the Hynes-Anderson or the Culp technique to meet the particular circumstances, and it should not be necessary to sever the isthmus or to perform a nephropexy (*Figures 13.5 and 13.6*). The concept of the isthmus itself as a cause of symptoms is not supported by the author's experience. Stone formation may result from stasis in the slightly dilated pelvis even in the absence of a true hydronephrosis.

Ureteric duplication may be seen in association with horseshoe kidney, and on a number of occasions an ectopic ureter has also been present (*Figure 13.7*). There are even two cases on record in which a retrocaval ureter was associated with a horseshoe formation. The anatomical arrangements of the blood supply of the horseshoe kidney have been described by Graves (1969). The radiological appearances, which are familiar to most urologists, have been reported in detail by Thieman and Wieners (1970).

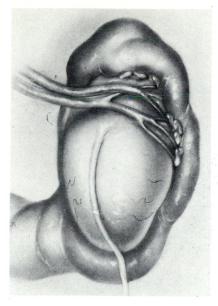

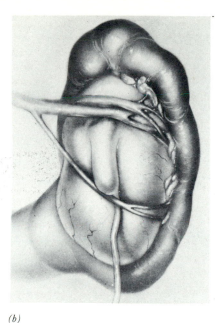

(a)   (b)

Figure 13.4. Horseshoe kidney. Diagram to show the form of hydronephrosis. *(a)* High insertion of the ureter into the dome-like pelvis. *(b)* Vascular obstruction to the ureter below the pelviureteric junction.

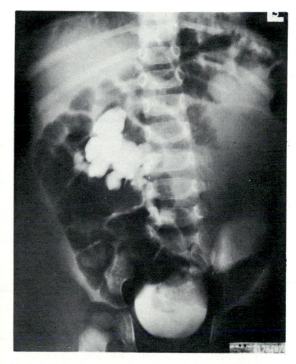

Figure 13.5. Horseshoe kidney with bilateral hydronephrosis in an 18-month-old boy with abdominal swelling as the presenting complaint. The intravenous urogram shows poor opacification on the left and hydronephrosis in a malrotated right kidney. The left renal element was removed and a pyeloplasty was performed on the right with satisfactory results.

Crossed ectopia

Where both kidneys lie on the same side of the abdomen they are almost always fused, and the crossed organ lies below and medial to the normal one (*Figure 13.8*). This condition is again likely to accompany multisystem anomalies and may be uncomplicated by any pathological process. However, in some cases it appears that due to the malformation of the crossed organ there is a relative inadequacy of nephron numbers and dysplastic changes are likely to be found (Marshall and Freedman, 1978). Pelviureteric obstruction is relatively uncommon but many patients have reflux and dilated ureters. Tanenbaum, Silverman and Weinberg (1970) have listed the common associations. Renal failure is inevitably a likely consequence of severe pyelonephritis where there is already dysplasia. From the surgical point of view, when one ureter is abnormal it is a relatively simple matter to perform a ureteroureterostomy at a high level where the two ureters are closely approximated and to excise the pathological channel.

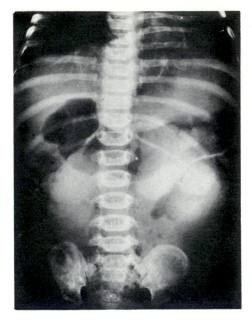

(a)

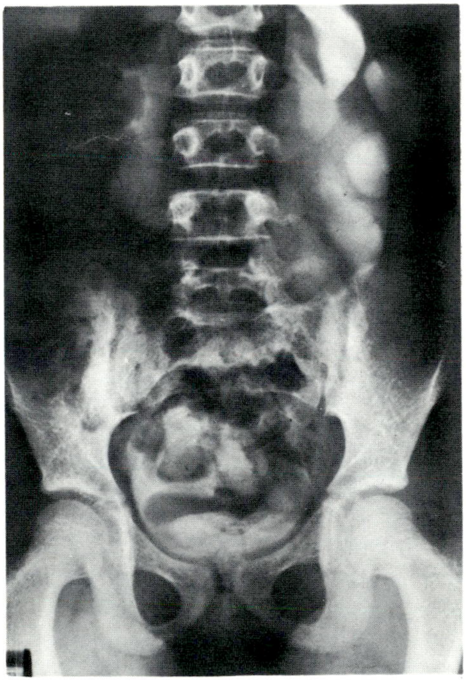

(b)

Figure 13.6. Horseshoe kidney with bilateral hydronephrosis in a neonate. The blood urea level was normal despite gross changes. *(a)* Intravenous urogram at presentation. *(b)* At 7 years after pyeloplasty.

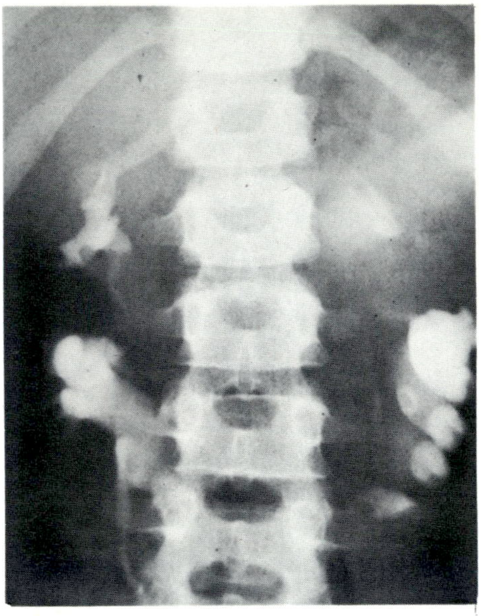

Figure 13.7. Horseshoe kidney with bilateral ureteric duplication and ectopic ureter from the left upper pole. Intravenous urogram in a girl with dribbling incontinence despite normal micturition.

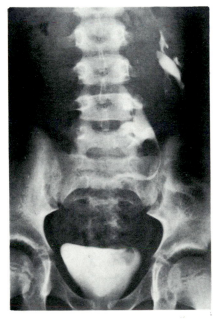

Figure 13.8. Crossed ectopia with fusion. Intravenous urogram in an uncomplicated case.

Dysmorphic kidney

In any large series of children's pyelograms there are some kidneys that are clearly abnormal in shape or have an unusual arrangement of the pelvicalyceal system while they do not fit into the standard categories already described. For instance the kidney in the prune belly syndrome may be dysmorphic in this sense, often having elongated infundibula with rounded calyces and yet no evidence of obstruction or scarring. In patients with a single ectopic ureter an irregularly shaped kidney is a common finding. Occasionally a kidney may appear to have

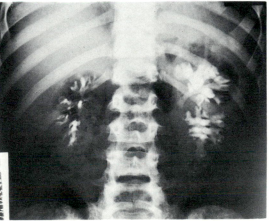

Figure 13.9. Polycalycosis. Intravenous urogram showing unusually numerous calyces with some obstruction to the left upper group.

an excessive number of calyces and this 'polycalycosis' (*Figure 13.9*) was recorded in the Rubinstein-Taybi syndrome by Béraud (1970). The kidney in the Laurence-Moon-Biedl syndrome is apt to be smaller than normal with rounded calyces but without evidence of obstruction. Extrarenal calyces, that is a renal

pelvis that breaks up into branches outside the renal hilum, are observed in some kidneys with or without hydronephrosis although their pathological significance is not apparent. While any of these kidneys may show histologically dysplastic changes it is not safe to deduce this from their shape alone, and it is perhaps therefore better to avoid the term dysplasia.

References

Béraud, C. (1970) Rein multicaliciel et syndrome de Rubinstein-Taybi. *Journal de Radiologie, d'Electrologie et de Médecine Nucléaire*, **51**, 197

Carleton, A. (1937) Crossed ectopia of the kidney and its possible causes. *Journal of Anatomy*, **71**, 292

Cook, W.A. and Stephens, F.D. (1977) Fused kidneys: morphological study and theory of embryogenesis. *In* Urinary Systems Malformations in Children. Birth Defects Original Article Series, Vol. 13, No. 5. (edited by Bergsma, D. and Duckett, J.W.). Liss, New York. p.327

Donahoe, P.K. and Hendren, W.H. (1980) Pelvic Kidney in Infants and Children. *Journal of Pediatric Surgery*, **15**, 486

Emanuel, B., Nachman, R., Aronson, N. (1974) Congenital solitary kidney: review of 74 cases. *Journal of Urology*, **111**, 394

Felix, W. (1912) *In* Manual of Human Embryology (edited by Keibell, F. and Malls, F.P.) Lippincott, Philadelphia and London. p.1140

Graves, F.T. (1969) Arterial anatomy of the congenitally abnormal kidney. *British Journal of Surgery*, **56**, 533

Gruenwald, P. (1943) Normal changes in the position of the embryonic kidney. *Anatomical Record*, **85**, 163

Kelalis, P.P., Malek, R.S. and Segura, J.W. (1973) Observations on renal ectopia and fusion in children. *Journal of Urology*, **110**, 588

Marshall, F.F. and Freedman, M.T. (1978) Crossed renal ectopia. *Journal of Urology*, **119**, 188

Potter, E.L. (1946) Facial characteristics of infants with bilateral renal agenesis. *American Journal of Obstetrics and Gynecology*, **51**, 885

Seipelt, H., Zoellner, K., Hilgenfeld, E. (1970) Morphological and functional studies in children with a single kidney. *Zeitschrift für Urologie und Nephrologie*, **63**, 349

Tanenbaum, B., Silverman, N. and Weinberg, J.R. (1970) Solitary crossed renal ectopia. *Archives of Surgery*, **101**, 616

Thieman, K.J. and Wieners, H. (1970) Problems in angiographic diagnosis of agenesis, aplasia and fusion anomalies of the kidney. *Radiologie*, **10**, 108

14 Hypoplastic, Dysplastic and Cystic Kidneys

D. Innes Williams and R.A. Risdon

Congenital disorders of renal parenchymatous tissue occur in a wide variety of conditions and our incomplete knowledge of the pathology is revealed by the confused nomenclature. The commoner genetic disorders such as polycystic kidneys have received full attention but the cystic dysplastic changes often encountered in urological practice and the cystic malformations accompanying the multiple anomaly syndromes are less well understood. Experimental evidence demonstrates that factors in the fetal environment can be responsible for cyst formation. Resnick, Brown and Vernier (1976) reviewed this topic. Ureteric obstruction (Bernstein, 1968) can certainly produce cystic dysplasia in the experimental animal and seems to do so in the human fetus. The embryology of the kidney is particularly relevant to the understanding of cystic disease and is therefore described in the following section, but the main emphasis in this chapter is on the diagnosis and the prognosis of the various forms of parenchymal disorder that may be encountered by the urologist.

Embryology

Three pairs of kidneys (the pronephros, the mesonephros and the metanephros) develop in the human embryo. The pronephros and the mesonephros are transient vestigial structures which form and rapidly regress in the early embryo. The definitive kidney (the metanephros) is derived in two parts: the nephrons from the metanephric blastema and the collecting system (the ureter, the renal pelvis, the calyces and the collecting ducts) from the ureteric bud. The latter forms as a hollow outgrowth from the mesonephric (wolffian) duct near the cloaca at about the 5 mm stage. When the tip of the ureteric bud impinges on the caudal end of the nephrogenic cord (the metanephric blastema) it undergoes a series of rapid dichotomous branchings. The first several generations of branches become distended when urine production starts and ultimately coalesce to form the renal pelvis and the major and minor calyces. Osathanondh and Potter (1964) identified two regions in each branch of the ureteric bud. The first is a slightly dilated tip or ampulla capable of branching and inducing nephron formation, and the second is an interstitial portion capable of elongation by cellular proliferation.

During the early phase of nephron production (the 5th–15th weeks) dichotomous branching of the ureteric bud continues. Oval condensations of metanephric blastema from which the nephrons develop become related to each ampullary tip. Every condensation rapidly develops a lumen which elongates and becomes S-shaped. At the proximal end a glomerulus forms and the intermediate portion becomes the convoluted tubule and the loop of Henle. The distal end soon attaches to the ampulla and the lumen becomes continuous with that of the ureteric bud, which is developing into a collecting duct. As the branching of the ureteric bud progresses ampullae with their associated nephrons are carried outwards, new nephrons forming and becoming attached with every branching.

After the 15th week branching of the ureteric bud ceases. Each ampulla is then capable of inducing the formation of a series of nephrons, each of which joins to the one immediately before it to produce a string or nephron arcade. In every arcade the innermost member is a nephron formed during the initial branching phase, and those added subsequently lie progressively nearer the surface of the developing kidney. This process continues until about the 22nd week when the ampullae advance beyond the zone where arcades are formed, the last member of each arcade becoming attached just behind the ampulla. Subsequently new nephrons are added singly and attached behind the ampulla between the 32nd–36th weeks when nephron formation ceases. These last-formed nephrons develop in the outer subcapsular cortex and can often be recognized as a nephrogenic zone in histological sections of the kidneys of premature infants.

Hypoplasia and the small kidney

The normal radiological dimensions and growth pattern of the normal child's kidneys have been recorded by Hodson *et al.* (1962). Where one or both kidneys fail to reach the expected size the term hypoplasia is sometimes employed but it is important to realize that very many factors (both congenital and acquired) may be involved and that on clinical, radiological and sometimes even pathological grounds it may be impossible to distinguish the original cause. Hypoplasia can be taken as a reasonable description of the miniature kidney with normal (although a smaller number of) reticuli, a normal renal parenchyma and a normal ureter. Such a miniature is occasionally seen as a unilateral phenomenon; however, it is very difficult to distinguish from the small kidney resulting from renal arterial stenosis (*see* Chapter 7) or from renal venous thrombosis which also may leave a kidney that is functional but diminutive. In both the above vascular disorders hypertension is a possible complication. Nevertheless the miniature kidney is sometimes observed in a child with normal blood pressure and in these circumstances probably requires no treatment.

If hypoplasia is bilateral, so that there is an overall shortage of nephrons, there is hypertrophy of the elements that are present and therefore gross distortion of the normal microscopic appearances. A disorder has been described of bilateral oligomeganephronic hypoplasia, which is a nonfamilial condition presenting early in childhood usually with vomiting and dehydration. On investigation such children are found to be suffering from polyuria and salt wasting. Urine concentration is poor, there may be slight proteinuria and there is progressive uraemia. The condition has been fully reviewed by Scheinman and Abelson (1970) and Carter and Lirenman (1970). Radiologically the kidneys are small although normal in shape. On intravenous pyelography urine concentration is found to be very poor while the urinary tract itself is normal. Microdissection studies by Fetterman and Habib (1969) demonstrated that there is a disproportionate enlargement of the proximal tubules within the hypertrophied nephrons. The treatment of these children is that of overall renal failure, but the disease is not necessarily progressive.

The term segmental hypoplasia is used in relation to the localized contraction of a segment of the kidney, particularly if it is associated with hypertension when the diagnosis of Ask-Upmark kidney is often applied. A number of authors have attributed this localized hypoplasia to an arterial anomaly with subsequent atrophy of the cortex (Reuterskiold and Wilbrand, 1971). Histologically in the segmental scars the glomeruli are absent or few in number, the tubules are atrophic or distended with colloid, the arterioles themselves are thick-walled and tortuous and there is little or no inflammatory cell infiltration. In the authors' practice the diagnosis of Ask-Upmark kidney has been very seldom substantiated. In cases where the radiological appearance is suggestive reflux has been the rule, and it seems likely that scarring resulting from an early infantile episode of pyelonephritis is responsible.

The great majority of kidneys that might be described as hypoplastic are more accurately termed dysplastic (see below) but pyelonephritis is much the commonest cause of a small contracted kidney in late childhood. The characteristic irregularity of scarring, the patchy loss of parenchyma, and the clubbing and elongation of the calyces are well known and fully described in Chapter 15. In some cases the kidney is more evenly affected with an overall shrinkage, but this as well as the irregular scarring is likely to be associated with reflux.

Obstructive atrophy is ordinarily responsible for loss of parenchyma in a hydronephrotic kidney that is larger than normal because of obstruction. Where there has been a transient acute obstruction, such as impaction of a calculus in the ureter or rarely very acute urine retention due to urethral valves, obstructive atrophy can lead to a small kidney with a smooth outline. Although all the calyces are then blunted, the regularity of the change usually distinguishes this condition from pyelonephritis.

Postirradiation atrophy can be seen in some children treated for malignant disease in whom the screening was inadequate.

Dysplasia

Dysplasia is a term loosely applied to widely varying conditions which, like so many portmanteau words, has now entered common usage to such an extent as to be irreplaceable. Originally it described a histological finding, although pathologists may differ as to the precise criteria for diagnosis. There is general agreement that a malformation characterized by the presence of cartilage cells and of primitive straight tubules surrounded by cuboidal epithelium and extending out into the cortex is dysplastic. Proglomeruli of fetal type may be present. There is diminished branching of the collecting ducts with cystic transformation of their terminal portions. Cysts are common but vary enormously in number and size, the multicystic kidney with an atretic ureter being one extreme. Risdon (1971) reviewed this topic and found that there was almost always a recognizable urinary tract anomaly in addition to the dysplasia. Others, for example Ericsson and Ivemark (1958), have suggested that dysplastic elements can be found in otherwise normal renal and ureteric systems and can themselves be responsible for a liability to infection.

In general dysplasia is not a familial condition although in our experience siblings have been affected. There are a number of multisystem anomaly syndromes (see below) which include renal pathology described as cystic dysplasia.

Congenitally misshapen kidneys that are not easily classified as fused or malrotated are sometimes described as dysplastic, but the histological features specified above are not necessarily found in such organs. Imperfect development of the ureter with irregularities of calibre and musculature, for instance in the prune belly syndrome, also attracts the use of the term dysplasia.

Renal dysplasia as encountered by the urologist is ordinarily associated with other urinary tract pathology in one of three forms.

Renal dysplasia with an atretic ureter

The upper part at least of the ureter is thread-like and impermeable. The kidney is very small and often described as aplastic, consisting of no more than a fibrocystic knob. Symptoms are unlikely to be related to the affected kidney, although contralateral pathology may be present. The multicystic kidney can also be included under this heading; clinically it presents different problems which merit separate consideration (see below).

Renal dysplasia with a patent but anomalous ureter

The most easily defined example of this is an ectopic ureter draining the upper moiety of a double kidney. The characteristic histology of dysplasia possibly accompanied by hydronephrosis and infection is confined to that moiety, while the lower pole is normal or involved only in acquired disease. The dysplasia in these cases has little or no effect on diagnosis and treatment, which are concerned with the ureteric problem.

The dysplastic kidney with a single but refluxing ureter constitutes a separate entity and one in which radiological differentiation from severe atrophic pyelonephritis may be impossible. However, a small dysplastic kidney may be observed in the neonate. Characteristically there is a cluster of closely packed clubbed calyces draining into a dilated renal pelvis that appears

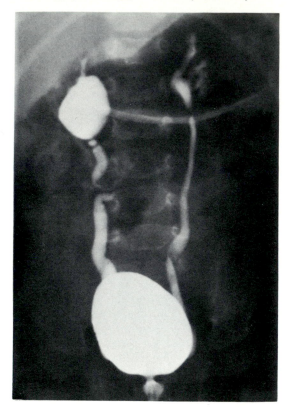

Figure 14.1. Renal dysplasia. Cystogram in an infant with severe uraemia but with sterile urine, no evidence of infection and no obstruction. Bilateral reflux outlines the kidneys. The left kidney is very small with crowded calyces and the right one is also small and obscured by an enlarged atonic renal pelvis.

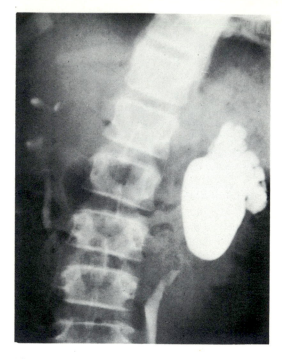

Figure 14.2. Atrophic kidney, probably dysplastic. Micturating cystogram outlining by reflux a small left kidney with bunched calyces and a dilated renal pelvis that empties slowly. The urine had been infected and the relative importance of congenital dysplasia and pyelonephritis cannot be assessed from this film.

to lie in the vertical plane (*Figure 14.1*). With reflux the dilatation increases and produces secondary kinking of the pelviureteric junction and an appearance of hydronephrosis. Such a kidney is easily infected and secondary pyelonephritis is common (*Figure 14.2*). Hypertension may follow. In bilateral disease there is often severe salt wasting in the neonatal stage and always a long-term problem of renal failure.

Renal dysplasia with urethral obstruction

Neonates with urethral valves or obliteration of the urethral lumen often present with severe dysplasia and multiple cortical cysts (Baert, 1978). When sufficient information is available reflux is always seen as an added factor. Children with a unilateral disorder often come to

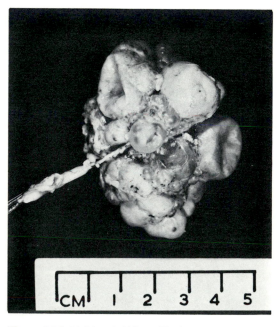

Figure 14.3. Multicystic kidney. Nephrectomy specimen showing the atretic upper ureter.

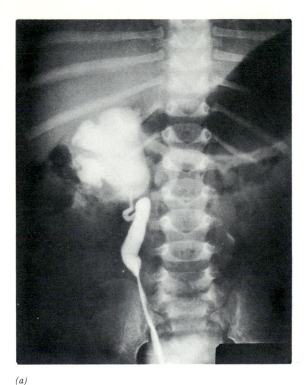

(a)

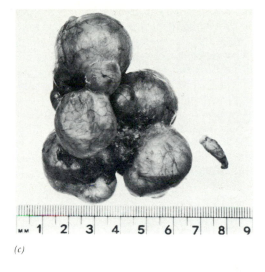

(c)

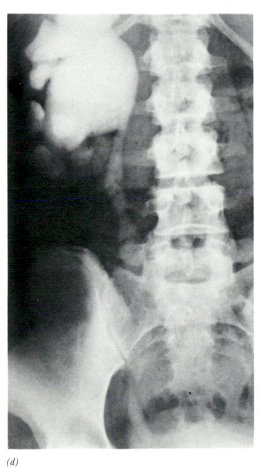

(b)

(d)

Figure 14.4. Left multicystic kidney with contralateral midureteric obstruction. *(a)* Cystogram showing reflux up to the atretic segment of the left ureter below the multicystic kidney. *(b)* Right retrograde pyelogram showing contralateral hydronephrosis. *(c)* Operative specimen showing left multicystic kidney. Ureteroplasty was performed on the right ureter. *(d)* Twenty-five year follow-up intravenous pyelogram showing recovery of right kidney.

nephrectomy when examination reveals the dysplasia; the opposite nonrefluxing kidney functions well and is therefore not available for histology. In neonates with urethral valves and bilateral reflux the overall renal function may be insufficient to maintain life and these patients almost always exhibit dysplasia.

Experimental work by Bernstein (1968) suggested that obstruction can itself produce dysplasia if it is operative at a particular stage of fetal development. This finding correlates well with the authors' experience of urethral valve cases.

The multicystic kidney

Although it is an easily recognizable clinical entity, multicystic kidney is pathologically an extreme form of dysplasia with an atretic ureter. The cysts are large and loosely bound together by a fibrous stroma containing a few primitive renal elements. The upper end of the ureter, the renal pelvis and the calyces are represented only by a fine thread without a lumen (*Figure 14.3*). The lower end of the ureter may be patent and of normal calibre, and may even allow reflux (*Figure 14.4*). As an occasional variant cases are seen in which the upper ureter is completely obliterated but a dilated renal pelvis is present, and while the renal tissue is almost completely replaced by cysts (*Figure 14.5*) the whole mass does bear some resemblance to the shape of a normal kidney.

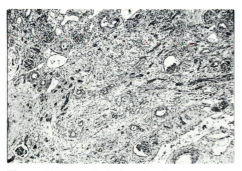

Figure 14.5. Histological section showing dysplastic elements in a multicystic kidney.

No effective function is present in the multicystic kidney, although claims are sometimes made that a radiologically faint and transient concentration of opaque medium can be demonstrated. The enlargement of the kidney is unlikely to be progressive, and in cases where no

operation is undertaken the mass becomes smaller in relation to the size of the child. Some examples are encountered in adult life, usually during investigation of a symptomless nonfunctioning kidney, and calcification of the cyst walls may be present. Hypertension was attributed to a multicystic kidney by Javadpour *et al.* (1970) but would certainly not be expected in these circumstances. However, the association of this apparently benign disorder with other urinary tract anomalies gives it added significance. On rare occasions it is bilateral; such cases are fatal soon after birth and may exhibit the stigmata of the oligohydramnios syndrome.

Cysts may affect one half of a horseshoe kidney or a crossed ectopic kidney, while in a series of 20 cases Pathak and Williams (1964) found the opposite kidney to be hydronephrotic in 11 and dysplastic in five. The hydronephrosis was due in some cases to ureterovesical obstruction and in others to a segmental narrowing of the ureter in the lumbar region where it had an appearance superficially resembling the atretic ureter associated with the multicystic kidney itself. It seems possible that aetiologically the ureteric disorder in these cases is primary. Some obstructed kidneys contain cysts and show a deterioration of renal function out of proportion to the degree of obstruction. There is in general no familial basis for the disorder, although in the authors' series one group of siblings was affected.

Characteristically the multicystic kidney presents as a mass in the abdomen of a newborn infant. There are no local symptoms but the child may well be under treatment for abnormalities of other systems. The coarsely lobulated nature of the swelling is strongly suggestive of the diagnosis, although clinically it may be difficult to distinguish from hydronephrosis with advanced destruction of the kidney. In the newborn period an ultrasound scan should be the first investigation, and in older infants an intravenous pyelogram usually precedes it. Ultrasound demonstrates the multicystic nature of the swelling, and in unilateral cases the normality of the opposite kidney. Radiologically the soft tissue mass may be evident (calcification is only present in later life). There is in general no concentration of contrast medium, although in the phase of total body opacification in the infant the cysts may show up as translucent areas.

In the otherwise fit child the above features alone may be sufficient for diagnosis. Nevertheless there is always concern as to the possibility of confusion with hydronephrosis due to pelvi-ureteric junction obstruction and many children require some further diagnostic procedure. Cyst puncture is readily performed. The injection of opaque medium does not produce an antegrade pyelogram in the multicystic kidney, since it outlines one or a few of the cysts only. However, this manoeuvre can make the diagnosis of hydronephrosis. In most cases a micturating cystogram is not required, but in some it shows reflux into the lower section of the obliterated ureter. At cystoscopy an orifice may or may not be present on the affected side. If it is, a retrograde ureterogram demonstrates the level of obliteration.

A very large multicystic kidney forming an easily palpable and visible swelling is best removed surgically. Smaller ones are harmless and may be left *in situ*. The operation is a simple procedure that may be undertaken through a small incision by collapsing the cysts. Contralateral ureteric disease must be sought and demands active surgical correction.

Development of polycystic disease

Kampmeier (1923) suggested that the first-formed generations of nephrons in the embryonic human kidney were vestigial structures that either failed to join the developing collecting ducts or did so only for a short time. He proposed that if they failed to regress then urine production in these closed vesicles might lead to cyst formation, extreme examples accounting for cases of congenital polycystic disease and minor ones explaining the common isolated cysts found in adult kidneys. Although it was popular for many years this theory is now discounted. Detailed microdissection studies of human fetal kidneys (Osathanondh and Potter, 1964) failed to substantiate Kampmeier's observations and established that cysts can arise in any part of the nephron or the collecting duct. Moreover they are generally not closed structures but communicating cystic dilatations or diverticula. Furthermore it is clear that there are many quite distinct varieties of cystic disease with different clinical, pathological and genetic

backgrounds, which cannot be regarded as variants of a single polycystic disorder.

It is evident that by no means all cysts are of developmental origin. Tubular blockage by deposition of material within the lumen or scarring of the adjacent interstitium may in the presence of continued urine production lead to cyst formation. This probably explains the simple or serous cysts frequently seen in a wide variety of acquired renal diseases and present in about half of all kidneys examined at postmortem in patients over the age of 50 years, particularly if the kidneys show arteriosclerotic change. Their rarity in children argues strongly for an acquired nature. Such cysts are seldom sufficiently widespread within the kidney to cause confusion with polycystic disease, although this difficulty occasionally arises in patients with end-stage chronic renal disease maintained on long-term haemodialysis (Dunnill, Millard and Oliver, 1977).

In many instances we are largely ignorant of the pathological mechanisms leading to renal cyst formation. Microdissection studies of various forms of cystic disease (Hooper, 1958; Osathanondh and Potter, 1964; Heggö and Natvig, 1965) have helped to clarify the position to some extent.

Infantile polycystic disease has been ascribed to hyperplasia of the interstitial portions of the ureteric bud branches leading to fusiform dilatation of the collecting ducts. The precise cause of this is unknown, but the disease is inherited as an autosomal recessive trait.

Microdissection in adult polycystic disease with autosomal dominant inheritance shows that in this condition cysts may occur in any segment of the nephron or the collecting duct and are intimately intermingled with normal structures. Abnormal nephron attachment and atypical branching of the collecting ducts are also seen and some ducts end in cystic dilatations as in cystic dysplasia. These findings suggest that the cysts are developmental defects, a conclusion supported by a report of adult polycystic disease occurring in a fetus from a family harbouring the abnormal gene (Carter, 1974). It has been proposed by Darmady, Offer and Woodhouse (1970) that patients who develop adult polycystic disease may merely inherit a metabolic defect that causes secondary changes in the kidney leading to cyst formation. Such a mechanism would explain the fact that adult polycystic disease usually presents in middle age.

Infantile polycystic disease

Infantile polycystic disease is the most clear-cut of all forms of cystic kidney, with pathological findings generally agreed by a variety of workers. It has been called 'hamartomous' by Osathanondh and Potter (1964) but this terminology is not widely accepted.

Pathologically both kidneys are grossly enlarged and in infantile cases seem to fill the entire abdomen. They are reniform and coarsely lobulated. Their surface is marked by numerous small cysts 1–2 mm across (*Figure 14.6*). The renal pelvis and calyces are enlarged and elongated. The cut surface of the kidney is honeycombed with elongated tubular cystic spaces with a generally radial arrangement, usually occupying the entire parenchyma (*Figure 14.7*)

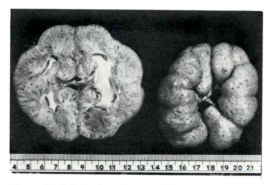

Figure 14.6. Infantile polycystic kidney. Autopsy specimen.

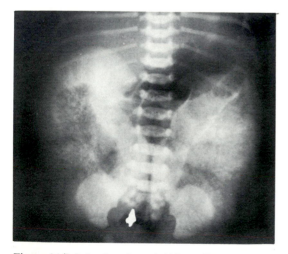

Figure 14.7. Infantile polycystic kidneys. Intravenous urogram in a newborn infant showing retention of contrast medium in the tubules throughout the parenchyma.

but sometimes sparing the medullary and immediate subcapsular zones. The cysts are derived from collecting tubules (Heggö and Natvig, 1965) which are diffusely enlarged and often saccular while remaining in continuity with the renal pelvis. There is no increase in the connective tissue elements of the kidney. Abnormalities of the lower urinary tract are unusual and constitute no part of the syndrome. Infantile polycystic disease is always bilateral and accompanied by proliferation of the bile ducts, and sometimes by cysts in the liver and pancreas. The hepatic cysts are associated with an excess of fibrous tissue and in later childhood hepatic fibrosis with portal hypertension may be the dominant feature in the clinical picture.

Blyth and Ockenden (1971) described four types corresponding to pathological and genetic differences. In the perinatal group they found that the kidneys were very large indeed and the child was either stillborn or succumbed soon after birth; at least 90 per cent of the renal tubules were affected by cystic dilatation. It is clear that very little treatment is possible for this group. In the second somewhat less severely involved group neonates presented with bilaterally enlarged kidneys associated with renal failure and in particular with salt wasting. Many of these children died 6 weeks or a little more following birth and proved to have involvement of about 60 per cent of the renal tubules. It is quite likely that some of them could be saved by aggressive biochemical management. In the third group infants were found to have enlarged kidneys and a palpable liver. A degree of renal failure was a feature but portal hypertension due to the hepatic involvement was an important cause of symptoms. These children survived a number of years and at postmortem were found to have involvement of about 25 per cent of renal tubules. Finally, in the juvenile form hepatomegaly was the presenting sign and the diagnosis of congenital hepatic fibrosis was often made. However, these children proved to have some 10 per cent of nephrons affected by cystic change with a radiological appearance that could be described as renal tubular ectasia. Genetic studies seemed to indicate that the four groups were separate and that a different gene mutation was responsible in each case. Other workers have not found so clear-cut a distinction. In general the pattern of inheritance is that of an autosomal recessive gene.

The diagnosis of infantile polycystic disease can often be made on clinical grounds, particularly when a second sibling is involved. It should, however, be confirmed at an early stage since bilateral hydronephrosis which is an essentially curable disease presents a somewhat similar clinical picture. High dose intravenous urograms (*Figure 14.8*) with late films and tomograms show the enlarged kidneys, the spreading

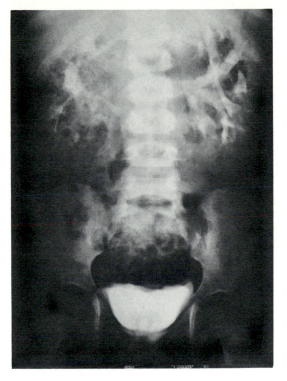

Figure 14.9. Infantile polycystic disease, juvenile form. Intravenous pyelogram in a child aged 5 years with a slight rise in the blood urea level but no significant symptoms. The liver was involved as demonstrated by biopsy. Opacification of elongated cystic spaces can be seen in the renal parenchyma.

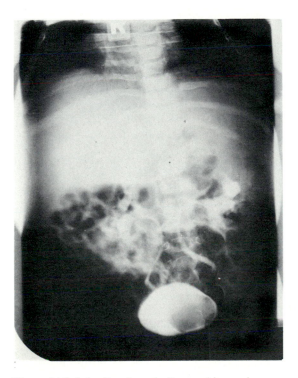

Figure 14.8. Infantile polycystic disease with ectopic ureterocele. Intravenous urogram in an infant with bilateral palpable kidneys and portal obstruction.

out of the calyceal pattern, and the opacification of multiple elongated cystic spaces throughout the parenchyma. Contrast medium may remain within these spaces for very long periods, often of several days in the neonate, although in the milder childhood and juvenile cases (*Figure 14.9*) the radiological signs are not so clear. Ultrasound scanning can give an immediate diagnostic picture.

Treatment is essentially the management of renal failure and especially the adjustment of the electrolyte balance. In children who are progressing satisfactorily the cysts do not appear to enlarge further with growth and equilibrium

may be reached. Ultimately renal transplantation may be required, provided that the condition of the liver warrants it. Genetic counselling is obligatory.

Adult polycystic disease

The adult form of polycystic disease is inherited as a dominant factor and appears in several generations of affected families. Cysts are believed to form very early in life, but they enlarge slowly (*Figure 14.10*) and do not usually present clinically until the third or fourth decade. A family history is obtained in just under 50 per cent of cases (Dalgaard, 1957) so that many must be due to new mutations.

Osathanondh and Potter (1964) found that multiple developmental anomalies are present and that cysts arise from the collecting tubules, Bowman's capsules and proximal convoluted tubules. A considerable increase in connective tissue is seen. All the cysts are likely to be in continuity with tubules in the first place, although this attachment may be lost with later expansion. The gross appearance of the kidney is highly irregular, with considerable distortion due to enlargement of individual cysts. The true form of the disease is bilateral, although asymmetry may occur and clinically the classic

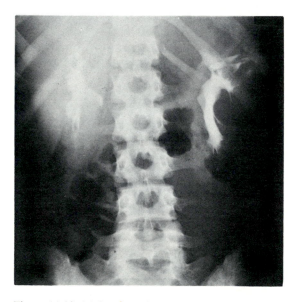

Figure 14.10. Adult polycystic disease. Intravenous urogram in a 12-year-old girl with asymmetrical cystic changes. Presentation was with left renal pain and a palpable kidney.

radiological appearance may seem to be unilateral. Liver involvement occurs in approximately one third of cases, with scattered cysts but no hepatic dysfunction in contrast to the infantile disorder. Blyth and Ockenden (1971) recorded this type of disease in childhood and even in the fetus. In general, however, there should be considerable reluctance to reach this diagnosis during childhood. Polycystic disease may be mimicked by bilateral multifocal nephroblastoma.

It is not unusual for adults suffering from polycystic disease to enquire whether their children are affected. It should be explained that a normal pyelogram during childhood does not exclude the presence of small cysts that will enlarge later. Regular ultrasound scans may elucidate this problem.

Medullary cystic disease and nephronophthisis

Gardner (1976) reviewed the literature on this subject. Over 200 cases have been reported with one or both of these diagnoses. Medullary cysts have been found in 73 per cent of those kidneys examined. They are confined to the medullary zone and usually remain rather small. Sporadic and familial cases have been described, the latter showing dominant or in childhood usually recessive types of inheritance. Children present during the first decade of life with some degree of renal failure. There is polyuria and polydipsia often associated with enuresis. Short stature with osteodystrophy is common. Anaemia and weakness are frequent complaints. On examination hypertension is often found and there is a severe urine-concentrating defect. Albuminuria, on the other hand, is unusual and neither cells nor casts are to be expected. Renal salt wasting is a prominent feature.

On intravenous pyelography the kidneys are found to be poorly opacified but of normal or decreased size, and only rarely are cysts demonstrated by distortion of the calyces or by translucent areas. Ultrasound scans may prove to be more efficient.

The prognosis of this disease is poor and involves hypertension and progressive renal failure. Ocular defects including retinitis pigmentosa may add to the child's misery. Rarely, hepatic fibrosis may be an accompanying feature (Delaney, Mullaney and Bourke, 1978).

Medullary sponge kidney

The so-called sponge kidney is typically a disease of adult life and has nothing in common with medullary cystic disease. Elongated tubular cysts are found in the pyramids and do not affect other parts of the kidney. Complicating calculus formation in the cystic spaces is very common, and passage of stones together with complicating urinary infection is the usual presenting complaint. The disease is usually but not always bilateral and can be associated with hemihypertrophy of the body (Harrison and Williams, 1971). It has rarely been described in childhood although Snelling, Brown and Smythe (1970) reported one case. The diagnosis is made radiologically from the presence of

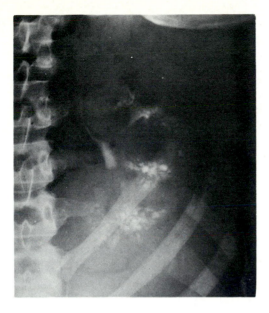

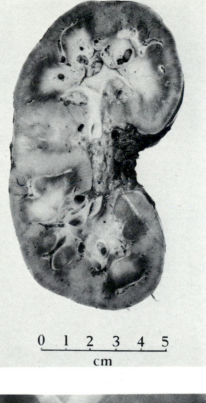

Figure 14.11. Sponge kidney. Intravenous pyelogram (left) and nephrectomy specimen (right) from an adolescent with unilateral disease.

calcium density opacifications in the papillae and on intravenous pyelography when filling of the cysts produces brush-like projections from the calyces (*Figure 14.11*). The cysts seldom fill in retrograde studies. The differential diagnosis is concerned with other causes of nephrocalcinosis as well as different forms of cystic disease. Treatment deals with the elimination of infection and occasionally the removal of obstructive calculi.

Serous cysts

The very common serous cysts found in adult life which frequently require differentiation from tumours are hardly ever encountered in childhood and appear to be an acquired disease. A few cases have, however, been collected by Siegel and McAlister (1980) and some of these appear to have a congenital basis. The case illustrated in *Figure 14.12* presented as a renal swelling provisionally diagnosed as a tumour. Rather more often large peripheral cysts are found in cases of urinary obstruction when the rest of the kidney is normal. Such examples have been seen in hydronephrosis and ectopic ureterocele, and the majority have occurred in boys with urethral valves. It has been suggested

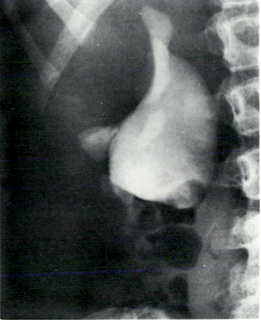

Figure 14.12. Solitary cyst. The intravenous pyelogram in a girl of 8 years with right renal pain. There is hydronephrosis due to pelviureteric obstruction and a mass in the upper pole of the right kidney, the capsule of which is faintly calcified.

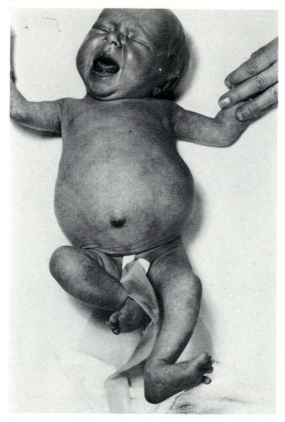

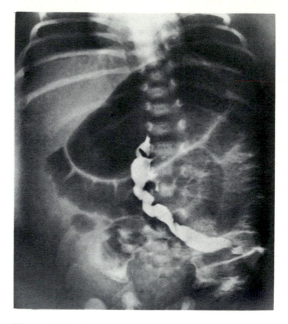

Figure 14.13. Solitary cyst in a case of urethral valves. A ureterostomy had been performed for severe obstruction with a functionless right kidney. The retrograde uretero-gram shows enormous displacement of the left kidney by a cyst which has probably formed by encapsulated extravasation. Clinically an abdominal mass is visible.

that some of these represent a partial rupture of the kidney with extravasation which becomes encysted (*Figure 14.13*). Treatment consists of aspirating or uncapping the cyst, which is solitary and has a good prognosis.

Multilocular cysts (cystadenomas)

The multilocular cyst is a rare condition closely simulating tumour, and its pathological differentiation from cystic and relatively benign forms of nephroblastoma is a matter of considerable difficulty. Pathological specimens show that multiple cysts are enclosed within a single capsule and are clearly distinguishable from the remainder of the kidney, but the cystic mass itself prolapses into the renal pelvis and can cause hydronephrosis. Histologically the cysts are lined by a simple flattened epithelium without renal elements. Radiologically and on ultrasound multilocular cysts can hardly be distinguished from nephroblastoma and therefore in

almost all cases nephrectomy is undertaken before diagnosis. The prognosis is excellent (Johnson *et al.*, 1973).

Pyelogenic cysts (calyceal diverticula)

Small and usually solitary cystic spaces in the normal parenchyma of the kidney communicating through a narrow track with a normal calyx are classified under this heading and are not uncommon. The cysts are lined by flattened epithelium and occasionally contain a stone. Some authors have emphasized the connection with pyelonephritis, although many examples are seen in apparently normal kidneys. Often the child has been investigated for recurrent infection or abdominal pain and the exact relationship between the cysts and the symptoms is obscure. Surgery is seldom required but with persistent infection or stone partial nephrectomy may be advised. This disorder should be distinguished from hydrocalycosis in which the infundibulum is obstructed and the calyx is dilated. These cases are further discussed in Chapter 17.

Microcystic disease

In the form of congenital nephrotic syndrome commonly seen in Finland cystic dilatation of the proximal tubule is found and referred to as microcystic disease. Clinically there is no suggestion of cysts and this disorder is not therefore discussed further.

Cystic disease and multiple anomaly syndromes

The Beckwith-Wiedemann syndrome characteristically causes exomphalos, macroglossia and gigantism (Irving, 1970). It may come to the notice of the urologist because of enlargement of the clitoris in a female or undescended testes in a male, and clinically there may also be exophthalmos and bony abnormalities of the metacarpals and the phalanges. Some patients have renal failure and a characteristic urographic appearance similar to that of the medullary sponge kidney but also associated with opacified cystic spaces in the parenchyma as seen in calyceal diverticula. The genital associations have been described by Charro Salgado *et al.* (1977).

In tuberose sclerosis multiple cysts or hamartomas are common and present a radiological appearance somewhat similar to that of adult polycystic disease. Other features of the syndrome which should enable a diagnosis to be made are epilepsy, mental deficiency, and adenoma sebaceum on the face.

There are rarer multiple congenital anomaly syndromes in which renal cysts are a feature. For example they are common in the autosomal trisomy syndromes (reviewed by Taylor, 1968). In Edward's syndrome (trisomy 18) cortical cysts are found in 15 per cent of cases and in Patau's syndrome (trisomy 13–15) in 33 per cent. The kidney lesion is a relatively unimportant feature of the total syndrome, which involves growth and developmental retardation with mental defect. Several other familial conditons often associated with renal cysts and believed to be due to autosomal recessive genes are described in the literature. These include the Zellweger cerebrohepatorenal syndrome, that is cerebral malformation and ocular and genital malformations with hepatic biliary dysgenesis (Bowen *et al.*, 1964; Jan *et al.*, 1970); Meckel's syndrome, namely microcephaly, occipital encephalocele, cleft lip and palate, and polydactyly (Hsia, Bratu and Herbordt, 1971); Jeune's syndrome of osteochondrodystrophic dwarfism with a small thorax (Herdman and Langer, 1968); the Laurence-Moon-Biedl syndrome of obesity, hypogonadism, retinitis pigmentosa and polydactyly (Alton and McDonald, 1973); chromosomal translocation syndromes (Talvik *et al.*, 1973); short rib polydactyly syndromes (Spranger *et al.*, 1974); Ehlers-Danlos syndrome (Imahori *et al.*, 1969); the oral-facial-digital syndrome (Doege *et al.*, 1964); and the lissencephaly syndrome (Dicker *et al.*, 1969). The renal cystic change is often, although by no means invariably, minor in extent. In Meckel's, Zellweger's and Jeune's syndromes pathological features of renal dysplasia may be present, and in the first it is bilateral and marked.

Similar cystic dysplastic changes have been described in association with the Dandy-Walker malformation of internal hydrocephalus with cystic dilatation of the fourth ventricle (D'Agnostino, Kernohan and Brown, 1963). It is of interest that in Meckel's and Zellweger's syndromes changes of congenital hepatic fibrosis indistinguishable from those associated with infantile polycystic disease are constantly found. Renal cysts are also recorded in the Von Hippel-Lindau syndrome with retinal angiomas and cerebellar haemangioblastomas.

References

Alton, D.J. and McDonald, P. (1973) Urographic findings in the Bardet-Biedl syndrome. *Radiology*, **109**, 659

Baert, L. (1978) Cystic kidneys, renal dysplasia and microdissection data in 5 children with congenital valvular urethral obstruction. *European Urology*, **4**, 382

Bernstein, J. (1968) Developmental abnormalities of the renal parenchyma: renal hypoplasia and dysplasia. *In* Pathology Annual (edited by Sommers, S.C.). Appleton-Century-Crofts, New York

Blyth, H. and Ockenden, B.G. (1971) Polycystic disease of kidneys and liver presenting in childhood. *Journal of Medical Genetics*, **8**, 257

Bowen, P., Lee C.S., Zellweger, H. and Lindenberg, R. (1964) Familial syndrome of multiple congenital defects. *Bulletin of the Johns Hopkins Hospital*, **114**, 402

Carter, C.O. (1974) Polycystic disease presenting in childhood. *In* 5th Conference on the Clinical Delineation of Birth Defects. Birth Defects Original Article Series, Vol. 10. Liss, New York. p.16

Carter, J.E. and Lirenman, D.S. (1970) Bilateral renal hypoplasia with oligomeganephronia: oligomeganephronic renal hypoplasia. *American Journal of Diseases of Children*, **120**, 537

Charro Salgado, A.L., Lopez Macia, A., Friere, P.P. and Fernandez-Cruz, A. (1977) Beckwith-Wiedeman syndrome with medullary sponge kidneys. *European Urology,* **3**, 108

D'Agnostino, A.N., Kernohan, J.W. and Brown, J.R. (1963) The Dandy Walker syndrome. *Journal of Neuropathology and Experimental Neurology,* **22**, 450

Dalgaard, O.Z. (1957) Bilateral polycystic disease of the kidneys: a follow-up study of 284 patients and their families. *Acta medica Scandinavica,* Suppl. 328

Darmady, E.M., Offer, J. and Woodhouse, M.A. (1970) Toxic metabolic defect in polycystic kidneys, evidence from microscopic studies. *Lancet,* i, 547

Delaney, V., Mullaney, J. and Bourke, E. (1978) Juvenile nephronophthisis, congenital hepatic fibrosis and retinal hypoplasia in twins. *Quarterly Journal of Medicine,* **47**, 281

Dicker, H., Edwards, R.H., Zukhein, G., Chou, S.M., Hartman, H.A. and Opitz, J.M. (1969) The lissencephaly syndrome. First Conference on the Clinical Delineation of Birth Defects. Birth Defects Original Article Series (edited by Bergsma, D.). Liss, New York. p.53

Doege, T.C., Thuline, H.C., Priest, J.H., Norby, D.E. and Bryant, J.S. (1964) Studies of a family with the oral-facial-digital syndrome. *New England Journal of Medicine,* **271**, 1073

Dunnill, M.S., Millard, P.R. and Oliver, D. (1977) Acquired cystic disease of the kidneys: a hazard of long-term intermittent maintenance dialysis. *Journal of Clinical Pathology,* **30**, 868

Ericsson, N.O. and Ivemark, B.I. (1958) Renal dysplasia and pyelonephritis in infants and children. *Archives of Pathology,* **66**, 255

Fetterman, G.H. and Habib, R. (1969) Congenital bilateral oligonephronic renal hypoplasia. *American Journal of Clinical Pathology,* **52**, 199

Gardner, K.D. (1976) Cystic Diseases of the Kidney. John Wiley and Sons, New York. p.173

Harrison, A.R. and Williams, J.P. (1971) Medullary sponge kidney and congenital hemihypertrophy. *British Journal of Urology,* **43**, 552

Heggö, O. and Natvig, J.B. (1965) Cystic disease of the kidneys: a microdissection study. *Acta Pathologica et Microbiologica Scandinavica,* **63**, 500

Herdman, R.C. and Langer, L.W. (1968) The thoracic asphyxiant dystrophy and renal disease. *American Journal of Diseases of Children,* **116**, 192

Hodson, C.J., Drewe, J.A., Karn, M.N. and King, A. (1962) Renal size in normal children. *Archives of Disease in Childhood,* **37**, 616

Hooper, J.W. (1958) Cystic disease of the kidneys in infants. *Journal of Urology,* **79**, 917

Hsia, Y.E., Bratu, M. and Herbordt, A. (1971) Genetics of the Meckel syndrome (dysencephalia splanchnocystica). *Pediatrics,* **48**, 237

Imahori, S., Bannerman, R.M., Grof, C.J. and Brennan, J.C. (1969) Ehlers-Danlos syndrome with multiple arterial lesions. *American Journal of Medicine,* **47**, 967

Irving, J.M. (1970) The EMG syndrome. *In* Progress in Pediatric Surgery, Vol. 1 (edited by Rickham, P.P., Hecker, W.C. and Prevot, J.). Urgan and Schwarzenberg, Munich

Jan, J.E., Hardwick, D.F., Lowry, R.B. and McCormick, A.Q. (1970) Cerebro-hepato-renal syndrome of Zellweger. *American Journal of Diseases of Children,* **119**, 274

Javadpour, N., Chelouhy, E., Moncada, L., Rosenthal, I.M. and Bush, I.M. (1970) Hypertension in a child caused by a multi-cystic kidney. *Journal of Urology,* **104**, 918

Johnson, D.E., Ayala, A.G., Medellin, H. and Wilbur, J. (1973) Multilocular renal cystic disease in children. *Journal of Urology,* **109**, 101

Kampmeier, O.F. (1923) A hitherto unrecognised mode of origin of congenital renal cysts. *Surgery, Gynecology and Obstetrics,* **36**, 208

Osathanondh, V. and Potter, E.L. (1964) Pathogenesis of polycystic kidneys. *Archives of Pathology,* **77**, 466

Pathak, I.G. and Williams, D.I. (1964) Multicystic and cystic dysplastic kidneys. *British Journal of Urology,* **36**, 318

Resnick, J.S., Brown, D.M. and Vernier, L. (1976) *In* Cystic Diseases of the Kidneys (edited by Gardner, K.D.). John Wiley and Sons, New York. p.221

Reuterskiold, G. and Wilbrand, H. (1971) The Ask-Upmark kidney. *Fortschritte auf dem Gebiete der Röntgenstrahlen,* **115**, 752

Risdon, R.A. (1971) Renal dysplasia. *Journal of Clinical Pathology,* **24**, 57

Scheinman, J.I. and Abelson, H.T. (1970) Bilateral renal hypoplasia with oligonephronia. *Journal of Pediatrics,* **76**, 369

Siegel, M.J. and McAlister, W.H. (1980) Simple cysts in Children. *Journal of Urology,* **123**, 75

Snelling, C.E., Brown, N.M. and Smythe, C.A. (1970) Medullary sponge kidney in a child. *Journal of the Canadian Medical Association,* **102**, 518

Spranger, J., Grimm, B., Weller, U., Weissenbacker, G., Hermann, J., Gilbert, E. and Krepler, R. (1974) Short rib polydactyly syndromes. *Zeitschrift für Kinderheilkunde,* **116**, 73

Talvik, T., Mikel'saar, A-V, Mikel'saar, R., Kaosaar, R. and Tuur, S. (1973) Inherited translocations in two families. *Humangenetik,* **19**, 215

Taylor, A.I. (1968) Autosomal trisomy syndromes. *Journal of Medical Genetics,* **5**, 227

15 Vesicoureteric Reflux

P.G. Ransley

Introduction

The normal ureterovesical junction allows free passage of urine in a prograde manner from the ureter into the bladder and prevents flow in the reverse direction even when the bladder is contracting. If this valvular mechanism is deficient, from whatever cause, the urine can flow back from the bladder into the ureter and the kidney creating the phenomenon of vesicoureteric reflux. A wide variety of factors can affect the ureterovesical junction and produce vesicoureteric reflux, which must not be considered as a single entity. Even in its most straightforward mode of occurrence and presentation vesicoureteric reflux remains one of the most controversial management problems in paediatric urology. Its chief consequence is the development of chronic pyelonephritic scarring which may lead to the secondary development of hypertension and to chronic renal failure.

The earliest recognition of the antireflux mechanism of the normal ureterovesical junction is attributed to Galen (150 AD) who noticed during postmortem studies that after tying off the urethra and filling the bladder no urine passed backwards up the ureters. Experimental studies confirming vesicoureteric reflux began at the end of the 19th century although the advent of contrast cystograms was necessary for detailed investigation. Gruber (1929) showed that there was species variation in the occurrence of reflux and that it was common in rabbits, less frequent in dogs and rare in pigs and humans. As early as 1924 Bumpus reviewed over 1000 cystograms in a wide variety of urological conditions, but the very variety of cases prevented recognition of the clear relationship between reflux and chronic pyelonephritis and at this stage reflux was regarded as a secondary phenomenon. The next 30 years saw little change in attitudes to vesicoureteric reflux, which was not regarded as a very serious problem.

During the 1950s there was renewed surgical interest with the development of antireflux procedures. At this time much more attention was paid to the bladder neck rather than the ureterovesical junction as the primary cause of the phenomenon and many unnecessary operations to relieve nonexistent bladder neck obstruction were performed. In 1958 there was the publication of what was to become one of the standard techniques for antireflux surgery by Politano and Leadbetter. Shortly afterwards the causative relationship between reflux and chronic pyelonephritis was established in a paper by Hodson and Edwards (1960) which remains one of the most important single contributions to this subject. Since that time a large number of clinical studies have been performed in relation to vesicoureteric reflux, urinary tract infection and renal scarring, yet there is still confusion about the correct method of management in any individual case.

The normal ureterovesical junction (*Figure 15.1*)

For most of its length the ureteric muscle exists in a loose irregular spiral and the fibres become parallel as the ureter penetrates the bladder wall. The intravesical ureter contains parallel longitudinal muscle fibres only and these fan out to form the muscle of the superficial trigone which extends down into the posterior urethra as far as the verumontanum. As the ureter

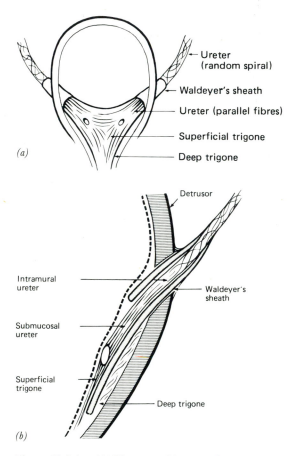

(a)

(b)

Figure 15.1 *(a and b)* Diagrams of the normal ureterovesical junction.

penetrates the bladder wall it becomes surrounded by a fibrous sheath (Waldeyer's sheath) fixed to the adventitia of the ureter just outside the bladder and extending downwards to gain attachment to the deep trigone. The ureter lies freely within the space enclosed by the sheath and so is able to move and adapt to different degrees of bladder filling. It continues onwards to lie submucosally within the bladder lumen.

The action of the ureterovesical valvular mechanism probably depends on the length of the submucosal intravesical segment and therefore indirectly on the ability of the trigonal

muscle to maintain this length. Providing there is adequate support from detrusor muscle behind the ureter the latter is compressed by any rise in intravesical pressure and reflux does not occur. Other mechanisms such as actual closure of the ureteric ostium and peristaltic activity probably also contribute since reflux can be demonstrated more easily in the dehydrated state when urine flow is reduced. The intravesical ureter grows longer with increasing age and this natural process may ultimately produce sufficient length to convert a primarily refluxing junction into a nonrefluxing one, that is spontaneous resolution of vesicoureteric reflux. Conversely any pathological process distorting the anatomy or normal function of the ureterovesical junction may result in secondary vesicoureteric reflux.

Pathogenesis and classification of vesicoureteric reflux

Primary reflux

Primary reflux is so called because it is thought to arise as the result of a primary failure of development of the ureterovesical junction mechanism. Such reflux is therefore thought to originate when urine production begins in the fifth month of intrauterine life. This description therefore includes all cases of vesicoureteric reflux without evidence of any other urological pathology. The great majority of children with reflux fall into this category.

Secondary reflux

Secondary reflux is defined as reflux that occurs as a result of other urinary tract pathology and therefore arises *de novo* at any time. The use of this classification is convenient because treatment for secondary reflux is usually dictated by the primary pathology, but the definitions should not be adhered to slavishly. For instance the ureter associated with a congenital paraureteric diverticulum and no outflow obstruction behaves much more like a primary case in terms of renal changes since bladder pressures are low. Conversely reflux occurring in response to detrusor instability without any obvious structural cause may be transient and resolve spontaneously while producing severe upper tract dilatation in the meantime. There has been much interest in recent years in the child who develops an unstable bladder and high voiding pressure and can be shown to void against a closed external sphincter (Allen, 1979). In many such children the bladder takes on the appearance of a neuropathic bladder, in the absence of any detectable neurological deficit. Although the disease may be transient, severe renal changes can occur in a short period of time.

Some ureters show reflux as the result of urinary infection and this is thought to be due to a combination of splinting of the ureterovesical junction by oedema and disturbed ureteric muscular activity. Such reflux can be classified as secondary because it occurs in response to a precipitating factor, but it is doubtful whether a completely normal junction can be made to behave in this manner and therefore there is an element of primary abnormality as well. Reflux in the ureter with a paraureteric diverticulum or in the lower moiety of a duplex system is clearly secondary while the clinical behaviour of the upper tract in these cases is very similar to that with primary reflux since the bladder is normal.

The most sinister forms of secondary reflux occur in high pressure bladders either due to outflow obstruction (commonly urethral valves) or spinal dysraphism producing a neuropathic bladder. The kidney subjected to reflux under these conditions is often severely damaged and may be nonfunctioning. Bilateral reflux in such circumstances may severely affect renal function.

Radiological features and grading of vesicoureteric reflux

Vesicoureteric reflux is of necessity diagnosed by radiological or radioisotopic techniques. The presence of reflux may be suspected from an intravenous pyelogram when there is classic pyelonephritic scarring or mild dilatation and tortuosity of the ureter (*Figure 15.2*) without evident obstruction, particularly if this dilatation increases with bladder filling during the course of the investigation. Longitudinal striation of the renal pelvis and the upper ureter

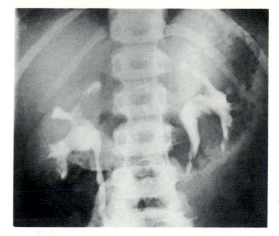

Figure 15.2. An intravenous pyelogram showing striation of the pelvis and upper ureter together with mild dilatation which is strongly suggestive of the presence of vesicoureteric reflux. The striation indicates that the system is subject to intermittent distension.

often indicates great distensibility and suggests the presence of reflux. However, these features may be misleading and a cystogram must be performed to confirm the diagnosis. The degree of ureteric dilatation on a cystogram may be much greater than that expected from the early films of a pyelogram series.

Grading of vesicoureteric reflux is convenient for communication but need not be applied too rigidly in an individual case. When comparing one case of reflux with another or sequential films in an individual case it is important to compare like with like. In other words the two images must be comparable and taken at the same stage of bladder filling or emptying. Trying to compare a cystogram at the end of filling with dense contrast medium and a subsequent 10-minute pyelogram with an empty bladder may lead to erroneous conclusions. One system of grading classifies reflux as mild, moderate and severe as follows (Rolleston, Shannon and Utley, 1970):

1. Mild, with reflux into the ureter only
2. Moderate, that is reflux filling the pelvicalyceal system without dilatation
3. Severe, namely reflux with calyceal dilatation.

Other methods divide a similar range of changes into four or five categories (Heikel and Parkkulainen, 1966). The time during cystography at which the exposure is made may considerably

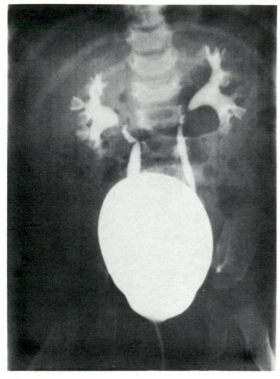

(a)

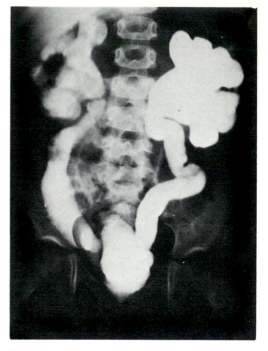

(c)

Figure 15.3. Grades of vesicoureteric reflux. *(a)* Mild; *(b)* moderate; *(c)* severe.

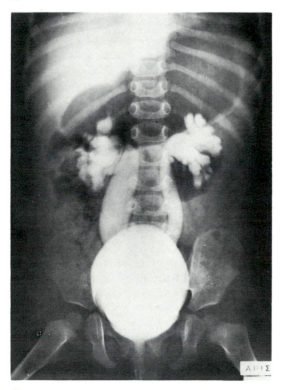

(b)

alter the radiographic appearance of the upper urinary tract dilatation, and overdistension of the bladder must be avoided. This generally occurs under anaesthesia and cystograms should ordinarily be obtained with the child awake. One of the problems with the simple grading system outlined above is that there are really many more categories beyond the 'severe' classification and at present we lack adequate criteria to differentiate between them.

Reflux may vary from a little wisp of contrast medium entering the lower ureter to massive dilatation of the whole upper urinary tract. In infants and young children this massive upper tract dilatation may be accompanied by a very large capacity thin-walled bladder and is then described as the megacystis-megaureter syndrome (*Figure 15.4*). This probably represents the extreme end of the reflux spectrum and indicates a degree of generalized urinary tract dysplasia.

The renal pelvis may distend considerably while reflux is occurring and together with the tortuosity of the upper ureter and a narrow pelviureteric junction this may give an appearance suggesting obstruction. Such secondary

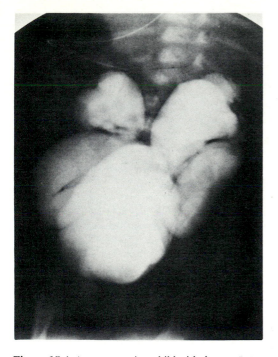

Figure 15.4. A cystogram in a child with the megacystis megaureter syndrome. The bladder has a smooth outline and is of very large capacity. The ureters and pelvicalyceal systems are massively dilated.

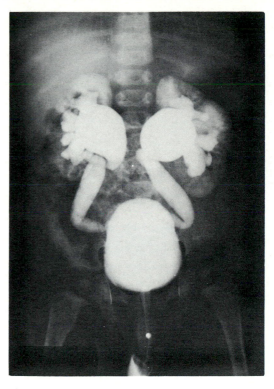

Figure 15.5. A cystogram demonstrating vesicoureteric and intrarenal reflux.

pelviureteric obstruction does occur, but it is uncommon.

Dilution of the contrast medium as it passes from a densely opacified bladder into a ureter distended with unopacified urine indicates that ureterovesical obstruction is present as well as reflux. The two phenomena can occur together as the result of either a stenosed orifice with a short tunnel or extravesical kinking of the ureter as it penetrates the bladder wall (Kesavan and Fowler, 1977).

Intrarenal reflux

When refluxed contrast medium has filled the pelvicalyceal system there is the potential for seeing the phenomenon of intrarenal reflux. This refers to the continued retrograde passage of contrast medium into the kidney along the collecting ducts and nephrons (*Figure 15.5*). A segment of renal parenchyma becomes opacified and linear streaks of contrast medium are seen radiating outwards from a calyx towards the capsule (Rolleston, Maling and Hodson, 1974; Ransley, 1977). By definition intrarenal reflux is

only seen during the course of a micturating cystogram when contrast medium is introduced from below. It has been of great interest in recent years, since this may be the mechanism by which bacteria gain access to the kidney or pressure is transmitted to the nephron itself.

Intrarenal reflux does not occur at every papilla and it is seen principally in the polar regions of the kidney where pyelonephritic scarring is also most common. The reason for this lies in the morphology of the renal papillae (Ransley and Risdon, 1975a). Intrarenal reflux only occurs where the papillae fuse together and lose their conical form to become larger structures presenting a flat or concave surface to the calyx (*Figure 15.6*). This fusion comes about predominantly in the poles of the kidney. The fact that the phenomenon of intrarenal reflux is seen only rarely even in a large series of cystograms has many possible explanations. For example the actual amount of contrast medium entering the kidney tubules is minute compared to the volume in the pelvicalyceal system and may escape X-ray detection. Alternatively the tubules may fill to capacity with the intrarenal

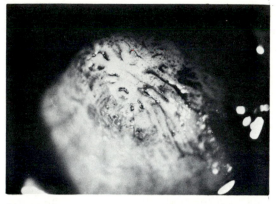

(a)

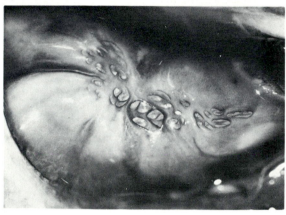

(b)

Figure 15.6. Two morphological variations of the renal papilla. *(a)* A conical papilla which is 'nonrefluxing', that is it does not allow intrarenal reflux to occur. *(b)* A compound papilla with large papillary ducts on a concave surface. This is a 'refluxing' papilla via which intrarenal reflux occurs when vesicoureteric reflux is present.

reflux of unopacified urine before the contrast medium arrives from the bladder. However, the most likely reason for the rarity with which intrarenal reflux is observed is that areas susceptible to this phenomenon develop scars before the first cystogram is performed and are therefore obliterated.

Dynamics of reflux

In a urinary tract with reflux bladder pressures are freely transmitted into the ureter and the pelvicalyceal system whether or not the ureter is dilated. Indeed the pressure is transmitted more freely by a dilated system (Ong, Ferguson and Stephens, 1974). With a normal bladder and a normal calibre ureter the intravesical pressure is low during filling and urine is conducted by ureteric peristalsis. When the bladder contracts during voiding the ureter distends and the pressure in the renal pelvis rises sharply, to return to normal a few seconds later. The kidney is probably little affected by such a short-term alteration in dynamics.

The situation is very different with a high pressure trabeculated bladder and a dilated ureter. Unstable bladder contractions occur during the filling phase, and towards the end of bladder filling there is a sustained pressure rise within the system as a whole so that the kidney has to produce urine against this elevated pressure, which is a situation more akin to urinary obstruction than to reflux. The incompetent ureterovesical junction is important because it allows the bladder pressure to be transmitted freely to the kidney all the time and results in obstructive changes. Peristalsis is generally ineffective under such circumstances and the kidney has to continue to secrete urine against a sustained back-pressure. In the absence of reflux the kidney does not show such extensive changes since the ureter continues to bear the brunt of the task of emptying into the high pressure bladder, and the kidney may continue to secrete urine into the renal pelvis at normal or only moderately elevated pressures.

Under conditions of bladder outflow obstruction the cystogram often shows dramatic vesicoureteric reflux. These appearances should not be taken to represent the fluid movements occurring naturally since the system is completely emptied by catheterization immediately prior to the cystogram and such complete emptying does not normally occur.

Residual urine is one of the most important consequences of vesicoureteric reflux. Even though the bladder may empty completely it partially refills with refluxed urine almost immediately and this residual volume may be important in the aetiology of recurrent urinary tract infection.

Reflux and urinary tract infection

Vesicoureteric reflux is generally detected as a result of investigation of urinary tract infection and is the commonest abnormality revealed. Between 30–50 per cent of girls suffering from urinary tract infection are found to have vesicoureteric reflux (Smellie and Normand, 1966), and this figure underlines the importance of the micturating cystogram in this group of patients. Interestingly a similar incidence is found among girls with asymptomatic bacteriuria.

Infants with severe vesicoureteric reflux and small shrunken kidneys that are often severely dysplastic may present with life-threatening infection, septicaemia, disseminated intravascular coagulation and acute-on-chronic renal failure. Such infection is assumed to be blood borne and affects males as often as females for the first few months of life after which girls dominate the clinical picture. The infection presumably occurs as the result of breakdown of the normal defence mechanisms in the urinary tract. Reflux may contribute to susceptibility by promoting residual urine but the volumes involved may be very small and this does not seem likely to be the only factor involved. It is not possible to separate children with reflux from those without simply on the basis of symptoms accompanying urinary tract infection, although fever and loin pain are more common in the former.

Urinary tract infection does not affect spontaneous resolution of reflux (Smellie and Normand, 1975). Conversely the resolution of reflux either spontaneously or following operation does not automatically mean the end of infections and some evidence suggests that they may continue to occur with the same frequency after surgery (Scott and Stansfeld, 1968). However, the symptoms accompanying any such infection may be decreased and this at least is of some benefit. If asymptomatic bacteriuria continues after the cessation of reflux then the patient should be treated with the same philosophy as a child who is found not to have reflux at the time asymptomatic bacteriuria is discovered. In general this means no antibiotic therapy. Parents of children with reflux should not receive a promise that the problem of urinary tract infection will disappear completely following reimplantation of the ureters because this may breed frustration and anxiety in the postoperative period.

Vesicoureteric reflux is one of the mechanisms by which bacteria can reach the kidneys and produce the clinical symptoms of acute pyelonephritis. Extension of the infection into the kidney by intrarenal reflux may be a crucial factor in the development of chronic pyelonephritic scarring.

Reflux and chronic pyelonephritis

The majority of children with vesicoureteric reflux have normal kidneys. When the kidney is abnormal and shows the classic features of chronic pyelonephritis it is generally assumed that it is expressing acquired disease. Nevertheless the change from normal to abnormal is rarely witnessed and one cannot be certain. The differentiation between congenital dysplasia and acquired pyelonephritis when the kidney is already scarred becomes quite impossible on radiological grounds. Histological examination may be able to help in the early stages, but specimens are never available for investigation. The only kidneys seen by the histopathologist are end-stage shrunken ones in which any pathological clues to causation have been destroyed.

In some severe cases, when infants present in chronic renal failure with massively dilated refluxing urinary tracts and tiny cystic dysplastic kidneys, it is quite evident that the renal state is derived from abnormal fetal development. What is not clear is whether or not reflux itself is an important factor in the genesis of the dysplasia or simply a phenomenon accompanying a poorly developed urinary tract. It is known that urinary tract obstruction *in utero* can produce renal dysplasia and it is possible that reflux acting in its obstructive mode may be causative. Mackie and Stephens (1975) have developed a rival theory in which the position of the ureteric orifice on the trigone is related to the degree of associated renal dysplasia. The position of the ureteric orifice indicates the site of origin of the ureteric bud which has to make contact with the adjacent mesoderm of the metanephros. The supposition of Mackie and Stephens (1975) is that the mesoderm is normal only in a small area overlying the normal ureteric position and that an abnormal ureteric bud arising too far cranially (laterally ectopic within the bladder) or caudally (in the bladder neck, the urethra or the vagina) makes contact with mesoderm lacking the capacity to develop into a normal kidney so that a dysplastic kidney results. This theory fits the common forms of duplex kidney in which one or other pole is dysplastic and associated with an ectopic orifice while the other is normal. However, the correlation is less clear with kidneys possessing a single orifice.

A kidney affected by chronic pyelonephritis

may demonstrate a range of changes. The commonest site for a single scar is in the upper pole when the calyx is dilated and drawn over to the midline, the papillary impression is lost and the overlying parenchyma is thinned, particularly along the medial border. A more severely affected kidney may show further areas of involvement with localized thinning and depression of the renal parenchyma overlying a dilated clubbed calyx. In its most severe form the kidney appears small and contracted and every

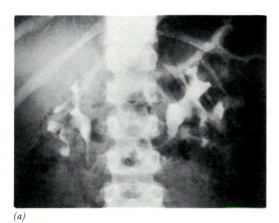

(a)

(b)

Figure 15.7. Severe chronic pyelonephritic scarring. *(a)* Unilateral. There is compensatory hypertrophy of the opposite normal kidney. *(b)* Bilateral widespread pyelonephritic change with accompanying calyceal dilatation.

calyx is involved (*Figure 15.7*). Lesions may be unilateral or bilateral and there is no recognizable pattern to the way in which pairs of kidneys are involved. A severely contracted kidney may have a contralateral fellow showing any of the whole range of changes from compensatory hypertrophy with a normal outline to similar severe involvement.

Chronic pyelonephritis is a very specific term which refers to the segmental lesion already described and is in practice a radiological diagnosis confirmed occasionally by histological examination. It is not a clinical diagnosis. The term reflux nephropathy has come into widespread use in recent years and is synonymous with chronic nonobstructive pyelonephritis.

The association between vesicoureteric reflux and chronic pyelonephritis was first clearly defined by Hodson and Edwards in 1960 but the precise mechanism of renal damage is still not completely resolved. The scars are segmental in nature and strictly related to a calyx. They occur most frequently at the upper pole of the kidney, less commonly at the lower pole and least often in the mid-zone. The parenchymal outline is often difficult to see even when scarring affects the lateral margins of the kidney, and the calyceal changes are much more apparent while less specific. Ultrasound and renal scanning with dimercaptosuccinic acid (DMSA) are becoming increasingly useful in the recognition and assessment of renal scars and may ultimately replace classic pyelography. Radioisotopic scanning with DMSA gives a particularly clear idea of the residual mass of functional renal parenchyma, which can be surprisingly less than may be inferred from the pyelograms. The individual kidney glomerular filtration rate determined by computerized diethylenetriaminepentacetic-acid (DTPA) scans allows assessment of the progress of a kidney with reflux whether or not it is scarred.

The overall incidence of renal scarring in vesicoureteric reflux depends on how cases are gathered, the quality of the radiology and the minimum accepted as a scar. Between 30–60 per cent of children with reflux who present with urinary tract infection have renal scarring. The most enigmatic feature is the fact that the formation of a scar in a previously normal kidney is very rarely documented radiologically. Those kidneys that have scars do not often change very significantly in the follow-up period and further new scarring is also an extremely rare event (Smellie *et al.*, 1975). Therefore, if a kidney is going to develop a scar then it usually does so in the period prior to the initial investigation, and conversely if it is normal at that time then it is likely to remain so during subsequent follow-up.

This curious behaviour has been explained by the persuasive theory that renal scarring is dependent on intrarenal reflux (Hodson *et al.*, 1975). Experimental work in pigs, which have multipapillary kidneys very similar to human ones, has shown that intrarenal reflux of infected urine results in rapid tubular destruction of the affected area. The human kidney is made up of 14 separate lobes each with its own individual papilla and these lobes fuse during development so that the mature kidney contains eight or nine papillae. The great majority of these are conical in form and do not allow intrarenal reflux to occur. In fact postmortem studies show that one third of children's kidneys possess only this nonrefluxing type of papilla and so intrarenal reflux cannot occur (Ransley and Risdon, 1975b). Most of the remaining two thirds have a single compound papilla at the upper pole only, the remainder being of the simple variety. Some have compound papillae at both upper and lower poles but the occurrence of kidneys with a majority of compound papillae is quite rare. This prevalence of papillary type fits in well with the observed pattern of renal scarring in any large series of cases.

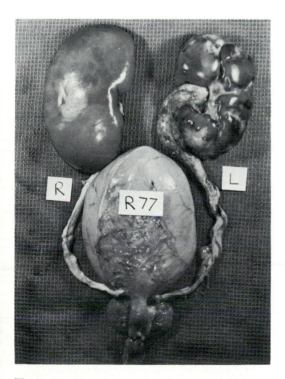

Figure 15.8. Experimental chronic pyelonephritic scarring. Unilateral vesicoureteric reflux and urinary infection have resulted in extensive scar formation on the refluxing side. There is no scarring in the nonrefluxing kidney in spite of chronic urinary infection.

It has been shown experimentally that when a kidney bearing compound papillae is subjected to vesicoureteric reflux so that intrarenal reflux occurs then the potential for scarring exists (Ransley and Risdon, 1978). If the urine remains sterile and the resting bladder pressure is normal, no parenchymal damage occurs and the kidney grows normally, that is sterile intrarenal reflux does not give rise to segmental renal damage. However, once urinary infection is established scarring may occur very rapidly (*Figure 15.8*). Although intrarenal reflux is the key factor and predetermines the areas in which scarring can occur, there are probably a number of factors that determine the speed of development and the extent of scarring within an area of intrarenal reflux. Given the right combination of pathogenic bacteria and bladder function dramatic and extensive scarring can occur in a matter of days and all kidneys studied experimentally have shown scars after only 2 weeks of reflux and urinary tract infection (Ransley and Risdon, 1980). Once scarring has occurred and involved all the areas capable of intrarenal reflux in a kidney, further episodes of urinary tract infection do not produce further damage since the remaining healthy renal parenchyma is *ipso facto* drained by simple papillae (*Figure 15.9*).

The nature of clinical investigation means almost certainly that children are investigated for reflux after one or more recognized or unrecognized urinary tract infections. It is therefore to be expected that no further change in the appearance of the kidney will occur in response to further episodes of infection.

This explanation of a common clinical observation leans heavily on a limited amount of experimental work and further clinical trials are required, but in the absence of any other evidence it is a useful hypothesis on which to base current treatment. The process of fibrosis and scar contraction together with growth of the surrounding parenchyma sufficient to render the scar visible on a pyelogram seems to take approximately 6 months and this must be taken into account when assessing an individual case.

Many other factors influence the scarring process. Prompt treatment may reduce the degree of permanent damage. The ability of the bacteria involved to adhere to mucosal surfaces due to the presence of fimbriae may be important. The roles of Tamm Horsfall protein, vascular changes and immune response are all

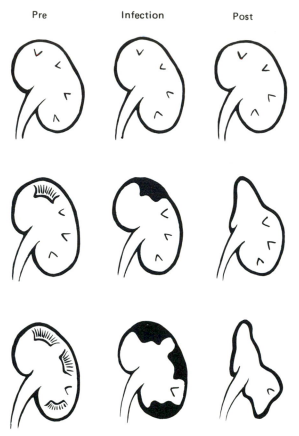

Pre   Infection   Post

Figure 15.9. Diagrammatic representation of the pathogenic mechanism of the formation of chronic pyelonephritic scars. The diagram is read from left to right. In each row the left hand kidney represents the situation with vesicoureteric reflux but no infection. The middle kidney shows the response to the combination of reflux and infection and the consequence of this is shown on the right. In the top row the kidney has no 'refluxing' papillae and there is no intrarenal reflux and no scar formation. The middle row represents the commonest situation of a single compound 'refluxing' papilla at the upper pole and the area of kidney subject to intrarenal reflux becomes scarred following an episode of infection. Note that only 'nonrefluxing' papillae remain once the area of intrarenal reflux has been destroyed. The bottom row indicates a kidney with a high proportion of compound 'refluxing' papillae and the combination of reflux and infection produces widespread parenchymal damage.

under investigation. Sterile reflux and intrarenal reflux appear to cause segmental renal damage only in association with generalized hydronephrotic changes under conditions of severe bladder outflow obstruction (Ransley and Risdon, 1978). This may be pertinent to renal pathology in patients with urethral valves but it is not likely to be important in primary vesicoureteric reflux.

Chronic pyelonephritis, hypertension and chronic renal failure

Chronic pyelonephritic scarring (reflux nephropathy) is one of the major causes of hypertension and chronic renal failure in childhood. Affected children are generally over 5 years old and it is common for the advent of hypertension to lead to a rapid deterioration of renal function which is often associated with proteinuria.

The development of hypertension is surprisingly common and as many as 18 per cent of children with severe bilateral renal scarring are affected on follow-up for 20 years or more (Wallace, Rothwell and Williams, 1978). The less the scarring the smaller is the risk of hypertension, and the incidence of unilateral disease of lesser extent is only 8 per cent. Nonetheless very severe hypertension may arise from a single pyelonephritic scar.

The correction of vesicoureteric reflux in a child with established pyelonephritic scarring and hypertension appears to have little influence on the outcome and hypertension may arise in a child with pyelonephritic kidneys many years after reflux has resolved spontaneously or been corrected surgically. It is therefore mandatory for any such child to have regular blood pressure measurements carried out indefinitely every 6 months–1 year.

The natural history of vesicoureteric reflux

In a case of primary vesicoureteric reflux defined by the categories in common use the general tendency is for improvement with time, probably due to a maturation process or growth of the intravesical, ureteric and trigonal musculature. Given sufficient time this may lead to complete cessation of reflux in a high proportion of cases. The latest figures from a series at University College Hospital, London, carefully followed up for 7–15 years show an overall spontaneous resolution rate for reflux of 79 per cent of ureters in 71 per cent of children (Normand and Smellie, 1979). Gross reflux was the least likely to disappear and resolution took place in 41 per cent of dilated ureters and 85 per cent of ureters of normal calibre. The occurrence of further urinary tract infection did not affect the rate. The presence of renal scarring does not directly influence the likelihood of reflux disappearing spontaneously but scarring is more commonly seen in the severer grades of reflux which themselves are less apt to resolve spontaneously. Nevertheless in the same series 63 per cent of ureters associated with scarred kidneys stopped refluxing spontaneously.

The natural history of the dynamic phenomenon of reflux is quite clearly that of improvement. The need to interfere with this natural process must depend upon the likely consequences of persistent vesicoureteric reflux while waiting for the changes at the ureterovesical junction to occur. Any such consequences need to be carefully considered from the point of view of possible harm to the child and the ease with which they can be controlled by treatment.

At present there is insufficient evidence available to make a dogmatic statement concerning the long-term consequences of vesicoureteric reflux. However, in children with normal kidneys at the outset of investigation reflux runs a very benign course and its continuation has very little effect on renal growth and function. Prophylactic chemotherapy is successful in the great majority of cases for controlling urinary tract infections and accompanying symptoms. This remains true for children with established scarring in whom the natural history of reflux follows a similar course to that in a child without scarring.

It is therefore necessary to separate the natural history of the reflux itself from that of established parenchymal damage. Scarred kidneys cannot be expected to follow normal renal growth curves and all that can be asked is that they grow to achieve their maximum potential given that the mass of parenchyma has been reduced. The renal size as measured on the intravenous pyelogram may be misleading since sinus fat may increase in bulk so that the overall measurement of renal length gives a false impression of true renal parenchymal dimensions.

The biggest problem in predicting the natural history in an individual case is the possibility of subtle changes of lower tract function. This is particularly true in younger children who may go through phases of bladder instability and dysfunctional voiding while gaining normal

urinary control. Close supervision of prophylactic therapy is required at this stage.

If children are managed conservatively and reach maturity still with reflux there is some pressure to correct this abnormality simply because it persists. This temptation should be resisted since the natural history of reflux in adult life is benign. Whether or not continuing reflux causes problems in pregnancy is unknown and as this information becomes available it will be necessary to try to separate the problems arising from pyelonephritic scarring from those due to reflux itself.

Reflux associated with bladder outflow obstruction may disappear following relief of the obstruction, but this occurs in less than half the cases. Reflux with severe bladder outflow obstruction is often accompanied by a nonfunctioning kidney that can be clearly defined by radioisotopic scanning; its treatment is by nephroureterectomy. The natural history of persistent reflux with reasonable renal function in such cases is generally benign and reflects changes in bladder function following relief of the obstruction. Intervention may be required if there is progressive upper tract dilatation, deterioration in renal function or demonstration of secondary obstructive phenomena at the ureterovesical junction. Reimplantation surgery has a much higher complication rate in the presence of a hypertrophied bladder and should not be undertaken lightly.

Investigation and treatment

The treatment of vesicoureteric reflux is complex. The era of wholesale reimplantation of ureters simply because they were refluxing has long since passed and attitudes are now generally much more conservative than they were 10 years ago. There is, however, no single plan of action that adequately copes with all the varied circumstances under which reflux occurs. Treatment depends a great deal on an understanding based on clinical experience of all the factors involved in an individual case.

Since it is known that with sterile urine and normal bladder function there is a high rate of spontaneous remission, the basic attitude may be conservative. In the presence of sterile urine there is little risk of renal scar formation, and even when recurrent infections occur most series and fundamental experimental studies indicate that there is little risk of sequential scarring. Renal growth and function may be followed during the course of treatment although they hardly ever influence the decision to operate.

A diagnosis of vesicoureteric reflux generally results from investigation of a child following a urinary tract infection. The intravenous pyelogram and the micturating cystogram are still the essential examinations and are now complemented and occasionally replaced by ultrasound and radioisotopic scanning. An early film in the pyelogram series and sufficient contrast medium are essential to see the renal outline which traditionally permits detection of renal scarring. However, scarring limited to the anterior and posterior surfaces may be more easily revealed by a DMSA renal scan which can also provide a measurement of differential renal function. The DTPA scan is less successful for imaging the renal parenchyma but can give estimations of individual kidney glomerular filtration rates and demonstrate whether or not there is free upper tract drainage. Techniques are being devised to detect vesicoureteric reflux at the completion of a DTPA scan with a voiding and postvoiding image showing retrograde movement of radioisotope. Such a method would be valuable during follow-up studies since it allows documentation of reflux or its cessation without the need for urethral catheterization. In less severe cases these radioisotopic studies are not necessary while in complicated situations both may be required to document upper tract morphology and function.

A micturating cystogram with contrast medium is essential as an initial examination to ascertain lower tract anatomy and in particular the presence of bladder diverticula and bladder outflow obstruction. Subsequent follow-up studies may utilize radioisotopic cystograms obtained either directly or indirectly since on these occasions the only question being asked is whether reflux is present or not. The requirement for a good quality contrast cystogram has been questioned in relation to older children (generally girls) in whom the pyelogram is normal. There is a great deal of support for the idea that if a girl over 5 years of age has a completely normal pyelogram then a micturating cystogram is not required. In other words, if she does have reflux then it is of a minor nature

and does not need treatment over and above that required for the control of symptoms.

Once these initial investigations have been completed prophylactic antibacterial chemotherapy is continued on an outpatient basis. Co-trimoxazole and nitrofurantoin are the commonly used agents and trimethoprim alone may prove useful, particularly in children allergic to sulphonamides. Twice-daily doses are generally advised at the outset, reducing to a single dose at night after 6 months or 1 year. The initial dose is calculated on the body weight at the beginning of treatment and if this dose is maintained it leads to an effective gradual reduction as the child grows.

Prophylactic chemotherapy may be maintained quite safely for many years and provided that the child remains well it is important not to repeat radiological investigations too often. The basic plan should be to aim at performing radiology after 2 years of conservative treatment for a child who is under 3 years at presentation and after 3 years for an older child. A proportion of cases resolve in the interim period while others continue to have reflux. If the latter remain well on prophylaxis this may be continued and a further period of conservative management planned. An interval of at least 3 years before further radiological examination during this second phase of treatment applies to all children.

How long to persist with conservative management is a matter of personal opinion. It has been shown that given sufficient time a very high proportion of cases of mild reflux resolve spontaneously and so do a significant proportion of more severe cases, especially in the younger age group. Most children seem to come to a natural decision point which usually coincides with the second follow-up examination about 6 years after presentation and before the age of 12 years. It is at this point that logic insists that either surgery should be undertaken or no further radiology is indicated. It is illogical to continue to visualize the presence of reflux while maintaining the same course of clinical action.

The author's practice, therefore, is to make a final decision in most cases at this stage. The prophylaxis should be stopped for 6 months or 1 year prior to the second set of X-rays in order to discover the clinical behaviour of the child off prophylaxis. If the cystogram continues to show reflux of minor degree then the decision can be made to stop further investigation and treatment. If the reflux is more severe, it is at this point that cystoscopy may assist coming to a decision as to whether or not surgery is required. In other words, when the evidence indicates that the reflux is of little consequence or likely to stop eventually then further unnecessary investigation and treatment can be halted. On the other hand, when it is clear from the golf-hole appearance of the ureteric orifice that the reflux is unlikely to stop spontaneously and when there have been several infections in the months after stopping prophylactic treatment then ureteric reimplantation is indicated. Surgery for reflux is a great deal easier to perform in childhood than after puberty.

This basic plan of treatment provides good care for the majority of patients with reflux, allows sufficient time for spontaneous remission in a large proportion of cases and selects those who require surgical correction. It inevitably leaves some asymptomatic children to go into adult life still with reflux. A proportion continue to resolve spontaneously through puberty but some girls inevitably continue to have reflux during reproductive life.

This protocol strictly limits the amount of radiation children with reflux receive without placing any of them at significant risk. It must be stressed that blood pressure monitoring must be continued if the child is known to have renal scars, even if further urological surveillance ceases.

Surgical management

At any stage along the path of conservative management the decision to stop and revert to surgery may be taken. A number of obvious factors quite clearly indicate when such a step is necessary and others in themselves are insufficient but over the years may gradually add up and provide an indication for reimplantation.

At the time of diagnosis of vesicoureteric reflux it is largely anatomical factors that confirm the need for surgery. A large paraureteric saccule, ectopic ureteric insertion, and the presence of both reflux and obstruction at the ureterovesical junction are the common conditions in this category. Later in the follow-up period social and functional factors become more important. Failure of medical treatment to control symptoms due to breakthrough infections is a clear indication that the programme is

failing to achieve its goal and operation is indicated. Poor compliance with drug treatment may be a factor in such cases but it should be noted that with devoted care infection can be reduced to an absolute minimum. Families who move frequently or live in isolated communities may be better served by early surgery. Strictly functional factors, such as a declining glomerular filtration rate or significant depression of renal growth, only affect the decision infrequently and such information is difficult to establish with certainty.

It should be clear from the outset that the presence of renal scars is not in itself sufficient indication for surgical treatment. The rare case of progressive scarring or new scar formation, however, is generally taken as an indication for surgery.

The most common situation is encountered in a child who gets several symptomatic infections while on prophylactic chemotherapy. In making a decision for surgery as a result of these infections it should be clear that the operation is being undertaken in order to reduce the symptomatology and not for any other reason. If the last cystogram was obtained more than 6 months prior to the decision for surgery it should be repeated before the operation.

The main surgical contribution to the management of reflux is reimplantation of the ureters or ureteroneocystostomy. In the very early stages of management other procedures may be necessary. For example in the infant with massively dilated upper tracts with reflux and a huge distended thin-walled bladder (megaureter-megacystis syndrome) a vesicostomy may be a valuable procedure to secure bladder drainage and allow urinary tract infection to be brought under control. The vesicostomy may be maintained for 1–2 years with very little inconvenience to mother or child because the urine drains directly into a nappy worn in the normal manner. If such cases are associated with very poor renal function and tiny cystic dysplastic kidneys then high urinary tract drainage may be necessary and this is best accomplished by the Y or ring ureterostomy. Such a diversion is again easy to manage with a large nappy rather than a collecting device and allows the nephrologist to concentrate on securing maximum renal function without the presence of any complicating urological factors.

Reimplantation of the ureter is a surgical procedure with few complications provided that the surgeon is familiar with the hazards and pitfalls of the various techniques. The most common complication is failure to prevent reflux and the most sinister is the occurrence of postoperative obstruction at the new ureterovesical junction. This may be due to stenosis from impairment of the ureteric blood supply or kinking at the new ureteric hiatus. Such obstruction may manifest itself early in the postoperative period and unusually prolonged postoperative vomiting must always be regarded with suspicion. However, obstruction may be delayed and insidious. For this reason follow-up radiological studies are mandatory following reimplantation. A child with early recurrence of infection and symptoms of urinary tract obstruction following surgery must be investigated without delay. In the normal course of events a DTPA scan at 3 months gives an early indication that there is satisfactory free drainage and should be followed by a repeat cystogram and intravenous pyelogram 1 year after surgery.

The surgical technique now most widely used in the UK is the Cohen advancement procedure in which the ureters are mobilized from within the bladder until sufficient length has been obtained. This entirely intravesical procedure has the dual advantages of limiting damage to the nerve supply of the bladder, which can follow extensive extravesical dissection, and avoiding any problems at the ureteric hiatus since the ureter continues to enter the bladder at the same point. Submucosal tunnels for each ureter are fashioned running across the bladder above the trigone. Each ureter therefore opens on the opposite side from the point of entry (*Figure 15.10*). This crossing over creates potential problems with retrograde pyelograms if these are required later in life but the advantages far outweigh this disadvantage and it is probably the safest method of reimplantation available today.

A modification of this technique has been described by Ahmed (1980) for dealing with megaureter. The ureter is transected at the bladder wall by a limited extravesical exposure and is then drawn through the original opening. This reduces the intravesical mucosal dissection and may be more easily combined with resection and remodelling of the ureter if required.

The Leadbetter-Politano method still enjoys wide popularity although the creation of a new entry point for the ureter higher in the bladder requires great care to avoid snaring the peri-

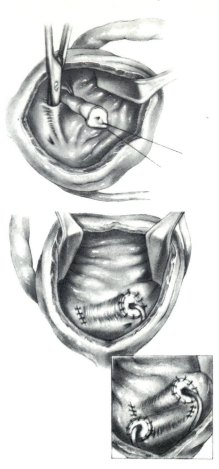

Figure 15.10. The Cohen operation.

toneum or placing the new ureteric hiatus too high or too laterally which could give rise to ureteric obstruction with a full or partially filled bladder.

Both techniques are capable of achieving successful results with correction of reflux and no obstruction in over 95 per cent of cases.

Remodelling or tapering of a grossly dilated ureter may be necessary to achieve a successful antireflux junction following reimplantation. It is generally agreed that a submucosal tunnel must be at least 2.5 times the ureteric diameter in order to prevent reflux. Since it is difficult to produce a tunnel greater than 3 cm in length it follows that ureters greater than 1 cm in collapsed 'diameter' must be considered for remodelling. In borderline cases the final decision generally rests on the quality of the ureteric musculature and peristalsis. With good active muscle there is obviously a chance that the ureter will contract further once reflux is prevented and so a larger ureteric diameter may be accepted in such circumstances. If tapering is performed, it is confined to the bottom 5–10 cm of ureter and there is no indication for extensive remodelling of the whole length of the ureter. Postoperatively remodelled ureters are drained with a small splint catheter for 10 days in addition to the bladder drainage.

Contraindications to reimplantation

In most cases reflux has a benign natural history and so it is clear that an operation to correct it must not carry any significant hazard. With normal calibre or only moderately dilated ureters and with an experienced surgeon using one of the standard techniques the risks are acceptably small. Reimplantation is contraindicated where the risks of surgical complications outweigh the potential benefit and this is a very difficult equation. The complication rate from the extensive remodelling required for reimplantation of grossly dilated ureters in the young infant is high and such cases can usually be managed conservatively without any problem in the early years. Attempted reimplantation of dilated ureters into thick-walled trabeculated bladders, for example in the case of urethral valves or neuropathic disease, also carries a greater risk and should be avoided. However, the more recent advancement procedures are considerably safer under these conditions than the traditional methods of reimplantation and the prospects for surgical intervention are being cautiously explored once more.

In general it remains true that the very poor kidney (a bad kidney), the big floppy ureter (a bad ureter) and the thick-walled trabeculated bladder (a bad bladder) both separately and particularly in combination are all significant contraindications to reimplantation surgery. The experience of the surgeon involved is an important factor and the temptation to perform a reimplantation procedure in a unit that does not regularly carry out such operations should be strongly resisted.

References

Ahmed, A. (1980) Transverse advancement ureteral reimplantation: pull-through alternative in megaloureter. *Journal of Urology*, **123**, 218

Allen, T.D. (1979) Vesicoureteral reflux as a manifestation of dysfunctional voiding. *In* Reflux Nephropathy (edited by Hodson, J. and Kincaid-Smith, P.) Masson, New York. p. 171

Bumpus, H.C. (1924) Urinary reflux. *Journal of Urology*, **12**,341

Gruber, C.M. (1929) A comparative study of the intravesical ureters (uretero-vesical valves) in man and in experimental animals. *Journal of Urology*, **21**, 567

Heikel, P.E. and Parkkulainen, K.V. (1966) Vesico-ureteric reflux in children, a classification and results of conservative treatment. *Annals of Radiology*, **9**,37

Hodson, C.J. and Edwards, D. (1960) Chronic pyelonephritis and ureteric reflux. *Radiology*, **2**,219

Hodson, C.J., Maling, T.M.J., McManamon, P.J. and Lewis, M.G. (1975) The pathogenesis of reflux nephropathy (chronic atrophic pyelonephritis). *British Journal of Radiology*, Suppl. 13

Kesavan, P. and Fowler, R. (1977) Vesico-ureteric reflux and ureterovesical obstruction. *Urology*, **10**,105

Mackie, G.G. and Stephens, F.D. (1975) Duplex kidneys: a correlation of renal dysplasia with position of the ureteral orifice. *Journal of Urology*, **114**,274

Normand, I.C.S. and Smellie, J. (1979) Vesicoureteric reflux: the case for conservative management. *In* Reflux Nephropathy (edited by Hodson, J. and Kincaid-Smith, P.). Masson, New York.p. 281

Ong, T.H., Ferguson, R.S. and Stephens, F.D. (1974) The pattern of intra-pelvic pressures during vesico-ureteral reflux in the dog with megaureters. *Investigative Urology*, **11**, 352

Politano, V.A. and Leadbetter, W.F. (1958) An operative technique for the correction of vesicoureteral reflux. *Journal of Urology*, **79**, 932

Ransley, P.G. (1977) Intrarenal reflux; anatomical dynamic and radiological studies. *Urological Research*,**5**,61

Ransley, P.G. and Risdon, R.A. (1975a) Renal papillary morphology and intrarenal reflux in the young pig. *Urological Research*, **3**, 105

Ransley, P.G. and Risdon, R.A. (1975b) Renal papillary morphology in infants and young children. *Urological Research*, **3**,111

Ransley, P.G. and Risdon, R.A. (1978) Reflux and renal scarring. *British Journal of Radiology*, Suppl. 14

Ransley, P.G. and Risdon, R.A. (1980) Reflux nephropathy: the effects of antibiotic treatment on the development of the pyelonephritic scar. *In* Pyelonephritis, Vol. 4 (edited by Losse, H., Asscher, A.W. and Lison, A.E.). Thieme, Stuttgart. p. 32

Rolleston, G.L., Shannon, F.T. and Utley, W.L.F. (1970) Relationship of infantile vesico-ureteric reflux to renal damage. *British Medical Journal*, i,460

Rolleston, G.L., Maling, T.M.J. and Hodson, C.J. (1974) Intrarenal reflux and the scarred kidney. *Archives of Disease in Childhood*, **49**,531

Scott, J.E.S. and Stansfeld, J.M. (1968) Treatment of vesico-ureteric reflux in children. *Archives of Disease in Childhood*, **43**,323

Smellie, J.M. and Normand, I.C.S. (1966) The clinical features and significance of urinary tract infection in childhood. *Proceedings of the Royal Society of Medicine*, **59**,415

Smellie, J.M. and Normand, I.C.S. (1975) Bacteriuria, reflux and renal scarring. *Archives of Disease in Childhood*, **50**,581

Smellie, J.M., Edwards, D., Hunter, N., Normand, I.C.S. and Prescod, N. (1975) Vesico-ureteric reflux and renal scarring. *Kidney International*, **8**,565

Wallace, D.M., Rothwell, D.L. and Williams, D.I. (1978) The long term follow-up of surgically treated vesico-ureteric reflux. *British Journal of Urology*, **50**,479

16 Ureteric Duplications and Ectopia

D. Innes Williams

Incidence

Duplication is one of the commonest malformations of the urinary tract and, although in many cases the function of both ureters and of their associated renal elements is normal, complications are common and present in a wide variety of forms. In children it is always important to bear in mind the possibility of duplication when reviewing pyelograms, remembering that one element may be nonopacified. Nation (1944) reviewed the incidence of duplication and found 109 cases in 16 000 autopsies while Campbell (1951) noted 342 cases in 51 880 autopsies, an approximately equal incidence of about 0.7 per cent. Duplication is more frequent in females, who are also more likely to exhibit pathological complications. The bifid ureter is commoner than complete duplication. Bilaterality is an important feature, but the type of duplication varies from one side to the other. There is an undoubted familial tendency. Whitaker and Danks (1966) found that there was a one-in-eight chance of duplication in siblings and parents.

Developmental anatomy

The ureter arises as an outgrowth from the wolffian duct. An understanding of the embryological process involved in bringing the ureteric orifice to its normal position in the bladder is essential for interpretation of the developmental anatomy of duplicated and ectopic ureters.

The wolffian ducts, which are mesodermal derivatives, are first formed in relation to the pronephric and mesonephric tubules in the dorsal wall of the coelom. The ducts grow caudally to reach the hind end of the embryo, where they turn sharply forward and at the 4–5 mm stage come in contact with the cloaca into which they open. From the angle in the wolffian duct the ureteric bud appears when the embryo reaches 5–6 mm and is soon capped by a condensation of mesenchyme from the lower end of the nephrogenic fold (*Figure 16.1*). This develops into the metanephric kidney. The ureteric bud then elongates and bifurcates repeatedly while the metanephros is carried upwards from the sacral to the lumbar region. From the ureteric bud are ultimately derived the collecting tubules, the calyces, the pelvis and the definitive ureter, and from the metanephrogenic cap the nephrons.

In the next stage of development the terminal segments of the wolffian ducts widen and are gradually absorbed into the wall of the newly formed urogenital sinus. The ureters then gain distinct orifices and are soon further separated from the wolffian ducts by the caudal movement of the latter, the intervening region giving rise to the trigone. The exact mechanism of this change has been a matter of some dispute. A full account of the development was given by Gyllensten (1949).

Normal

Duplication with ectopic ureter

Bilateral single ectopic ureter

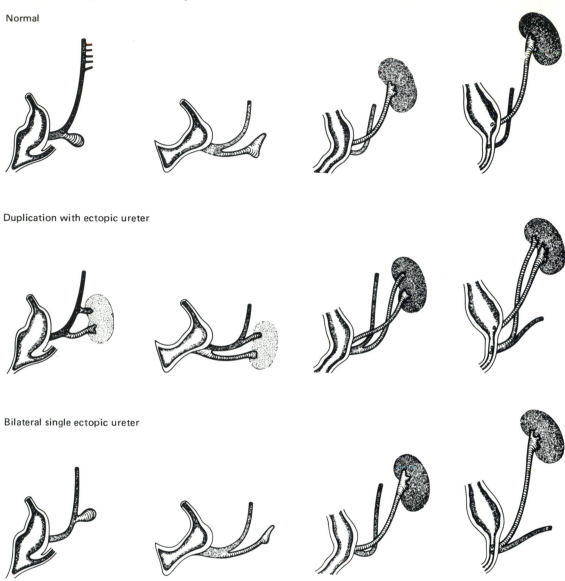

Figure 16.1 The embryology of the lower end of the ureter. The diagrams on the top line (normal) show the development of the ureteric bud on the wolffian duct, the gradual absorption of the terminal segment of the duct into the urogenital sinus, the separation of the ureter from the wolffian duct and finally the development of the bladder neck between the definitive openings of the ureter and the wolffian duct derivatives. The second line shows the corresponding situation with a ureteric duplication in which an ectopic bud is formed high up on the wolffian duct and ultimately comes to open along with the wolffian duct derivatives into the urethra. Since the lower pole ureter reaches its normal position, the development of the bladder neck is normal. The third line shows the situation in which a single ureteric bud is in the ectopic position. This retains its connection with the wolffian duct and the bladder neck is not properly formed.

In the 10 mm embryo the terminal segment of the wolffian duct opens as a funnel into the dorsolateral horn of the urogenital division of the cloaca. At the 10–14 mm stage the funnel gradually disappears, largely as a result of outgrowth of the urogenital sinus epithelium into it; although a part of the wolffian duct may be taken up in the sinus wall its epithelium is soon replaced. In this way the ureter achieves a separate opening into the sinus, but no sooner has it accomplished this than its orifice is obliterated by a heaping up of epithelial cells. A definite membrane is formed from these cells which continues to occlude the ureter until the embryo reaches 35 mm, that is to say throughout the period during which the trigonal area is being formed.

In the meantime the wolffian ducts with their widened ends form caudomedial loops immediately proximal to their entry into the sinus. Each loop is so placed that the final cranially directed limb is pressed against the wall of the sinus, and as the loop lengthens the intervening tissue between the lumen of the duct and the sinus atrophies and disappears. This process continues so that the actual opening of the duct moves caudally away from the ureteric orifice, leaving a groove in the dorsal wall of the sinus lined with wolffian duct epithelium. The groove is soon undermined by ingrowth of the sinus epithelium and obliterated. Thus the vertical extent of the trigone is formed. Its breadth is accounted for by dilatation of the upper part of the sinus to form the bladder, and the ureters do not move apart until this dilatation is evident.

Further changes then occur at the site where the wolffian ducts open into the urogenital sinus. The müllerian or paramesonephric ducts develop like the wolffian ones on the dorsal wall of the coelom, grow caudally and fuse with one another. At about the 30 mm stage their fused tip pushes up between the orifices of the wolffian ducts to form the müllerian tubercle. In the male the wolffian ducts remain as the ejaculatory ducts and Müller's tubercle as the verumontanum, and the utriculus masculinus may represent the remnant of the müllerian ducts. However, in the female the wolffian ducts atrophy in the normal embryo, while the müllerian tubercle is obliterated by the outgrowths of the sinovaginal bulbs from the urogenital sinus which form the lower part of the vagina.

Ureteric duplications come about as a result of the appearance of an accessory ureteric bud, either on the side of the normal ureter or on the wolffian duct itself. The exact site of origin of this accessory bud is of great importance in determining the ultimate anatomical relationships. Nevertheless there can be little doubt that the same embryonic inductor is responsible for all types of duplication, since the bifid ureter and the complete duplex are frequently found on opposite sides of the same subject and there is a continuous series bridging the gap between the two extremes of double pelvis and complete duplication with ectopia.

It follows from the double nature of the bud that all its derivatives are separate. Accordingly a double ureter is accompanied by a double renal pelvis, and the calyces of the two systems scarcely ever communicate. On the other hand the mass of metanephric tissue may remain single although the nephrons are differentiated in relation to two systems of collecting tubules. Thus the double kidney, while commonly longer than the normal one, shows on its surface very little evidence of its duplicity. There may be a sulcus indicating the junction of the two segments, and very rarely there is complete separation when the smaller mass is referred to as a supernumerary kidney. The blood supply to the two segments is very variable.

Figure 16.1 shows the formation of the bifid ureter that results from an accessory bud arising on the cranial side of the normal one. This accessory bud comes into contact with the upper pole of the metanephros, and in the definitive kidney the upper calyces drain into the small upper pelvis; the lower and more normal pelvis is formed from the original bud. The site of bifurcation of the ureter depends on the origin of the accessory bud so that there may be simply a bifid pelvis or the fork may lie at any lower point along the length of the ureter and even actually within the bladder wall. In the latter case the two ureters may lie parallel to one another; more often crossing in the frontal plane can be seen.

In the common type of complete duplex the accessory bud forms on the wolffian duct immediately cranial to the angle. So placed, the bud makes contact with the upper pole of the metanephros causing a kidney indistinguishable from that found in association with the common type of bifid ureter. From *Figure 16.1* it can be seen that the caudomedial loop of the wolffian duct brings the orifice of the accessory ureter into a position caudal and medial to the normal, that is to a position on the trigone nearer the internal meatus. Again the ureters may lie parallel, but frontal crossing in two places is the rule. The two ureters are bound together by a loose sheath throughout their length, although in the lowest half-inch besides being enclosed in the common sheath of Waldeyer they are much more closely adherent and can only be separated by sharp dissection.

If the accessory bud arises from the wolffian duct at some little distance cranial to the angle, it does not make a satisfactory junction with the metanephros. The resulting calyces are poorly formed and the associated parenchyma is dysplastic while the lower pole is left free to develop along almost normal lines. The loop on the wolffian duct carries this bud further caudally so that the ectopic ureter may open at the bladder neck or in the posterior urethra, or may fail to reach the urogenital sinus altogether. Thus in the male this ectopic ureter may end in the ejaculatory ducts, the seminal vesicle or the vas deferens (derivatives of the wolffian duct). In the female the degeneration of the parent duct may leave the ureter to open into the vestibule or to form a fistulous connection with the vagina, the uterus or even the rectum.

The musculature of these abnormally derived ureters is often defective, and in clinical cases the ectopic ureter is always dilated at least in part. On occasions the ectopic ureter is the only ureter on that side and presumably no bud arose in the normal position at the angle.

The lower end of the ectopic ureter may lie very close to the trigone and to the lumen of the urethra. In other instances it ends blindly or through a narrow orifice and the dilated lower end bulges into the bladder as a ureterocele.

If an accessory bud on the wolffian duct develops caudal to the angle as described in a 10 mm embryo by Chwalla (1927), it is unlikely to reach the metanephros. Accordingly the author has been unable to find a description of a complete duplex in which the cranial pole is the main formation. It may be argued that an accessory bud in this position is responsible for the development of a congenital vesical diverticulum behind and lateral to the normal ureteric orifice. However, since the section of the wolffian duct caudal to the angle disappears as a result of widening out and being taken up into the urogenital sinus and takes no part in the loop formation, the author believes that an accessory bud in this position is lost altogether and cannot attain a site outside the trigonal area.

Mackie and Stephens (1977) suggested that a single bud in this abnormal position on the wolffian duct could be responsible for lateral ectopia of the ureter, that is a very wide trigone, and correlated this with dysplasia of the corresponding kidney. It should be noted that such lateral ectopia is likely to be complicated by reflux, a process that could itself be responsible for the dysplasia.

It is evident that the bladder neck and trigonal mechanisms are developed in the section of the urogenital sinus that lies between the ureteric orifice and the final situation of the wolffian duct opening. Where the only ureter is ectopic in its termination and retains its connection with the wolffian duct there is thus no differentiation in the urogenital sinus of a bladder neck zone. The full consequences are seen in cases of bilateral single ectopic ureters when there is no discernible bladder neck and no bladder continence. To a lesser extent a similar defect may be found in association with unilateral single ectopic ureter.

As it ascends to its normal situation in the loin the metanephros obtains its blood supply from the aorta according to the level reached. In the case of a double kidney there is therefore no strict correlation between vascular supply and urinary drainage. The arterial system does not differ significantly from that found in the normal kidney, although in most cases the upper renal element is supplied by the apical artery and the upper branch of the main renal artery.

Incomplete duplication (the bifid ureter)

In this common group the kidney is drained by two renal pelves but the ureters unite at some point between the pelviureteric junction and the bladder. This bifurcation most often occurs at or

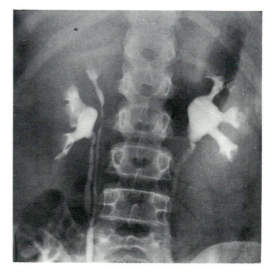

Figure 16.2. Bifid ureter. Intravenous urogram showing bifurcation at L4–L5.

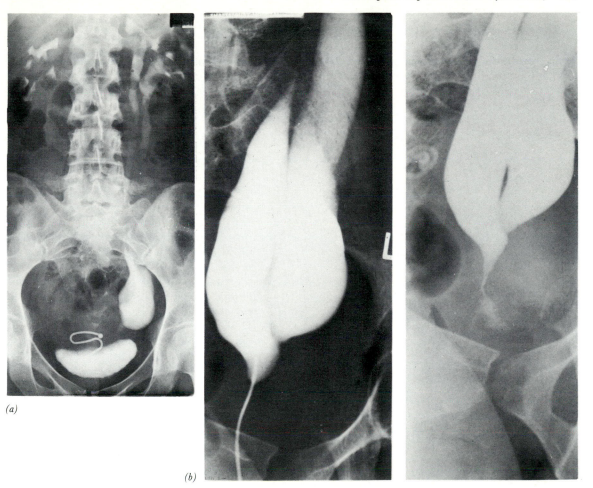

(a)

(b)

Figure 16.3. Bifid ureter with ureteroureteric reflux and dilatation. *(a)* Intravenous urogram showing pyelonephritic scarring of both renal elements and dilatation of the lower ureters. *(b)* Retrograde pyelogram showing unobstructed terminal common channel but free reflux between one ureter and the other, producing hydroureter.

below the level of the sacroiliac joint (*Figure 16.2*) and may occasionally be within the intramural segment.

The point of union between the ureters is a region where disorders of peristalsis may occur, and the urine is apt to be propelled from one branch into the other rather than down the common stem. This results in a mild and variable dilatation of the two branches (*Figure 16.3*) but seldom in serious hydronephrosis. Although such disorders can undoubtedly give rise to renal pain and predispose to urinary infection, in the author's experience treatment is seldom required and vague abdominal pain should not be too readily attributed to a bifid ureter if the urine is sterile. When symptoms are severe and persistent and the abnormality can be confirmed by video studies of the pyelogram, the bifurca-

tion should be eliminated surgically (*Figure 16.4*). Where the junction occurs near the lower end it is a simple matter to excise the common stem and reimplant both ureters into the bladder. Where the junction is at a higher level it is preferable to convert the bifid ureter into a bifid renal pelvis, anastomosing the upper ureter to the lower renal pelvis and excising the complete length of redundant ureter while ensuring that no blind stump is left at the point of bifurcation. Heminephrectomy is very seldom necessary in these circumstances.

Vesicoureteric reflux is observed in the bifid ureter and enters both limbs. Pyelonephritic scarring when present affects both halves of the kidney, although not always to the same extent. If reimplantation is undertaken for the prevention of reflux in a ureter with a low bifurcation,

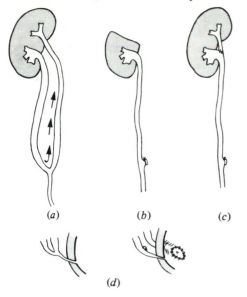

(a)   (b)   (c)

(d)

Figure 16.4. Operation for bifid ureter with complications. *(a)* Anatomy. *(b)* Heminephrectomy and ureterectomy. *(c)* Ureteropyelostomy and ureterectomy. *(d)* Reimplantation of both ureters through separate orifices.

the two branches should be implanted separately so that subsequent ureteroureteric reflux cannot occur.

Bifid ureter may be associated with pelviureteric obstruction; usually only the lower element is involved, because this alone has a well formed pelviureteric junction. Hydronephrosis so extreme that concentrating ability is lost in the lower element may give rise to a diagnostic problem, because only the upper ureter with two distorted calyces is visible and the condition may be confused with renal tumour. At pyeloplasty in cases of bifid ureter it is often convenient to incorporate the upper pole ureter into the side of the repair of the pelviureteric junction.

A caudal bifurcation in which a ureter is single at the upper end and bifurcates lower down is an extremely rare malformation. Phokitis (1954) reviewed 11 reported cases. Some of these were open to question since the anatomy of the lower end of an obstructive megaureter is sometimes hard to determine unless the excised terminal segment is carefully pinned out and fixed without kinks, and unless the concomitant vesical saccule is identified it may be easy on transverse section to imagine that there is a double ureter. There have been reports of one branch from a caudal bifurcation entering the

bladder and another the vagina, causing a dribbling incontinence. However, in these cases there is a possibility of the vaginal opening being an epithelialized fistula following previous surgery or trauma.

Complete duplication with vesical ureteric orifices

The developmental anatomy has already made it clear that in complete duplication the ureter from the upper pelvis enters the bladder nearer to the bladder neck than its fellow. In the uncomplicated case the orifice at the normal position on the corner of the trigone corresponds to the lower renal pelvis while a slit-like orifice on the ridge running downwards and medially drains the upper ureter. Some variation in this position is possible (Stephens, 1963). Both ureters may open together, presenting a double-barrelled appearance, and on rare occasions there may even be a slight upward shift of the upper ureteric orifice.

Reflux is the most common complication of complete ureteric duplication. Where both orifices are very close together reflux may occur into both ureters, although almost always to a lesser extent into the upper one (*Figure 16.5*). In the common anatomical situation the longer course of the upper ureter completely protects it whereas the lower ureter has a right-angled junction with the bladder or is involved in a paraureteric saccule. Reflux into only the lower element of the duplication is then the characteristic finding and is associated with pyelonephritic scarring of the lower half of the kidney (*Figure 16.6*).

In cases of reflux there is the possibility of a conservative or an operative approach to treatment. For minor degrees it is customary in the author's unit to adopt an entirely expectant attitude, with chemoprophylaxis and regular supervision in anticipation that reflux will cease spontaneously. This approach is adopted in the case of double or single ureters. When there is dilatation of the ureter, persistent infection, immediate reinfection following cessation of medication, or severe pyelonephritic scarring then surgery is undertaken.

Operative treatment takes several forms. In

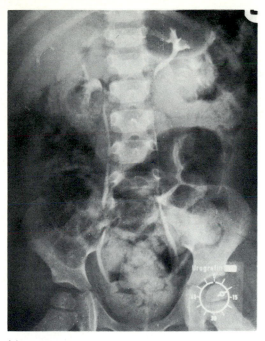

(a)

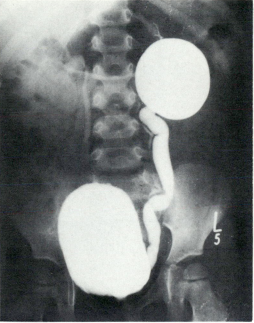

(b)

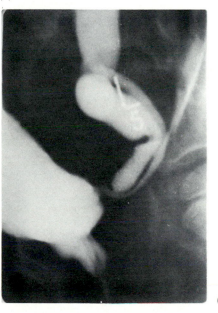

(c)

Figure 16.5. Complete duplication with both ureteric orifices opening at the corner of the trigone. (*a*) Intravenous urogram showing left duplex system with normal upper and hydronephrotic lower pole. (*b*) Cystogram showing reflux into both ureters. (*c*) Cystogram showing possible element of ureterovesical obstruction to the lower pole ureter.

lower-pole ureter was easily dissected from it and reimplanted by a Cohen technique (*see* Chapter 15). An alternative approach is anastomosis of the two ureters so that the whole kidney is drained by the nonrefluxing upper pole ureter. This anastomosis is best made at the renal level with excision of the redundant length of ureter, and should not be made immediately above the bladder level.

The most radical approach to the problem of lower pole pyelonephritis is heminephrectomy, and this was performed in 53 out of a total of 185 duplications requiring operation. When the kidney is exposed the distinction between the upper and lower renal elements is easily made because of the severity of the pyelonephritic scarring. It is often a surprise to find that the well preserved upper pole, even though drained by only two calyces, occupies at least two thirds of the bulk of the kidney while the lower pole, possessing numerous calyces, is shrivelled and fibrotic. Lower pole vessels are as numerous as normal with the middle, lower and posterior branches of the renal artery involved. After preliminary ligature of the blood vessels heminephrectomy

the simplest the refluxing ureter is reimplanted. However, since the two ureters are normally closely bound together at the lower end it is usually convenient to reimplant both en bloc. This was the method adopted in 82 out of 100 cases of reimplantation for duplex systems in the author's series. In the remaining 18 subjects the upper pole channel was left *in situ* and the

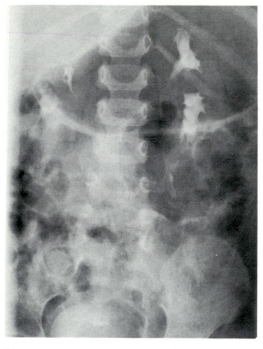

(a)

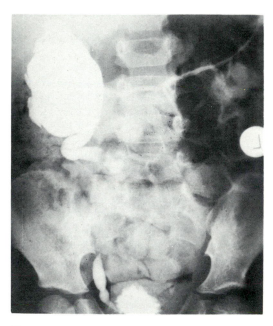

(b)

Figure 16.6. Complete duplication with lower pole reflux on the right, uncomplicated on the left. (*a*) Intravenous urogram showing poorly functioning lower pole element on the right; the other calyces are normal. (*b*) Cystogram showing reflux into grossly dilated lower renal pelvis on the right.

can be undertaken by a wedge-shaped incision through healthy tissue adjacent to the upper edge of the pathological segment. The length of the lower pole ureter is then excised. At the end of the operation it may be useful to perform a nephropexy since the upper element may have a long and tenuous arterial supply.

Blind-ending duplications

One branch of a bifid ureter or one ureter derived from the bladder may terminate blindly at its upper end (Albers, Geyer and Barnes, 1968). Sometimes there is an atretic thread leading upwards from the blind end towards the kidney; more often none can be found. The anomaly is usually recognized on the intravenous pyelogram because opaque medium passed down the complete ureter refluxes into the blind bifurcation. Such a bifurcation is scarcely distinguishable from a true ureteric diverticulum and Culp (1947) reviewed the literature on this subject, presenting 11 cases of which two were found in childhood. Most of these patients do not require any treatment at all, and excision of the blind end in duplications where severe dilatation has occurred presents no technical problems. Many instances in which a pouch opens out from the bladder were formerly regarded as cases of blind accessory ureters but are now taken to be examples of the common saccule pushing out through the ureteric hiatus.

Supernumerary kidneys

Accessory renal elements entirely separate from the normal kidney are very rare. Carlson (1950) was only able to find 51 cases presenting at all ages, some in childhood. This supernumerary organ almost always has some additional malformation such as hydronephrosis or hypoplasia; it is most often found in the iliac fossa or the pelvis and its ureter joins that from the normal kidney above the bladder. The hydronephrotic sac may present as a mass in the abdomen causing partial obstruction to the normal kidney. Rubin (1948) recorded a supernumerary kidney lying above the normal organ and drained by an ectopic ureter.

Triplications of the ureter

Three or more ureters may drain a single kidney. They may unite with one another or two may enter the bladder separately. The kidney itself is almost always anomalous, very often malrotated and dysplastic, and very liable to complications of pyelonephritis (Scott, 1970).

Ectopic ureter

It has been shown above that if the ureteric bud on the wolffian duct is far from the normal site then the ureteric opening is not taken up into the bladder but remains in the bladder neck area, in the posterior urethra, or in the wolffian duct derivatives in the male, or may break through into the müllerian duct derivatives in the female. Usually, although not always, ectopic buds are accessory and the ectopic ureter is found in association with a duplex kidney.

As already described the ureter from the upper pelvis of a duplex kidney opening low on the trigone may be protected by its anatomy from the reflux affecting its fellow. If it opens further away and is unquestionably ectopic, the ureter is almost always dilated (sometimes severely) and the renal element that it drains is often dysplastic or pyelonephritic. The complications and therefore the mode of presentation vary with the sex of the child and the position of the opening.

Ectopic ureter with duplication in the female

When the orifice in the more common female case is at or immediately below the bladder neck, persistent or recurrent pyuria is usually the first evidence of the abnormality. Incontinence is not a notable feature, although obviously some urge incontinence can occur in any girl with pyuria. The ureter shows reflux and is dilated; it is almost always demonstrable on micturating cystography and the opening is identifiable endoscopically.

When the ureter opens into the lower urethra, the vestibule or the vagina then dribbling incontinence is the rule and infection is less common. The characteristic complaint is one of continual slight wetting despite normal micturition at normal intervals. Sometimes incontinence occurs only during the day and this appears to be related to the reservoir effect of the grossly dilated ureter when the child is in a recumbent position. One feature of the history that may be misleading is the statement that the child went through a period of being completely dry. Where the opening of the ectopic ureter is in the lower urethra or very close to it, it seems likely that the urethral musculature can maintain a precarious continence until the ureter above has dilated.

Although frequency and urgency are absent from the classic history, frequency can be induced by repeated exhortations to the child to pass urine in the hope of keeping her dry. Moreover, in one case seen by the author a girl appeared to be able to retain urine in her vagina for a short period by strenuous contraction of her pelvic musculature; her efforts were similar to those of a child trying to restrain an urgent desire to micturate.

In the case of urethral ectopia the dribbling incontinence may be due to the return of urine refluxed into the ureter during micturition, and the symptom may therefore be present even when the upper part of the ectopic ureter is atretic and the renal element without function. Such an ectopic ureter is functionally a diverticulum of the urethra and it seems likely that all congenital diverticula of the female urethra have this basis. A thread-like ureter is found at the upper end. When the urine from an ectopic ureter is infected the presenting symptom may be vaginal discharge and the urinary tract should always be investigated when this complaint is made in infancy.

The diagnosis of low ectopic ureter in the female can be suspected from the history and from the dampness of the vulva. The exact source of the urine leak is often hard to find (*Figure 16.7*). An opening in the lower urethra can be identified with the urethroscope while one at the meatus can be found with a probe, but a high vaginal opening may defy a long search. This process cannot be assisted by the

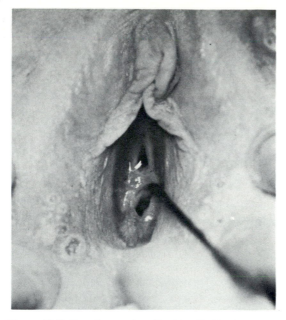

Figure 16.7. Ectopic ureteric orifice identified beside the urethra in a girl with dribbling incontinence.

intravenous injection of dye substances because the renal element is incapable of concentrating the dye. However, it may be valuable to fill the bladder by catheter with a coloured fluid and then apply a pad to the vulva. If the pad rapidly becomes wet with clear fluid it is evident that the leak does not occur from the bladder.

Failing direct identification and catheterization of the ectopic ureter the diagnosis can usually be made radiologically. With high doses of contrast medium the renal element drained by the ectopic ureter, almost always the upper pole of a duplex kidney, is faintly opacified but is seen to be abnormal in the formation of its calyces (*Figure 16.8*). It may be hydronephrotic and is often very small. A duplex system with a normal lower pole and an abnormal upper one is usually associated with ectopic ureter. If there is no visualization of the upper element, its presence should be recognized from features in the lower element as follows:

1. The calyces are fewer in number than in the normal kidney and the uppermost is further

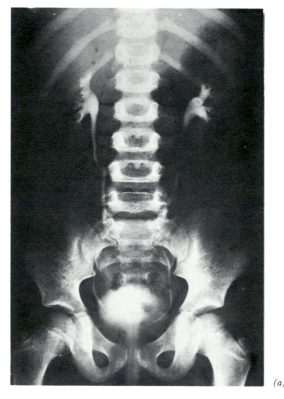

(a)

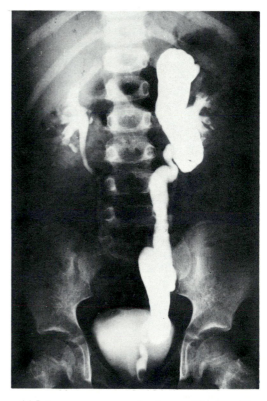

(b)

Figure 16.8. Left ectopic ureter in a girl with dribbling incontinence. (*a*) Intravenous urogram showing opacification of the lower pole only on the left side, with evidence of external pressure on the bladder by the nonopacified ectopic ureter. (*b*) Combined intravenous urogram and retrograde ureterogram showing the dilated ectopic upper-pole ureter with its opening into the urethra.

from the upper limit of the renal outline than the lowest is from the lower limit. Where the opposite kidney has an uncomplicated duplication a direct comparison of calyces is available.

2. The upper pole of the kidney appears to be rotated downwards and outwards, giving the pyelogram something of the appearance of a drooping flower. (A similar picture may be seen occasionally in renal tumours.)
3. The upper calyx is short and although the cups of the calyces may be directed upwards or medially they are close to the pelvis and have no long neck like the lower calyces. Occasionally the pelvis is malrotated.
4. The pelvis is displaced laterally away from the vertebral column, and the ureter instead of running vertically downwards forms with the pelvis one gentle curve that gradually approaches the paravertebral region at the level of the fourth or fifth lumbar vertebra.
5. The ureter, being adherent to an unseen dilated ureter, is not straight but exhibits a series of scalloped curves.
6. An ultrasound scan may show the upper element as separate from the lower one.

A duplex kidney with a nonopacified upper renal pelvis strongly suggests the presence of an ectopic ureter, although the precise anatomy is not evident. A micturating cystogram often clarifies the issue since most high level ectopic orifices allow free reflux, and good oblique views of the urethra show the exact site. There is always a possibility that reflux also occurs into the lower pelvis on the same side.

Single ectopic ureter in the female

Symptoms of infection or incontinence are found with unilateral single ectopic ureter as well as with duplication, but the diagnosis may present greater difficulty since dysplasia affects the whole kidney which therefore may not opacify on the intravenous urogram. Cystoscopy shows no ureteric orifice on the corresponding side of the bladder, and the distinction must be made between an absent kidney and an ectopic ureter. However, the small kidney should be demonstrable by scans with ultrasound or ^{99m}Tc-dimercaptosuccinic acid, although its position within the abdomen may be unusual.

Occasionally with the unilateral single ectopic ureter there is deficient bladder neck continence,

as discussed in relation to the bilateral condition (*see* below).

Ectopic ureter in the male

The ectopic ureter may enter the posterior urethra or the ejaculatory duct, or may join with the vas deferens (Cendron and Bonhomme, 1968). In boys it is more common to find that the ureter is single and the kidney it drains is dysplastic or ectopic. Incontinence may occur, usually through reflux into the dilated ureter, but severe pyuria is more often seen. Sometimes the ureter becomes enormously dilated and together with the cystic seminal vesicles forms a palpable swelling in the pelvis evident on bimanual examination (*Figure 16.9*).

Because of the junction with the vas deferens and the urinary reflux into the common terminal segment (*Figure 16.10*) epididymitis is the first sign of trouble in a number of boys. The diagnosis is established by the same radiological methods as in high level ectopic ureter in the female. A cystogram is therefore routine in suspected cases and gives the diagnosis more often than the pyelogram. Johnson and Perlmutter (1980) reported the association of single-system ectopic ureterocele with anomalies of the genital tract.

Treatment

In most cases the ectopic ureter is treated by heminephrectomy, or nephrectomy in the case of the unilateral single anomaly, together with ureterectomy. The alternative is conservative surgery by reimplantation of the lower end of the ectopic ureter into the bladder or by anastomosis of the two ureters with excision of the distal segment of the ectopic one. This has the advantage of preservation of all functioning renal tissue, although as already noted the renal element associated with the ectopic ureter is small and the output of urine from it is seldom a significant proportion. An additional factor in conservatism is the avoidance of an incision and subsequent scar in the lumbar region since most of the children involved are girls. In favour of heminephrectomy is the improbability of obtaining anything like a normal renal or ureteric system. The renal tissue is dysplastic or

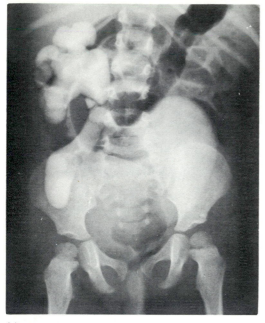

(a)

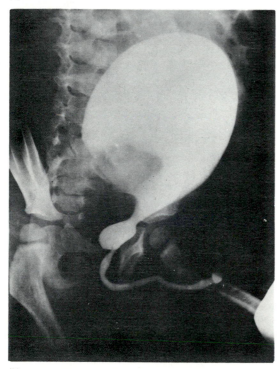

(b)

Figure 16.9. Left single ectopic ureter in a boy with extravesical dilatation of the terminal segment. (*a*) Intravenous urogram showing right hydronephrosis, nonopacified left kidney and displacement of the bladder by the unseen dilated ureter. (*b*) Micturating cystogram showing the bladder displacement.

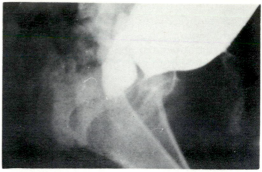

(a)

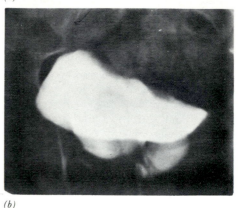

(b)

Figure 16.10. Ectopic ureter in a boy presenting with epididymitis and a functionless right kidney on intravenous urography. These cystourethrograms show reflux into the dilated lower end of the urethral ectopic ureter.

pyelonephritic, and the ureter is dilated and frequently defective in its musculature. In the author's series of 101 duplicated ureters with simple ectopia a conservative approach was chosen for only 12 children.

When there is ureteric duplication with a simple ectopic ureter the lower pole of the kidney is ordinarily normal. Occasionally it is involved in reflux and pyelonephritis, and out of the above 101 examples a total nephrectomy was performed in six. Commonly an inspection of the exposed kidney shows a pathological upper pole with scarring and hydronephrosis and a normal lower pole thus indicating an easy line of incision.

The technique of heminephrectomy requires some brief comment. It is usually possible to identify and ligature vessels supplying the upper pole but it is seldom possible to cut through an entirely bloodless area. The operation should commence with dissection of the renal pedicle. First to be identified is the small apical artery that leaves the aorta or the renal artery high up and courses directly to the substance of the upper pole. Once this has been divided mobilization of the upper part of the kidney is more easily effected. The upper pole renal artery is then identified in a position similar to that in an anatomically normal kidney. It may lie above or in front of the ectopic ureter and not infrequently has a branch going behind it. Below the ureter in the renal sinus between the two renal pelves there are seldom more than a few small veins. The main lower pole arteries should be identified before the upper pole vessels are ligatured and divided. Difficulties in this dissection occur only when there is considerable dilatation of the ectopic ureter, particularly if it has been infected for a long period when surrounding fibrosis makes separation of the vessels from the pelvis difficult and may hazard the integrity of the lower pole vessels.

The scarring and the hydronephrosis of the upper segment usually make it difficult to raise an intact flap of renal capsule in the manner often employed for simple partial nephrectomy, and heminephrectomy is best undertaken by a wedge-shaped incision into the renal tissue immediately below the area indicated by the pathological changes on the surface. The cut should therefore be made into the normal tissue of the lower half of the kidney; if the line of incision is correctly chosen no calyces are encountered. However, some degree of malrotation of the kidney is common with an overlap of calyces so that they are opened during excision. Their closure with catgut suture causes no problems. Small bleeding vessels exposed in the parenchyma can be underrun with a fine catgut suture, and the two flaps of renal tissue created by the wedge-shaped incision are then brought together with a few vertical mattress sutures which maintain haemostasis very satisfactorily. It is rarely necessary to employ any additional manoeuvre to control bleeding. The ureter is gently dissected free from the vessels supplying the lower pole and from the second ureter. It is traced downwards as far as the bladder, a second suprapubic incision being required to remove the lower end. Even in apparently unilateral cases the second incision should be used to inspect the opposite side since bilateral ectopic ureters have too often been overlooked.

Postoperative progress in these children is generally very smooth, although urine drainage from the wound may persist for 24–48 hours.

Intravenous pyelograms performed after a few months show that the upper calyx of the lower pole of the kidney rotates inwards towards the midline, but function is ordinarily well preserved.

In the male, when the ectopic ureter and the vas deferens join in a multilocular cystic mass involving the seminal vesicle, complete excision may be very difficult. The mass should be removed as far as possible without damaging the posterior urethra and the vas should be tied. It is not possible to secure normal function in the vas and this must be sacrificed if further attacks of epididymitis are to be avoided.

Bilateral single ectopic ureters

When associated with duplex kidneys bilateral ectopic ureters present no special problems other than the multiple operations required. If there are bilateral single ectopic ureters an entirely different situation arises. As already pointed out, where there has been no separation of the ureters from the wolffian ducts by caudal migration of the latter no true trigone can be formed and no normal bladder neck mechanism is present. Thus incontinence has a dual basis

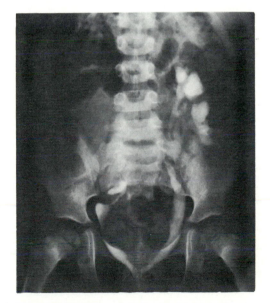

Figure 16.11. Bilateral single ectopic ureters. Intravenous urogram in a girl with continuous dribbling incontinence and absent micturition. Both kidneys are abnormally formed and the right is ectopic. The two ureters are dilated and open into the urethra.

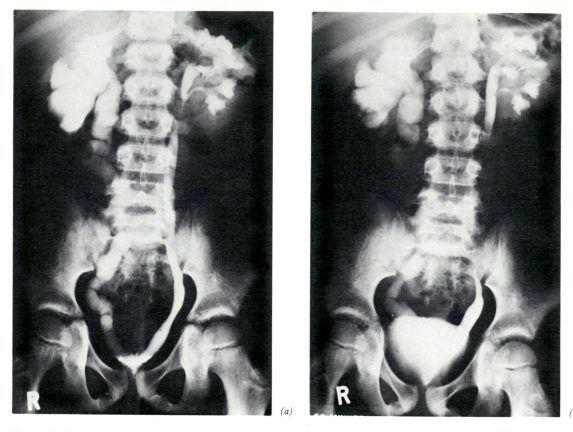

(a)   *(b)*

Figure 16.12. Bilateral single ectopic ureters in a boy. (*a*) Intravenous urogram showing dilated ureters with low termination. (*b*) Later film showing tapering bladder outflow.

and is due not only to the position of the ureteric orifices but also to the incompetent bladder neck. In girls there is the additional problem that the urine does not flow into the bladder which therefore remains very small in capacity.

The diagnosis of bilateral ectopic ureters in the female may be suspected from the clinical findings of dribbling incontinence, absent micturition, a normal urethral meatus and no neurological disturbance.

Intravenous urograms show some degree of abnormality in both kidneys, perhaps only as a minor proportion of dysmorphism or maybe severe hydronephrosis. The low termination of the ureters is often discernible and there is variable filling of the bladder (*Figure 16.11*). Micturating cystograms demonstrate the absence of a clearly defined bladder neck and usually show reflux into moderately dilated ureters. On endoscopy in girls the orifices are found at a variable distance within the urethral meatus. They are often asymmetrical in position

although rarely terminating outside the urethra. Concomitant vaginal abnormalities may occur. In boys the orifices lie a short distance above the verumontanum (*Figure 16.12*; Williams and Lightwood, 1972). In this group simple reimplantation of the ureters leaves the incontinence unchanged due to a sphincteral weakness. However, there is clearly considerable variability in the exact level of the ureteric ectopia and therefore in the possibilities of reconstruction.

The author's series of 14 cases included four girls with very small bladder capacities accompanied by hydronephrotic dysplastic kidneys. In one of the four reimplantation of the ureter and bladder neck tightening alone resulted in upper tract dilatation due to a small capacity bladder with persistent reflux which subsequently demanded diversion. The other three had a colocystoplasty or caecocystoplasty to enlarge bladder capacity but the result was satisfactory in only one case. There were five girls with bladders of fair capacity who were treated by reimplantation and some form of bladder neck support. Four of these had moderately good results although continence was imperfect at first. The last girl's condition was unimproved and diversion was advised. There were five boys whose bladders were much better formed than the girl's; all had a bladder neck tightening procedure with reimplantation. Continence was very much improved while still somewhat imperfect in two until puberty solved this problem.

Ectopic ureterocele

Ectopic ureterocele is an important anomaly that can present in many ways during infancy and childhood. Because of its complications it was seldom recognized in adult practice until the anatomy was fully defined by Ericsson (1954). Girls are affected more often than boys in a ratio of about 7:1. Both kidneys are equally likely to be involved and almost always show ureteric duplication. Bilaterality occurs in about 10 per cent of cases.

Functional anatomy

The ectopic ureter derived from the upper pole of a duplex kidney typically has its opening in the upper urethra a short distance below the bladder neck. The opening itself is of variable size but immediately proximal to it the ureter is grossly dilated to form a ureterocele-like swelling beneath the mucosa of the trigone (*Figure 16.13*). At this point the ureter retains some of its muscular coat, which gradually thins out, and its own longitudinal blood supply. Sometimes the ureterocele is relatively small and almost spherical, lying at the bladder neck well clear of the ureteric orifices (*Figure 16.14*). More often it is large, filling and stretching the trigonal area so that the other orifices are drawn up on to its slopes.

Sometimes it is evident that the bulge is composed of a coiled dilated ureter rather than a spherical cystic dilatation. In general the ectopic orifice itself is not stenotic while in a few cases it is wide enough to allow reflux; very occasionally it is either sealed off or so small as to be undiscoverable, when it is associated with a

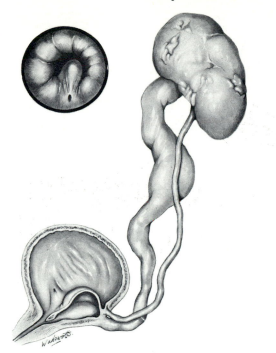

Figure 16.13. Ectopic ureterocele. Drawing to show the characteristic anatomy of the common form with inset to show the urethroscopic appearance. (Reproduced by permission of the editor, *British Journal of Urology*.)

dysplastic renal element. The ectopic orifice occasionally opens into the lower urethra where it causes dribbling incontinence in girls. In these cases the dilated terminal ureter distends the urethral wall, often rendering the bladder neck incontinent, and the ureteric lumen is only separated from the urethral lumen by a paper-thin membrane that is easily ruptured. In boys the low opening is still above the verumontanum and the terminal ureter exhibits behind the

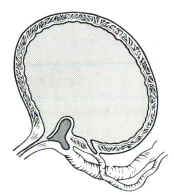

Figure 16.14. Ectopic ureterocele, small variant. (Reproduced by permission of the editor, *British Journal of Urology*.)

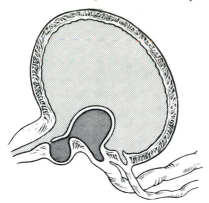

Figure 16.15. Ectopic ureterocele with posturethral extension. (Reproduced by permission of the editor, *British Journal of Urology*.)

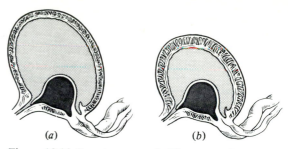

Figure 16.16. Ectopic ureterocele. Diagrams to show a tense ureterocele with a narrow orifice. (*a*) At rest. (*b*) During micturition. There is no change in the size of the ureterocele. The ipsilateral lower pole orifice remains valvular and may well be obstructed. (Reproduced by permission of the editor, *British Journal of Urology*.)

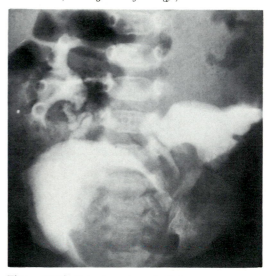

Figure 16.17. Ectopic ureterocele. Intravenous urogram in a girl with severe urinary infection. On the left side there is duplication, only the hydronephrotic lower pole being opacified. It is displaced downwards by the enormous upper-pole ectopic ureter. The filling defect in the bladder corresponds to the nonopacified ureterocele. (Reproduced by permission of the editor, *British Journal of Urology*.)

urethra a cystic dilatation distinct from the ureterocele swelling within the bladder (*Figure 16.15*). The caecoureterocele described by Stephens (1971) corresponds to this type.

The tension within a ureterocele varies with the degree of stenosis of the ectopic orifice, the function of the renal element, and the presence or absence of infection. A very tense ureterocele draws up the ipsilateral lower pole ureter, stretching and obstructing its orifice, and lower pole hydronephrosis is therefore likely to be a complication (*Figures 16.16 and 16.17*). A lax ureterocele that empties readily does not obstruct the lower pole ureter but rather undermines its support so that reflux takes place into it (*Figure 16.18*) and with this condition lower pole pyelonephritic scarring is to be expected (*Figure 16.19*; Williams, Fay and Lilley, 1972). Also, the lax ureterocele may evert during micturition (Weiss and Spackman, 1974) producing a very confusing radiological appearance.

The integrity of the detrusor coat is inevitably breached by the entry of the dilated ureter, and the muscular backing of the ureterocele may be deficient. Thus when the ureterocele is tense and inadequately backed it can be displaced outwards through the bladder wall during micturition, carrying with it a sulcus of bladder mucosa which is opacified on the micturating cystogram. Some possible radiological consequences are illustrated in *Figures 16.20 and 16.21*. Furthermore if the poorly backed ureterocele is uncapped, either spontaneously following rupture or by operation, the weak area of the detrusor bulges outwards during micturition and throws up a distal lip that can obstruct the bladder neck.

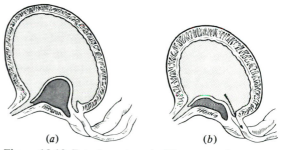

Figure 16.18. Ectopic ureterocele. Diagrams to show compressible ureterocele. (*a*) At rest. (*b*) During micturition. The ureterocele is flattened and does not support the ipsilateral lower pole orifice which therefore allows reflux. (Reproduced by permission of the editor, *British Journal of Urology*.)

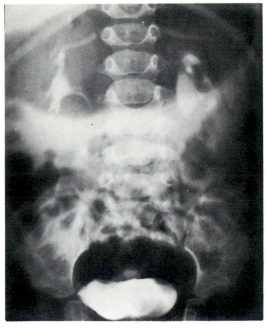

(a)

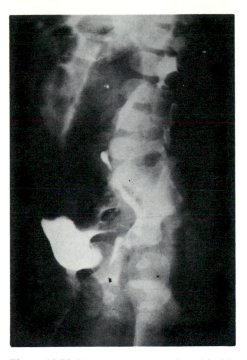

Figure 16.20. Intravenous urogram in a girl with ectopic ureterocele showing on lateral view the posterior projection of the circumferential sulcus. (Reproduced by permission of the editor, *British Journal of Urology*.)

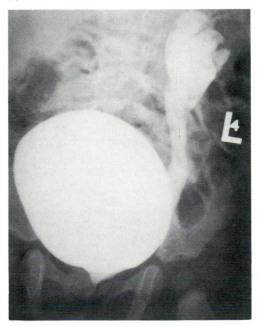

(b)

Figure 16.19 Ectopic ureterocele with lower pole pyelonephritis. (*a*) Intravenous urogram showing a small scarred left kidney. Certain features of the pyelogram suggest duplication of the ureter and there is a faint filling defect in the bladder corresponding to the nonopacified upper pole. (*b*) Cystogram showing lower pole reflux and the characteristic beak deformity due to the ureterocele at the bladder neck. (Reproduced by permission of the editor, *British Journal of Urology*.)

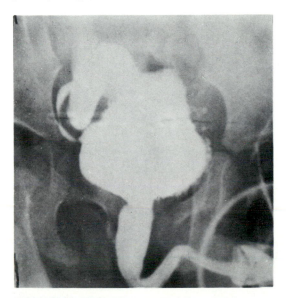

Figure 16.21. Micturating cystogram in a severely obstructed boy with a tense ectopic ureterocele which is totally displaced outside the bladder during micturition and outlined only by the circumferential sulcus. Reflux takes place into the ipsilateral lower pole ureter. (Reproduced by permission of the editor, *British Journal of Urology*.)

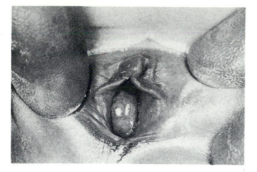

Figure 16.22. Prolapsed ectopic ureterocele in an infant girl.

An ectopic ureterocele may prolapse through the bladder neck. In boys it is forced down only as far as the membranous urethra, but being wedged there produces a severe degree of obstruction. In girls the ureterocele may prolapse through the external urinary meatus either acutely during micturition or on a chronic basis (*Figure 16.22*). The latter form must be differentiated from the low opening ureterocele which can also distend the urethrovaginal septum.

Sloughing and spontaneous rupture may follow prolapse. The remaining mucosal tags can be obstructive and free reflux takes place into the ectopic ureter as well as into the unsupported ipsilateral lower pole ureter (*Figure 16.23*).

Presentation and diagnosis

Ectopic ureterocele is remarkable for the variety of ways in which it can present. The greatest number of cases are found during investigation of severe urinary infection without evident localizing signs. The infection involves the dilated ectopic ureter most severely and this is sometimes converted into a pyoureter, producing extremely severe constitutional signs in the infant. Other parts of the urinary tract are also involved in the infection, particularly the ipsilateral lower pole with its refluxing ureter, and this sometimes dominates the picture. In infants with a sealed-off ureterocele one may find sterile urine within the ectopic ureter and heavily infected urine in the bladder.

The ureterocele may obstruct the bladder neck and cause retention. It is perhaps the most common cause of retention in infant girls although it can bring about severe degrees of upper tract dilatation in both sexes.

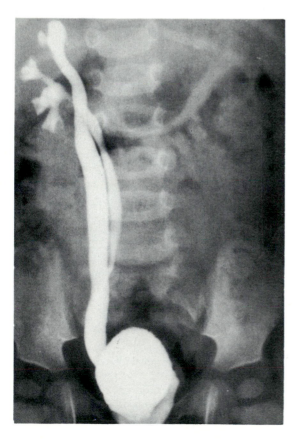

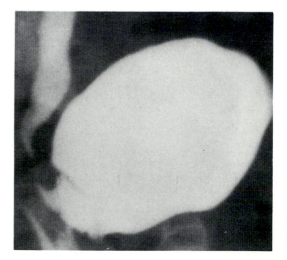

Figure 16.23. Ruptured ectopic ureterocele in a girl. Cystograms showing free reflux into both ureters. (Reproduced by permission of the editor, *British Journal of Urology*.)

Incontinence is seldom due to the position of the ectopic ureter itself but is simply a complication of the cystitis. Colicky abdominal pain due to acute obstruction of an enormously dilated ectopic ureter is another mode of presentation. In this case the ureter itself is often palpable as an elongated cystic mass in the abdomen.

Prolapse presents as a pink swelling at the external urinary meatus. While a bulging hydrocolpos produces a somewhat similar appearance it is easily distinguished by closer inspection. However, the rare paraurethral cyst in an infant girl can be very confusing and one must rely chiefly on the radiograms to make the differential diagnosis. Apart from prolapse the diagnosis cannot be made clinically, although it may be suspected in a girl with retention and a tense tortuous ureter palpable in the abdomen.

The intravenous pyelogram characteristically shows a duplex kidney with a nonopacified upper pole on one or both sides and a bladder with a large rounded filling defect in the base (*Figure 16.24*). High dose pyelograms may reveal some function in the upper pole and the size of

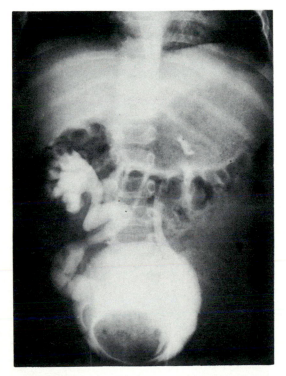

Figure 16.24. The characteristic pyelogram of an ectopic ureterocele. There is a nonopacified upper pole on the right side. The lower pole is obstructed and the bladder shows a filling defect due to the ureterocele.

the ectopic ureter can vary enormously. The ureterocele itself may almost fill the bladder or may appear as a scalloped defect at the bladder neck no more than 1–2 cm across. The outline of the defect is characteristically smooth and rounded but if the ureterocele is very lax, oedematous or ruptured it becomes irregular. The ipsilateral lower pole and the contralateral ureters are often dilated and a cystogram is important to demonstrate or exclude reflux. In cystograms with a dense opaque medium the defect of the ureterocele is obscured in the anteroposterior view but well demonstrated in the lateral view of the bladder.

Endoscopically the diagnosis is best made with the urethroscope when the prolongation of the ureterocele along the posterior urethral wall can be seen together with the ectopic orifice itself.

Treatment

Ectopic ureterocele is a complex anomaly in which treatment is required not only for the ureterocele itself and for the corresponding renal element in the upper pole of the kidney but also for the obstructed or refluxing lower pole and the opposite ureter, and occasionally for reconstruction of the bladder neck. Each element in this treatment must be considered before the overall plan can be discussed (Hendren and Montford, 1971; Belman, Filmer and King, 1974).

The ectopic ureterocele may be incised endoscopically, uncapped surgically, excised completely or left untouched. Endoscopic incision is appropriate only in those acutely infected cases with an urgent requirement for drainage of a pyoureter and pyonephrosis. It is then valuable but should be regarded as a temporary expedient only and the bladder should be drained by catheter to minimize reflux until the next operative step is taken.

Uncapping of the ureterocele through the open bladder has been the standard treatment for many years and is appropriate when the detrusor backing is firm so that it does not leave a weak trigonal area. The procedure must be meticulous to avoid leaving mucosal tags at the bladder neck and to protect the lower pole ureter. Haemostasis requires attention by diathermy or by a running suture along the cut edge. Complete excision across the trigone of the lower end of the ectopic ureter including its ureterocele is preferable where uncapping would leave a considerable deformity. Reconstitution of the detrusor layer and reimplantation of the lower pole ureter are essential stages in this operation (*Figure 16.25*).

When there is a ureterocele opening low in the urethra, uncapping alone leaves the child incontinent with a double-barrelled urethra and a relaxed bladder neck. In such cases, as in those where there is a considerable dilatation behind the urethra, excision is essential and must be combined with some reconstruction of the bladder neck and the posterior urethral wall. Access is always difficult particularly in older and obese children.

In infants a transperitoneal approach to the back of the bladder and the urethra is useful. The bladder is first mobilized anteriorly by section of the obliterated umbilical arteries. It is then drawn upwards out of the pelvis and the plane between the vagina and the urinary tract is developed and opened up as far as possible. The ectopic ureter is dissected from its fellow and followed downwards where it is found to constitute the posterior wall of the bladder neck and the urethra in the midline. When it is excised the urethra is left as a strip anteriorly and must be resutured to form a tube. Perhaps surprisingly, this reconstruction can restore normal continence.

Finally the small flat ureterocele can be left untouched if heminephrectomy has removed the renal element and the ureter above it. This has the great advantage of avoiding any disturbance of normal micturition. If, however, a large ureterocele is not excised then the redundant tissue is apt to fall into the bladder neck and produce retention or a predisposition to infection.

As with the simple ectopic ureter, heminephrectomy is usually required and only where there is an overall nephron deficiency is it desirable to preserve the dysplastic upper pole. In a very few children the ectopic ureter is of near normal calibre and reimplantation may be justifiable; this occurs more often when the ureterocele, although associated with duplication, is completely within the bladder. On the other hand total nephrectomy is indicated more often than with simple ectopic ureter because of the frequency of secondary lower pole pathology. Thus in the author's series of 184 examples heminephrectomy was performed in 117,

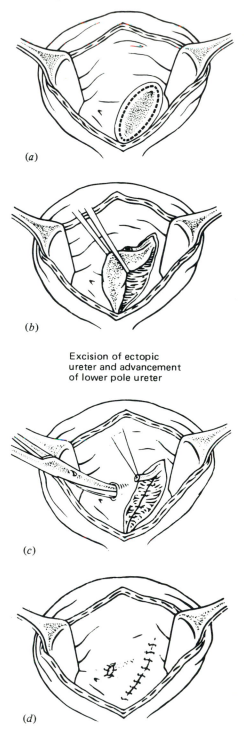

Ectopic ureterocele with double ureter

(*a*)

(*b*)

Excision of ectopic ureter and advancement of lower pole ureter

(*c*)

(*d*)

Figure 16.25. Operation for ectopic ureterocele. Excision of ectopic ureter, reconstitution of detrusor layer and reimplantation of ipsilateral lower pole ureter.

nephrectomy in 36 and conservative surgery in 31.

In summary the standard treatment for a child diagnosed as having ectopic ureterocele is heminephrectomy, ureterectomy with uncapping or excision of the ureterocele, and reimplantation of the ipsilateral lower pole ureter. All these procedures can be undertaken at one operation, or as a staged programme for infants. For the small ureterocele and for the low opening ureter with incontinence heminephrectomy should first be undertaken alone and the desirability of bladder surgery determined later. In the acutely infected case endoscopic incision of the ureterocele and drainage should be the primary measure. If this is indequate, surgical uncapping of the ureterocele together with a temporary terminal cutaneous ureterostomy may be useful, with heminephrectomy later.

Postoperative complications of ectopic ureterocele are usually due to failure to totally correct the reflux or obstruction in the lower pole ureter, or to bladder outflow problems.

References

Albers, D.D., Geyer, J.R. and Barnes, S.D. (1968) Blind ending branch of bifid ureter. *Journal of Urology*, **99**, 160

Belman, A.B., Filmer, R.B. and King, L.R. (1974) Surgical management of duplications of the collecting system. *Journal of Urology*, **112**, 316

Campbell, M.F. (1951) *Clinical Paediatric Urology*. Saunders, Philadelphia

Carlson, H.E. (1950) Supernumerary kidney. *Journal of Urology*, **64**, 224

Cendron, J. and Bonhomme, C. (1968) Uretère à termination ectopique extravésicale chez des sujets de sexe masculin. *Journal d'Urologie et Néphrologie*, **74**, 31

Chwalla, R. (1927) The process of formation of cystic dilatation of the vesical end of the ureter and of diverticula at the ureteral ostium. *Urologic and Cutaneous Reviews*, **31**, 499

Culp, O.S. (1947) Ureteral diverticula. *Journal of Urology*, **58**, 309

Ericsson, N.O. (1954) Ectopic ureterocele in infants and children. *Acta Chirurgica Scandinavica*, Suppl. 197

Gyllensten, L. (1949) Contributions to the embryology of the human bladder: the development of the definitive relations between the openings of the Wolffian duct and the ureters. *Acta Anatomica*, **7**, 305

Hendren, W.H. and Montford, G.J. (1971) Surgical correction of ureteroceles in children. *Journal of Paediatric Surgery*, **6**, 235

Johnson, D.K. and Perlmutter, S. (1980) Single system ectopic ureteroceles. *Journal of Urology*, **123**, 81

Mackie, G.G. and Stephens, F.D. (1977) Duplex kidneys: a correlation of renal dysplasia with the position of the ureteric orifice. *In* Urinary System Malformations in Children (edited by Bergsma, D. and Duckett, J.W.). Birth Defects: Original Article Series Vol. 13, No. 5. Liss, New York. p. 313

Nation, E.F. (1944) Duplication of the kidney and ureter: a statistical study of 230 new cases. *Journal of Urology*, **51**, 456

Phokitis, M. (1954) L'uretère bifide caudale. *Journal d'Urologie médicale et chirurgicale*, **60**, 45

Rubin, J.S. (1948) Supernumerary kidney with ectopic ureter. *Journal of Urology*, **60**, 405

Scott, R. (1970) Triplication of the ureter. *British Journal of Urology*, **42**, 150

Stephens, F.D. (1963) Congenital malformations of the rectum, anus and genito-urinary tract. Livingstone, Edinburgh

Stephens, F.D. (1971) Aetiology of ureteroceles and effects of ureteroceles on the urethra. *British Journal of Urology*, **40**, 483

Weiss, R.M. and Spackman, T.J. (1974) Everting ectopic ureteroceles. *Journal of Urology*, **111**, 538

Whitaker, J. and Danks, D.M. (1966) A study of the inheritance of duplication of the ureters and kidneys. *Journal of Urology*, **95**, 176

Williams, D.I. and Lightwood, R.G. (1972) Bilateral single ectopic ureters. *British Journal of Urology*, **44**, 269

Williams, D.I., Fay, R. and Lillie, J.G. (1972) The functional radiology of ectopic ureterocele. *British Journal of Urology*, **44**, 417

17 Upper Urinary Tract Obstructions

J.H. Johnston

The functional disorder

Pelvis and ureter

Pelviureteric peristalsis begins with the onset of electrical activity at pacemakers in the urinary collecting system. The precise position of the pacemakers differs among species and in man they appear to be in the region of the papillary attachment of each minor calyx (Gosling and Dixon, 1974). Electron microscopy has shown that there may be additional sites at the pelviureteric junction and in the ureter (Hanna *et al.*, 1976). From the pacemaker a wave of depolarization and propulsive ureteric contraction progresses distally as the impulse is transmitted from one muscle cell to the next. The pacemakers are stimulated to activity by stretching which results from calyceal distension consequent on urine flow. However, stretch is not essential for ureteric activity since peristalsis can persist in the absence of urine excretion.

The electrical properties of the ureter are determined by the distribution of ions on either side of the cell membrane and by the relative permeability of the membrane to the ions (Weiss, 1978). Movement of sodium and calcium ions into the cell produces muscular contraction and their movement out of the cell causes relaxation. Alpha-adrenergic and beta-adrenergic sympathetic receptors exist in the ureteric wall and probably influence ureteric function, but it is uncertain whether cholinergic parasympathetic fibres have a significant action. The ureter can act without any nervous attachments as shown by its effective function when transplanted.

Transport of urine from the calyces to the bladder is partly active, due to pyeloureteric peristalsis, and partly passive, resulting from the hydrostatic pressure generated by urine excretion (Rose and Gillenwater, 1978). When a sudden complete ureteric obstruction occurs the kidney continues to produce urine and there is a proximal build-up of pressure which distends the system. The immediate responses are a rise in wall tension due to enhanced muscle tone and an increase in the force and frequency of peristaltic waves. Soon afterwards peristalsis weakens and later the ureter no longer generates significant contractions and active transport of urine ceases.

With a long-standing obstruction the glomerular filtration rate (GFR) falls, there is reabsorption of sodium and water in the proximal tubules, and pyelotubular, pyelovenous and pyelolymphatic backflow occurs. As a result the pressure in the obstructed system decreases, often to normal levels, and the ureter regains its ability to generate contractions; nevertheless, these have less propulsive power than normal since they are less forceful and do not coapt the walls of the dilated system. Pyeloureteric contractility may be retained indefinitely, especially if there is muscular hypertrophy, although secondary complications, in particular infection, may modify the situation. Infection alone can impair ureteric muscular activity by the direct action of bacterial endotoxins (Teague and Boyarsky, 1968). Such effects are reversible but invasive infection, which is a common complication of obstruction, can lead to fibrous replacement of the musculature so that contractility is permanently lost. The position is further complicated by the fact that in practice many chronic pelviureteric obstructions are intermittent or variable in degree of completeness. Thus raised intraluminal pressures and/or dilatation of the system may exist only when the urinary excretion rate is unusually high. Conversely (see below) a dilated upper urinary tract is not necessarily obstructed.

The age of the patient at the time of onset of urinary obstruction greatly influences the pathological anatomy. In the fetus, and to a lesser degree in the young infant, obstruction produces much more severe degrees of dilatation than in the older child or adult and in addition ureteric lengthening and tortuosity are commonly seen. It is likely that these effects are due to the occurrence of obstruction before the ureter has obtained its full complement of muscle cells and elastic tissue or before there is full maturation of the musculature. Incomplete development of the sympathetic nervous system may also be relevant (Weiss, 1978).

Kidney parenchyma

Renal structure

The effects of urinary obstruction on the renal parenchyma depend upon the degree and the duration of the obstruction and, in cases of obstruction originating prenatally, upon the level of maturation of the developing kidney at the time of onset. Whether the renal pelvis is intrarenal or extrarenal also appears to be significant.

Knowledge of the mechanisms by which kidney structure and function are affected has been largely obtained from experimental animal studies. From investigations in the pig Matz, Craven and Hodson (1969) considered that with a persisting obstruction loss of renal substance is initiated by a direct pressure effect on and within the renal papillae. As a result of rupture and atrophy of the ducts of Bellini and the collecting tubules there is progressive loss of pyramidal tissue. The cortical changes are secondary to the papillary lesions and consist mainly of tubular atrophy within the individually affected nephron units. Compression of the renal venous tributaries by raised intrarenal pressure may contribute to furthering the kidney damage. Renal arterial blood flow is well maintained to begin with but later is reduced so that

parenchymal ischaemia with further atrophy and fibrosis results. In a histological study of hydronephrotic kidneys in children Winterburn and France (1972) showed that there were degenerative changes in the interlobular and arcuate arteries consisting of intimal elastic cushions and breaks in the internal elastic lamina; the severity of the changes was directly proportional to the degree of hydronephrosis.

Renal dysplasia characterized mainly by the persistence of primitive tubules and the presence of foci of cartilage is a common finding in children with congenital urinary obstruction. The anomaly ranges in degree from focal areas within a functioning kidney to an afunctional aplastic or multicystic organ. It is presumed to be caused by prenatal interference with urine flow preventing normal development of the metanephros. Beck (1971) was able to reproduce renal dysplasia by inducing ureteric obstruction in fetal lambs.

Renal function

During the early stages of an acute urinary obstruction the GFR falls as the tubular pressure rises. With increasing duration of the obstruction and a progressive decrease in the number of functioning nephrons the GFR becomes permanently reduced. Chisholm and Osborn (1976) pointed out that when discussing changes in tubular activity it is necessary to consider function both during and after the obstructive episode. While obstruction exists the urine increases in osmolality and there is reduced sodium excretion due partly to tubular cell damage with altered permeability and partly to changed transit times. The combined effect of diminutions in haemodynamics and in tubular transport interferes with the osmotic gradient and the concentrating power of the kidney, resulting in a decrease in the maximum urinary concentration. Long-standing partial obstruction may present as nephrogenic diabetes insipidus with polyuria unresponsive to antidiuretic hormone.

Following the relief of obstruction both GFR and renal blood flow may be reduced. Impaired urine concentration often persists but acidification and alkalinization of the urine may be unaffected. Increased excretion of water results from the lack of the normal osmolar gradient which depends on the counter-current system. On occasions postobstructive diuresis occurs and causes profuse losses of salt and water which may have serious clinical effects if the patient has a solitary kidney or bilateral disease. The mechanisms responsible vary and urea-mediated osmotic diuresis, natriuresis due to the elimination of sodium retained during the obstructed phase, tubular deficiency interfering with sodium reabsorption and lack of renal response to antidiuretic hormone may play differing roles in individual cases (Peterson *et al.*, 1975).

Recoverability of renal function

The question of whether or not an obstructed kidney is worth preserving is a common clinical problem in cases of unilateral disease. In an acutely obstructed system intravenous urography may show a dense nephrogram due to retention of contrast medium within the renal tubules and this appearance presages good postoperative recovery of renal function. However, the nephrogram caused by obstruction must be distinguished from that due to renal tubular necrosis and also from the shock nephrogram seen in children recovering from trauma or exhibiting a hypotensive reaction to the contrast medium. In the former the radiological appearance is the result of leakage of contrast medium from necrotic tubules into the interstitium while in the latter it is caused by tubular stasis which permits excessive reabsorption of salt and water; both these nephrograms occur bilaterally. On the nephrogram obtained in obstruction it is often possible to see dilated calyces as relatively radiolucent filling defects. Sometimes an acute ureteric obstruction, such as may result from an impacted stone, causes calyceal rupture in the region of the papillary fornix and perirenal extravasation of contrast medium.

Where there is chronic obstruction intravenous urography may demonstrate a shell nephrogram caused by retention of contrast medium in papillary tubules stretched around the circumference of dilated calyces. Tomography may allow an assessment of parenchymal thickness. However, even with high doses of contrast medium and delayed films nonvisualization can occur and it may not be possible to decide whether this is due to complete and irreversible nonfunction or to temporarily impaired contrast-medium excretion and/or dilution in a dilated system with the possibility of useful renal recovery. Hypertrophy of the con-

tralateral kidney is indicative of severe renal malfunction starting at an early age.

Several methods of determining function in an obstructed kidney before operation have been employed. Ultrasound is of value in demonstrating the thickness of the parenchyma. Radioisotopic renography and renal scintiscans with the gamma-camera computer system can be used to indicate individual kidney function and allow comparison between the two sides (Bueschen, Evans and Schlegel, 1974). Ibrahim and Asha (1978) reported that in the absence of urea-splitting organisms a urinary pH of less than 6 in the obstructed system forecasted good recovery whereas one of 7.3 or more was an indication for nephrectomy. Nanninga and O'Conor (1976) used tetrazolium as a biochemical assay of mitochondrial activity from a biopsy specimen of kidney tissue. Beaman, Gillenwater and Hatcher (1974) recorded that the relative concentrations of inulin and para-aminohippuric acid in the plasma and in the urine in the renal pelvis correlated well with the degree of impairment of kidney function. Aron, Tessler and Morales (1973) found arteriography to be of prognostic significance and noted that loss of the arcuate and interlobular arteries indicated little likelihood of functional recovery.

Most of the above methods are measures of renal function when obstruction is still present and they are not therefore necessarily indicative of the prospects for postoperative recovery. Preliminary drainage of the kidney may be warranted for this purpose, or when the kidney is to be exposed surgically the decision whether to conserve or to excise may of necessity have to be made at operation. Gross cystic dysplasia is a clear indication for nephrectomy but otherwise an assessment should be made of the overall bulk of stretched kidney tissue rather than its thickness alone. In the young child it is justifiable to preserve a doubtful kidney rather than remove it since good recovery with restoration of growth can occur in what appeared initially to be an unpromising situation. Hinman's (1926) theory of renal counterbalance postulated that once a kidney established dominance over its mate the decline of the diseased kidney progressed even if the causative factors were eliminated. However, Allen (1974) has shown that this concept is invalid and that once the injurious lesion has been removed the two kidneys stabilize at their own levels of activity without further change.

Calyceal diverticulum

A calyceal diverticulum is a spherical cavity lined by transitional epithelium which communicates by a narrow neck with a normal minor calyx (*Figure 17.1*). The lesion may be solitary, or multiple diverticula may affect one or both kidneys. It is a common incidental finding on intravenous urography in infants and young children and is therefore presumed to be of developmental origin. It has been suggested to result from failure to degenerate of the third and fourth order divisions of the ureteric bud (Middleton and Pfister, 1974).

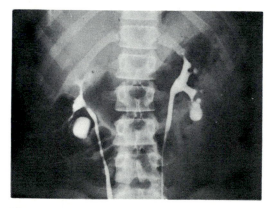

Figure 17.1. Bilateral asymptomatic calyceal diverticula.

As a rule the diverticulum is symptomless and nonprogressive and no surgical treatment is needed. Complications are rare. Nicholas (1975) described a case in which a calyceal diverticulum in a 4-year-old girl formed over a period of 8 years a large palpable solitary noncommunicating cyst. The commonest complication and the main indication for surgery is the formation within the diverticulum of calculi which are generally small and multiple. The operative technique required depends upon the pathological anatomy. Formal partial nephrectomy is indicated when a large diverticulum occupies the upper or lower kidney pole. A small diverticulum communicating with a nonpolar calyx must be approached through the renal parenchyma. The diverticular lining may be dissected out and removed and the communication with the calyx ligated; however, this technique leaves a dead space and the possibility of reformation of the diverticulum. Alternatively the existence of the diverticulum may be accepted and its

neck widened or dilated and subsequently splinted for some weeks so as to eliminate intradiverticular stasis by allowing free emptying into the calyx.

Hydrocalyx

In this condition one or more calyces are dilated as a result of infundibular obstruction which may be intrinsic or extrinsic. With intrinsic obstruction, which is generally considered to be due to a developmental anomaly, the affected infundibulum is lengthened and severely narrowed. One or both kidneys may be involved. If the lesion is responsible for symptoms or if complications such as calculi develop, surgery is needed. Partial nephrectomy is indicated if one dilated calyx is localized to one or other pole of the kidney. For more diffuse renal involvement with several affected calyces treatment is difficult and although intubated infundibulotomy has been employed the long-term results have not been satisfactory (Williams, 1977). Acquired hydrocalyx resulting from fibrosis of the infundibulum is an unusual complication of pyelolithotomy for staghorn calculus (*see* Chapter 29).

Extrinsic infundibular obstruction causing hydrocalyx involves the upper kidney pole and is the result of an unusually long superior infundibulum, or less often the upper moiety of a duplex ureter or pelvis, being compressed or angulated by blood vessels within the renal

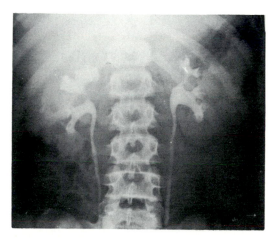

Figure 17.2. Right superior infundibular obstruction due to vascular compression with dilated upper pole calyces and a filling defect in the infundibulum.

hilum (*Figure 17.2*). The precise vascular anatomy varies. The infundibulum may be compressed by the artery to the posterior renal
segment or between this vessel and the main
renal vein. Alternatively, it may be compressed
between an artery and posterior veins or caught
in a fork in the artery to the upper renal pole. In
the child the presenting symptom is flank pain.
Urography shows dilatation and delayed
emptying of the upper calyces and there is often
a transverse filling defect in the infundibulum.
The calyceal dilatation is rarely more than
moderate.

Asymptomatic minor degrees of upper pole
hydrocalyx presumed to be due to vascular
infundibular compression are common findings
on intravenous urography in children and operative intervention is indicated only if the lesion
can be clearly shown to be responsible for
significant and persisting symptoms. In doubtful cases high dose urography and delayed films
are valuable. Selective arteriography has been
advocated to delineate the exact anatomy but
this investigation is rarely warranted because
the obstruction is demonstrable by routine urological techniques and the causative anatomical
details are readily determined at operation.
Since the calyceal dilatation is rarely severe and
the overlying parenchyma is generally well preserved, polar partial nephrectomy is unjustified
and surgery aims at relieving the obstruction by
intrahilar dissection. Division of intrarenal
arteries, which would lead to devascularization
of kidney tissue, must be avoided. Fraley (1966)
and Johnston and Sandomirsky (1972) employed dismembered infundibulopyeloplasty by
which the infundibulum is detached from the
pelvis, mobilized to avoid the obstructing vessels
and reanastomosed. Although operation is effective in relieving symptoms, postoperative
urography generally shows no significant
change in the degree of calyceal dilatation.

Hydronephrosis due to pelviureteric obstruction

Pathology

Pelviureteric junction

The most common findings at operation in cases
of pelvic hydronephrosis are various kinks and
angulations at the pelviureteric junction. There
is no doubt that these are themselves obstructive
but differing opinions have been expressed as to
whether they represent the primary pathology
or are secondary developments resulting from
some less overt obstructive lesion of either functional or organic nature in the upper ureter.
Several lesions have been described and several
theories offered.

HIGH INSERTION OF THE URETER
In this common situation the ureter has its
origin high on the anteromedial aspect of the
renal pelvis instead of at its most dependent
part. Diuresis produces spherical distension of
the pelvis which carries the pelviureteric junction even higher and compresses the ureter
against the pelviureteric fascia so that a valvular
form of obstruction is induced. In the early
stages it is probable that spontaneous correction
occurs when the rate of urine excretion returns
to normal but later adhesions form, the deformity is maintained and the obstruction becomes
persistent. Rarely a mucosal flap valve crosses
the interior of the pelviureteric junction and
reinforces the extrinsic obstruction.

OVERDISTENSIBLE RENAL PELVIS
Whitaker (1975) suggested that hydronephrosis
may be due to a congenitally overdistensible
pelvis. When the pelvis dilates as a result of
diuresis the peristaltic wave is unable to coapt
the pelvic walls and obliterate the lumen so that
urine cannot be expelled into the ureter.

ABERRANT VESSELS
The anterior division of the renal artery may
bifurcate near its origin, the inferior branch
crossing anterior to the ureter about 2 cm below
the pelviureteric junction on its way to enter the
renal hilum. This artery, which is usually
accompanied by small veins, causes pelviureteric angulation which increases in degree
and obstructive effect as the distended pelvis
drops into the gap between the upper and lower
hilar vessels. A high ureteric insertion often
coexists. Johnston *et al.* (1977) and Uson, Cox
and Lattimer (1968) found aberrant vessels to
be involved in respectively 59 (24 per cent) of
238 cases and 28 (18 per cent) of 154 cases of
hydronephrosis in children.

URETERIC STENOSIS AND DYSKINESIA
A fibrous stricture causing severe stenosis at the

pelviureteric junction is an uncommon finding but frequently the proximal 1–2 cm of the ureter are relatively narrow and thin-walled. This may be an isolated lesion or may be associated with pelviureteric angulations with or without aberrant vessels. The hypoplastic segment of ureter has been considered to be the site of disordered or absent peristalsis although different authors have found different histological changes and have produced different interpretations of the obstructive mechanisms involved. Murnaghan (1958) noted a preponderance of longitudinally arranged muscle fibres which could prevent the propulsion of urine. Foote *et al.* (1970) found either complete absence of muscle or small abnormal fibres which they considered would halt transmission of the peristaltic wave. Notley's (1968) electron-microscopic studies revealed an excess of collagen which without narrowing the lumen could prevent normal ureteric distension and so interfere with pelvic emptying.

PERSISTING FETAL FOLDS
During prenatal life the ureter, particularly in its proximal portion, contains invaginations of the musculature and the mucosa (Ostling, 1942). These infoldings are bridged by the adventitia and may not be immediately apparent on external inspection of the ureter. Fetal folds commonly persist after birth and may be seen on urography in infants and young children. Ordinarily they disappear with growth and are not obstructive. However, excessively developed persisting fetal folds are an occasional cause of pelvic hydronephrosis. Typically in such cases the renal pelvis retains its conical shape and dependent exit and its degree of dilatation is less than that of the calyces (*Figure 17.3*; Johnston, 1969).

URETERIC POLYP AND URETERIC PAPILLOMA
A polyp arising in the upper ureter is a rare cause of hydronephrosis. The lesion consists of narrow finger-like fronds composed of connective tissue covered by transitional epithelium. The diagnosis may be made when urography shows an irregular filling defect, but more often the polyp is found unexpectedly at surgery when a palpable thickening is noted in the ureter. The lesion is of hamartomatous rather than neoplastic nature and requires only local excision of the involved segment of ureter followed by pyeloureteroplasty. Benign ureteric papilloma is an extremely rare cause of hydronephrosis in children. Cases have been recorded by Johnston *et al.* (1977) and Mirandi and De Assis (1975). Management is the same as that of ureteric polyp. Multiple ureteric polyps may occur in the Peutz-Jegher syndrome of intestinal polyposis and perioral and intraoral pigmentation.

DISCUSSION
In order to determine whether pelviureteric angulations were the primary cause of hydronephrosis or secondary to a pre-existing intrinsic obstruction in the ureter Johnston (1969) performed urodynamic studies during operation on 32 hydronephrotic kidneys in children. Using a constant inflow of saline into the renal pelvis the intrapelvic pressure was measured before and after releasing the angulations. In 24 instances the obstruction was entirely relieved by unkinking the pelviureteric junction. In the other eight the obstruction persisted because of ureteric stenosis, a mucosal flap across the pelvic exit or an intrinsic obstruction presumably of functional nature. Whether these anomalies preceded the pelviureteric kinking or were caused by it could not be decided. It is apparent that a variety of obstructive lesions can lead to pelvic hydronephrosis during childhood and that the primary agent may be reinforced yet obscured by secondary developments so that it may not be possible to determine which preceded which.

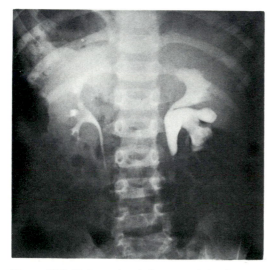

Figure 17.3. Hydronephrosis due to persisting fetal folds. The dilatation of the calyces is greater than that of the renal pelvis which retains its conical shape and dependent exit.

Secondary pelviureteric obstruction

Pelviureteric obstruction and mild degrees of vesicoureteric reflux can occur coincidentally, but massive reflux that rapidly distends the upper tract can lead to pelviureteric angulation and subsequently slow pelvic emptying. Often the angulations are transient and pelvic dilatation does not occur at physiological rates of urine excretion, and in these cases surgery is needed only to cure the reflux. On occasions the obstructive kinks become permanent as a result of adhesions and in such circumstances pyeloureteroplasty is necessary as well as ureteric reimplantation. Similar secondary obstructions at the pelviureteric junction may be found with megaureter due to dyskinesia of the lower ureter and with hydroureter caused by lower urinary tract obstruction.

Other congenital anomalies of the contralateral kidney

During childhood and especially in infancy pelvic hydronephrosis is often bilateral although generally the two kidneys are unequally affected. Both kidneys were involved in 19 of 219, 20 of 109 and 24 of 130 cases respectively in the series of Johnston *et al.* (1977), Kelalis *et al.* (1971) and Uson, Cox and Lattimer (1968). In children under 6 months of age bilateral hydronephrosis was found by Robson, Rudy and Johnston (1976) in 10 of 33 cases and by Williams and Karlaftis (1966) in 10 of 26 cases. With unilateral hydronephrosis the opposite kidney is frequently congenitally absent or the site of cystic dysplasia and nonfunctioning. Johnston *et al.* (1977) noted hydronephrosis of a solitary functioning kidney in nine of 219 cases.

Pelvic hydronephrosis and other urinary tract abnormalities are common coincidental findings in children with developmental lesions elsewhere, in particular congenital heart disease, imperforate anus and myelodysplasia. Investigation of the urinary tract should be routine in such cases.

Complications

Trauma

An enlarged diseased kidney is more susceptible to closed injury and more readily ruptured than a normal one. Many cases of pelvic hydronephrosis first present following trauma and Johnston *et al.* (1977) had eight such cases in their 219 patients. For this reason all renal injuries in children, even when apparently mild, require assessment by intravenous urography. Sometimes rupture involves the pelvis only, with no parenchymal injury, and in these circumstances haematuria may be slight or absent. Spontaneous perforation of a pelvic hydronephrosis is a rare cause of urinary ascites in the newborn (Johnston and Hood, 1969).

Calculi

Stones form in some 4.5 per cent of pelvic hydronephroses. They are usually composed of calcium phosphate and generally small and multiple. The staghorn stone that occurs with urinary infection caused by urea-splitting organisms is rarely associated with pelviureteric obstruction.

Pyonephrosis

Although positive bacterial cultures may be obtained from the urine in a hydronephrotic pelvis, severe infection leading to pyonephrosis and inflammatory destruction of the parenchyma is very rare.

Hypertension

Hypertension is an uncommon complication of hydronephrosis during childhood. It is encountered mainly when the disease involves a solitary kidney (Davis *et al.*, 1973). Increased renin secretion occurs chiefly in the early stages of pelviureteric obstruction and in chronic cases hypertension is the result of sodium retention. When the opposite kidney is anatomically normal some subtle defect in its ability to excrete sodium has been postulated (Vaughan, Buhler and Laragh, 1974). Normotension can generally by restored by pyeloureteroplasty. Presto and Middleton (1973) reported hypertension in a child with hydronephrosis who also had intrinsic stenosis of the ipsilateral renal artery.

Clinical features

Pelvic hydronephrosis in childhood is commoner in the male and in unilateral cases the left kidney is more often involved. In the series of Johnston *et al.* (1977) the male:female ratio was 154:65 and the left:right ratio 139:61.

In babies a very frequent mode of presentation is with a palpable and often visible abdominal tumour. The mass is commonly found on routine examination of the newborn child. In the series of Robson, Rudy and Johnston (1976) the hydronephrosis produced an obvious swelling in 18 of 33 cases. Other symptoms include fever, anorexia, failure to thrive and haematuria. If there is bilateral disease or a solitary kidney, acidaemia and azotaemia may be apparent clinically or on biochemical evaluation. With the increasing use of fetal ultrasound the diagnosis of hydronephrosis has been made prenatally in several instances.

After infancy pain, frequently accompanied by vomiting, is the commonest presenting complaint. The toddler often indicates the umbilical region as the site of his discomfort so that gastrointestinal disease may be simulated. In the older child pain is referred to the loin. On occasions there is a history of fever and of painful micturition suggestive of urinary infection, but documented bacilluria is uncommon and occurred in only 39 of the 219 cases seen by Johnston *et al.* (1977). Haematuria may occur even in the absence of such complications as trauma or stone and it is considered to be due to rupture of mucosal vessels caused by pelvic distension. Rarely hypertension is the presenting feature, either because of its effects or because of its detection at routine school medical examination.

Hydronephrosis may be quite symptomless and may be found unexpectedly on pyelography carried out for disorders of micturition or on the gratuitous pyelogram obtained following angiography in children with congenital heart disease. Genetic factors are undoubtedly concerned in the causation of hydronephrosis (Finn and Carruthers, 1974; Cohen *et al.*, 1978) and when a strong family history of the disorder exists pyelography is warranted in an asymptomatic child.

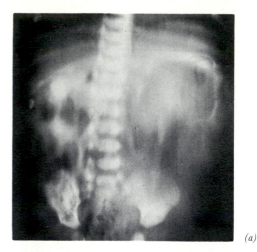

(a)

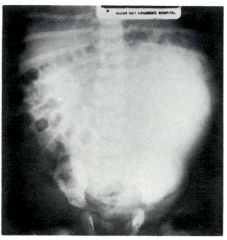

(b)

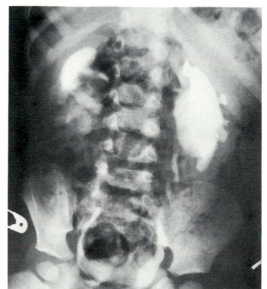

(c)

Figure 17.4. Intravenous pyelograms in a newborn boy with bilateral hydronephrosis due to pelviureteric obstruction and with a large abdominal mass. *(a)* Preoperative 20 minutes exposure showing calyceal dilatation on the right and a shell nephrogram on the left. *(b)* Preoperative 4 hours exposure demonstrating a large left hydronephrosis. *(c)* Twenty-two months after bilateral pyeloureteroplasty.

Diagnosis

As already discussed, in a long-standing hydronephrosis standard contrast-medium doses and exposure times during intravenous urography may fail to show the dilated system. However, with delayed films and, if necessary, a supplementary injection most hydronephroses can be demonstrated (*Figure 17.4*). Since the contrast medium sinks to the bottom of a pool of urine the pelviureteric obstruction is more obvious in the prone than in the supine position. If a normal-sized ureter is not visible below the dilated pelvis on the intravenous pyelogram, cystography is needed to exclude vesicoureteric reflux. In the absence of reflux retrograde ureterography is required to eliminate the possibility of the pelviureteric obstruction being secondary to an obstruction in the ureter or at the ureterovesical junction. This investigation is conveniently performed under anaesthesia immediately before operation. When there is no concentration on intravenous urography and when a distended kidney is evident on ultrasound the pathological anatomy can be shown by percutaneous needling and prograde pyelography.

Renal arteriography may be of prognostic value as regards the potential of the kidney to recover function (Aron, Tessler and Morales, 1973) but the investigation is not needed routinely. It is indicated if hypertension exists since hydronephrosis may coexist with renal arterial stenosis (Presto and Middleton, 1973).

Intermittent and equivocal hydronephrosis

With intermittent hydronephrosis the pelviureteric junction readily allows the transfer of urine when the urinary excretion rate is normal, but under conditions of diuresis it is unable to cope with the extra load so that pelvic dilatation occurs and pain results. Between attacks the pyelogram may be normal although a rather large pelvis and a high ureteric insertion are suggestive. The diagnosis may be made on intravenous urography or radioisotopic renography (O'Reilly *et al.*, 1978) when the patient is overhydrated or has received a diuretic such as frusemide. It is important to vary the patient's position during examination since obstruction may be demonstrable only in the erect posture. Fluoroscopy with urography is of particular value. Whitfield *et al.* (1977) considered that

obstruction was proven when with frusemide the area of the renal pelvis increased by more than 22 per cent. Sometimes investigations under diuresis give false-negative results and when uncertainty exists the most valuable technique is intravenous urography during an attack of pain.

When urography shows only mild pelvicalyceal dilatation or when calyectasis exists with an undilated pelvis a question arises as to whether or not obstruction exists. Useful information in such equivocal cases can be obtained from the investigations described above for intermittent hydronephrosis and also from retrograde pyelography with fluoroscopic observation of the over-filled pelvis. Whitfield *et al.* (1978) employed gamma-camera renography and reported that measuring radioisotopic transit times through the kidney parenchyma could determine if an obstructive nephropathy was present. Whitaker (1978) performs pressure-flow studies following percutaneous puncture of the renal pelvis and instillation of saline in cases of doubtful obstruction. The intravesical pressure is monitored through a catheter passed *per urethram*. An intrapelvic inflow rate of 10 ml/min is employed. The sum of pressure produced by the resistance in the pelvic tube and the intravesical pressure is subtracted from the intrapelvic pressure to provide the pressure required for saline to pass from the pelvis to the bladder. In the absence of obstruction this should not exceed 12 cm of saline.

Treatment

In adults pelvic hydronephrosis can be a stable condition in which the radiological appearance and the renal function remain unchanged for long periods (Bratt, Aurell and Nilsson, 1977). In children the lesion is more likely to be progressive because of increasing urine output with growth and there is always the risk of complications such as trauma, stone formation and infection. The author's view is that operative intervention is indicated in unequivocal cases whether or not symptoms exist.

Nephrectomy

Nephrectomy is required when the renal parenchyma is irredeemably damaged and the kidney can make no useful contribution to total renal function. As already discussed preoperative assessment of the degree of recovery possible can be extremely difficult and the decision between nephrectomy and pyeloplasty often has to be made at operation. In young infants it is commonly found that a large abdominal mass clinically suggestive of an irreversible lesion consists of a very dilated pelvis with a well preserved kidney perched on its periphery. Severe cystic dysplasia is a clear indication for nephrectomy. Otherwise an assessment should be made, after the pelvis has been emptied, of the total volume of kidney tissue present rather than of its thickness alone. Generally one should err on the side of preserving a doubtful kidney rather than removing it since useful restoration of function can occur in what appeared initially to be an organ of little value.

Nephrostomy

Nephrostomy as a preliminary to definitive surgery may be useful for allowing assessment of the prospects for functional recovery in a kidney of uncertain value. From the therapeutic viewpoint nephrostomy has few indications. It may be required as a very temporary measure when there is a tense hydronephrosis and operation must be delayed because of intercurrent disease or the need for surgery to a better-preserved contralateral kidney. The preferred technique is percutaneous insertion of a fine polyethylene catheter into the renal pelvis through a needle.

Pyeloureteroplasty

The release of local angulations is often sufficient to relieve pelviureteric obstruction, but except in some cases of hydronephrosis due to persisting fetal folds the kinks inevitably reform after operation so that some form of pyeloplasty is nearly always needed. Dismembered pyeloureteroplasty of the Anderson-Hynes (Anderson, 1963) type is applicable to most cases (*Figure 17.5*). Because of the small calibre of the ureter in infants and young children it may be impossible to produce a water-tight pelviureteric anastomosis and at the same time avoid the possibility of early postoperative obstruction due to oedema. For this reason it is the author's practice to splint the anastomosis by a fine polyethylene catheter and provide nephrostomy drainage for some 10 days. The calamitous effects of drainage predicted by Anderson (1963)

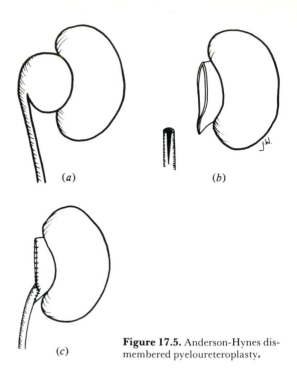

(a)   (b)

(c)

Figure 17.5. Anderson-Hynes dismembered pyeloureteroplasty.

have not occurred. Nephrostomy, even with a closed drainage system, must carry a small risk of allowing the introduction of infection but this remote possibility seems preferable to disruption of the suture line with prolonged urine leakage and to the possible consequences of scarring and recurrent obstruction when splinting and nephrostomy are omitted. Nephrostomy drainage without splintage may allow transverse healing and obstruction at the pelviureteric anastomosis (Rickwood and Phadke, 1978).

For obstruction associated with an aberrant renal artery Stewart (1947) fixed the upper and lower kidney poles in apposition so that the aberrant vessel was brought upwards clear of the pelviureteric junction. Hellstrom (1927) mobilized the artery and either sutured its adventitia to the pelvis or buried it in a tunnel in the anterior pelvic wall. With both methods obstructing angulations must be freed in addition. Neither technique is essential since the obstructive effect of an aberrant artery is readily eliminated during a dismembered pyeloureteroplasty simply by performing the anastomosis anterior to the vessel.

With bilateral hydronephrosis both kidneys may be dealt with at the same operative session, employing either a transverse transperitoneal approach or separate extraperitoneal anterior abdominal incisions. Alternatively each kidney can be treated separately with an interval of 2 weeks between operations.

Duplex, horseshoe and ectopic kidneys

Pelviureteric obstruction may occur in the lower component of a double ureteric system. Pyeloureteroplasty can often be performed by the usual dismembered technique but if the two ureters unite a short distance below the kidney it may be necessary to anastomose the pelvis of the lower hemikidney to the side of the ureter from the upper one. The latter is usually very narrow so that a meticulous technique is needed to avoid ureteric stenosis or devascularization.

Pelviureteric obstruction in malrotated kidneys such as horseshoe and pelvic ectopic organs is generally associated with a high ureteric insertion on a high sited pelvis, and employing the dismembered operation it may not be possible to construct a funnel-shaped pelvis coning straight into the ureter. Correction of the malrotation, which requires division of the bridge of a horseshoe kidney, may improve the anatomical arrangement but this is often prevented by an anomalous renal blood supply. The difficulty is

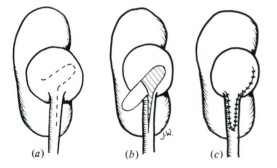

(a)   *(b)*   *(c)*

Figure 17.6. Culp-DeWeerd pyeloureteroplasty.

best resolved by the use of the pelvic-flap pyeloplasty technique of Culp and DeWeerd (1951; *Figure 17.6*). This allows the construction of a low pelviureteric junction without the need to alter the position of the kidney.

Results

In general pyeloureteroplasty for pelvic hydronephrosis produces excellent clinical results such that the operative mortality should be nil,

the morbidity rate is small, complications are uncommon and symptoms are nearly always completely relieved. Reoperation was needed in only seven of 214 kidneys in the series of Johnston *et al.* (1977). In three cases calculi had formed and in four there was persistent or recurrent obstruction; no secondary nephrectomies were needed. On the other hand the pyelographic result is often disappointing in that the calyceal outlines rarely return to normal except when obstruction was intermittent or very recent. Johnston *et al.* (1977) studied the pyelograms of 140 kidneys before and after pyeloureteroplasty and found that calyceal dilatation had deteriorated in five, was unaltered in 53 and had improved in 82. Maximum improvement is reached within 6 months of operation. Johnston and Kathel (1972) assessed the results of operation in 32 hydronephrotic kidneys in children by comparing preoperative and postoperative isotopic renograms assessed by analogue-computer simulation. Even in the absence of pyelographic change it was found that 23 kidneys had improved tubular function and 29 had increased emptying rates after operation. Tveter, Nerdrum and Mjolnerod (1975) also found that improved renal function and drainage could be shown by renography in 75 per cent of cases after pyeloureteroplasty.

Lengthy follow-up is advisable for children who have had bilateral hydronephrosis or hydronephrosis involving a solitary kidney because of the possibility of failure of kidney growth and the consequent onset of renal insufficiency. In patients with unilateral disease prolonged review and repeated pyelography are particularly necessary if nephrectomy has been performed since the increased workload imposed on the contralateral kidney may lead to the later development of hydronephrosis even after an interval of several years.

Megacalycosis

In this relatively common condition all the major and minor calyces of the affected kidney show various degrees of dilatation; the overlying parenchyma is thinned but the pelvis is undilated and cones normally into a normal ureter (*Figure 17.7*). As a rule the lesion is unilateral.

Urinary stasis in the dilated calyces may be apparent on radiography and renography although there is no demonstrable urinary obstruction and the pelvis is seen at fluoroscopy to empty freely into the ureter. Gittes and Talner (1972) considered megacalycosis to be due to a developmental hypoplasia of the renal pyramids of unknown causation. Johnston (1973) pointed out the similarity of the pathological changes to those seen in cases of hydronephrosis caused by persisting fetal ureteric folds and suggested that the condition may be the result of a burnt-out

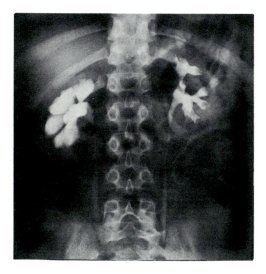

Figure 17.7. Megacalycosis of the right kidney. Intravenous pyelogram showing uniformly dilated calyces and a normal unobstructed pelvis.

obstruction in which fetal folds led to obstructive changes in the kidney and then involuted, as they normally do, so that only the effects of the obstruction remained. This concept is supported by the occasional finding of a true obstructed hydronephrosis in the opposite kidney and by the occurrence of cases with minor degrees of fold obstruction which lie midway between megacalycosis and fully developed hydronephrosis.

Unobstructed megacalycosis calls for no operative treatment. Vesicoureteric reflux must be excluded since it may be associated with a similar pyelographic picture, and the possibility of intermittent pelviureteric obstruction may need consideration and appropriate investigation.

Ureteric aplasia, hypoplasia, stenosis and atresia

If the ureteric bud fails to form then the ipsilateral hemitrigone is absent, and since the differentiation of the metanephros depends upon contact with a ureter the kidney does not develop. In the male the derivatives of the mesonephric duct may be absent or anomalous.

Hypoplasia, stenosis and atresia of the ureter may take several forms. The entire ureter including the pelvis may be absent or there may be a narrow thin-walled tube or a solid threadlike structure. The ureter may taper to an atretic end a few centimetres below the kidney. In some instances there is an atretic gap with an intact ureter above and below. Such gross abnormalities are associated with severe renal dysplasia of aplastic or multicystic type. It is likely that the ureteric obstruction is responsible for the renal malformation since Beck (1971) was able to produce renal dysplasia by obstructing the ureter in fetal lambs. The ureteric lesion itself may be the result of some intrinsic fault in the embryonic bud but the pathological appearances, in particular that in which a localized segment of ureter is missing, suggest that the ureter may have developed normally but was then subjected to ischaemic or other adverse influences. Gross ureteric anomalies with renal dysplasia often coexist with contralateral hydronephrosis due to lesser degrees of congenital obstruction.

When associated with a functioning kidney localized ureteric hypoplasia and luminal narrowing is seen most often just below the pelviureteric junction in cases of hydronephrosis. As stated above it remains uncertain whether the lesion is the primary cause of the obstruction or a secondary development consequent on pelviureteric angulations. Rarely stenosis affects the middle third of the ureter. Allen (1970) described its occurrence at the pelvic brim and considered that a defect in the ureteric musculature might be caused by vascular compression during fetal life. Severe annular constriction of the midureter causing hydroureteronephrosis was described by Johnston (1968) and is generally associated with a more severely anomalous contralateral ureter with renal dysplasia and lack of function. Radiologically stenosis of the middle portion of the ureter may be simulated

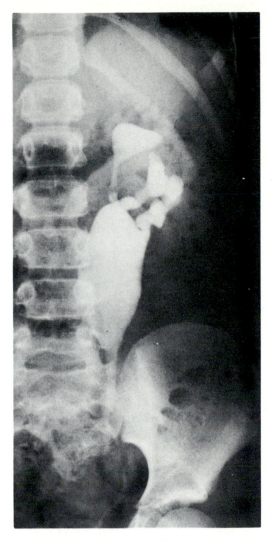

Figure 17.8. Extrarenal pelvis with a low sited pelvi-ureteric junction simulating ureteric stricture. The infundibula are also extrarenal.

by a low sited pelviureteric junction (*Figure 17.8*). The absence of obstruction with the latter is readily demonstrable by fluoroscopy.

Vascular obstruction of the ureter

An aberrant renal artery crossing the ureter just below the pelviureteric junction is a well recognized factor in the causation of pelvic hydronephrosis (see above). Vascular obstruction of the ureter at lower levels is uncommon. Young and Kiser (1965) reported cases of compression of the juxtavesical ureter by the obliterated umbilical artery, but since division of the vessel did not improve ureteric emptying it is likely that these were examples of obstructed megaureter and that the abnormal artery was not the essential aetiological factor. However, in the patients of Greene *et al.* (1954) and Javadpour, Solomon and Bush (1972) division of anomalous vessels crossing the lower ureter was effective in relieving ureteric dilatation. Compression and obstruction of the right ureter by the ovarian vein has been described in women during and after pregnancy. Although the ovarian vein syndrome is occasionally invoked to explain recurrent right lower quadrant pain in postpubertal girls, proof of its occurrence in this age group is lacking and indeed some authors (Coolsaet, 1978) have questioned whether at any age it exists at all.

Circumcaval ureter

A circumcaval position of the ureter is the result of abnormal development of the abdominal venous system and not of the urinary tract. The commonest form of the condition, in which the right ureter encircles the inferior vena cava from behind forwards, is due to persistence of the right posterior cardinal vein or the right subcardinal vein instead of the supracardinal vein as the definitive vena cava. In spite of its anomalous derivation the vena cava is generally of normal anatomical appearance. Kenawi and Williams (1976) recognized two types of resulting urological abnormality. In the first the renal pelvis and the upper ureter are directed medially and almost horizontally, and in these patients there is little or no urinary obstruction. In the second variety the proximal ureter descends from the renal pelvis and then curves upwards and medially as a reversed J to pass behind the vena cava at about the level of the third lumbar vertebra (*Figure 17.9*). Obstruction with dilatation of the upper ureter results from venous compression of the ureter against the vertebra and local ureteric fibrosis and stenosis may develop secondarily. In addition obstructive kinks may occur at the junction of the descending and ascending limbs of the J and sometimes also at the pelviureteric junction.

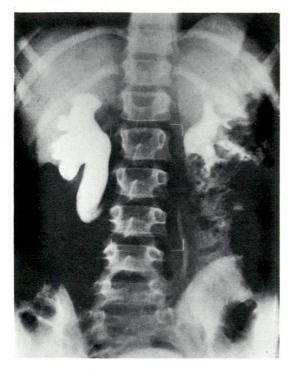

Figure 17.9. Circumcaval ureter with obstruction at the ureteric angulation.

Abnormalities of the contralateral kidney such as agenesis, hydronephrosis, ectopia and hypoplasia may be present. Other congenital anomalies involving the cardiovascular system commonly coexist. Circumcaval ureter occasionally presents during childhood but more often symptoms do not occur until the third or fourth decade. The diagnosis is made from intravenous and/or retrograde urography which demonstrates the spiral course of the ureter, its close proximity to the vertebral column and the dilated supracaval segment.

At operation the ureter is preferably divided through its dilated portion; the lower end is then brought from behind the vena cava and reanastomosis is performed. If the retrocaval part of the ureter is stenotic or closely adherent to the caval wall, division of the undilated infracaval portion may be unavoidable. The ureteric anastomosis should be made obliquely and temporary splintage is advisable.

Other variations on the theme of circumcaval ureter are rare. Murphy (1963) described a right ureter lying behind bilateral venae cavae. The left ureter may be circumcaval in association with situs inversus abdominis (Brooks, 1962).

Hanna (1972) reported cases in which the ureters passed posterior to the common iliac vessels.

Ureteric valves

Multiple transverse folds produced by invaginations of the musculature occur in the ureter as a normal phase of fetal development (Ostling, 1942). They often persist postnatally and may be seen, particularly in the upper ureter, on pyelograms in infants (*Figure 17.10*). Ordinarily

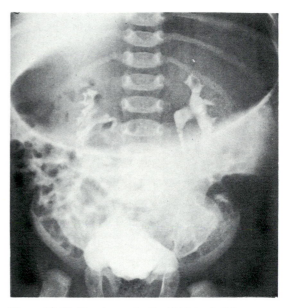

Figure 17.10. Nonobstructive fetal folds in the left ureter below the pelviureteric junction. Intravenous pyelogram in a newborn girl.

the folds are not obstructive and disappear with growth, but in some instances (see above) they occur in an exaggerated valvular form and may cause pelvic hydronephrosis. Folds that obstruct and later involute have been considered to be responsible for megacalycosis (Johnston, 1973).

Valvular obstructions in the middle and lower ureter are rare; they were described by Busch *et al.* (1963). Ureteric valves must be distinguished from the angulations commonly seen in a dilated and lengthened ureter and also from the kink that may occur at the junction of the dilated and undilated segments of an obstructed megaureter.

Fowler and Kesavan (1977) reported what they termed a tilt valve in the lower ureter. The condition is characterized by a sharp angulation between the dilated proximal ureter and a short undilated extravesical segment. The anatomy is very similar to that of an obstructed megaureter although the undilated portion is not obstructive and side-to-side anastomosis between it and the dilated ureter effectively allows the latter to drain into the bladder.

Acquired extrinsic ureteric obstruction

Displacement and obstruction of the ureter may result from retroperitoneal inflammatory conditions such as may complicate vertebral osteomyelitis or a perforated appendix. Neoplastic disease, for example neuroblastoma, teratoma, the various types of lymphoma and secondary lymph-node involvement from a testicular tumour, may have a similar effect.

Retroperitoneal fibrosis

Idiopathic retroperitoneal fibrosis is essentially a disease of adult life but several cases have been reported during childhood (Farrer and Peterson, 1962; Peterson, Besecker and Hutchison, 1974). The fibrosis begins in the region of the great vessels at the level of the sacral promontory and extends laterally to envelop the ureter. The inferior vena cava or the aorta may be partly occluded. Obstruction of the ureters occurs as a result of fibrotic compression interfering with peristalsis and as a rule there is no invasion of the ureteric wall.

Nonidiopathic retroperitoneal fibrosis in children, producing effects similar to those seen in the idiopathic type, has been reported from a variety of causes. Vasculitis following Henoch-Schoenlein purpura, rheumatoid arthritis, retroperitoneal haemorrhage, extravasation of urine, lymphangitis secondary to leg infections and systemic lupus erythematosus has been cited (Cerny and Scott, 1971; Lloyd *et al.*, 1974; Wacksman, Weinerth and Kredick, 1978). Some cases have followed the administration of methysergide bimaleate, an antiserotonin drug used in the treatment of migraine. The time interval between the initial pathological lesion and the onset of symptoms due to fibrosis may be some months or even years.

The symptomatology of retroperitoneal fibrosis is often vague. Pain in the back or the gluteal region, immobility of the hip and oedema or ischaemia of the legs may result from fibrous involvement of the posterior abdominal musculature or from compression of the great vessels or the retroperitoneal lymphatics. Loin pain may occur because of ureteric obstruction, and polyuria and polydipsia simulating diabetes insipidus may develop because of interference with renal tubular function. On occasions oliguria or anuria of sudden onset occurs without previous symptoms. Weight loss, fever and an elevated erythrocyte sedimentation rate are often present. Pyelography demonstrates hydronephrosis and dilatation of the proximal ureter and characteristically the lower ureter is displaced medially. Ultrasound reveals a smooth-bordered and relatively echo-free mass in front of the sacral promontory. This investigation is valuable for diagnosis and also for following the response to treatment (Sanders *et al.*, 1977).

Treatment depends upon the pathogenesis. In nonidiopathic cases the fibrosis may resolve with antibiotic control of inflammation, discontinuation of methysergide bimaleate when it is incriminated, and steroid therapy when collagen diseases are responsible and the erythrocyte sedimentation rate is raised. Ureteric obstruction may need emergency nephrostomy drainage prior to operative freeing of the ureters from the fibrous plaque. Recurrent obstruction after ureterolysis can be prevented by placing the ureters intraperitoneally or wrapping them in pedicle grafts of omentum.

Diverticula of the pelvis and the ureter

These anomalies are rare. Myers and DeWeerd (1972) described a very large diverticulum of a normal renal pelvis which produced an abdominal mass in a 7-week-old boy. Such a lesion is presumed to represent one moiety of a duplex pelvis, or possibly a supernumerary infundibulum, which failed to establish communication with the developing renal blastema. Ureteric diverticula diagnosed during childhood occur as muscle-coated tubular protrusions extending upwards from and almost parallel to the ureter itself. The size of the diverticular lumen is generally similar to that of the ureter and there is little doubt that the diverticulum represents a blind-ending branch of a bifid ureter. Complications such as infection or calculus formation are uncommon and surgery is not needed in their absence. Multiple tiny ureteric diverticula may be encountered in adults (Norman and Dubowy, 1966). They are seen on retrograde but not intravenous urography and are considered to be due to small mucosal herniations between the muscle fibres caused by an abnormally high intraureteric pressure. Such diverticula are of no clinical significance.

Transient ureteric dilatation in infancy

Moderate dilatation of the ureter without demonstrable obstruction or vesicoureteric reflux and with spontaneous resolution is occasionally encountered in the newborn and in young babies who have undergone excretory urography because of failure to thrive or suspected urinary infection. Otherwise the ureterectasis may be discovered fortuitously in infants having routine pyelography because of some nonurological congenital abnormality with which urinary tract lesions are commonly associated; for example Rickwood (1978) reported its occurrence in cases of imperforate anus. The aetiology of the ureteric dilatation is obscure. Low grade infection or delayed maturation of ureteric function may be significant. Alternatively maternal hormones may have a similar dilating effect on the fetal ureter as they do on that of the mother. As a rule the ureteric dilatation involves mainly the lumbar spindle and in most cases calyectasis is absent or minimal.

The obstructed megaureter

Pathology

In this condition, also termed primary, idiopathic and nonrefluxing megaureter, the intravesical and intramural parts of the ureter and

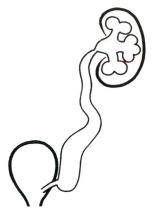

Figure 17.11. Diagram of the anatomy of obstructed megaureter.

sometimes also a short length of the extravesical ureter are of normal calibre but constitute an obstruction to the flow of urine (*Figure 17.11*). Although some authors (Allen, 1970) have designated the lesion as a stricture, in the vast majority of cases there is no ureteric stenosis and a ureteric catheter or a probe at operation can be passed easily. At fluoroscopy and at surgery the undilated part of the ureter can be seen to

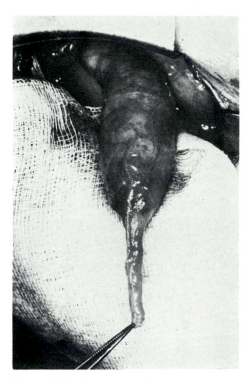

Figure 17.12. Operation photograph of obstructed megaureter showing the junction of the dilated and undilated segments.

produce a functional block in that it fails to transmit the peristaltic wave from the dilated portion (*Figure 17.12*). The precise pathogenesis is disputed and different authors have described different histological changes in the inert ureteric segment. It is possible that more than one lesion may be responsible. Murnaghan (1957) noted an abnormal muscular arrangement with an excess of circular in proportion to longitudinal fibres. Tanagho (1974) confirmed this observation and postulated that the anomaly resulted from a failure of the normal process of elongation of the lower ureter during embryogenesis because of compression by blood vessels or the vas deferens. Mackinnon *et al.* (1970) found a muscular deficiency in the obstructive segment which would explain its failure to conduct peristalsis. Notley (1972) recorded an excess of collagen that might lead to obstruction by preventing normal ureteric distension without causing luminal narrowing. Cussen (1977) showed that the wall of the dilated portion of the ureter exhibited both muscular hypertrophy and hyperplasia since there was an increase in the number and the size of the muscle cells.

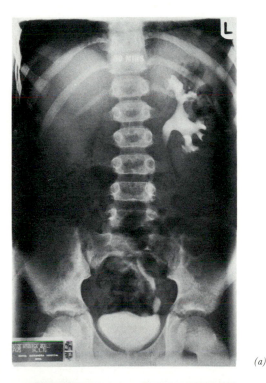

(a)

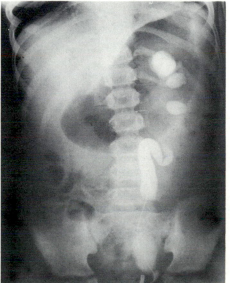

(b)

Figure 17.13. Late onset dilatation in a boy with obstructed megaureter affecting a solitary left kidney. (*a*) Intravenous pyelogram at 9 years with left flank pain. The pyelogram is normal with slight dilatation of the lower ureter. (*b*) Retrograde pyelogram 6 months later and following 2 days of anuria showing typical obstructed megaureter. (*c*) Intravenous pyelogram 6 months after ureteric reimplantation. Normal anatomy restored.

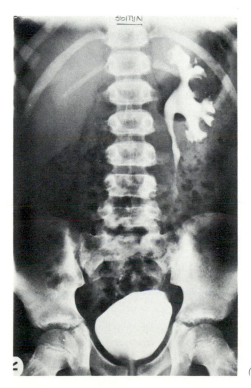

(c)

Typically the ureteric dilatation resulting from the obstruction is maximal immediately above the dysfunctional segment and often the ureter is somewhat lengthened and tortuous. Calyectasis of variable degree is generally present but as a rule the pelvis remains relatively undilated unless there is a secondary obstruction at the pelviureteric junction. Rarely the ureteric dilatation is minimal even though the obstruction leads to well marked calyceal clubbing and parenchymal thinning. It is important to recognize that although the causative pathology in the lower ureter is of congenital origin, the proximal ureter is not necessarily dilated at birth or in early childhood and that symptoms of ureteric obstruction may exist before decompensation of the musculature occurs and dilatation develops (*Figure 17.13*).

Obstructed megaureter may occur bilaterally. However, the ureters are often asymmetrically affected and dilatation may be severe on one side before it is apparent on the other. In unilateral cases the left ureter is more often affected and the contralateral kidney is frequently abnormal. Tiburcio and Lima (1978) reviewed 80 cases of obstructed megaureter. They found that the condition was bilateral in seven and that in unilateral cases the left:right proportion was 41:32. The opposite kidney was congenitally absent in 10 patients, dysplastic and nonfunctioning in two and associated with severe reflux in one.

Complications

The most common complication is infection. Association with Proteus infection may lead to calculus formation and this complication occurred in eight of the author's cases. Typically facetted stones form a cast of the dilated ureter and a staghorn calculus may develop in the kidney in addition (*Figure 17.14*). In adults with long-standing megaureter a transitional cell carcinoma may develop in the dilated portion (Heal, 1973).

Clinical features

Obstructed megaureter is significantly commoner in boys and in the author's series the male:female ratio was 65:15. The series of Williams and Hulme-Moir (1970) and Hanna and

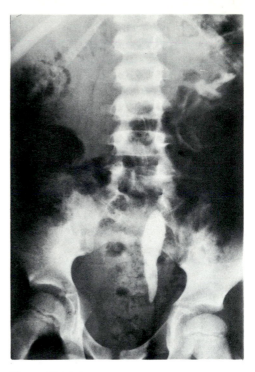

Figure 17.14. Straight film showing ureteric and renal calculi complicating obstructed megaureter.

Jeffs (1975) also showed a male preponderance and a similar higher incidence of involvement on the left side. Presentation is often in early childhood and 26 of the author's cases were seen in the first year of life. The symptoms are usually those of urinary infection with fever and abdominal or flank pain. Haematuria may occur even in the absence of stones and is presumed to be due to the tearing of mucosal vessels as a result of ureteric distension. When a solitary functioning kidney is affected there may be features of either acute or chronic renal insufficiency.

Diagnosis

The diagnosis of obstructed megaureter is usually first suggested from the intravenous urogram which typically shows calyectasis and ureteric dilatation with a rounded lower extremity in the dilated segment; occasionally a thin wisp of contrast medium is seen in the undilated part. However, quite often impaired renal concentration and contrast-medium dilution prevent clear demonstration of the pathological anatomy on the excretion pyelogram so that confirmation of the diagnosis and adequate assessment require retrograde or prograde urography. At endoscopy the ureteric orifice is usually of normal appearance while sometimes it is raised on a nipple. Fluoroscopy following injection of contrast medium usually reveals that the dilated ureter undergoes vigorous peristalsis although the contractions do not obliterate the lumen. As the wave descends the terminal ureteric segment fails to open adequately, if at all, and the contrast medium is squeezed back within the contraction ring towards the kidney. Marked delay in ureteric emptying is characteristic. In some instances, particularly when there has been an acute exacerbation of obstruction, the dilated ureter is aperistaltic and inert. This does not necessarily mean that the situation is irreversible and such ureters are often capable of recovering activity when they are decompressed. Usually cystography reveals the absence of vesicoureteric reflux. Infrequently reflux does occur, but it is of minor degree and does not resemble the free massive reflux seen with the refluxing megaureter.

Treatment

Occasionally the kidney drained by an obstructed megaureter has already been destroyed by back-pressure or infection or both at the time of presentation so that nephroureterectomy is unavoidable. If any doubt exists as to the potential of the kidney, a short period of nephrostomy drainage is indicated because useful recovery of function can occur in an apparently unpromising case when obstruction is relieved and infection is controlled. At the other extreme there are mild degrees of obstructed megaureter with minimal ureteric dilatation and little or no calyectasis. Such cases, which are encountered mainly in the older child or adult, may be managed by observation alone and the condition can remain unaltered for many years. Nevertheless, there is always the possibility of sudden deterioration with the development of acute-on-chronic obstruction, severe infective complications or calculus formation. In the great majority of cases of obstructed megaureter presenting during childhood reconstructive surgery is indicated.

Ureteric reimplantation

The Politano-Leadbetter (Politano and Leadbetter, 1958) transvesical technique of

ureteric reimplantation can be employed following resection of the adynamic ureteric segment when the ureter is only mildly or moderately dilated and without significant redundancy and tortuosity. When the latter exist my own preference in unilateral cases is an extravesical approach, modified from Paquin (1959), in order to ensure preservation of the ureteric blood supply.

The ureter is exposed extraperitoneally through an oblique incision in the appropriate iliac fossa and is ligated and divided at its entry to the bladder. Tortuosities are released as far as the ureteric blood supply allows and the resulting redundant part of the ureter along with any extravesical aperistaltic segment is excised. The extremity of the remaining ureter is narrowed over a length of some 50 mm by excision with resuture of a wedge of ureteric wall. The wedge must be taken from the antimesenteric aspect of the ureter, preserving the main longitudinally running blood vessels. The temptation to produce a normal ureteric calibre must be resisted to avoid jeopardizing the blood supply. There is no necessity for extensive remodelling of the ureter and only the part that is to form the new intravesical ureter need be narrowed surgically. Through an oblique incision in the superolateral bladder wall the narrowed ureter is reimplanted to lie in a submucosal tunnel that brings the new ureteric orifice very close to the original one.

To prevent subsequent vesicoureteric reflux the new intravesical ureter must be of sufficient length relative to its diameter. Since the narrowed ureteric segment is still wider than normal a longer than normal intravesical ureter is

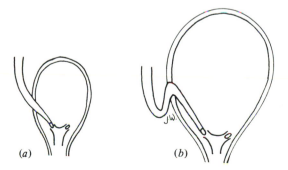

Figure 17.15. Possible effects of reimplanting the ureter high in the bladder. (*a*) With the bladder empty the ureter has a straight course. (*b*) When the bladder fills and the ureteric hiatus rises, the ureter becomes angulated. This complication can be avoided by suturing the bladder musculature below the new hiatus to the psoas muscle so that the ureteric entry is rendered immovable.

needed. The new ureteric hiatus must therefore be high in the bladder wall and this may lead to the late complication of ureteric angulation and obstruction when the bladder fills (*Figure 17.15*). Such a possibility can be averted by suturing the detrusor musculature to the psoas muscle so that the new hiatus is a fixed immovable point.

Secondary pelviuretic obstruction

Although secondary angulations are commonly present in a tortuous megaureter they are not themselves obstructive and any remaining after ureteric reimplantation straighten out spontaneously with time. However, interference with pelvic emptying can occur when the ureter angulates on the renal pelvis. In such instances the pelvis is more dilated than with lower ureteric obstruction alone and on occasions the intravenous urogram fails to demonstrate the dilated ureter so that a misdiagnosis of primary pelvic hydronephrosis may be made. Secondary pelviureteric obstruction may resolve spontaneously after ureteric reimplantation. More often it does not and pyeloureteroplasty is then needed.

Results

The obstructed megaureter and its related kidney generally show a great capacity for recovery and reconstructive surgery gives highly satisfactory results. Often the ureter returns to a virtually normal calibre and there is obvious lessening of calyceal dilatation (*Figure 17.13*). Tiburcio and Lima's (1978) review of the author's cases recorded postoperative pyelographic improvement in 86 per cent of renal-ureteric units and deterioration in 6 per cent, mainly because of vesicoureteric reflux. Similar results have been reported by Williams and Hulme-Moir (1970) and Hanna and Jeffs (1975).

Orthotopic ureterocele

In children a simple or orthotopic ureterocele involving the termination of a single ureter is less commonly encountered than an ectopic ureterocele sited on the ureter draining the upper moiety of a duplex kidney. In the author's experience (Snyder and Johnston, 1978) the latter exceed the former in a proportion of about 4:1.

The orthotopic ureterocele represents a cystic dilatation of the intravesical portion of the ureter which occurs as a result of stenosis of the ureteric orifice. The cyst extends between the superficial and deep muscle layers of the trigone so that it is restricted to the trigonal area. Often the ureteric enlargement is asymmetrical and the orifice may then be sited on the superior or medial aspect of the ureterocele. The wall is composed of connective tissue and stretched muscle fibres covered externally by bladder mucosa and lined by ureteric mucosa. The size of the ureterocele depends upon the length of the intravesical ureter and the size of the orifice. With severe meatal stenosis the cyst is large and permanently distended and with lesser degrees of obstruction it remains small, fills only with the arrival of each urine bolus and collapses after it has emptied into the bladder.

The degree of upper urinary tract dilatation varies. Snyder and Johnston (1978) reported significant hydroureteronephrosis in 13 of 20 childhood cases in four of which the affected kidney failed to concentrate contrast medium on intravenous urography and in one of which the upper end of the ureter ended blindly in the pelvis without any kidney tissue present. Amar (1971) reported a similar case of a ureterocele draining a blind-ending ureter. A large ureterocele may encroach upon and obstruct the opposite ureteric orifice. Not uncommonly ureteroceles occur bilaterally. There is a high incidence of associated congenital abnormalities, and imperforate anus, vaginal agenesis and spina bifida were seen in the author's series.

Ureteroceles are believed to result from obstruction of the developing ureter during embryogenesis. Tanagho (1972) suggested that there is delayed and incomplete canalization of the ureteric bud at its origin from the mesonephric duct. The concept of a prenatal obstruction implies that the dilatation of the system is caused by distension with urine. This is difficult to reconcile with absence of the kidney although it is possible that there is in such cases transient urine production by a renal unit that subsequently vanishes.

Diagnosis

A ureterocele is generally demonstrable by intravenous urography. It may appear as a positive cobra-headed dilatation surrounded by a thin contrast-free halo within the cystogram (*Figure 17.16*) or, when renal function is impaired, as a round radiolucent filling defect. In

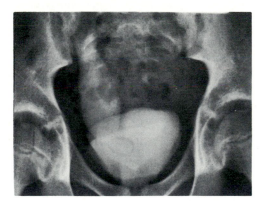

Figure 17.16. Intravenous pyelogram showing right orthotopic ureterocele with a halo surrounding a 'cobra-head' and a dilated ureter.

the latter situation it is important by careful endoscopic scrutiny to exclude the possibility of an ectopic ureterocele draining a small nonfunctioning upper hemikidney and causing secondary obstruction of the twin ureter and the lower hemikidney. The ureterocele is usually readily recognized at cystoscopy as a persistent or intermittent cyst and its narrow urine jet may be visible. However, a lax ureterocele may be compressed and emptied by high intravesical pressure and sometimes it becomes everted into the extravesical ureter so that a diverticulum is simulated. Similar eversion may occur during micturating cystography and in these circumstances vesicoureteric reflux may be seen.

Treatment

In the unusual case of an orthotopic ureterocele in which there is no upper tract dilatation an expectant attitude is warranted. The existence of hydroureteronephrosis necessitates surgery. Simple incision of the ureterocele either endoscopically or at open operation has been reported to give satisfactory results in adults (Wines and O'Flynn, 1972). This method carries a good chance of allowing subsequent ureteric reflux,

even when the incision is restricted to the inferior aspect of the cyst, and is inadvisable in young children except as a temporary measure to allow drainage of a severely infected system. The optimum treatment is excision of the ureterocele and reimplantation of the ureter into the bladder. When the ureteric dilatation is no more than moderate the Politano-Leadbetter (Politano and Leadbetter, 1958) transvesical technique is satisfactory. With severe dilatation an extravesical approach with ureteric tailoring similar to that described for megaureter is preferable. It is often necessary to strengthen the thinned vesical bed of the ureterocele by approximating strong musculature from either side.

Differential diagnosis: obstruction or stasis?

Many types of pelviureteric dilatation resulting from obstruction have characteristic anatomical features and their radiological and endoscopic demonstration allows the causative pathology to be determined without difficulty. However, it is important to make a full clinical and urological assessment if diagnostic errors are to be avoided. For example obstruction at the pelviureteric junction may be secondary to lower ureteric obstruction or gross vesicoureteric reflux, and a primary pelvic hydronephrosis may be misdiagnosed if the anatomy and the function of the ureter and the ureterovesical junction are not investigated. Also, in some infravesical obstructions the most obvious radiological feature is bilateral upper tract dilatation and delayed ureteric emptying into the bladder so that the omission of adequate examination of the bladder and the urethra may suggest an obstruction at the ureterovesical juntion.

It cannot be assumed that every dilated non-refluxing ureter is obstructed. Other pathogenic factors such as infection, pre-existing but no longer active obstruction, primary or secondary impairment of ureteric muscular activity and polyuria must be considered.

Bacterial ureteritis has been shown to cause paresis of the ureteric musculature and luminal dilatation involving mainly the lumbar spindle by the direct action of endotoxins (Teague and Boyarsky, 1968). Such ureteritis is probably responsible for the reversible ureteric dilatation commonly seen on intravenous urography when the kidney contains a staghorn infection stone.

Megacalycosis has been considered to be the result of a transient ureteric obstruction caused by fetal folds in the upper ureter. The folds subsequently disappear, leaving only the residue of their obstructive effects (Johnston, 1973).

Defective muscularization of the pelviureteric wall, often with fibrous replacement, may be a primary developmental abnormality as with ectopic ureter or in cases of the prune belly syndrome. Moderately dilated hypodynamic ureters of this type are commonly encountered in children with anorectal anomalies. Alternatively, in an initially normal ureter impaired muscular activity may be secondary to long-standing dilatation consequent on obstruction, especially when this is complicated by invasive infection.

Polyuria increases the workload of the renal pelvis and the ureter and if it is of sufficient degree then even a normal system may be unable to cope so that dilatation and impaired peristaltic activity result. Such effects are seen with diabetes insipidus of hypothalamic-pituitary or nephrogenic origin. The latter may be a primary inherited anomaly or secondary to a variety of renal lesions including obstructive nephropathy (Shapiro *et al.*, 1978) in which case obligatory polyuria exacerbates the degree of pelviureteric dilatation due to the obstruction. In a normal child the diuretic effect of intravenous contrast medium in a high dose can cause moderate upper tract dilatation if the bladder is full during the investigation.

Differentiation of a true urinary obstruction from urinary stasis resulting from one or more of the above factors may be difficult, especially since obstruction can produce these effects secondarily. As already discussed valuable information can be obtained from high dose intravenous urography or from retrograde or prograde urography with fluoroscopy. Radioisotopic and scanning techniques under conditions of diuresis may also be helpful. However, the answer may only be obtained when the pressures in the system are measured during maximal rates of flow (Whitaker, 1978) and this investigation must be regarded as the final arbiter (see Hydronephrosis due to pelviureteric obstruction).

Pyeloureteritis, impaired muscular activity and polyuria require consideration not only as primary causes of pelviureteric dilatation and urinary stasis but also as regards their secondary roles of increasing the severity of dilatation and stasis in cases of undoubted obstruction. In the latter event the existence of one or more of these factors and the possibility of its improvement or reversal clearly modifies the results obtainable from surgical relief of obstruction and may influence the technique employed. When the secondary effects are minimal simple relief of the obstruction should be sufficient to restore normal pyeloureteric function and adequate emptying of the upper tract. When they are of severe degree so that dilatation may persist when the obstruction is eliminated, operative narrowing of the system may be needed in addition to allow the peristaltic wave to coapt the pelviureteric walls and effectively propel the urine bolus. Even in the absence of obstruction pelviureteric tailoring may improve the emptying of a decompensated system (Hendren, 1972). Hanna *et al.* (1977) found that the capability of an obstructed ureter to recover effective function can be predicted by electron-microscopic study of the proportion of muscle cells to collagen in its wall.

Ureteric substitutes

The possibility of replacing an afunctional, diseased or traumatized ureter in whole or in part by an effective substitute has long been a urological philosopher's stone and much animal experimental work has been carried out in the attempt to find a satisfactory prosthesis. The subject has been reviewed by Boxer, Johnson and Ehrlich (1978).

Nonbiological prostheses composed of vitallium, tantalum, polyethylene, Ivalon, Dacron, Teflon, Silastic or polyvinyl chloride have been unsuccessful in the long term because of migration of the foreign body, reflux, leakage, anastomotic stricture and phosphate encrustation. Even in the absence of such complications lack of peristalsis generally leads to hydronephrosis. Ferry (1961) and Djurhuis *et al.* (1974) incorporated mechanical plastic valves into Silastic prostheses to prevent reflux and although some success was obtained in animals the valves were ineffective in humans mainly because of encrustation.

Various biological ureteric substitutes have been used. The appendix and the fallopian tube have limited clinical application because of their shortness. Free grafts of autologous artery or vein, lyophilized homologous ureter and grafts of fascia and skin have all proved unsuccessful. The most commonly employed ureteric substitute has been a segment of ileum interposed in an isoperistaltic direction between the renal pelvis and the bladder. Enhanced peristaltic efficiency and a more effective antireflux technique of ileocystostomy can be obtained if the ileal segment is narrowed by excision of its antimesenteric aspect. Middleton (1977) found the method to be effective in two of three patients. Fritzche *et al.* (1975) reported 47 implantations of ileal ureter in adults followed up for periods of up to 17 years; there was no kidney deterioration in any patient but reflux from the bladder to the ileum was invariably present. The author's limited experience of ileal replacement of the ureter in children has been less sanguine and accords with that of Tanagho (1975) who recorded ileal dilatation, redundancy and progressive worsening of renal function. Because of stasis, absorption of urinary constituents may lead to hyperchloraemic acidosis, particularly in patients with impaired kidney function.

Loss of one or other extremity of the ureter can generally be managed successfully without the use of a ureteric substitute. When the vesical end is traumatized or has to be resected urinary tract continuity can be restored by transureteroureterostomy, a bladder psoas-hitch procedure or a Boari bladder flap. When the ureter is undilated it may be implanted under the mucosa of the Boari flap to prevent subsequent reflux. A gap at the proximal end of the ureter can be bridged by a flap raised from the renal pelvis. Alternatively autotransplantation of the kidney to the iliac fossa may be performed (DeWeerd *et al.*, 1976).

Hirschhorn (1964) made use of ileal peristalsis to promote kidney drainage in cases of aperistaltic megaureter by wrapping the renal pelvis and the ureter in a bowel segment from which the mucosa had been removed. Politano, Lynne and Small (1972) found the ileal sleeve to be effective in six cases. In the author's experience a megaureter that has permanently lost peristaltic activity is rarely associated with a useful kidney and the method appears to have very limited clinical applications.

References

Allen, T.D. (1970) Congenital ureteral strictures. *Journal of Urology*, **104**, 196

Allen, T.D. (1974) Compensatory renal hypertrophy. *In* Reviews in Paediatric Urology (edited by Johnston, J.H. and Goodwin, W.E.). Excerpta Medica, Amsterdam. p.411

Amar, A.D. (1971) Simple ureterocele at the distal end of blind-ending ureter. *Journal of Urology*, **106**, 423

Anderson, J.C. (1963) Hydronephrosis. Heinemann, London

Aron, B., Tessler, A. and Morales, P. (1973) Angiography in hydronephrosis. *Urology*, **2**, 231

Beaman, C.R., Gillenwater, J.Y. and Hatcher, J. (1974) Prediction of irreversible damage from hydronephrosis. *Transactions of the American Association of Genito-Urinary Surgeons*, **66**, 32

Beck, A.D. (1971) The effect of intra-uterine urinary obstruction upon the development of the fetal kidney. *Journal of Urology*, **105**, 784

Boxer, R.J., Johnson, S.F. and Ehrlich, R.M. (1978) Ureteral substitution. *Urology*, **12**, 269

Bratt, C.G., Aurell, M. and Nilsson, S. (1977) Renal function in patients with hydronephrosis. *British Journal of Urology*, **49**, 249

Brooks, R.J. (1962) Left retrocaval ureter associated with situs inversus. *Journal of Urology*, **88**, 484

Bueschen, A.J., Evans, B.B. and Schlegel, J.U. (1974) Renal scintillation camera studies in children. *Journal of Urology*, **111**, 821

Busch, F.M., Weibel, D.C., Morns, W.E. and Pohl, C.E. (1963) Ureteral valves. *Journal of Urology*, **90**, 43

Cerny, J.C. and Scott, T. (1971) Non-idiopathic retroperitoneal fibrosis. *Journal of Urology*, **105**, 49

Chisholm, G.D. and Osborn, D.E. (1976) Pathophysiology of obstructive uropathy. *In* Scientific Foundations of Urology, Vol. I (edited by Williams, D.I. and Chisholm, G.D.). Heinemann, London.p.65

Cohen, B., Goldman, S.M., Kopilnick, M., Khurana, A.V. and Salik, J.O. (1978) Ureteropelvic junction obstruction: its occurrence in 3 members of a single family. *Journal of Urology*, **120**, 361

Coolsaet, B.L.R.A. (1978) Ureteric pathology in relation to right and left gonadal veins. *Urology*, **12**, 40

Culp, O.S. and DeWeerd, J.H. (1951) A pelvic flap operation for certain types of ureteropelvic obstruction. *Proceedings of the Staff Meetings of the Mayo Clinic*, **26**, 483

Cussen, L.J. (1977) Quantitation of muscle cells of the ureter. *In* Urinary System Malformations in Children (edited by Bergsma, D. and Duckett, J.W.). Birth Defects Original Article Series, Vol. 13, No. 5. Liss, New York.p.11

Davis, R.S., Manning, J.A., Branch, J.L. and Cockett, A.T.K. (1973) Renovascular hypertension secondary to hydronephrosis in a solitary kidney. *Journal of Urology*, **110**, 724

DeWeerd, J.H., Paulk, S.C., Tomera, F.M. and Smith, L.H. (1976) Renal autotransplantation for upper ureteral stenosis. *Journal of Urology*, **116**, 23

Djurhuis, J.C., Gyrd-Hansen, N., Herstrom, R. and Svendsen, O. (1974) Total replacement of ureter by a Scurasil prosthesis in pigs. *British Journal of Urology*, **46**, 415

Farrer, J. and Peterson, C.G. (1962) Idiopathic retroperitoneal fibrosis: report of first case observed in a child. *Pediatrics*, **30**, 225

Ferry, C.A. (1961) Ureteral plastic valves in dogs. *Journal of Urology*, **85**, 525

Finn, R. and Carruthers, J.A. (1974) Genetic aspects of hydronephrosis associated with renal agenesis. *British Journal of Urology*, **46**, 351

Foote, J.W., Blennerhasset, J.B., Wiglesworth, F.W. and Mackinnon, K.J. (1970) Observations on the ureteropelvic junction. *Journal of Urology*, **104**, 252

Fowler, R. and Kesavan, P. (1977) Extravesical reconstruction for ureterovesical obstruction in childhood. *Journal of Urology*, **118**, 1050

Fraley, E.E. (1966) Vascular obstruction of the superior infundibulum causing nephralgia – new syndrome. *New England Journal of Medicine*, **275**, 1403

Fritzche, P., Skinner, D.G., Craven, J.D., Cahill, P. and Goodwin, W.E. (1975) Long-term radiographic changes of the kidney following the ileal ureter operation. *Journal of Urology*, **114**, 843

Gittes, R.F. and Talner, L.B. (1972) Congenital megacalices versus obstructive hydronephrosis. *Journal of Urology*, **108**, 833

Gosling, J.A. and Dixon, J.S. (1974) Species variation in the location of upper urinary tract pacemaker cells. *Investigative Urology*, **11**, 418

Greene, L.F., Priestley, J.T., Simon, H.B. and Hempstead, R.H. (1954) Obstruction of the lower third of the ureter by anomalous blood vessels. *Journal of Urology*, **71**, 544

Hanna, M.K. (1972) Bilateral retroiliac artery ureters. *British Journal of Urology*, **44**, 339

Hanna, M.K. and Jeffs, R.D. (1975) Primary obstructive megaureter in children. *Urology*, **6**, 419

Hanna, M.K., Jeffs, R.D., Sturgess, J.M. and Barkin, M. (1976) Electron microscopy – pale muscle cells at pelviureteric junction and throughout the ureter – may represent the pacemaker cell population. *Journal of Urology*, **116**, 718

Hanna, M.K., Jeffs, R.D., Sturgess, J.M. and Barkin, M. (1977) Ureteral structure and ultrastructure: the dilated ureter, clinico-pathological correlation. *Journal of Urology*, **117**, 28

Heal, M.R. (1973) Primary obstructive megaureter in adults. *British Journal of Urology*, **45**, 490

Hellstrom, J. (1927) Relation of abnormally running renal vessels to hydronephrosis and an investigation of the arterial condition of 50 kidneys. *Acta Chirurgica Scandinavica*, **61**, 289

Hendren, W.H. (1972) Restoration of function in the severely decompensated ureter. *In* Problems in Paediatric Urology (edited by Johnston, J.H. and Scholtmeijer, R.J.). Excerpta Medica, Amsterdam.p.1

Hinman, F. (1926) Renal counterbalance. *Archives of Surgery*, **12**, 1105

Hirschhorn, R.C. (1964) The ileal sleeve: first case report with clinical evaluation. *Journal of Urology*, **92**, 113

Ibrahim, A. and Asha, H.A. (1978) Prediction of renal recovery in hydronephrotic kidneys. *British Journal of Urology*, **50**, 222

Javadpour, N., Solomon, T. and Bush, I.M. (1972) Obstruction of the lower ureter by aberrant vessels in children. *Journal of Urology*, **108**, 340

Johnston, J.H. (1968) Hydroureter and megaureter. *In* Paediatric Urology (edited by Williams, D.I.). Butterworths, London. p.166

Johnston, J.H. (1969) The pathogenesis of hydronephrosis in childhood. *British Journal of Urology*, **41**, 724

Johnston, J.H. (1973) Megacalicosis: a burnt-out obstruction? *Journal of Urology*, **110**, 344

Johnston, J.H. and Hood, P.A. (1969) Spontaneous perirenal extravasation and urinary ascites in the newborn infant. *Urology Digest*, **8**, 20

Johnston, J.H. and Kathel, B.L. (1972) The results of surgery for hydronephrosis as determined by renography with analogue computer simulation. *British Journal of Urology*, **44**, 320

Johnston, J.H. and Sandomirsky, S.K. (1972) Intra-renal vascular obstruction of the superior infundibulum in children. *Journal of Pediatric Surgery*, **7**, 318

Johnston, J.H., Evans, J.P., Glassberg, K.I. and Shapiro, S.R. (1977) Pelvic hydronephrosis in children: a review of 219 personal cases. *Journal of Urology*, **117**, 97

Kelalis, P.P., Culp, O.S., Stickler, G.B. and Burke, E.C. (1971) Ureteropelvic obstruction in children: experiences with 109 cases. *Journal of Urology*, **106**, 418

Kenawi, M.M. and Williams, D.I. (1976) Circumcaval ureter; a report of four cases in children with a review of the literature and a new classification. *British Journal of Urology*, **48**, 183

Lloyd, D.D., Balfe, J.W., Barken, M. and Gelfand, E.W. (1974) Systemic lupus erythematosus with signs of retroperitoneal fibrosis. *Journal of Pediatrics*, **85**, 226

Mackinnon, K.J., Foote, J.W., Wiglesworth, F.W. and Blennerhasset, B. (1970) The pathology of the adynamic distal ureteral segment. *Journal of Urology*, **103**, 134

Matz, L.R., Craven, J.D. and Hodson, C.J. (1969) Experimental obstructive nephropathy in the pig: pathology. *British Journal of Urology*, **41**, Suppl.

Middleton, A.W. (1977) Tapered ileum as ureter substitute in severe renal damage. *Urology*, **9** 509

Middleton, A.W. and Pfister, R.C. (1974) Stone-containing pyelocaliceal diverticulum: embryogenic, anatomical, radiologic and clinical characteristics. *Journal of Urology*, **111**, 2

Mirandi, D. and De Assis, A.S. (1975) Transitional cell papilloma of ureter in young boy. *Urology*, **5**, 559

Murnaghan, G.F. (1957) Experimental investigation of dynamics of normal and dilated ureter. *British Journal of Urology*, **29**, 403

Murnaghan, G.F. (1958) The dynamics of the renal pelvis and ureter with reference to congenital hydronephrosis. *British Journal of Urology*, **30**, 321

Murphy, L.J.T. (1963) Retrocaval ureter: a report of two cases. *Australian and New Zealand Journal of Surgery*, **33**, 23

Myers, R.P. and DeWeerd, J.J. (1972) Congenital diverticulum of the renal pelvis: report of a case. *Journal of Urology*, **108**, 330

Nanninga, J.B. and O'Conor, V.J. (1976) The use of tetrazolium to determine hydronephrotic damage in human kidneys. *Journal of Urology*, **116**, 286

Nicholas, J.L. (1975) An unusual complication of calyceal diverticulum. *British Journal of Urology*, **47**, 370

Norman, C.H. and Dubowy, J. (1966) Multiple ureteral diverticula. *Journal of Urology*, **96**, 152

Notley, R.G. (1968) Electron microscopy of the upper ureter and the pelvi-ureteric junction. *British Journal of Urology*, **40**, 37

Notley, R.G. (1972) Electron microscopy of the primary obstructive megaureter. *British Journal of Urology*, **44**, 229

O'Reilly, R.H., Testa, H.J., Lawson, R.S., Farrer, D.J. and Edwards, E.G. (1978) Diuresis renography in equivocal urinary tract obstruction. *British Journal of Urology*, **50**, 76

Ostling, K. (1942) Genesis of hydronephrosis. *Acta Chirurgica Scandinavica*, **72**, Suppl.86, p.5

Paquin, A.J. (1959) Ureterovesical anastomosis: description and evaluation of a technique. *Journal of Urology*, **82**,573

Peterson, A.S., Besecker, J.A. and Hutchison, W.A. (1974) Retroperitoneal fibrosis and gluteal pain in a child. *Journal of Pediatrics*, **85**, 228

Peterson, L.J., Yarger, W.E., Schocken, D.D. and Glenn, J.F. (1975) Post-obstructive diuresis: a varied syndrome. *Journal of Urology*, **113**, 190

Politano, V.A. and Leadbetter, W.F. (1958) An operative technique for the correction of vesicoureteral reflux. *Journal of Urology*, **79**, 932

Politano, V.A., Lynne, C. and Small, M.P. (1972) Ileal sleeve for the dilated ureter. *Journal of Urology*, **107**, 31

Presto, A.J. and Middleton, R.G. (1973) Cure of hypertension in a child with renal artery stenosis and hydronephrosis in a solitary kidney. *Journal of Urology*, **109**, 98

Rickwood, A.M.K. (1978) Transient ureteric dilatation in neonates with imperforate anus: a report of 4 cases. *British Journal of Urology*, **50**, 16

Rickwood, A.M.K. and Phadke, D. (1978) Pyeloplasty in infants and children with particular reference to the method of drainage postoperatively. *British Journal of Urology*, **50**, 217

Robson, W.J., Rudy, S.M. and Johnston, J.H. (1976) Pelviureteric obstruction in infancy. *Journal of Pediatric Surgery*, **11**, 57

Rose, J.G. and Gillenwater, J.Y. (1978) Effects of obstruction on ureteral function. *Urology*, **12**, 139

Sanders, R.C., Duffy, T., McLoughlin, M.G. and Walsh, P.C. (1977) Sonography in the diagnosis of retroperitoneal fibrosis. *Journal of Urology*, **118**, 944

Shapiro, S.R., Woener, S., Adelman, R.D. and Palmer, J.M. (1978) Diabetes insipidus and hydronephrosis. *Journal of Urology*, **119**, 715

Snyder, H.M. and Johnston, J.H. (1978) Orthotopic ureteroceles in children. *Journal of Urology*, **119**, 543

Stewart, H.H. (1947) A new operation for the treatment of hydronephrosis in association with lower polar (or aberrant) artery. *British Journal of Surgery*, **35**, 43

Tanagho, E.A. (1972) Anatomy and management of ureteroceles. *Journal of Urology*, **107**, 729

Tanagho, E.A. (1974) The pathogenesis and management of megaureter. *In* Reviews in Paediatric Urology (edited by Johnston, J.H. and Goodwin, W.E.). Excerpta Medica, Amsterdam. p.85

Tanagho, E.A. (1975) A case against incorporation of bowel segments into the closed urinary system. *Journal of Urology*, **113**, 796

Teague, N. and Boyarsky, S. (1968) The effect of coliform bacilli upon ureteral peristalsis. *Investigative Urology*, **5**,423

Tiburcio, M.A. and Lima, S.V.C. (1978) Functionally obstructed megaureter. *Brazilian Journal of Urology*, **4**, 36

Tveter, K., Nerdrum, H.J. and Mjolnerod, O.K. (1975) The value of radioisotope renography in the follow-up of patients operated upon for hydronephrosis. *Journal of Urology*, **114**, 680

Uson, A.C., Cox, L.A. and Lattimer, J.K. (1968) Hydronephrosis in infants and children. *Journal of the American Medical Association*, **205**, 323

Vaughan, E.D., Buhler, F.R. and Laragh, J.H. (1974) Normal renin secretion in hypertensive patients with primarily unilateral chronic hydronephrosis. *Journal of Urology*, **112**, 153

Wacksman, J., Weinerth, J.L. and Kredick, D. (1978) Retroperitoneal fibrosis in children. *Urology*, **12**, 438

Weiss, R.M. (1978) Ureteral function. *Urology*, **12**, 114

Whitaker, R.H. (1975) Some observations and theories on the wide ureter and hydronephrosis. *British Journal of Urology*, **47**, 377

Whitaker, R.H. (1978) Clinical assessment of pelvic and ureteral function. *Urology*, **12**, 146

Whitfield, H.N., Britton, K.E., Fry, I.K., Hendry, W.F., Nimmon, C.C., Travers, P. and Wickham, J.E.A. (1977) The obstructed kidney: correlation between renal function and urodynamic assessment. *British Journal of Urology*, **49**, 615

Whitfield, H.N., Britton, K.E., Hendry, W.F., Nimmon, C.C. and Wickham, J.E.A. (1978) The distinction between obstructive uropathy and nephropathy by radioisotope transit times. *British Journal of Urology*, **50**, 433

Williams, D.I. (1977) Personal communication

Williams, D.I. and Hulme-Moir, I. (1970) Primary obstructive megaureter. *British Journal of Urology*, **42**, 140

Williams, D.I. and Karlaftis, C.M. (1966) Hydronephrosis due to pelvi-ureteric obstruction in the newborn. *British Journal of Urology*, **38** 138

Wines, R.D. and O'Flynn, J.D. (1972) Transurethral treatment of ureteroceles: a report of 45 cases mostly treated by transurethral resection. *British Journal of Urology*, **44**, 207

Winterburn, M.H. and France, N.E. (1972) Arterial changes associated with hydronephrosis in infants and children. *British Journal of Urology*, **44**, 96

Young, J.D. and Kiser, W.S. (1965) Obstruction of the lower ureter by aberrant blood vessels. *Journal of Urology*, **94**, 101

18 Investigation of bladder function

J.H. Johnston and Neville Harrison

Clinical features

The investigation of disorders of bladder function in children begins with the history. Indeed, a careful account of the symptomatology obtained from an intelligent, observant and interested parent may elucidate the problem completely.

In the patient who has difficulty in voiding, painful micturition suggestive of infection should be distinguished from true dysuria associated with a slow dribbling stream. This may result from an obstructive lesion, from defective detrusor function or occasionally from free reflux to severely dilated ureters where the urine follows the path of least resistance up the ureters rather than down the urethra.

When faced with the common situation in which the child presents with diurnal wetting, often in association with nocturnal enuresis, it is important to determine whether the complaint is of more or less continual involuntary leakage indicative of sphincteral weakness or overflow from a full bladder or whether the symptom is accompanied by frequency and preceded by urgency, indicating bladder instability. Wetting precipitated by laughing or giggling, which is a benign condition that can be confidently predicted to resolve as the patient's sense of humour becomes more sophisticated, must be distinguished from true stress incontinence. In the absence of other symptoms the latter is rare in childhood but may be encountered with posterior urethral anomalies or neurogenic disease. In boys dribbling of urine after a normal act of voiding may be caused by a urethral diverticulum or an ectopic ureter opening into the urethra. Both these lesions fill during micturition and subsequently empty their contents back into the urethra and thence to the exterior. In girls continual diurnal leakage in addition to normal micturition is highly suggestive of an ectopic ureter opening in the lower urethra, the vulva or the vagina.

Acute retention of urine is an occasional occurrence in boys of toddler age as a consequence of ammoniacal irritation of the preputial or urethral meatus. It generally resolves promptly following the application of a local anaesthetic cream and the traditional warm bath. Rarely in children of either sex acute retention with strangury carries a more ominous significance because it may be the first symptom of a botryoid sarcoma of the bladder. Due to prolapse of a portion of the tumour into the urethra. The benign posterior urethral polyp of boys often produces temporary interruption of the stream but it seldom causes total retention.

Whether the symptoms are lifelong or acute, and constant or intermittent is clearly important. Enquiry about the child's general health, his drinking and bowel habits and the family history may provide useful diagnostic clues.

A distended bladder is generally obvious on clinical examination but since the bladder is mainly an abdominal organ in the child the finding is not necessarily indicative of pathology. Re-examination after voiding is needed in such circumstances and if the child is a boy it may be helpful to watch him micturate. However, caution is required in interpreting the child's performance. Not infrequently modesty inhibits a normal boy from micturating at all in front of spectators, or he produces a deceptively substandard flow because of inadequate sphincteral relaxation of psychogenic origin. Conversely the observation of an apparently normal act of voiding does not exclude organic disease. Boys with posterior urethral valves can sometimes produce a strong sustained stream as a result of vigorous contraction of the hypertrophied detrusor.

Suprapubic compression may demonstrate that a bladder is expressible because of sphincteral insufficiency and it is often helpful to examine the child standing or during straining since these may induce a urine leak not evident on recumbency. Relevant genital anomalies such as epispadias are generally obvious provided that they are looked for and in this respect it is clearly important to examine the vulva in girls. Inspection and palpation of the spine, especially the sacral segments, and examination of the perineum for anal tone and cutaneous sensation are required to exclude neurogenic lesions. Ammoniacal excoriation of the skin and wet underpants in a child well past the napkin age are indicative of a severe degree of incontinence and often of organic disease. Urine microscopy and culture are needed routinely and in some cases the urinary pH is significant. A highly acid urine, particularly if it is concentrated, is occasionally the only detectable cause of painful micturition in young children.

The newborn infant

Normal neonates show considerable variation in the time interval between birth and the first voiding of urine. Sherry and Kramer (1955) observed 500 full-term babies and noted that 67 per cent micturated during the first 12 hours of life and 25 per cent within the following 12 hours. In 7 per cent voiding was delayed for more than 24 hours and in 0.6 per cent it did not occur until after 48 hours. However, in clinical practice precise information can often be lacking. An infant may micturate unnoticed during or soon after birth. Also, since the urine output during the first days of life is small and ranges from 15–60 ml/day it is possible that a small quantity of urine may be passed and may evaporate from the napkin.

The maximum urinary flow rate in infancy was measured by Kroigaard (1967), who found it to be 6–8 ml/s, and also by O'Donnell and O'Connor (1971), who noted it to be significantly less at under 3 ml/s. Ordinarily the normality or otherwise of the urine stream is interpreted subjectively on the basis of the observer's experience. A newborn boy can produce a sustained and forceful stream that can be projected over a distance of some 60–90 cm when he is supine. In some infants micturition occurs as intermittent spurts rather than an uninterrupted flow. Sometimes voiding is induced by crying, indicating that a rise in intra-abdominal pressure can initiate the act. Similarly suprapubic compression may bring about micturition and give a false impression that the bladder is expressible because of sphincteral incompetence. In some boys the bladder remains palpable after voiding and the frequent occurrence of incomplete bladder emptying in the male but not the female neonate has been shown by radiological studies (O'Donnell and O'Connor, 1971).

Radiology

Adequate radiological examination of the bladder generally requires retrograde cystography. In boys local anaesthesia of the urethra avoids the more unpleasant aspects of the procedure and helps to ensure a cooperative patient. If the child micturates immediately before catheterization, an accurate measure of the residual volume can be obtained. The preferred radiological technique is fluoroscopy with spot films or, in selected cases, with videotape recording.

During intermittent viewing the bladder is filled continuously by an intravenous drip set to a little beyond the point at which the patient declares a wish to void. The bladder capacity is noted. Anteroposterior and oblique viewing, with films if necessary, is performed before the catheter is removed and the general shape of the bladder and the existence of trabeculation, sacculation or diverticula are noted. After the catheter is withdrawn and before voiding begins involuntary filling of the posterior urethra indicative of proximal sphincteral insufficiency may be evident. During micturition a radiolucent plastic receptacle is used and one must ensure in boys that its neck is not tightly pressed against the penoscrotal junction so that it partially obstructs the urethra. The position of the patient relative to the X-ray tube depends upon the centre of interest. For the bladder outlet and the urethra oblique and lateral views are generally most informative, while anteroposterior observation is needed in addition if vesicoureteric reflux is suspected. A cooperative child may be able to interrupt the urine stream and demonstrate the efficiency of his external sphincter and his urethral milk-back mechanism, but failure to achieve this is not necessarily abnormal. At the conclusion of voiding an estimation can be made of the residual urine. If a significant volume exists, the patient is encouraged to try again. It is often helpful, and enjoyable for the patient, to let him watch his performance on the television monitor.

Endoscopy

The advent of modern fibreoptic instruments has revolutionized endoscopy in children and clear viewing of the bladder and the urethra is now possible even in newborn infants. However, endoscopy tends towards subjective interpretation, especially as regards lesser degrees of pathological change, and different opinions concerning the appearances may be obtained from different observers. Whether or not a bladder neck is unduly prominent or abnormally wide open may be disputed, as may also the significance of a submontanal urethral fold in a boy or the existence or otherwise of mild bladder trabeculation.

Although gross pathological changes are obvious to all viewers, they must be interpreted cautiously as regards vesicourethral function. For example a thickened bladder neck was formerly considered to be indicative of primary bladder neck obstruction but this is now recognized to be rare, if it exists at all (*see* Chapter 19). Secondary bladder neck hypertrophy, which is sometimes itself obstructive, can occur if there is urethral obstruction at a lower level. An unusually wide-open vesical outlet is generally suggestive of a deficiency in the proximal sphincteral mechanism resulting from a neuropathic lesion or a local developmental anomaly such as epispadias or bilateral single ectopic ureters. Nevertheless, this appearance may simply be caused by passive opening of the bladder neck from overfilling of the viscus or by the pharmacological effect of anaesthetic agents such as thiopentone or halothane.

Bladder trabeculation with or without diverticula or saccules has long been considered diagnostic of outflow obstruction. However, such changes can develop as a result of uninhibited detrusor contractions in an unstable bladder in the absence of any obstruction to voiding of either an anatomical or a functional nature (*see* Chapter 19).

Reduction in bladder capacity due to contracture resulting from organic changes is apparent at endoscopy, but diminished capacity of functional origin may not be detected since the examination in children is generally performed under general anaesthesia and often with neuromuscular blocking agents. Drugs also influence the volume of fluid the bladder can accommodate; Doyle and Briscoe (1976) found that the bladder capacity was reduced by the administration of diazepam and increased by halothane.

Urodynamics

Not only for small boys do the dynamics of micturition hold a fascination and, although the term urodynamics is relatively new, bladder pressure measurements have been made in humans for nearly a century, beginning with the pioneering work of Mosso and Pellicani in the 1880s (Doyle, 1975). Modern improvements in urodynamic methods have been made possible by advances in electronics which allow pressures and flow rates to be measured and recorded with relative ease. Some authorities feel that the techniques which have been developed and used mainly in adults are unsuitable for children and it is true that extrapolating from adults to children can be misleading. Nevertheless with some modifications in technique and interpretation urodynamic measurements can be just as valuable for the investigation of selected bladder disorders in children as in adults.

Techniques

Cystometry

Cystometry is the technique of measuring the pressure-volume relationships within the bladder. In the past this was confined to bladder filling but now the complete voiding cycle is usually studied and can be conveniently divided into filling and voiding phases.

For the filling phase fluid is instilled into the bladder through a 6 or 8 F catheter. In children under 4 years a suprapubic catheter may be more satisfactory and some investigators prefer this method routinely. Normal saline or radiographic contrast medium at room temperature is used. A medium filling rate is usual (*Table 18.1*) and it should be recorded. Although the normal bladder is remarkably little influenced by variations in the filling rate, fast filling may unmask

Table 18.1   Cystometry filling rates

Slow filling	Up to 10 ml/min
Medium filling	10–100 ml/min
Rapid filling	Over 100 ml/min

abnormalities that might otherwise be missed. Air or carbon dioxide cystometry is quicker than fluid cystometry but has the disadvantage that the voiding phase cannot be studied.

To measure pressure within the bladder a separate fine catheter (an epidural catheter with an external diameter of 1 mm is very suitable) is passed alongside the filling catheter and connected to a suitable chart recorder. Alternatively it is possible to fill and to record pressure through a single catheter provided that allowance is made for the zero error resulting from the filling pressure, and this method is needed when the urethra is too narrow to accommodate two catheters.

Changes in intra-abdominal pressure due to movement, straining or coughing are transmitted to the bladder and recorded on the cystometrogram. To distinguish pressure changes due solely to detrusor contractions intra-abdominal pressure may be recorded by measuring rectal pressure through a fine fluid-filled catheter passed through the anus. Rectal pressure can then be electronically subtracted from total bladder pressure to give the important intrinsic or detrusor pressure. If the patient is unable to tolerate the additional tube in the rectum, a somewhat less precise but generally satisfactory technique is to distinguish intra-abdominal pressure rises visually and record their occurrence on the tracings. Another method is to employ electromyography to detect contractions of the abdominal muscles.

Filling is continued until the patient expresses a strong desire to micturate or involuntary voiding occurs. For the voiding phase of cystometry the filling catheter is removed, or clamped if it is suprapubic, while the fine recording catheter is retained. Cooperative children are asked to cough, strain and then micturate. During voiding the bladder pressure, the abdominal pressure and the urinary flow rate are measured. The latter is usually recorded by determining the weight of urine passed per second and deriving the flow electronically.

Cystometry should be performed with the child awake in order to obtain important information about bladder sensation. Children over the age of 3 years usually have proprioceptive function as shown by their awareness of fullness, the desire to micturate and the sensation of voiding as well as complete emptying. Younger children show characteristic reactions such as toe-curling to bladder filling, indicating a sensory input from the bladder. General anaesthesia or sedation should not be used

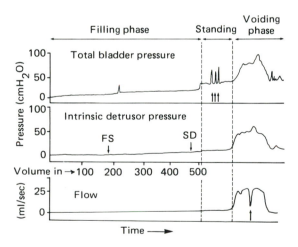

Figure 18.1. Normal filling and voiding cystometry. FS = first sensation of bladder filling, SD = strong desire to void. The arrows on standing indicate coughing and the arrow during voiding indicates where the child is asked momentarily to stop voiding. (Reproduced by permission of the editor, *British Journal of Hospital Medicine*.).

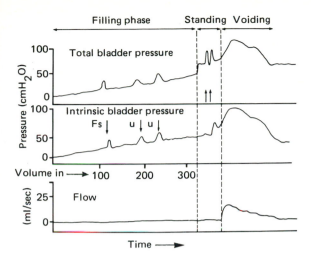

Figure 18.2. Diagram of an abnormal cystometrogram. FS = first sensation of bladder filling, U = urgency. The arrows on standing indicate coughing which precipitates a voiding contraction. The abnormal features are uninhibited detrusor contractions, a steep filling slope also indicating abnormal detrusor activity and a high voiding pressure with a poor flow rate indicating outflow obstruction. (Reproduced by permission of the editor, *British Journal of Hospital Medicine*.).

ordinarily for cystometry as it makes it impossible to assess the sensory aspects of the investigation and in addition may alter bladder behaviour by suppressing detrusor contractions.

Examples of normal and abnormal cystometrograms are shown in *Figures 18.1 and 18.2.*

THE BETHANECHOL OR DENERVATION HYPERSENSITIVITY TEST

This is a supplementary test used to distinguish infranuclear from supranuclear neurological lesions. It is based on the fact that denervated smooth muscle is hypersensitive to cholinergic stimulation. The technique is to measure the intravesical pressure, with the bladder filled to 20 per cent of its capacity, before and 20 minutes after a subcutaneous injection of bethanechol. A denervated bladder shows a pressure rise greater than 15 cmH$_2$O. The main value of the investigation is in the diagnosis of the occult neuropathic bladder (Williams, Hirst and Doyle, 1974) but grey areas between normal and obviously abnormal readings are common so that the test is often indeterminate. A false-positive result may be obtained in a child with a normally innervated bladder and uninhibited detrusor contractions resulting from functional immaturity.

COMBINED X-RAY AND PRESSURE STUDIES

Until the advent of urodynamics micturating cystography was the main method of studying voiding. By combining the pressure recordings of cystometry with fluoroscopy the value of both investigations is enhanced. The bladder pressure tracings and the flow rate can be superimposed on the X-ray monitor so that both can be

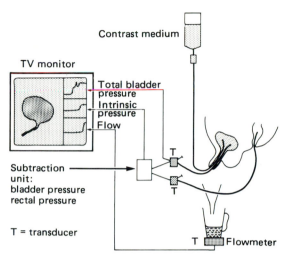

Figure 18.3. Schematic diagram of the apparatus for combined X-ray pressure cystogram (after the method of Bates, Whiteside and Turner-Warwick, [1970]). (Reproduced by permission of the editor, *British Journal of Hospital Medicine*.).

seen simultaneously and events coordinated (*Figure 18.3*). If the investigation is recorded on videotape, there is the added advantage of an action replay during which the case can be discussed or reviewed.

Urethral pressure profile

The urethral pressure profile is a graphic record of the intraluminal pressure exerted by the urethral wall on a recording catheter as it is withdrawn from the bladder to the external meatus. The profile quantifies the urethral closing forces during filling and provides information about the sphincter mechanism. It does not measure, nor necessarily reflect, urethral resistance during voiding (Harrison, 1976). The simplest and most commonly used method of obtaining the pressure profile uses an 8F catheter with a closed extremity and with side holes through which there is a flow of fluid at a rate of at least 2 ml/min (Brown and Wickham, 1969). Pressure changes in the system are measured by

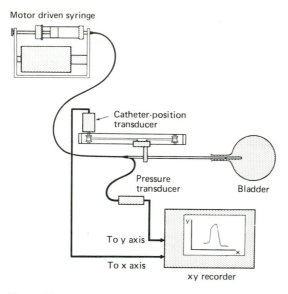

Motor driven syringe

Figure 18.4. Diagram of apparatus for recording urethral closure pressure profile by the method of Harrison and Constable (1970). (Reproduced by permission of the editor, *British Journal of Hospital Medicine*.)

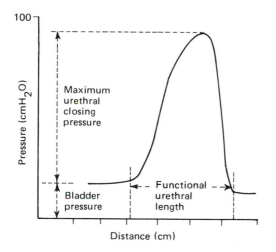

Figure 18.5. Diagram of a normal urethral pressure profile in a girl. (Reproduced by permission of the editor, *British Journal of Hospital Medicine*.)

a transducer and recorded on a chart recorder (*Figure 18.4*). A typical profile is shown in *Figure 18.5* together with some of the measurements that can be made. The maximum urethral closing pressure is the difference between the maximum point on the profile and the bladder pressure. Functional urethral length is the length of the urethra over which the profile pressure exceeds the bladder pressure.

Electromyography

Although electromyography of smooth muscle has been attempted, it is striated muscular activity that is usually recorded. The most common technique involves inserting fine monopolar wire electrodes into the anal sphincter or alongside the urethra into the urethral sphincter. Anal plug or adhesive tape electrodes are alternative methods of obtaining EMGs. Electromyography combined with cystometry is particularly useful for demonstrating detrusor-sphincter dyssynergia characterized by continuing contraction of the external urethral sphincter during voiding (Firlit, Smey and King, 1978). In the neurologically intact individual the anal sphincteral EMG reflects the activity of the external urethral sphincter but this does not necessarily apply in the child with neuropathy caused by myelodysplasia. In such cases detrusor-sphincter dyssynergia may coexist with a lax totally paralysed anus.

Noninvasive techniques

Any technique that avoids the discomfort catheterization can cause is particularly desirable especially when, as is often the case, repeated tests are required over a period of time.

UROFLOWMETRY
Urinary flow rate during micturition is the simplest noninvasive dynamic investigation. The peak flow rate is the most useful measurement. In addition the overall voiding pattern as regards intermittency or continuance of flow may be of diagnostic importance.

ULTRASOUND RESIDUAL URINE AFTER MICTURITION
One residual urine measurement in isolation is of little value. In children under the age of 4 years residual urine appears to be quite common and probably reflects physiological immaturity. A reduction in the vesical residue is often one of the main objectives of treatment and following changes in its volume is a useful way of monitoring this achievement. Ultrasound has the advantage over catheterization after voiding since it is quick, simple, harmless and well tolerated (Harrison, Parks and Sherwood, 1976). Although this method cannot be used for accurate quantitative measurement, progressive changes can be readily followed (*Figure 18.6*).

Neuropathic bladder

Residual: before treatment with
           phenoxybenzamine

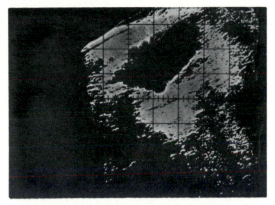

After treatment

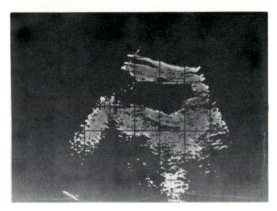

Figure 18.6. Ultrasound residual urine estimations in a girl aged 4 years with a myelomeningocele. Midline sagittal bladder scans before and after treatment with phenoxybenzamine representing residual volumes of 160 ml and 40 ml respectively. (Reproduced by permission of the editor, *British Journal of Urology*.)

Combining uroflowmetry with ultrasound residual urine estimations provides a useful noninvasive method of following voiding disorders which is appreciated by both the child and the investigator.

Comments on methodology

The value of the information obtained from any investigation is directly proportional to the care with which the test is performed, and in no situation is this more true than in the study of voiding disorders in children. Urodynamic evaluations are not easy and require considerable time, understanding and patience. However,

once the investigator has gained sufficient confidence and experience of the techniques most children who are capable of comprehending what is required of them can be successfully studied.

In a child with normal sensation, especially a boy, introduction of the urethral catheter can present difficulties. Catheterization is best done in the ward at least 30 minutes before the urodynamic tests are carried out. If the patient undergoes endoscopy, the opportunity can be taken to insert urethral or suprapubic catheters and electromyographic electrodes under anaesthesia, and the urodynamic studies are then performed the following day. However, on occasions the presence of a draining catheter even for a period of only a few hours can induce bladder irritability, reduce the functional capacity and give misleading results on cystometry.

Sedation of the patient for urodynamic studies is undesirable because the drug may influence bladder and urethral function and also because children tend to become more fractious as they become sleepy. The emphasis must be on a relaxed atmosphere obtained by simple explanation, reassurance and privacy. Some children are intrigued by the apparatus and the readings as they are obtained while others prefer diverting activities.

Interpretation of urodynamic results

In interpreting urodynamic studies both bladder and urethral function must be considered. The bladder shows two complementary but conflicting phases. During filling it must act as a leak-proof reservoir without associated awareness or discomfort and during voiding it must become a pump to expel its contents completely. The former depends as much on the absence of detrusor activity as on bladder neck and urethral competence while the latter relies on coordinated muscular contraction and adequate outflow opening. The whole cycle is dependent on neuropharmacological control at both local and higher levels. All these aspects of bladder function must be taken into account when interpreting the results obtained from urodynamic investigations.

Detrusor instability

Bladder capacity depends not only on the physical size of the reservoir but also on the suppression of detrusor activity to allow this capacity to be reached before the desire to void occurs. The term detrusor instability was introduced as an extension of the concept of an uninhibited detrusor (Bates, 1971). Uninhibited detrusor contractions are involuntary contractions which the patient cannot suppress, occurring during filling cystometry. Unstable detrusor contractions are also involuntary but are induced by such provocations as rapid filling, standing, coughing or straining. Thus the terms uninhibited and unstable are similar but not synonymous. Detrusor hyper-reflexia is detrusor overactivity due to a neurological disorder.

Under the age of 10 uninhibited contractions appear to be quite common, occurring in over 50 per cent of children, and must be considered normal. Over the age of 10 they are unusual and in adults they are abnormal.

Pressure and flow

Several urodynamic studies in children with apparently normal bladder function have been carried out although the numbers, particularly in the under 3 age group, are understandably small (Gierup, 1970; Hjalmas, 1976). There is considerable lack of agreement on normal values which probably reflects not only a wide range of normality but also artifacts and variations due to differences in technique. Each investigation unit must therefore to some extent define its own values. In general the emphasis should be more on the overall pattern of the urodynamic features correlated with the behaviour and the reaction of the child at the time of the examination and less on absolute figures. The most useful objective measurements are the maximum detrusor pressure, the maximum flow rate during micturition and the detrusor pressure at maximum flow. A guide to normal levels is given in *Table 18.2*. Voiding pressures tend to be somewhat higher in boys and increase with age. Flow rates also increase with age in both sexes. Girls appear to void differently from boys in that they are more dependent on urethral changes than on detrusor activity (Hjalmas, 1976).

Formulae designed to calculate urethral resistance are all derived from the hydrodynamics of rigid tubes. The urethra is clearly not a rigid tube and such calculations have tended to confuse rather than clarify so they are not recommended. *Table 18.3* shows various pressure-flow relationships that should be identifiable from the overall pattern of the urodynamic study.

Residual urine

A residual urine measurement of more than 10 per cent of the total bladder volume is suggestive of some voiding disorder, but the finding is of lesser significance in younger children. Large residual volumes may indicate detrusor failure or outflow obstruction, or may result from psychological inhibitions under test conditions. If vesicoureteric reflux is present, there is the possibility of misinterpretation as a result of

Table 18.2 Normal values for urodynamic parameters

Cystometrogram	Residual urine	Less than 10% bladder capacity
	Bladder capacity	Increases with age or height, e.g. 250 ml at age 10
	Pressure rise during filling	Up to 25 cmH$_2$O
	Detrusor pressure at maximum flow	Up to 75 cmH$_2$O
	Maximum flow	More than 15 ml/sec
Urethral pressure profile	Maximum urethral closing pressure	More than 50 cmH$_2$O

Table 18.3 Pressure-flow relationships

Voiding pressure	Peak flow	Other features	Indications
Low	High		No obstruction
High	Low		Outflow obstruction
Low	Low	Intermittent flow and abdominal pressure rises	Detrusor failure
Normal	Low		Relative obstruction
High	Normal		Compensated obstruction
Fluctuating	Variable	No abdominal activity	Sphincter-detrusor dyssynergia

urine re-entering the bladder from the ureters. The absence of residual urine is a significant observation, although without pressure-flow studies vesicourethral dysfunction cannot be excluded.

Urethral pressure profile

The maximum urethral pressure shows a wide scatter in normal individuals and is related to age. The high values found in children decline with increasing years. A single measurement is seldom of diagnostic significance by itself, except at the extremes of the range (*Figure 18.7*).

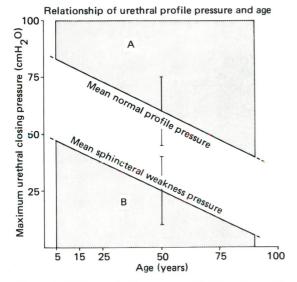

Figure 18.7. The urethral pressure profile. The relationship between age and urethral closure pressure compared in normal controls and patients with incompetent sphincters. Values in area A are likely to be associated with competent closure mechanisms and those in area B with sphincteral weakness. (Reproduced by permission of the editor, *British Journal of Hospital Medicine*.)

The shape of the profile may be characteristic and changes due to voluntary contraction of the pelvic floor, electrical stimulation, drug administration or alterations in posture often give useful information and add another dimension to bladder studies (Harrison, 1976). Urethral profilometry is an unpleasant investigation for the conscious patient with normal sensation and, providing atropine and muscle relaxants are avoided, the investigation can be carried out under light general anaesthesia to gain useful therapeutic indications. The effect of adrenergic drugs on the involuntary urethral sphincter can be determined and the possible value of electrical stimulation of the pelvic diaphragm by an electronic implant can be evaluated.

The place of urodynamic investigations

Many disorders of micturition can be diagnosed and treated without urodynamic testing. For example the clinical, radiological and endoscopic features of outflow obstruction due to posterior urethral valves are quite characteristic. However, when urethral dilatation, residual urine or recurrent infection persist after resection of the valves it is important to know whether an obstructive element remains, and in such circumstances urodynamic evaluation is indicated.

Straightforward nocturnal enuresis and daytime urgency and wetting associated with a morphologically normal urinary tract do not require pressure studies. If there is persistent incontinence with anatomical abnormalities, urodynamic investigations can provide useful information and guides to therapy.

In the neuropathic bladder neither the anatomical level of the spinal lesion nor the overt neurological signs may correlate with the type of bladder behaviour. To refer to upper or lower motor neurone lesions can be misleading and the bladder dysfunction must be described in urodynamic terms.

In the investigation of bladder disorders the type and the extent of the tests carried out must be selected according to the clinical problem. The urodynamic findings should always be assessed together with the clinical features and the routine urological measurements. The objective, which is summarized in *Figure 18.8*, is to define the bladder disorder in functional terms and so provide a rational basis for successful management. It must be emphasized that a young child who is incapable of responding to reassurance and explanation cannot be expected to endure or cooperate in the elaborate urodynamic investigations possible in adults. It is always necessary to modulate the studies within the patient's tolerance level and to stop short of causing pain or acute discomfort. This is not only for obvious humanitarian reasons but also because once the child becomes distressed the usefulness of the investigation is necessarily at an end.

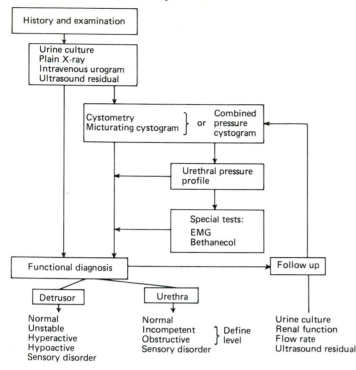

Figure 18.8. Flow-chart for investigation of bladder function.

In children with voiding disorders who are intolerant of urodynamic investigations when awake Koff *et al.* (1980) found that useful information could be obtained concerning detrusor function and external sphincteral activity by cystometry and electromyography performed under light anaesthesia. This has the advantage that it eliminates such artifacts as voluntary contraction of the sphincter simulating true detrusor-sphincter dyssynergia.

References

Bates, C.P. (1971) Continence and Incontinence. *Annals of the Royal College of Surgeons of England*, **49**, 18

Bates, C.P., Whiteside, C.G. and Turner-Warwick, R. (1970) Synchronous cine/pressure/flow cystourethrography with special reference to stress and urge incontinence. *British Journal of Urology*, **42**, 714

Brown, M. and Wickham, J.E.A. (1969) The urethral pressure profile. *British Journal of Urology*, **41**, 211

Doyle, P.T. (1975) History of urodynamics. *In* Urinary Incontinence (edited by Caldwell, K.P.S.) Secior, London.p.45

Doyle, P.T. and Briscoe, C.E. (1976) The effects of drugs and anaesthetic agents on the urinary bladder and sphincters. *British Journal of Urology*, **48**, 329

Firlit, C.F., Smey, P. and King, L.R. (1978) Micturition urodynamic flow studies in children. *Journal of Urology*, **119**, 250

Gierup, J. (1970a) Micturition studies in infants and children: normal urinary flow. *Scandinavian Journal of Urology and Nephrology*, **4**, 191

Gierup, J. (1970b) Micturition studies in infants and children: intravesical pressure, urinary flow and urethral resistance in boys without infravesical obstruction. *Scandinavian Journal of Urology and Nephrology*, **4**, 217

Harrison, N.W. (1976) The urethral pressure profile. *Urological Research*, **4**, 95

Harrison, N.W. and Constable, A.R. (1970) Urethral pressure measurement: a modified technique. *British Journal of Urology*, **42**, 229

Harrison, N.W., Parks, C. and Sherwood, T. (1976) Ultrasound assessment of residual urine in children. *British Journal of Urology*, **47**, 805

Hjalmas, K. (1976) Micturition in infants and children with normal lower urinary tract: a urodynamic study. *Scandinavian Journal of Urology and Nephrology*, Suppl. 37

Koff, S.A., Solomon, M.H. Lane, G.A. and Lieding K.G. (1980) Urodynamic studies in anaesthetized children. *Journal of Urology*, **123**, 61

Kroigaard, N. (1967) Micturition cinematography with simultaneous pressure flow study in infancy and childhood. *Journal of Pediatric Surgery*, **2**, 523

O'Donnell, B. and O'Connor, T.P. (1971) Bladder function in infants and children. *British Journal of Urology*, **43**, 25

Sherry, S.N. and Kramer, I. (1955) The time of passage of the first stool and the first urine by the newborn infant. *Journal of Pediatrics*, **81**, 570

Williams, D.I., Hirst, G. and Doyle, P.T. (1974) The occult neuropathic bladder. *Journal of Pediatric Surgery*, **9**, 35

19 Bladder disorders

J.H. Johnston

Agenesis

Agenesis of the bladder is very rare and its precise embryogenesis is uncertain. Faulty cloacal development may be responsible when there are associated anorectal anomalies; otherwise, failure of the lower portions of the mesonephric ducts to form the trigone and the proximal urethra is the likely mechanism. Palmer and Russi (1969) reviewed the literature and found 34 examples had been recorded. Of the affected infants 27 were stillborn and six of the live patients were female. In surviving girls the ureters open onto the vestibule or into the vagina and the presenting symptom is continual urine leakage. Hydroureteronephrosis and persistent urinary tract infection are usually present. Treatment requires urinary diversion either by ureterosigmoidostomy or to the abdominal surface.

Hypoplasia

An extremely small thin-walled bladder is found in association with severe degrees of epispadias and also with bilateral single ectopic ureters opening into the lower urethra in girls. The bladder remains underdeveloped since it has never been called upon to perform the normal vesical functions of retaining and evacuating urine. However, if urinary control can be achieved by bladder neck reconstruction then the bladder is generally capable of appreciable enlargement and of improvement in muscularity.

Duplication and related anomalies

These include a variety of congenital anomalies which were reviewed by Abrahamson (1961). With complete vesical duplication each hemi-bladder has its own ureter and urethra, and reduplication of the genitalia, the lower alimentary tract (Ravitch, 1953) and the lower part of the vertebral column (Dutta *et al.*, 1974) may coexist. In cases of incomplete duplication the two portions of the bladder communicate and there is a single urethra. A complete sagittal septum on one side of the midline shuts off one bladder chamber and the obstructed ipsilateral kidney is aplastic (Tacciuoli, Laurenti and Racheli, 1975). An incomplete sagittal septum with a free lower margin has been described in boys with covered exstrophy of the cloaca (Johnston and Koff, 1977). When there is an incomplete coronal septum the bladder is partially subdivided into anterior and posterior portions. The hour-glass bladder has a horizontal constriction partially separating upper and lower compartments. This condition can be simulated radiologically by a urachal diverticulum or a fundal contraction ring which can be well developed in a hypertrophied infected bladder. On occasions a grossly dilated posterior urethra in boys may during cystourethrography closely resemble an hour-glass bladder, particularly in cases of bilateral single ectopic ureters opening into the urethra. A multiseptate bladder is divided by septa into several compartments, some of which communicate.

The management of bladder duplication and similar abnormalities depends on the individual circumstances. Upper tract anomalies commonly coexist and the correction of these and the elimination of urinary obstruction are the essential aspects of treatment.

Trigonal cyst

Tacciuoli, Laurenti and Racheli (1976) described a 7-year-old girl in whom a cyst on the posterior aspect of the bladder neck interfered with bladder emptying and caused upper tract dilatation. The endoscopic appearance was that of an ectopic ureterocele but the cyst had neither ureteric nor urethral openings. It was lined by transitional epithelium and was considered to be derived from Von Brunn's epithelial nests. Marsupialization of the cyst into the bladder relieved the obstruction.

Diverticula

A bladder diverticulum is a herniation of the mucosa through a defect in the detrusor musculature. Unlike a saccule, which in the unhypertrophied bladder may not be evident at all except during a voiding contraction, a diverticulum forms a permanent protrusion. Vesical diverticula, most commonly projecting through the ureteric hiati, are seen in children with severe infravesical obstruction and also in cases of neuropathic bladder associated with detrusor-sphincter dyssynergia. However, diverticula and similar protrusions of various types are often encountered in the absence of obstruction or neurological disorders.

Inguinal protrusions

Inguinal protrusions or bladder ears are bilateral pouches seen in infants, especially boys, which lie anterolaterally in relation to the deep

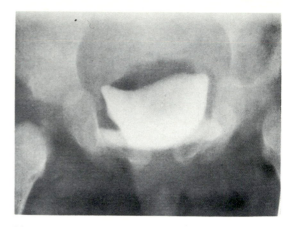

Figure 19.1. Bladder ears. Cystogram in a baby girl.

inguinal rings. They are seen as lateral extensions on the cystogram (*Figure 19.1*). They disappear spontaneously and neither investigation nor treatment is needed.

Paraureteric saccule

The paraureteric (Hutch, 1958) saccule is often encountered in children with primary vesicoureteric reflux. As a result of muscular deficiency of the ureteric insertion into the trigone the

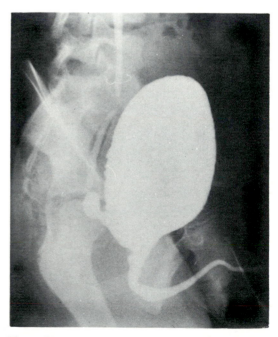

Figure 19.2. Micturating cystogram in a boy showing a paraureteric saccule associated with vesicoureteric reflux.

intravesical part of the ureter, carrying with it its overlying mucosa, recedes through the ureteric hiatus during a detrusor contraction. The then extravesical mucosal pouch becomes distended and vesicoureteric reflux occurs (*Figure 19.2*). As a rule the saccule is transient, existing only during reflux, but occasionally a small persistent pouch may require excision during ureteric reimplantation.

Congenital diverticulum

This type of diverticulum occurs almost exclusively in the male. As a rule the lesion is solitary although sometimes bilateral diverticula are seen. The diverticular neck is sited on the posterolateral bladder wall above the ureteric hiatus. There is no pre-existing obstructive uropathy and the condition is considered to be due to a developmental defect in the detrusor musculature through which the mucosa herniates as a result of normal rises in intravesical pressure during voiding. The sac wall consists of mucosa covered by compressed perivesical tissues and in some cases a few muscle fibres are present. As the diverticulum enlarges it may compress and obstruct the ureter or the ureter may come to open within it so that ureteric reflux occurs. Occasionally the diverticulum extends downwards and displaces the bladder outlet forwards

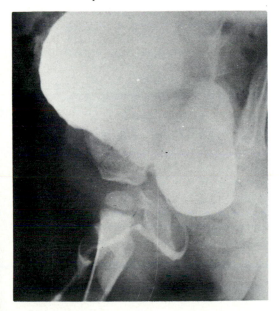

Figure 19.3. A large vesical diverticulum in a boy displacing the bladder outlet forwards during micturition.

when interference with bladder emptying and upper tract dilatation commonly follow (*Figure 19.3*). Less often a very large diverticulum allows such accumulations of residual urine as to produce, passively, intravesical pressures sufficiently high to cause hydroureteronephrosis (Johnston, 1960).

In most cases the presenting symptoms are those of urinary tract infection or haematuria. Rarely an exceptionally large diverticulum causes a palpable abdominal swelling or a bilobed mass results from retained urine in the bladder and the diverticulum. Diagnosis requires cystography with oblique views. The diverticulum often appears small when the bladder is relaxed and exposures during micturition are needed to evaluate its full dimensions. Cystoscopy reveals the round relatively narrow diverticular neck and its relationship with the ureteric orifice.

Diverticulectomy is indicated if urinary tract infection is occurring because of the accumulation of residual urine in the sac, if the pouch is interfering with bladder emptying or if the diverticulum is involving the ureter and causing either obstruction or reflux. A small diverticulum can be excised from within the bladder but a larger one is more conveniently exposed and removed from without, if necessary by a transperitoneal approach. Ureteric reimplantation to the bladder is needed if the ureter is densely adherent to or opens into the diverticulum.

With a relatively small diverticulum that causes only transient symptoms an expectant policy may be adopted. However, this must take into consideration the liability of a vesical diverticulum to develop a carcinoma and, if this occurs, the poor prognosis that exists because of the likelihood of rapid extravesical infiltration by the growth (Montague and Boltuch, 1976). Ostroff, Alperstein and Young (1973) described a squamous cell carcinoma developing in a congenital solitary diverticulum in a man aged 21 years.

Bladder saccules and diverticula in enuresis

In the majority of enuretic children with or without daytime symptoms of frequency, urgency and urge incontinence the urine is sterile and

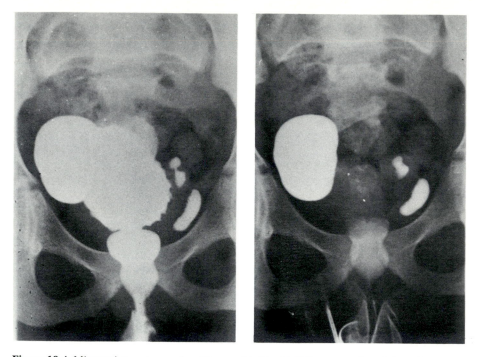

Figure 19.4. Micturating cystogram in a 10-year-old girl with lifelong enuresis and diurnal urgency and wetting. Coliform bacilluria was present. During voiding (left) the cystogram shows several diverticula and a spinning-top urethra. After voiding (right) the bladder is empty but there is residual urine in the diverticula.

routine urological investigations reveal no causative urinary tract pathology. In a minority with the same lifelong symptomatology the urine is commonly infected and although the bladder empties completely urography and endoscopy demonstrate features suggestive of an infravesical obstruction, bladder saccules or diverticula (mainly paraureteric in position) exist and vesicoureteric reflux may develop (*Figure 19.4*). Radiological and urodynamic investigations reveal no obstructive lesion of either organic or functional nature (Johnston, Koff and Glassberg, 1978). Detrusor-sphincter dyssynergia is excluded by sphincteric electromyography but cystometry demonstrates an unstable uninhibited bladder musculature and it is this disorder, with infection as a secondary exacerbating factor, that is the essential pathology.

When an uninhibited detrusor contraction occurs the child resists the sudden unexpected urge to void by inducing a strong voluntary contraction of the external urethral sphincter. Little girls often supplement the sphincteric contraction by squatting on the heel, that is the curtsey sign described by Vincent (1966). The effect of the voluntarily resisted detrusor contraction is to produce an abnormally high intravesical pressure which persists until either the detrusor relaxes or the volume of the bladder content is reduced by urine leakage, as commonly occurs, or micturition. Ultimately the frequently repeated pressure rises produce the pathological changes in the bladder and reflux may develop as a result of both the functional disorder and the anatomical alterations at the ureterovesical junction.

Treatment involves control of infection by chemotherapy. Symptomatic management of the uninhibited bladder is difficult in the short term. Propantheline may be effective but often has to be given in doses sufficiently large to produce anticholinergic side effects. Alternatively emepronium or dicyclomine may be employed. In the author's experience vesical distension under anaesthesia is ineffective. In the vast majority of cases the bladder disorder represents a temporary immaturity of function and the symptoms improve and ultimately resolve completely. Reflux may then stop spontaneously and saccules become less conspicuous although well developed diverticula generally persist.

However, while symptoms and infection continue reflux from the high tension bladder can rapidly lead to pyelonephritic scarring in the kidney and operation may be needed if there is evidence of this development. Diverticulectomy is seldom required on its own account, but established diverticula may be excised when ureteric reimplantation is needed to cure reflux.

The dysfunctional bladder (bladder bulge)

This condition, which is encountered almost entirely in girls, is characterized by a slow dribbling stream and diurnal wetting. Examination shows a persistently full bladder. The urinary flow rate is low and the stream is intermittent, leaving a large residual urine volume. Urinary tract infection is generally present. On pyelography the upper urinary tract is normal or only mildly dilated. Cystoscopy and cystography commonly demonstrate a unilateral outward bulge or wide-mouthed diverticulum due to a thinned area of bladder musculature lying lateral to the ureteric orifice and extending to the bladder neck; the right side is more often affected (*Figure 19.5*). There may be mild bladder trabeculation elsewhere but no anatomical

urethral obstruction is demonstrable. Neuropathic disease and detrusor-sphincter dyssynergia can be excluded by urodynamic, cystometric and electromyographic investigations.

It has generally been considered that the bladder bulge is secondary to the emptying disorder and that the latter, which corresponds to the dysfunctional lazy bladder described by de Luca, Swenson and Fisher (1962), is probably of psychogenic origin. Campbell (1970) carried out psychometric testing in children with voiding difficulties and infection and found that they suffered from emotional disturbances such as timidity, insecurity and shyness. That a functional disorder can be responsible is shown by the fact that the condition often responds, albeit slowly, to encouragement to micturate at regular specific intervals and to ensure complete evacuation by multiple voidings. The use of drugs such as carbachol to enhance detrusor tone and phenoxybenzamine to lower urethral resistance is often helpful.

In some instances the bladder bulge itself is the main factor responsible for the vesical dysfunction. The situation is very similar to that which can follow the uncapping of a poorly backed ectopic ureterocele (Williams, Fay and Lillie, 1972) where the localized detrusor defect prevents normal opening of the bladder neck. Excision of the weakened area of musculature responsible for the bladder bulge can then lead to normal bladder emptying.

A diffuse bladder bulge due to thinning of an area of detrusor musculature may be encountered in the neuropathic bladder (*Figure 19.6*).

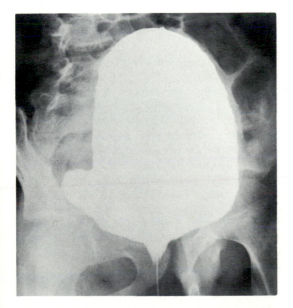

Figure 19.5. Bladder bulge. Cystogram in a 10-year-old girl with slow stream, diurnal wetting and large residual urine after voiding.

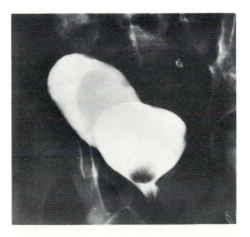

Figure 19.6. Large bladder bulge on superolateral aspect of a neuropathic bladder. Cystogram in a 3-year-old boy with spina bifida.

Resection of the involved portion of the bladder may be required to eliminate residual urine if the bladder dysfunction is to be managed conservatively.

Wide bladder neck

The wide bladder neck syndrome is a condition of uncertain pathogenesis presumed to be of congenital origin, although symptoms do not necessarily date from early childhood. Both males and females may be affected. The complaint is of diurnal leakage of urine, particularly on exertion, and in some cases bed-wetting also occurs. The upper urinary tract is normal. Cystography with fluoroscopy shows that at rest the bladder neck is open and there is filling of the proximal urethra. On voiding the bladder outlet and the proximal urethra dilate widely (*Figure 19.7*) and when the child voluntarily interrupts

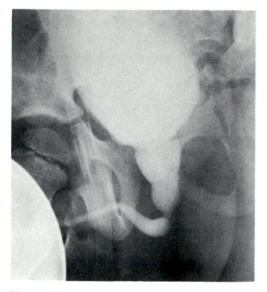

Figure 19.7. Wide bladder neck syndrome. Micturating cystogram in a boy with diurnal stress incontinence.

the stream there is incomplete milk-back from the urethra to the bladder. Urethral pressure profilometry shows a low maximum pressure and a short functional sphincteral length. Cystometry demonstrates no abnormality of sensation or detrusor function and there are no uninhibited contractions. Mild cases generally respond to voiding at 2-hourly or 3-hourly intervals and the use of ephedrine or imipramine, if necessary combined with an anticholinergic such as propantheline. Perineal faradism to increase the muscular tone in the pelvic diaphragm is often helpful. Spontaneous symptomatic improvement occurs with time and operative intervention is seldom needed. In the author's experience the Young-Dees operation (Young, 1922; Dees, 1949) is effective. Williams and Morgan (1978) found that the Marshall-Marchetti suspension technique (Marshall, Marchetti and Krantz, 1949) gave the best results. The margins of the wide bladder neck syndrome are difficult to define precisely and with lesser degrees of the anomaly the diagnosis becomes disputable.

Megaureter-megacystis syndrome

The megaureter-megacystis syndrome is characterized by a very large capacity, and on clinical assessment an apparently persistently full, bladder. It is encountered in association with primary reflux to a dilated upper tract, which is either bilateral or much less often unilateral. The bladder is thin-walled and untrabeculated and the trigone appears large because of the laterally placed and generally wide open ureteric orifices. Formerly it was considered by some authorities that such cases showed a functional defect of the detrusor as well as of the ureters and that operative enlargement of the vesical outlet was needed to encourage bladder emptying (Paquin, Marshall and McGovern, 1960). This concept is supported by the not uncommon finding of a slow urine stream and by the occasional occurrence of acute retention of urine. However, cystography with fluoroscopy demonstrates that during voiding the bladder content tends to follow the line of least resistance up the ureters rather than down the urethra and that even in the child with acute retention the bladder empties completely (*Figure 19.8*). At the conclusion of voiding the bladder promptly refills from the dilated upper tract so that on clinical evaluation it appears to be perpetually distended. The large bladder capacity is a consequence of the large volumes

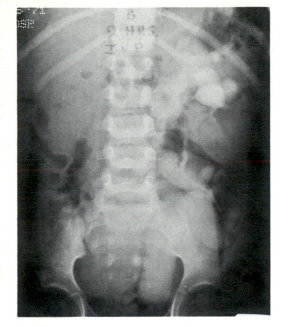

(a)

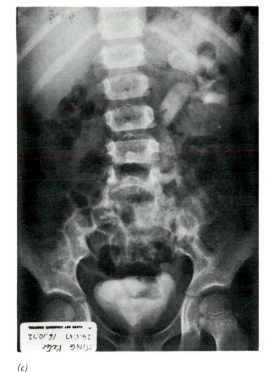

(c)

Figure 19.8. Megaureter-megacystis syndrome in a 4-year-old boy who developed retention of urine. (*a*) Intravenous pyelogram showing gross left hydro-ureteronephrosis and no concentration by the right kidney. (*b*) Cystogram showing bilateral reflux. (*c*) Intravenous pyelogram 16 months following right nephroureterectomy and reimplantation of left ureter into bladder. The patient is micturating normally.

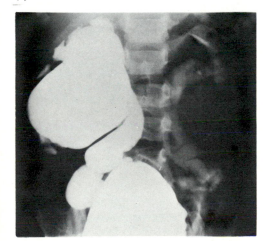

(b)

the organ is required to accommodate as a result of urine regurgitating to and from the capacious ureters and, often, of polyuria caused by impaired renal function.

The treatment of megaureter-megacystis syndrome is that of the associated refluxing megaureters which is dependent upon the degree of impairment of ureteric and renal function. The bladder itself requires no specific measures. When reflux is cured normal micturition becomes established and the high false residual volume after voiding is eliminated.

Occult neuropathic bladder

Lapides (1967) first suggested that vesical dysfunction could occur as a consequence of neurological disease confined in its effects to the lower urinary tract. Such terms as subclinical neurogenic bladder, occult neurological bladder, isolated neurogenic dysfunction and non-neurogenic neurogenic bladder were later employed although different authors have applied them to quite different clinicopathological states (Mix, 1977). Lapides (1967) described a condition characterized by an uninhibited low capacity bladder which caused urge incontinence but did not lead to upper tract dilatation. Kamhi, Horowitz and Kovetz (1971) considered occult neuropathy to be the essential causative factor

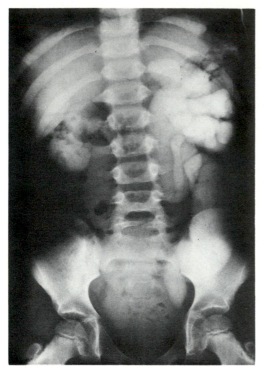

(a)

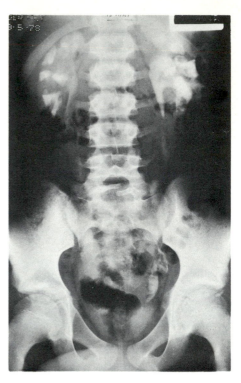

(c)

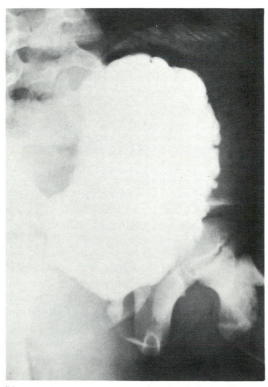

(b)

Figure 19.9. Occult neuropathic bladder. (*a*) Intravenous pyelogram in an 8-year-old boy with urine retention and overflow incontinence showing gross bilateral hydroureteronephrosis. *(b)* Cystourethrogram showing bladder trabeculation and dilated posterior urethra. Patient treated by endoscopic sphincterotomy, phenoxybenzamine and bladder training. (*c*) Intravenous pyelogram at age 14 showing improved upper tract dilatation; there was normal voiding without medication.

in children with recurrent urinary tract infection. The term occult neuropathic bladder is preferably restricted to cases that in the absence of an anatomical infravesical obstruction exhibit vesical retention and various degrees of upper tract dilatation and kidney damage. Some children suffer from severe rectal dyschezia in addition but apart from that no neuropathic lesion is evident elsewhere. The urological picture is precisely similar to that seen in the child with overt neurological disease due to spina bifida or sacral agenesis.

The patient presents with urinary incontinence of the dribbling overflow type. Symptoms of urinary tract infection are common. In some cases presentation is delayed until azotaemia develops as a result of severe hydroureteronephrosis. The bladder is persistently distended and usually inexpressible. Routine neurological examination reveals no abnormality, and radiology of the spine and myelography show normal results. The bladder is severely trabeculated and sacculated and various degrees of upper tract dilatation and renal parenchymal atrophy are evident with or without vesicoureteric reflux (*Figure 19.9*). Urodynamic studies reveal a slow intermittent urine flow with incomplete bladder emptying and a high urine residue after voiding. Electromyography of the external urethral sphincter combined with cystometry demonstrates high intravesical voiding pressures with failure of the sphincter to relax during a detrusor contraction.

The diagnosis of occult neuropathic bladder is essentially a negative one based on the exclusion of organic infravesical obstruction and overt neuropathic disease. Expert neurological advice is essential since bladder dysfunction may be the first evidence of spinal cord tethering or dysraphism, or of compression of the cord or the cauda equina by a tumour or cyst. Williams, Hirst and Doyle (1974) found the Lapides (Lapides *et al.*, 1962) denervation supersensitivity test to be positive in some cases of occult neuropathy. However, this test cannot be accepted as diagnostic since it can, in the author's experience, be negative in cases of neuropathic bladder caused by spina bifida.

The aetiology of the occult neuropathic bladder is disputed and hence the therapeutic approach has varied. Hinman and Baumann (1973) and Allen (1977) considered that psychological disorders were the basis. They found that most affected children had an abnormal personality in that they were unusually shy and withdrawn and there was often a history of parental domination, family disruption and other social problems. They employed bladder retraining whereby the child was instructed to void every 3 hours during the day and to ensure that the bladder was completely emptied. Hypnosis was found to be helpful in the early stages and often benefit was obtained from biofeedback methods in which the patient watched his own urodynamic performance on the recording instruments and his voiding on the fluoroscope.

In the author's experience children with occult neuropathy have not shown any obvious emotional disturbances apart from those to be expected as a result of urinary incontinence, and discussions with parents have not revealed any **evidence** of unusual family stress. On the assumption that the condition is caused by a subtle but true neuropathic lesion affected children have been treated along lines applied successfully to many cases of overt neuropathy (Johnston and Farkas, 1975). These have aimed at facilitating bladder emptying by lowering urethral resistance. Phenoxybenzamine is often effective. If alpha-adrenergic blockade is shown by urethral pressure profilometry to be ineffective, endoscopic external sphincterotomy is employed. Vesicoureteric reflux may need operative cure. In addition the child is encouraged to micturate at regular 3-hourly intervals, to perform multiple voidings and to aid evacuation by straining or manual abdominal compression in order to achieve complete emptying. If such measures are not effective, a regimen of intermittent catheterization like that employed for overt neuropathy may be successful. Constipation often requires treatment with laxatives, suppositories or in some instances enemas.

The function of the occult neuropathic bladder often improves with time and in several cases in the author's experience affected children have ultimately achieved normal micturition habits while at the same time their upper tract dilatation has shown improvement (*Figure 19.9*). In some patients with gross upper tract damage urinary diversion may be unavoidable but otherwise conservative management should be pursued. There can be no indication in the early stages of treatment for urinary diversion purely to control incontinence.

The occult neuropathic bladder and the so-called dysfunctional bladder may have certain similarities at a clinical level. However, full investigation generally allows a clear distinction to be made. In the dysfunctional bladder there is little trabeculation and upper tract dilatation, if present at all, is never more than mild. Urodynamic studies demonstrate no incoordination between detrusor and sphincter activity. On the other hand in the occult neuropathic bladder obstructive bladder changes, and often the degree of upper tract dilatation, are severe and detrusor-sphincter dyssynergia can be shown to exist by cystometry and sphincteric electromyography. Koff (1980) pointed out that external sphincteric electromyography with the patient asleep and awake can distinguish between involuntary and voluntary contraction. Dyssinergia during sleep implies organic neuropathy while, if it is only present while awake, it suggests a psychosomatic lesion.

Urachal anomalies

The urachus or median umbilical ligament extends from the apex of the bladder to the umbilicus. It is composed of a fibromuscular cord that even in the adult may have a narrow tubular lumen lined by modified transitional epithelium or by columnar mucosa similar to that in the intestine. The urachus is derived in part from the ventral portion of the cloaca and in part from the allantois lying in the body stalk; how much each component contributes is uncertain.

Patent urachus

If the urachus is patent, the allantois remains open and urine escaping from the bladder before birth may lead to the umbilical cord becoming distended. After the cord sloughs off leakage of urine from a mucosa-covered nipple may be evident or alternatively there may be a fistula in the depths of a normal-looking umbilicus. Patent urachus may occur as a consequence of a congenital infravesical obstruction. It is seen particularly in boys with the prune belly syndrome when there is atresia or stenosis of the membranous urethra; it may also be encountered in infants with neuropathic bladder due to spina bifida. More commonly congenital urachal fistula occurs as an isolated anomaly. Herbst (1937) noted that obstruction was present in only 14 per cent of reported cases. Schreck and Campbell (1972) pointed out that the urachus is ordinarily closed before a prenatal infravesical obstruction is effective. The diagnosis of urachal fistula is confirmed by cystography which is also needed to exclude an obstructive lesion. Treatment requires excision of the fistulous tract and closure of the bladder.

Urachal cyst

In this condition the two extremities of the urachal canal close while the intervening portion between the bladder and the umbilicus remains unobliterated and becomes distended by its mucosal secretions and by desquamated cells. The cyst may present clinically as an abdominal tumour or more often remains symptomless until infection, usually by staphylococci, occurs. The patient is most commonly an infant and has a tender infraumbilical swelling with reddening of the overlying skin. Drainage of pus may occur spontaneously through the umbilicus and may persist intermittently in the form of a urachal sinus. Rarely an infected cyst ruptures into the peritoneal cavity (McMillan, Schullinger and Santulli, 1973) or intestinal obstruction occurs from bowel adherence (Irving and Rickham, 1978). An uninfected urachal cyst is treated by excision. When, as is usually the case, infection exists then excision *in toto* is generally impossible. Incision, curettage of the cyst lining and drainage are effective.

Urachal diverticulum

In this disorder the vesical end of the urachus remains open as a bladder diverticulum. The size of the communication with the bladder varies and when it is small an intradiverticular calculus may form. A wide-mouthed urachal diverticulum is seen typically in the prune belly syndrome and in some cases calcification of the diverticular wall is present at birth. Diverticulectomy is needed if a stone is present or, in prune belly syndrome, if the diverticulum is a source of significant residual urine.

Urachal carcinoma

This takes the form of a mucus-secreting adenocarcinoma that involves the bladder apex. As a rule the condition occurs during adult life but Cornil, Reynolds and Kickham (1967) reported an example in a 15-year-old girl.

Vesicourethral anomalies in incomplete prune belly syndrome

Genitourinary anomalies in boys with the prune belly syndrome are discussed in Chapter 24. On occasions one or more of the same abnormalities

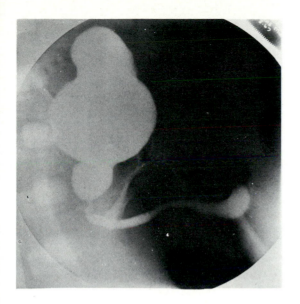

Figure 19.10. Pseudo-prune belly. Micturating cystourethrogram in a clinically normal boy with dysuria showing urachal diverticulum, dilated posterior urethra and megalourethra of the penile portion.

are encountered in boys with a normal abdominal wall. Most commonly such pseudo-prune-belly cases present with impalpable testes, megalourethra or urinary tract infection resulting from urinary stasis. Less often voiding difficulty is the main complaint. The clinically normal 7-year-old boy whose micturating cystourethogram is shown in *Figure 19.10* complained of dysuria and a slow urine stream. Radiography showed the urachal diverticulum and dilated proximal urethra characteristic of the prune belly syndrome. Normal voiding followed internal urethrotomy just below the dilated segment.

Vesicovaginal fistula

A congenital fistula between the bladder and the vagina in the presence of a normal urethra is extremely rare. An example with a pin-hole communication was reported by Swinney (1951). In the author's own experience of one case the fistula took the form of a narrow incompetent accessory urethra lying posterior to the main one and extending from the bladder trigone to the anterior wall of the vagina.

A considerable number of iatrogenic vesicovaginal fistulas were produced in the heyday of bladder neck obstruction when surgeons overdid endoscopic resection or open wedge excision of the posterior margin of the vesical outlet. The accident has also occurred in the author's experience by a surgeon fulgurating endoscopically the stump of an ectopic ureter left behind after nephroureterectomy. Repair of a vesicovaginal or vesicourethrovaginal fistula can be exceedingly difficult. An abdominal transperitoneal approach is needed with the patient in the lithotomy position to allow access to the vagina. The aim is to separate the bladder and the urethra entirely from the vagina both above and below the fistula and to close each viscus separately. A bougie passed through the vaginal introitus helps to define the margins of the fistula and by pushing the vagina upwards improves access. If there is a shortage of tissue, the bladder and the urethra must take precedence over the vagina. It is often valuable to reinforce the repair by a omental pedicle graft inserted between the two suture lines.

Persistence of the urogenital sinus produces what is in effect a congenital vesicovaginal fistula in which a very short wide incompetent urethra opens high on the anterior wall of the vagina. Continence can be achieved by the construction of a neourethra from the trigone or the anterior bladder wall. A similar bladder outlet anomaly often exists with persistence of the cloaca when the incontinent urethra opens into the common evacuating channel.

Bladder neck obstruction

Some years ago the urological and paediatric journals contained many articles on primary bladder neck obstruction in children, most of them advocating its surgical correction. Now the condition is never mentioned. This is naturally a source of great satisfaction to those of us who never believed in the existence of the disease (Johnston, 1960), but women who now suffer from various degrees of urinary incontinence and men who now ejaculate retrogradely as a result of overenthusiastic resection or widening of the bladder outlet during childhood may take a less complacent view. The misconception concerning bladder neck obstruction in children arose in the 1950s when surgeons tried to apply the principles of adult urology to paediatric disorders. Marion's disease, characterized by a fibrous contracture of the vesical neck and accepted as a pathological entity in men, was considered to cause bladder diverticula, refluxing megaureters and megacystis in boys. Later, lesser degrees of bladder neck obstruction were thought to be important in children of both sexes in the aetiology of recurrent urinary tract infection, vesicoureteric reflux and enuresis.

Since primary bladder neck obstruction has no distinctive local diagnostic features its existence or otherwise has been very much a matter of opinion. The endoscopic assessment of a prominent posterior margin to the vesical outlet and of minor degrees of bladder trabeculation is highly subjective. In girls a spinning-top shape on the micturating urethrogram was originally believed to be pathognomonic of the condition and subsequently the same urethrographic outline was considered to demonstrate the existence of distal urethral stenosis. In fact the spinning-top urethrogram is a normal appearance in little girls with high voiding rates and is indicative simply of the differing degrees of distensibility of different parts of the urethra (Johnston, Koff and Glassberg, 1978). Bladder-neck biopsies in cases of presumed obstruction have been reported to show muscular hypertrophy with or without fibrosis but lacking any gross deviation from the normal. Bodian (1957) considered that fibroelastosis characterized by an excess of periurethral fibrous and elastic tissue was the basic lesion in boys, but confirmation of the existence of the condition requires histological examination of the entire posterior urethra and the bladder base.

The greater use of urodynamic methods of investigation and also clinical experience have now convinced most urologists that bladder neck obstruction as a primary lesion in children is extremely rare, if it exists at all. The diagnosis can only be considered to be established when in a case of an unquestionably obstructed bladder other disorders, in particular neuropathic disease or external sphincteral dysfunction of organic or emotional origin, have been confidently excluded by the appropriate investigations.

Secondary bladder neck obstruction may be encountered following the relief of a urethral obstruction at a lower level. The thickened bladder neck, being part of the generalized detrusor hypertrophy, can then cause the persistence or the later reappearance of outflow obstruction. Such an occurrence is occasionally seen after the fulguration of urethral valves in boys; it is readily relieved by endoscopic incision of the posterior margin of the bladder outlet. Similarly, although the primary obstructive lesion in cases of detrusor-sphincter dyssynergia of either overt or occult neuropathic origin is in the external urethral sphincter, secondary changes at the bladder neck may continue to interfere with vesical emptying after the sphincteral malfunction has been corrected. However, in both these conditions it is important not to anticipate the existence or later development of secondary bladder neck obstruction by resecting the vesical outlet at the time of treating the urethral pathology. An intact vesical neck is important in the maintenance of full urinary control, especially following the fulguration of urethral valves in boys.

References

Abrahamson, J. (1961) Double bladder and related anomalies: clinical and embryological aspects and a case report. *British Journal of Urology*, **33**, 195

Allen, T.D. (1977) The non-neurogenic neurogenic bladder. *Journal of Urology*, **117**, 232

Bodian, M. (1957) Some observations of the pathology of congenital idiopathic bladder neck obstruction. *British Journal of Urology*, **29**, 393

Campbell, W.A. (1970) Psychometric testing with the human figure drawing in chronic cystitis. *Journal of Urology*, **104**, 930

Cornil, C., Reynolds, C.T. and Kickham, L.J.E. (1967) Carcinoma of the urachus. *Journal of Urology*, **98**, 93

Dees, J.E. (1949) Congenital epispadias with incontinence. *Journal of Urology*, **62**, 513

de Luca, F.G., Swenson, W. and Fisher, J.H. (1962) The dysfunctional "lazy" bladder syndrome in children. *Archives of Disease in Childhood*, **37**, 117

Dutta, T., George, V., Meenakshi, P.K. and Das, G. (1974) Rare combination of duplication of genito-urinary tract, hindgut, vertebral column and other associated anomalies. *British Journal of Urology*, **46**, 577

Herbst, W.P. (1937) Patent urachus. *Southern Medical Journal*, **30**, 711

Hinman, F. and Baumann, F.W. (1973) Vesical and ureteral damage from voiding dysfunction in boys without neurologic or obstructive disease. *Journal of Urology*, **109**, 727

Hutch, J.A. (1958) The ureterovesical junction: the theory of extravesicalisation of the intravesical ureter. University of California Press, Berkeley

Irving, I.M. and Rickham, P.P. (1978) Umbilical abnormalities. *In* Neonatal Surgery, 2nd edn (edited by Rickham, P.P., Lister, J. and Irving I.M.). Butterworths, London. p.309

Johnston, J.H. (1960) Vesical diverticula without urinary obstruction in childhood. *Journal of Urology*, **84**, 535

Johnston, J.H. and Farkas, A. (1975) Congenital neuro-pathic bladder: practicalities and possibilities of conservational management. *Urology*, **5**,719

Johnston, J.H. and Koff, S.A. (1977) Covered cloacal exstrophy: another variation on the theme. *Journal of Urology*, **118**, 666

Johnston, J.H., Koff, S.A. and Glassberg, K.I. (1978) The pseudo-obstructed bladder in enuretic children. *British Journal of Urology*, **50**, 505

Kamhi, B., Horowitz, M.I. and Kovetz, A. (1971) Isolated neurogenic dysfunction of the bladder in children with urinary tract infection. *Journal of Urology*, **106**, 151

Koff, S.A. (1980) Personal communication

Lapides, J. (1967) Cystometry. *Journal of the American Medical Association*, **201**, 124

Lapides, J., Friend, C.R., Ajemian, E.P. and Reus, W.F. (1962) Denervation supersensitivity as a test for neurogenic bladder. *Surgery, Gynecology and Obstetrics*, **114**, 241

McMillan, R.W., Schullinger, J.N. and Santulli, T.V. (1973) Pyourachus: an unusual surgical problem. *Journal of Pediatric Surgery*, **8**, 387

Marshall, V.F., Marchetti, A. and Krantz, K.E. (1949) Correction of stress incontinence by simple vesico-urethral suspension. *Surgery, Gynecology and Obstetrics*, **88**, 509

Mix, L.W. (1977) Occult neuropathic bladder. *Urology*, **10**,1

Montague, D.M. and Boltuch, R.L. (1976) Primary neo-plasms in vesical diverticula: report of 10 cases. *Journal of Urology*, **116**, 41

Ostroff, E.B., Alperstein, J.B. and Young, J.D. (1973)

Neoplasm in vesical diverticula: report of 4 patients, including a 21 year old. *Journal of Urology*, **110**, 65

Palmer, J.M. and Russi, M.F. (1969) Persistent urogenital sinus with absence of the bladder and urethra. *Journal of Urology*, **102**, 590

Paquin, A., Marshall, V.F. and McGovern, J.H. (1960) The megacystis syndrome. *Journal of Urology*, **83**, 634

Ravitch, M.M. (1953) Hindgut duplication: doubling of colon and genital urinary tracts. *Annals of Surgery*, **137**,588

Schreck, W.R. and Campbell, W.A. (1972) The relation of bladder outlet obstruction to urinary-umbilical fistula. *Journal of Urology*, **108**, 641

Swinney, J. (1951) A case of congenital vesico-vaginal fistula. *British Journal of Urology*, **23**, 64

Tacciuoli, M., Laurenti, C. and Racheli, T. (1975) Double bladder with complete sagittal septum. *British Journal of Urology*, **47**, 645

Tacciuoli, M., Laurenti, C. and Racheli, T. (1976) Trigonal cyst in childhood. *British Journal of Urology*, **48**, 323

Vincent, S.A. (1966) Postural control of urinary inconti-nence: the curtsey sign. *Lancet*, ii, 631

Williams, D.I. and Morgan, R.C. (1978) Wide bladder neck syndrome in children: a review. *Journal of the Royal Society of Medicine*, **71**, 520

Williams, D.I., Fay, R. and Lillie, J.G. (1972) The function-al radiology of ectopic ureterocele. *British Journal of Urology*, **44**, 417

Williams, D.I., Hirst, G. and Doyle, D. (1974) The occult neuropathic bladder. *Journal of Pediatric Surgery*, **9**, 35

Young, H.H. (1922) An operation for the cure of inconti-nence associated with epispadias. *Journal of Urology*, **7**, 1

20   Male urethral anomalies

D. Innes Williams

Embryology

The primitive cloaca is divided in the coronal plane between the 9mm and the 15 mm stages by downgrowth of the urorectal septum from the junction of the hindgut and the allantois (*Figures 20.1 and 20.2*). The ventral compartment so formed becomes the urogenital sinus and the ventral section of the cloacal membrane the urethral membrane which ruptures soon after it has been defined, that is, when the embryo measures 16–17 mm.

The lower segment of the urogenital sinus below the vesical dilatation is a roughly L-shaped cavity. The vertical limb is the pars pelvina which receives the wolffian ducts and forms all the urethra down to the orifices of Cowper's glands in the bulb. The horizontal limb, the pars phallica, consists of that forward

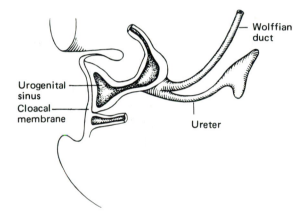

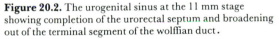

Figure 20.2. The urogenital sinus at the 11 mm stage showing completion of the urorectal septum and broadening out of the terminal segment of the wolffian duct.

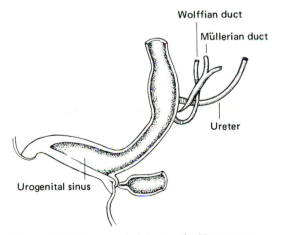

Figure 20.3. The urogenital sinus at the 25 mm stage demonstrating the loop on the wolffian duct and the formation of the urethral plate.

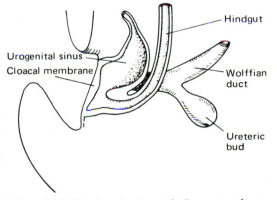

Figure 20.1. The cloacal region at the 9 mm stage demonstrating the downgrowth of the urorectal septum.

prolongation of the cloaca which has from a very early stage extended up into the genital tubercle. Its caudal wall is formed by the urethral (formerly the cloacal) membrane until the 16–17 mm stage when this ruptures, laying the sinus wide open to the amniotic cavity (*Figure 20.3*).

Müller's tubercle is a hillock in the posterior wall of the pars pelvina formed at about the 30 mm stage by the fused tip of the müllerian ducts pushing up between the orifices of the wolffian ducts. Caudal to this the sinus shows a well marked crista urethralis posteriorly and a variable number of lateral submontanal folds. The prostatic tubules appear in the upper part after the embryo reaches 60 mm, by which time condensation of the surrounding mesenchyme already shows evidence of the formation of the external urinary sphincter. The wolffian ducts remain as the ejaculatory ducts and Müller's tubercle as the verumontanum, and the utriculus masculinus perhaps represents the remnant of the müllerian ducts. More probably it results chiefly from the sinovaginal bulbs which are outgrowths of the sinus epithelium and in the female form the lower part of the vagina. The disappearance of the müllerian duct system in the normal male is dependent upon the production by the fetal testis of the antimüllerian hormone (*see* Chapter 35). Persistence of part of the system in male intersex cases is not unexpected but sometimes a lack of this specific hormone results in the development (often unilaterally) of a uterus and a fallopian tube in an otherwise normal male. Utricular cysts may result from premature closure of the opening of the müllerian duct or of the sinovaginal bulbs before the cranial portions have atrophied.

At the time of rupture of the urethral membrane the cavity of the pars phallica of the urogenital sinus does not extend as far as the tip of the genital tubercle, although a solid lamella of cells continuous with the epithelium of the sinus is prolonged into the region beginning to differentiate as the glans. In the shaft of the penis the open urogenital sinus shows as a groove which at the 40 mm stage is transformed into a tube by fusion of its lateral margins, that is the urethral folds. Within the glans, however, the solid lamella of cells known as the urethral plate remains (*Figure 20.4*) and canalizes at a later stage to form the glandular urethra (Williams, 1951). Minor degrees of duplication of the urethra, particularly of the hypospadiac variety, probably originate from partial canalization of

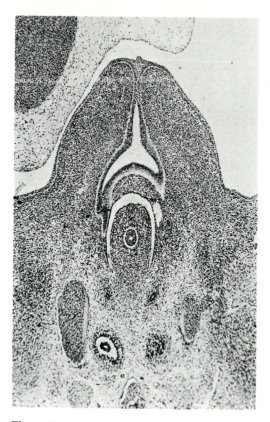

Figure 20.4. Transverse section of a 25 mm embryo showing in the centre the hindgut suspended upon its mesentery in the coelomic cavity. Anteriorly is the urogenital sinus cut so that it shows the entry of the ureters into the pars pelvina and the anterior prolongation of the pars phallica, reaching out into the phallus as the solid urethral plate. Posteriorly the ureters are cut across again and reach the metanephric condensations shown between the umbilical arteries.

this urethral plate. Epispadiac duplications must have an origin similar to that of bladder exstrophy (*see* page 299) while collateral urethras follow the pattern of duplication of the bladder.

Posterior urethral diverticula and utricular cysts

A number of abnormalities may present the appearance of a diverticulum in the posterior urethra. A pouch that opens below the verumontanum is characteristic of the stump of the rectourethral fistula in imperforate anus (*see*

Chapter 22). The diagnosis is evident from the history. The pseudodiverticulum may require treatment because of the reservoir of urine that forms during micturition and empties afterwards, causing dribbling incontinence. Stone formation is also a complication. Depending upon the size of the pouch, excision should be undertaken transperitoneally, transtrigonally or pararectally.

An ectopic ureter in the male may open at or above the verumontanum. If its lower extremity is dilated, it is effectively a urethral diverticulum and requires excision.

In intersex cases a vagina entering the posterior urethra is not unusual and varies considerably in size and to some extent in position. The more severe the degree of the external abnormality the greater is the likelihood of vaginal development although there is no strict correspondence. Usually the opening is found surrounded by mucosal tags in the membranous region without any development of a verumontanum. In lesser examples the opening has the appearance of an enlarged prostatic utricle. In most cases the urine flows freely in and out of the vaginal cavity and causes no

symptoms (*Figure 20.5*). However, when the distal urethra is obstructed, perhaps as a result of surgery for hypospadias, infection in the residual vaginal urine can cause considerable problems. Epididymitis may complicate the infection since the vasa are closely associated with the vaginal wall and open somewhere near its orifice. Incontinence due to the reservoir effect occurs as in other posterior urethral diverticula and may necessitate excision of the vagina.

Some intersex patients have persistent müllerian duct structures which are usually unilateral and open through an apparently normal prostatic utricle. The latter may become obstructed and a utricular cyst may develop (Morgan, Williams and Pryor, 1979). Such a cyst forms a mass in the pelvis associated with pain and perhaps recurrent pyuria. Its enlargement can cause pressure on the urethra and retention of urine. The cyst is ordinarily palpable on bimanual pelvic examination and is not demonstrable radiologically unless the communication with the urethra is patent. An example of partial obstruction with infection is shown in *Figure 20.6*. Operative excision of the vagina or utricle is only required in symptomatic cases. A transperitoneal approach after mobilization of the bladder is effective for babies, while in older children it may be preferable to make a midline

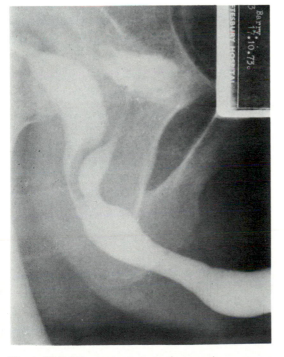

Figure 20.5. Micturating cystourethrogram in a young man with slight stricture following hypospadias repair showing free filling of the vagina.

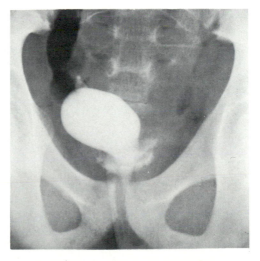

Figure 20.6. Micturating cystogram in a 14-year-old boy with recurrent infection and incontinence following hypospadias repair. The bladder is almost empty, leaving a dilated utricular cyst. At operation this cyst lay entirely retroperitoneally and was without either uterus or fallopian tubes. Both the vasa were involved in its wall.

incision across the trigone of the bladder in order to reach the cyst.

A tubular utricular diverticulum is characteristic of the prune belly syndrome and seldom requires treatment.

Urethral duplications

The two chief types of double urethra are sagittal and collateral. The great majority of cases fall into the first category, in which the two channels are in the same sagittal plane one above the other. Not all are complete duplications. The accessory channel is more likely to be found in the distal part of the penis than in the prostatic section of the urethra. A minority of cases are collateral, the two channels lying side by side. This is the characteristic arrangement in diphallus, but incomplete forms of this anomaly are seen where the penis is not completely split (Williams and Kenauri, 1975).

Epispadiac duplications

In this group the accessory channel lies on the dorsum of the penis (*Figure 20.7*). Most cases of complete duplication fall into this category. Incomplete varieties are rare but abortive examples with a dorsal penile sinus are relatively common. The accessory opening may be at any point on the dorsum of the penis from the glans to the base. In some patients it is a vertical cleft and in others a transverse slit as in true epispadias. An upward curvature of the penis is often associated. The channel runs backwards above the corpora cavernosa and then passes deep to

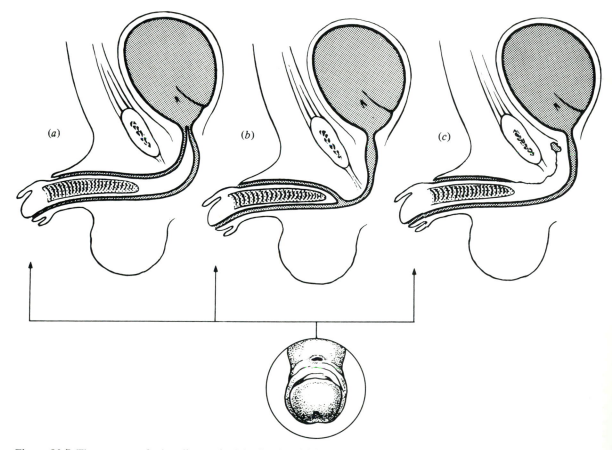

Figure 20.7. The anatomy of epispadiac urethral duplication. (*a*) Complete: both channels enter the bladder. (*b*) Incomplete: bifid urethra. (*c*) Abortive: the posterior extremity is atretic. (Reproduced by permission of the editor, *European Urology*.)

the pubic symphysis to join the bladder anterior to the normal bladder neck. Where the opening is wide there is incontinence in spite of normal micturition. Those presenting in adult life complain of difficulty in achieving normal intercourse due to the upward chordee (*Figure 20.8*) as well as of some urinary incontinence.

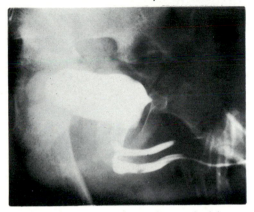

Figure 20.8. Incomplete epispadiac urethral duplication. Urethrogram to show the anatomy and the forward kinking of the normally placed channel as a result of the shortening of the accessory urethra.

Most common in this category are abortive duplications, that is blind dorsal penile sinuses, usually with a slight serous or purulent discharge and also the upward chordee characteristic of the more complete forms. In general the sinus extends back as far as the region of the pubic symphysis and can be traced no further although it is not unlikely that an atretic cord extends upwards. In one of the author's cases and in others described by Mogg (1968) such a cord could be traced upwards to the ventral surface of the bladder where it became distended to form a minute cyst with a tenuous connection to the umbilicus. This type therefore has the appearance of an abortive sagittal duplication of the bladder although there is no connection to the ureters or kidneys.

Within the epispadiac group of disorders there are seldom major anomalies elsewhere in the body. However, in a few as in true epispadias the pubic symphysis is not fully united. There is no abnormality of the normally placed urethra and continence is normal after the accessory channel has been excised.

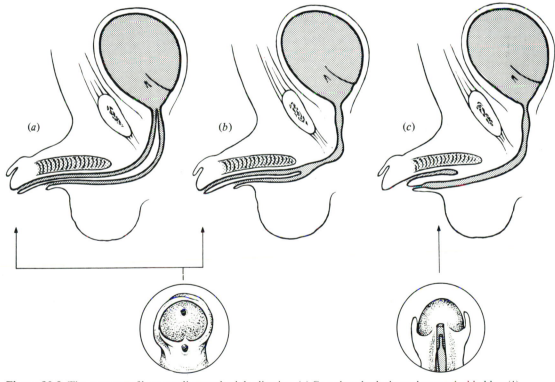

Figure 20.9. The anatomy of hypospadiac urethral duplication. (*a*) Complete: both channels enter the bladder. (*b*) Incomplete: bifid urethra. (*c*) Abortive: the common blind accessory channel is dorsal to the hypospadiac urethra. (Reproduced by permission of the editor, *European Urology.*)

Hypospadiac duplications

In these conditions (*Figure 20.9*) both channels lie ventral to the corpora cavernosa and one opening is in the position of hypospadias while the other lies on the glans in the normal position or slightly dorsal to it.

Incomplete duplication, that is forked urethra, may follow the same pattern. A single posterior urethra splits to form two channels from that point forwards.

Treatment may be required for obstruction but penile curvature is not a feature and incontinence is uncommon. Therefore in most cases there seems no necessity to remove the two channels, although an operation that excises the septum between them may succeed in removing the obstructive effect.

Abortive duplications that fall into this category are extremely common. In hypospadias where the opening of the urethra is a little short of the coronal sulcus it is not at all uncommon to find a second opening in the groove on the glans distal to the hypospadiac urethra. This sinus extends backwards for 2–3 cm dorsal to the urethra. At times the sinus extends a good deal further proximally to the base of the penis and even to the membranous area and in such circumstances the track may become infected.

Attention is usually drawn to its presence by the accidental introduction of a sound or catheter into the accessory channel rather than the complete one.

Spindle urethra

This deformity (*Figure 20.10*) in which the urethral channel splits into two just below the bladder neck and reunites in the region of the penoscrotal area is rare. The author has seen three clear-cut examples in all of which a posterior urethral obstruction was present. Stenosis of one channel caused it to dilate and press upon the other, thus impeding the flow through both. An operation to unite the two channels should be curative.

Bifid urethra with pre-anal accessory track

In the author's experience this is the commonest form of duplication. The characteristic features are bifurcation of the urethra at approximately the level of the verumontanum, an anatomically normal channel passing forward from this point that is atretic to a greater or lesser extent and a posterior channel that is often wide, supple and well controlled, and opens at the anal margin or in the perineum (*Figure 20.11*). There have been suggestions that the posterior channel is a fistula

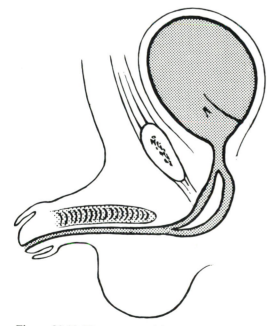

Figure 20.10. The anatomy of the spindle urethral duplication. (Reproduced by permission of the editor, *European Urology*.)

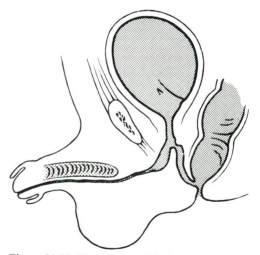

Figure 20.11. The anatomy of the bifid urethra with pre-anal accessory track. (Reproduced by permission of the editor, *European Urology*.)

rather than a urethral duplication. However, in the majority the mucosa of the aberrant channel is healthy and surrounded by an adequate muscularis. Some patients pass urine satisfactorily from the perianal opening and do not demand

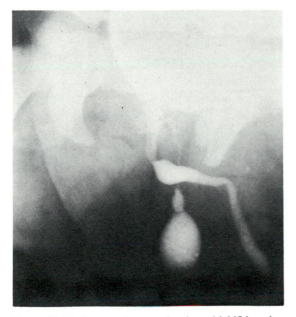

Figure 20.12. Cystourethrogram in a boy with bifid urethra and pre-anal accessory track. The anomalous channel arises at one side of the verumontanum and reaches down to the perineum with a terminal dilatation. Unusually for this anomaly there is no constriction of the penile urethra.

treatment. Others have a degree of urinary obstruction causing some upper tract damage.

In the anterior channel the stenosis usually affects the urethra from the bulb to a point 1–2 cm short of the external meatus. The meatus itself is ordinarily normal but even the finest bougies cannot be introduced for more than 2–3 cm. Exploration of the atretic zone demonstrates that it is surrounded by fibrofatty tissue without evidence of a corpus spongiosum and if an attempt is made to cut back the urethra, laying it open to the skin as in the Johanson procedure, the lumen is lost a short distance back from the tip of the penis. The pathology of the stenosis is not clear but one of the author's cases presented with a hard mass in the penoscrotal and inguinal region that proved to be extravasation of urine which had occurred spontaneously in spite of the fact that urine was being passed from the anal urethral opening. This suggests that there was some intrinsic defect of the wall of the urethra and a pathological process commencing during fetal development.

There may be accompanying abnormalities in the urinary tract apart from the effects of obstruction and a vesical diverticulum, reflux and an ectopic ureter have all been encountered (*Figure 20.12*). Externally the scrotum may be bifid with a smooth strip in the midline that incidentally facilitates repair. Several reported cases possessed tracheo-oesophageal fistulas or had rectal abnormalities (*Figure 20.13*).

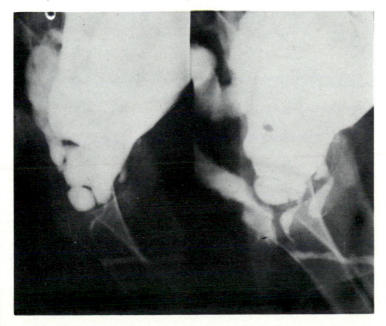

Figure 20.13. Cystourethrogram in a boy with urethral duplication and pre-anal accessory track associated with urethral diverticulum and ectopic ureter. The X-ray shows on the right the normally placed channel ending abruptly at the root of the penis; the accessory channel lies posteriorly and some opaque medium is discharged into the rectum. The posterior urethral diverticulum is also shown.

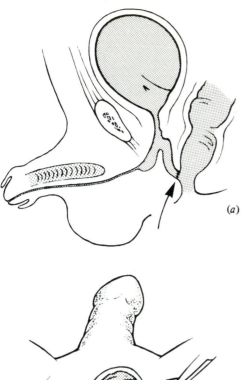

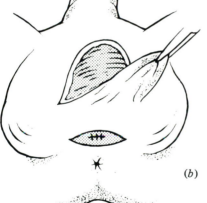

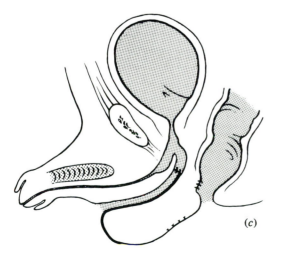

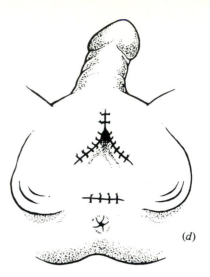

Figure 20.14. Operation for bifid urethra with pre-anal accessory track, first stage. The posterior channel is mobilized and detached from its external orifice and a scrotal pedicle is formed, canalized and anastomosed to the proximal cut end of the accessory urethra. In this way the functional urethral meatus is brought to the midscrotal point. At a second operation, as for hypospadias, a distal meatus can be constructed. The normally placed but stenotic urethra is untouched. (Reproduced by permission of the editor, *British Journal of Urology*.)

In undertaking reconstructive surgery the aim is to produce a second complete urethral channel to the tip of the penis. The atretic state of the anatomically normal channel together with its surrounding fibrosis seems to make any attempt at simple urethroplasty impossible. In the series reported by Williams and Bloomberg (1976) a staged procedure was adopted. First the anal opening was transferred to a point in the anterior perineum under the protection of a colostomy. Secondly a buried strip of skin extending from the perineal opening to the tip of the penis was formed into a tube and covered as in hypospadias repair. In each case a good functioning urethra was produced with normal continence although the urethral opening was not quite terminal on the penis. Two cases were treated by scrotal flap urethroplasty without preliminary colostomy. The anal urethral opening was first divided and the posterior channel mobilized. A flap from the anterior part of the scrotum was then outlined and turned back to be anastomosed to the proximal cut end of the posterior urethral channel. The anal defect was closed and at a second operation the division of the flap was accompanied by penile urethroplasty (*Figure 20.14*).

Collateral duplications

Complete diphallus with consequent urethral duplication is a rare abnormality and in most examples one penis contains only an impermeable urethral cord. Two such cases have been observed in the author's practice but it is not intended to describe them in detail here. There are incomplete examples of diphallus where the penis forms a single column while the glans has a lobed appearance representing partial formation of a second organ. In such cases there may

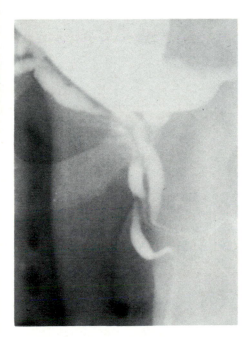

Figure 20.15. Double bladder with four urethras. Cystogram showing two bladders of which the left is only partly full. Three of the four urethras are outlined. The fourth enters the anal canal and is obscured. There is reflux into the seminal vesicles and vas on the right side.

be a complete urethra or an abortive channel (Oudard and Jean, 1921). In one remarkable case reported by Woodhouse and Williams (1979; *Figure 20.15*) a boy was found to have a collateral duplication of the bladder with four urethral channels. One of them was a short duct with an opening into the anus and the other three traversed the penis, lying in the same sagittal plane but obstructed by partial atresia. By excising the anal opening and running the penile channels into one a normal urine flow and normal continence were obtained.

Cowper's duct dilatation

Micturating cystourethrograms not infrequently show Cowper's duct as a short channel running backwards from the bulb of the urethra. This is not necessarily an abnormal finding and should not be mistaken for a urethral duplication. At times the orifice appears to become obstructed when a small cystic swelling can be observed radiologically or endoscopically in the floor of the bulb. This cyst may then rupture accompanied by slight dysuria or bleeding after which reflux into the duct is inevitable and complicating infection a possibility. Surgical treatment is very unlikely to be required.

Anterior urethral diverticula

Although they are easily overlooked, anterior urethral diverticula are not uncommon and should always be borne in mind in cases of bladder outflow obstruction. Several distinct forms may be encountered. An anterior urethral valve is almost always the distal lip of a diverticulum.

Wide-mouthed diverticula

Wide-mouthed diverticula are found in the bulb or at the penoscrotal junction. Characteristically the opening has a valvular distal lip that obstructs the urethra. Most of the author's cases have presented in infancy or during the first 3 years but a few with long-standing symptoms have turned up later in childhood. They had signs of lower urinary tract obstruction of a varying degree, often with severe upper tract dilatation and reflux. Infection was a common complication. Some incontinence is the rule, partly due to the emptying of the diverticulum after micturition and partly due to bladder overflow. The sac is occasionally large enough to show as a swelling in the scrotal area and pressure in this region always produces a little urine at the external urinary meatus.

The micturition or expression urethrogram shows a trabeculated bladder, some dilatation of the posterior urethra with perhaps a slight collar at the bladder neck and some dilatation again in the bulb. The diverticulum itself is distinct from the bulb and shallow and wide mouthed while the distal urethra is narrow, demonstrating the obstructive effect of the distal lip (*Figure 20.16*). Injection urethrograms show the distal urethra to be normal so that the cause of obstruction may well be overlooked.

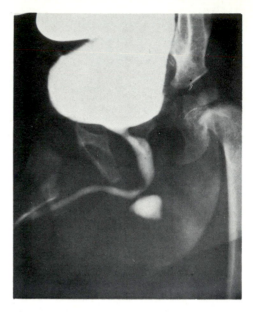

Figure 20.17. Narrow-necked urethral diverticulum. Micturating cystogram in an 8-year-old boy with pain and infection.

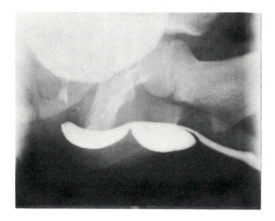

Figure 20.16. Wide-mouthed anterior urethral diverticulum. Micturating cystogram in a boy with difficult micturition.

Treatment normally consists of endoscopic incision of the distal obstructive lip followed by a period of catheter drainage. Very large diverticula may be excised surgically and rarely, in the infected and uraemic infant, a staged procedure may be required as in the Johanson urethroplasty for stricture. Vesicoureteric reflux may require treatment as well. Although the bladder is hypertrophied it is seldom so enormously thickened as in posterior urethral obstruction and is therefore much more amenable to surgery. The prognosis naturally depends upon the state of the upper tract at the time of surgery but in general it is good.

Narrow-necked diverticula

Narrow-necked diverticula occur in the bulb of the urethra. A spherical cavity communicates with the urethra through a narrow neck like a cherry on a stalk (*Figure 20.17*). While there is no obstructive element, considerable stasis exists in the diverticulum and stone formation is common. The symptoms are local pain and dysuria and the treatment is simple excision.

Dorsal diverticulum of the fossa navicularis

Sommer and Stephens (1980) reported a series of boys suffering from quite severe penile pain and dysuria with urethral bleeding who were found to have a small diverticulum on the dorsal urethral wall at the level of the base of the glans. These sacs apparently arose from the fossa navicularis. Such a diverticulum is apt to be missed on routine urethrography or even urethroscopy but is easily found once suspected. The symptoms are readily relieved by cutting the septum between the diverticulum and the urethral lumen with scissors introduced through the external meatus.

Traumatic diverticula

An indwelling catheter, particularly when traction is applied to it in the treatment of rupture of the posterior urethra, damages the ventral wall of the urethra at the penoscrotal junction. This may result in a periurethral abscess or in simple overstretching of the urethral wall, either of which can lead to a wide-mouthed diverticulum. Fistula formation may be a complication.

Anterior urethral fistula

Fistulas of the urethra may be congenital (*Figure 20.18*) with a large defect in the floor of the urethra. However, most cases result from operative trauma. Hypospadias repair is the most

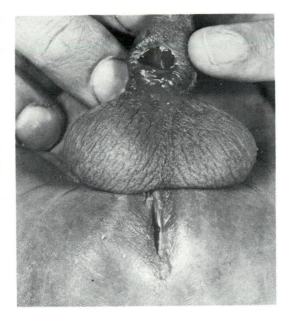

Figure 20.18. Congenital urethral fistula with wide urethral channel. Possibly the result of fetal rupture of a megalourethra.

notorious offender. Sometimes at circumcision a deeply placed suture at the frenum includes the urethral wall and produces a fistula. Fistulas in the penile urethra are easily treated by dissecting the skin away from the fistula and uniting the edges with a double-stop suture as in hypospadias repair. The postcircumcision fistula is on the edge of the glans so that skin around it cannot be mobilized. It is then preferable to bare an area of glans around and distal to the hole and then to draw forwards and over it a curtain of skin from the shaft of the penis.

Megalourethra

In this condition there is an enormous expansion of the anterior and especially the penile

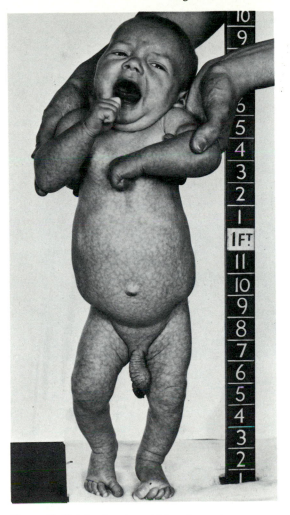

Figure 20.19. Megalurethra with long lax penis.

urethra. The penis is huge and lax (*Figure 20.19*) and urine distends it during micturition (*Figure 20.20*) and dribbles away afterwards. Megalourethra appears to be due to a defect of the cavernous tissue and occurs in two forms. In the milder type, which was called scaphoid by Stephens (1963), there is a loss of the corpus spongiosum in the distal urethra, the corpora cavernosa are intact but somewhat elongated and the glans is normal while the distal urethra is wide. Excision of the redundant urethral tissue restores the penis to something like a normal appearance, although some elongation remains.

In the other category, namely fusiform (Stephens, 1963), the corpora cavernosa are also deficient so that the whole penis is without

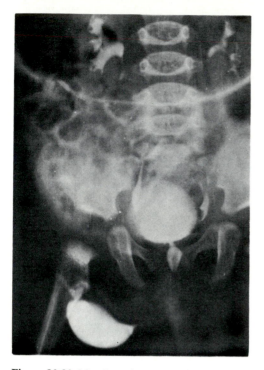

Figure 20.20. Megalourethra. Intravenous urogram showing normal upper tract and huge dilatation of distal urethra.

supporting structures and repair can never be very satisfactory.

This anomaly seldom occurs alone and may be accompanied by agenesis of the abdominal muscles and severe upper urinary tract anomalies.

References

Mogg, R.A. (1968) Congenital anomalies of the urethra. *British Journal of Urology*, **40**, 638

Morgan R.J., Williams, D.I. and Pryor J.P. (1979) Müllerian duct remnants in the male. *British Journal of Urology*, **51**, 488

Oudard, M. and Jean, G. (1921) Canaux urétérales accessoires. *Journal d'Urologie et Néphrologie*, **11**, 177

Sommer J.T. and Stephens F.D. (1980) Dorsal diverticulum of the fossa navicularis. *Journal of Urology*, **124**, 94

Stephens, F.D. (1963) Congenital Malformations of the Rectum, Anus and Genito-urinary Tract. Livingstone, London.

Williams, D.I. (1951) The development and abnormalities of the penile urethra. *Acta Anatomica*, **15**, 176

Williams, D.I. and Bloomberg, S. (1976) Bifid urethra with pre-anal accessory track (Y duplication). *British Journal of Urology*, **47**, 877

Williams, D.I. and Kenawi, M.M. (1975) Urethral duplications in the male. *European Urology*, **1**, 209

Woodhouse, C.R.J. and Williams, D.I. (1979) Duplications of the lower urinary tract in childhood. *British Journal of Urology*, **51**, 481

21   Male urethral obstructions

D. Innes Williams

Some of the most interesting and challenging problems in paediatric urology arise from the consequences of male congenital urethral obstructions and acquired urethral stenosis. Restoration of an unobstructed urethra with preservation of continence is the primary objective, but often the secondary changes in the upper urinary tract require as much attention if renal function is to be preserved. The physiological effects of obstructive uropathy have been discussed in Chapter 17 in relation to upper tract lesions and they occur equally with lower tract obstructions. These renal and ureteric disorders are most clearly exemplified by cases with urethral valves, and this chapter therefore includes a full discussion under this heading. It should be appreciated that comparable problems can be encountered with other causes of chronic retention of urine. However, the acute disorders with a sudden onset of painful retention are usually due to minor lesions that are readily corrected.

In children acute retention with complete inability to pass urine and a tense and painfully distended bladder is often due to transitory causes. A meatal ulcer with a scab covering the external orifice may be so painful that micturition is inhibited and urine is passed only when the child has fallen asleep from exhaustion. A very concentrated urine, along with oxaluria, can cause pain and inhibition. Constipation and distension of the rectum with hard faeces exacerbates this condition and can cause retention. In these circumstances a sedative, an enema and copious alkaline fluids are sufficient treatment.

Acute retention can also be the culmination of a chronic process, particularly in urethral stricture. Impacted urethral calculi naturally produce retention and in areas of endemic stone disease this is much the commonest cause. Lobules of bladder tumour prolapsing into the urethra cause extreme strangury, while most tumours and most congenital urethral anomalies are more likely to cause chronic than acute retention. The presence of a vesical diverticulum pushing down into the pelvis and compressing the urethra may exacerbate the obstruction due to the long-standing urethral lesion.

In the newborn acute retention has a somewhat different significance and must be distinguished from anuria. The dehydrated infant who is otherwise normal may pass no urine for 24–48 hours; the bladder does not become palpable and no treatment is required other than the administration of fluids. Anuria is rarely due to renal agenesis and if it is then the diagnosis can usually be made from associated signs (*see* Chapter 20). True retention at this age is most often due to temporary obliteration of the urethral meatus, usually with coronal hypospadias. More severe atresia of the posterior urethra and urethral valves are occasional causes of acute retention.

Investigation of urethral obstruction

In major disorders the presence of obstruction is seldom in doubt from clinical examination but careful investigation is required to determine the level of the lesion and for this purpose radiology and endoscopy provide the most important evidence and are described here. In minor disorders the obstructive nature of the complaint may not be so obvious and urodynamic methods may be required in addition. These procedures are described in Chapter 18.

The urethra may be outlined radiologically by micturating cystourethrography or injection urethrography. The technical details of both these procedures are familiar but certain points relevant to the infant should be noted. Catheterization must be scrupulously sterile and gentle. An 8 F polythene catheter or feeding tube is often appropriate. The opaque medium must be properly diluted since a concentrated solution may irritate the neonatal mucosa and produce bladder spasm with the appearance of trabeculation and sacculation. The urethra must be observed fluoroscopically during active micturition since films during simple filling or restrained voiding can give a misleading impression. In the infant with retention true micturition cannot be obtained but contrast medium flows back around the catheter when the bladder is tensely distended.

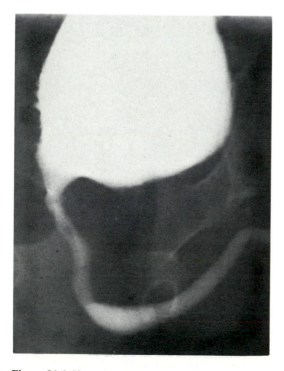

Figure 21.1. Normal cystourethrogram in a boy.

The form of the urethra as seen on cysto-urethrograms can vary within normal limits (*Figures 21.1 and 21.2*). Slight narrowing at the bladder neck, widening of the posterior urethra and a definable external sphincteral region are the rule. The bulb is wide and tapers towards the penile section. An angle is seen at the penoscrotal junction when micturition takes place in the erect position and this can be misinterpreted as an obstruction. If the boy is nervous and passing urine into a bottle, there can be external pressure at this point. Moreover if the urine bottle is plastic and radiolucent then the source of pressure is not evident on the X-ray so that a stricture may be wrongly suspected (*Figure 21.3*). Opposite the verumontanum there is often an anterior indentation that is not pathological and is thought by some to represent the crossing of the striated muscle fibres extending upwards from the external sphincter. Below the verumontanum there may be some transverse linear filling defects representing soft and nonobstructive folds of mucosa and sometimes the posterior urethra has a 'baggy trousers' appearance as if it is not fully stretched (*Figure 21.4*). In the bulb of the urethra there may be a slight constriction due to the nuda muscle (Kjellberg, Ericsson and Rudhe, 1957). All these features can create diagnostic problems in the interpretation of possible obstructive symptoms (Moorman, 1973).

The injection urethrogram using a viscous medium is useful only for outlining the anterior urethra. It gives a very clear picture of strictures. However, injection urethrography should not be performed within 48 hours following any other instrumentation, both because there is a danger of extravasation and because the stricture sought may have been dilated by the instruments.

Endoscopically the urethra is best inspected through the direct-viewing telescope and where there is any possibility of an anterior urethral lesion the obturator should not be used. The cystoscopist should observe the passage as the instrument is advanced through the urethra for the first time. The calibre of good cystoscopes has been progressively reduced so that inspection through a 9 F instrument is almost always possible even in the neonate. Diathermy or a cold knife requires a larger calibre, but only on rare occasions is it necessary to perform a perineal urethrostomy to allow access. The greatest gentleness must be exercised in any

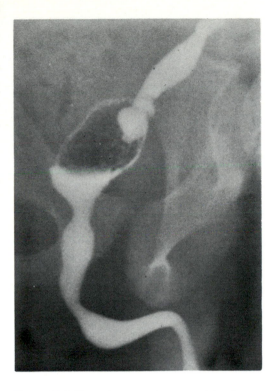

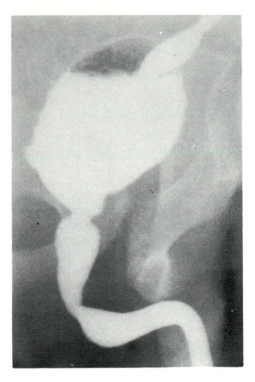

Figure 21.2. Normal cystourethrogram with reflux.

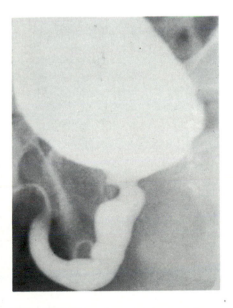

Figure 21.3. Normal cystourethrogram in a boy with simulated obstruction due to a plastic urine bottle.

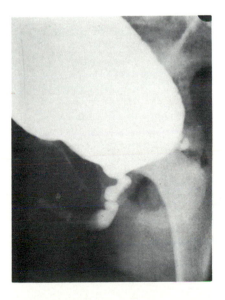

Figure 21.4. Multiple urethral folds of doubtful obstructive significance.

attempt at dilatation of an infant's urethra because even apparently minor damage can produce a subsequent stricture.

Congenital valves in the posterior urethra

The disorder known as urethral valves is the commonest obstructive anomaly of male children that can produce both an immediate threat to life and a long-term risk of chronic renal failure. Its high incidence has only been recognized since paediatricians became aware of the necessity for full investigation of infected and uraemic infants and since the misleading urological diagnosis of bladder neck obstruction was largely discarded for the prepubertal child. In clinical practice the incidence varies enormously with the criteria for diagnosis of minor cases. Thus Hendren (1971) found a large number of minor obstructions in older boys and believed the lesion to be relatively common. If only severe examples where hydronephrosis is a feature are included, most reported series are relatively small. In the author's personal experience it required 9 years practice to find 100 new cases with hydronephrosis. Rattner, Meyer and Bernstein (1963) described 21 postmortem cases in 2569 necropsies over a 12-year period. Sibling involvement has been observed in some families but no pattern of inheritance has emerged.

Pathology

The classic appearance of urethral valves is as folds of mucosa with a scanty fibrous stroma in the posterior urethra below the verumontanum. They appear to be exaggerations of the ridges commonly observed in this area, namely the plicae colliculi. Normally below the verumontanum there is a short midline crest from which spring these low ridges, coursing downwards and laterally to be lost before encircling the urethra. Ridges in this position are particularly prominent in 100 mm embryos where they appear to link the müllerian tubercle with Cowper's glands, although their relationship to other structures in the urogenital sinus remains obscure. It must be assumed that the persistence

of this prominence together with the anterior fusion of the folds produces the obstructive valve. Many years ago Bazy (1903) suggested that the valve represented a persistence of the cloacal membrane, and Kaplan (1976) believed that this could account for some cases where a diaphragmatic appearance is found. Embryologically the disorder appears to be a relatively late development because it is unusual for valve formation to be accompanied by other major anomalies, for example absent kidney, imperforate anus or tracheo-oesophageal fistula, which are often seen in conditions such as urethral duplication.

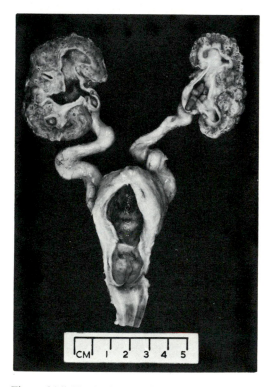

Figure 21.5. Urethral valves. Postmortem specimen from a neonate with renal failure despite bilateral nephrostomy. The posterior urethra is opened in the anterior sagittal plane and shows the valves to be bicuspid. The bladder is grossly hypertrophied, the ureters are dilated and the renal parenchyma is cystic.

A postmortem specimen of urethral valves prepared by opening the urinary tract down the midline produces the classic appearance described by Young, Frontz and Baldwin (1919) as type I, in which the valves are bicuspid with one on either side (*Figure 21.5*). However, in infants particularly the anterior membrane is the most important element of the obstruction and the sagittal slit-like lumen is confined to its posterior limits. Dissections reported by Robertson and Hayes (1969) also showed that the severely obstructive valve is more like a diaphragm with a small opening posteriorly, as was perhaps suggested by Young's type III (*Figure 21.6*). Radiologically the bulging anterior wall of the urethra is readily visualized on true lateral views (*Figures 21.7 and 21.8*) while the individual ridges running up to the verumontanum on each side of the posterior channel are best seen on anteroposterior films. Endoscopically the lateral lips of this channel are more easily appreciated than the anterior membrane which can hardly be brought into view through the foreoblique lens. Field and Stephens (1974) suggested that there is a variation of this diaphragmatic type of obstruction in which the membrane balloons out into the bulb of the urethra in the form of a wind-sock. This type has not been encountered by the author. The anatomy of the fully developed urethral valve can therefore be defined, although the lesser folds and ridges seen radiologically and of doubtful obstructive function have not been subjected to pathological investigation.

It should be noted that other forms of obstruction can occur at approximately the same level as urethral valves. For instance in the prune belly syndrome (*see* Chapter 24) the urethra tapers to a relative narrowing in this region, although only normal urethral ridges are seen. Occasionally with ectopic ureter and very rarely with congenital rectourethral fistula there is a firm stenotic ring below the opening that is evidently obstructive. Hypertrophy of the verumontanum was originally described as a cause of obstruction and this structure often appears enlarged in cases of urethral valves, but it is doubtful whether it can itself be responsible for symptoms. Bodian (1957) described urethral fibroelastosis as a lesion that he believed to be responsible for severe bladder outflow obstruction. The normal simple prostatic glandular structures were scanty and replaced by a thick sheath of fibrous and elastic tissue surrounding the whole length of the urethra and reaching right down to the bulb. Some such changes may be observed in severe examples of urethral valves and the pathological diagnosis of a specific lesion has not been confirmed by other observers.

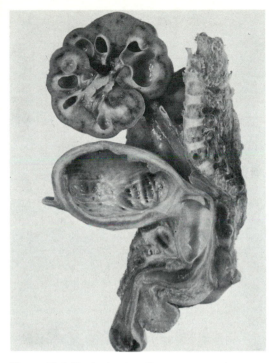

Figure 21.6. Urethral valves. Postmortem specimen from a neonate who died untreated at 3 days. Sagittal section shows the valves as a diaphragm bulging anteriorly. The renal parenchyma is surprisingly well preserved.

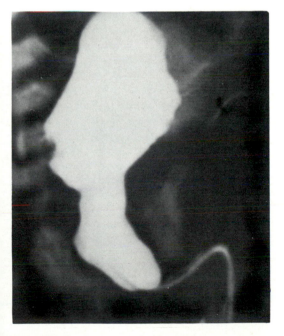

Figure 21.7. Urethral valves. Micturating cystourethrogram in a neonate showing the dilated posterior urethra and anterior bulge.

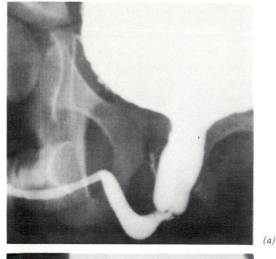

(a)

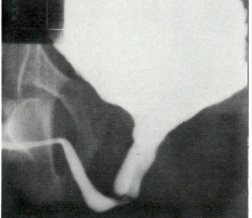

(b)

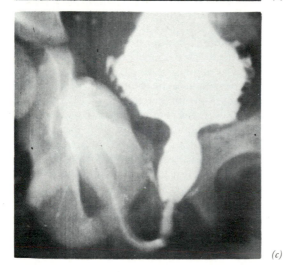

(c)

Figure 21.8. Urethral valves. Serial micturating cystourethrograms in a boy of 2 years with difficult micturition.

Consequential pathology

Urethral dilatation above the valves is an obvious consequence of the obstruction, as is the hypertrophy of the detrusor muscle. The bladder neck often remains as a prominent ring and the urethral dilatation below excavates the subtrigonal zone leaving fibrous ridges radiating upwards and outwards from the verumontanum. In Young's original description folds in this position were depicted as type II valves. It is difficult to see how they could be obstructive and it is now generally believed that they represent only a consequence of the classic valvular obstruction. Although the bladder neck is prominent, it is seldom rigid and does not itself obstruct bladder outflow. It is possible that in some late cases where fibrosis has occurred the secondary changes may demand a bladder neck plasty; this must be unusual.

Massive detrusor hypertrophy is common and is accompanied by sacculation. Often para-ureteric saccules reach considerable dimensions but individual large diverticula above the trigonal area are rare, while not unexpected. Involvement of the ureter in a saccule or a wide dilatation of the ureteric orifice allows reflux. However, the trigone frequently remains small and hypertrophied so that the ureters are drawn downwards and reflux is prevented in spite of the severe degree of outflow obstruction. Pathological changes at the ureterovesical junction may assume considerable importance once the urethral valves have been destroyed. Although reflux may cease spontaneously in mild examples it is likely to persist if there is a paraureteric saccule. Some degree of secondary ureterovesical obstruction is seen at times, particularly if the massively hypertrophied bladder has been allowed to contract as a result of suprapubic cystostomy or vesicostomy drainage. It is then presumably due to the bulk of thickened muscle around the intramural ureter. In other cases the obstruction appears to be analogous to that found in simple megaureter.

The ureters are dilated and tortuous, the renal pelvis is hydronephrotic and in severe examples dysplastic changes may be seen in the renal parenchyma. Even in cases presenting shortly after birth there is considerable variation in the degree of secondary upper tract pathology and this is at least partly correlated with the presence or absence of reflux. Some infants appear to have suffered an acute exacerbation of obstruction shortly after birth while the trigonal mechanism has been preserved; the ureters are dilated but not greatly elongated and retain their elasticity, and the kidneys are hydronephrotic but not dysplastic. The condition is therefore reversible, although death may occur as a result of an acute biochemical upset or infection, as in the case illustrated in *Figure 21.6*. Left untreated these infants undergo progressive renal destruction with chronic irreversible changes in the ureters. In other infants the chronic condition appears to be established at birth. There are less acute signs in the bladder while the ureters are grossly thickened and tortuous, and the kidneys show dysplasia with or without cyst formation. This change may be such as to preclude any chance of normal survival beyond early infancy.

As already described in Chapter 17 there is good evidence that fetal ureteric obstruction can produce renal dysplasia, while in the context of bladder outflow obstruction it appears that dysplasia is only likely where reflux complicates the situation. Not infrequently reflux is unilateral and then major dysplastic changes are invariably present in the refluxing kidney while the other, although hydronephrotic, is well preserved and capable of efficient function. This is the basis of successful nephrectomy for unilateral reflux in cases of urethral valves. Henneberry and Stephens (1980) believed that the dysplasia is constantly associated with a laterally placed ureteric orifice resulting from a low origin of the ureteric bud.

Extravasation of urine from the kidney is a complication that has been increasingly recognized in the neonate with urethral valves although it does not seem to occur in later infancy. Characteristically the extravasation occurs from the better of the two kidneys where there is asymmetry correlated with unilateral reflux. The leak may occur through a recognizable, while minute, defect in the renal parenchyma but often the site cannot be found and is assumed to be at the calyceal fornix. Sometimes the extravasation forms an accumulation of urine under the capsule and when it is contained within this layer it may become walled off and stable, having the appearance of a solitary renal cyst. These cysts are apt to be diagnosed later in the course of the disease and their origin from extravasation is not always appreciated. In other cases the urine escapes through the capsule to form a urinoma, at first confined within

Gerota's fascia, which may reach considerable proportions and may ultimately break through into the peritoneum with resultant urinary ascites. The source of the ascitic fluid is often not identified at the time of surgery and the bladder is occasionally suspected. The cause of extravasation is unknown, but since it is a feature of neonates it is possible that birth trauma is involved, and it is noticeable that haematuria has been present on occasions.

Presentation

Urethral valves can present at any stage in childhood and a few even come to notice during early adult life. In a referral centre receiving cases from alert paediatricians the majority are brought for treatment during the first 6 months of life and many during the first 2 weeks. The signs in early presentation are retention with a palpably distended bladder, urinary tract infection and uraemia, in various combinations. Later in childhood infection is still an important cause for complaint and investigation may reveal obstruction of any grade of severity. In older children incontinence may be the symptom that brings the child to hospital. It may be of a minor degree and little more than enuresis due to a minor urethral abnormality or occasionally it may be a major urinary obstruction with uraemia.

There are certain characteristic patterns that deserve some discussion. During the first few days of life an apparently fit boy may become rapidly distressed with vomiting and refusal of feeds. He may then be found to have a tensely distended bladder and to pass only an intermittent dribble of urine. This is the acute form of retention with hydronephrosis which is rapidly reversible. Chronic retention with more severe upper tract changes often presents a few days or weeks later. Such infants suffer vomiting, failure to thrive or loss of weight and bowel disturbance, and the bladder is palpably distended but softer and overflowing. Some infants with severe obstruction have such fully developed detrusor hypertrophy that they can pass urine in a good stream and empty the bladder with only a small residue in spite of having massive hydronephrosis and renal failure.

Fever due to urinary tract infection is the first sign of urethral valves in many infants, especially after the first week of life. It is often septicaemic and accompanied by meningism. The enlarged kidneys may be a more prominent feature than the distended bladder and the renal parenchyma is swollen, almost hard to the touch, and contains multiple small abscesses. Abdominal enlargement may be due to intestinal distension rather than dilatation of the urinary tract, and some children reach the urologist only after barium investigations for suspected bowel disorder. These signs are particularly associated with multiple coils of dilated ureters, which are sometimes infected, distending the retroperitoneal space. Perirenal extravasation produces a loin mass and ascites, which is a generalized abdominal enlargement with characteristic signs. Haematuria is a rare feature occurring especially in the neonate.

Later in childhood urinary tract infection presents with the nonspecific signs and symptoms that might be associated with any urinary tract abnormality. A poor stream is seldom a complaint from the child, who is accustomed to it, but it may be obvious to his parents or friends. Incontinence in mild degree may take the form of urgency by day or bed-wetting or finally continuous overflow. Even in older children chronic renal failure, perhaps with renal rickets, may lead to the investigation that reveals the urethral valves.

Diagnosis

The definitive anatomical diagnosis of urethral valves is made radiologically or endoscopically, the former method giving the more reliable evidence. Cystography must be performed during micturition or expression of urine from the distended bladder when the dilatation of the

posterior urethra is evident, with cut-off at the membranous level and a thin stream in the bulb. In infants particularly lateral or oblique views demonstrate the forward bulge of the supra-membranous zone (*Figures 21.7 and 21.8*). In older children with less severe obstruction the diagnosis may not be so clear-cut. The valves appear as linear filling defects and to demonstrate obstruction convincingly there should be a difference in calibre between the urethra above and below them. It is in these circumstances that films during micturition with maximum detrusor effort are so important because simple filling obscures the differential calibre.

Endoscopically valves are best seen with the direct-viewing telescope or failing that with the foreoblique device. As the instrument is withdrawn from the bladder with irrigation flowing the hypertrophied bladder neck is first seen as a prominent lip posteriorly (*Figure 21.9*) and the dilated urethra then comes into view below, with ridges radiating upwards from the verumontanum. This itself is tilted backwards by the dilatation and from its lower slopes spring the two folds which course downwards and outwards around the circumference to fuse anteriorly. As the instrument passes through the gap between these folds they snap together to form a slit in the sagittal plane. Transversely placed folds with concentric closure are suspect and are not usually obstructive. In doubtful cases urodynamic methods may be required to demonstrate a high voiding pressure and a low flow rate, but these techniques are appropriate only in older children in whom the radiological or endoscopic appearances have left some doubt.

Radiologically the disorders that must be considered in the differential diagnosis are

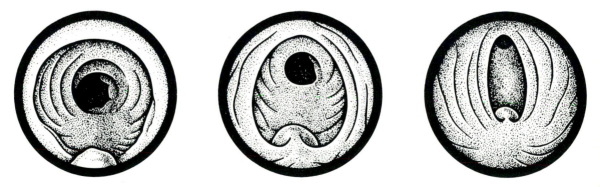

Figure 21.9. Urethral valves. Diagrams of endoscopic appearance showing hypertrophied bladder neck, dilated proximal urethra and urethral valve closure.

prune belly syndrome, in which the dilatation of the posterior urethra ordinarily tapers to a narrow section in the membranous area without the cut-off characteristic of urethral valves (*see* Chapter 24), and neuropathic bladder, in which external sphincteral spasm may also cause dilatation of the same region. Interestingly, dilatation of the prostatic utricle evident on cystograms is seen in the prune belly syndrome much more often than with urethral valves, while filling of the prostatic ducts in older boys is characteristic of the infected neuropathic bladder but not of congenital obstruction. Some reflux into the vas deferens is not impossible in any of these situations. In doubtful cases full X-ray of the spine is of value in identifying neuropathic disease.

The anatomical diagnosis of urethral valves is of course only a part of the investigation required. An intravenous urogram is obligatory in all except neonatal cases and those with severe uraemia, and in most instances precedes the micturating cystogram. Urinalysis and haemoglobin, plasma creatinine and electrolyte measurements are routine laboratory tests. In neonates and uraemic infants intravenous urograms may be noncontributory and even hazardous because of severe dehydration, and the full gamut of other imaging techniques should be employed both for immediate diagnosis and to constitute a baseline for follow-up investigations. Renal swellings at birth are often best investigated by ultrasound scanning, which also identifies the degree of bladder distension, and subsequent scans show the degree to which bladder drainage has deflated the hydronephrosis. In this way it may be possible to postpone intravenous urography until bladder drainage and correction of dehydration have been accomplished. Radioisotopic scanning using ^{99m}Tc-dimercaptosuccinic acid gives reliable serial estimations of differential renal function. Since in many instances one kidney is virtually destroyed even before birth, this information is of great value. Diethylenetriaminepentacetic-acid scans provide data on the clearance of radioisotope from the renal pelvis and from the ureter.

Management

As is evident from the previous discussion, the author believes that endoscopic treatment should only be undertaken where the diagnostic criteria have been strictly observed and that the enuretic child with doubtfully obstructive folds should be treated medically. Where clear-cut obstruction exists, however, the results of surgery are dramatic.

In the older child with well preserved renal function diagnosis may be followed by endoscopic urethral valve ablation without any special preoperative preparation. Where infection is present antibiotics should be administered, if necessary with a period of urethral catheter drainage. In younger children the catheter must be of small calibre, that is 6–8 F according to age. A simple feeding tube is often the most appropriate instrument. Catheters can usually be introduced with ease, although they occasionally curl up in the posterior urethra and cannot negotiate the lip of the bladder neck. As an alternative, suprapubic needle puncture with introduction of a polythene catheter is acceptable for a few days.

In the uraemic infant much more intensive preoperative care is required, with full cooperation from the paediatric nephrologist. These infants are usually dehydrated and acidotic on admission and require fluid and electrolyte replacement. Severe infections are often present and it may be necessary to administer antibiotics in an emergency before sensitivities are available. Currently gentamicin is used in this situation. Urethral catheter drainage may be required for longer periods in such infants and provided that a catheter of suitable dimensions is properly secured in place and allowed to drain freely this system can be safely maintained for 2–3 weeks. Nevertheless it is preferable to proceed to valve ablation at an early stage to obtain catheter-free micturition.

At times it becomes apparent that bladder drainage has not secured adequate upper tract deflation. Fever persists and the kidneys are still enlarged on palpation and on ultrasound scanning. In such circumstances bilateral nephrostomy should be performed as an emergency procedure. Following this upper tract drainage most infants rapidly improve so that it is possible to proceed to urethral valve ablation with subsequent removal of the nephrostomy catheters. However there are some children in whom renal function fails to improve, infection persists and radiology shows grossly dilated tortuous ureters. In these circumstances there may be a case for instituting long-term upper tract drainage by cutaneous ureterostomy before considering any operation on the valves. As will be seen later, upper tract reconstruction may well be required at a subsequent stage and some authors (Hendren, 1970) have advocated early total remodelling and reimplantation of ureters with resection of the urethral valve at the same procedure. The author's preference is for a less hazardous staged approach, since at times there is an altogether unexpected improvement following simple valve resection which obviates the need for further treatment.

Valve ablation

There have been reports from time to time of valves that have disappeared after very prolonged urethral catheter drainage (Cendron, Deburge and Karlaftis, 1969). Most urologists have found this a disappointing procedure and prolonged instrumentation is unsatisfactory, being particularly liable to infection. The advent of reliable miniature endoscopes has in general eliminated the need for any other approach to the destruction of urethral valves. In older children the loop resectoscope is the easiest instrument to use; a bite of tissue can be removed from each valve's edge in the posterolateral position and preferably also from the anterior midline. With infants the resectoscope loop may involve too deep a destruction of tissue and it is preferable to use either a cold knife passed through the direct-viewing urethroscope, which can incise the valve edge in the same situations, or a simple pointed diathermy electrode that can be pushed against the valve margins from below to produce diathermy coagulation of the obstructing edge. No attempt should be made to resect the prominent lip of the bladder neck in the early stages of the management of urethral valves, and such treatment needs to be considered only very rarely in the long term.

Postoperatively the urethral catheter may be left *in situ* for 3–4 days after which satisfactory micturition is normally resumed. Possible local complications include stricture and incontinence. The former may arise from too severe a diathermy burn at the site of the urethral valves or from instrumental damage to the anterior urethra in the penoscrotal area. Signs of such stricture appear within a few weeks or months of the original procedure and this possibility should not be forgotten in any child whose postoperative progress is unsatisfactory. Urinary incontinence is particularly liable to be a long-term complication in infants with severe obstruction and may follow any method of valve resection. It is accentuated by bladder neck resection (Whitaker, Keeton and Williams, 1972) and usually improves spontaneously. Almost all cases are cured by the onset of pubertal changes in the posterior urethra, but in the meantime they may be helped by imipramine.

Other immediate complications of valve resection include haematuria and the onset of a fresh infection requiring better antibiotic control. In infants who had an acute obstruction a postoperative diuresis with sodium loss may be observed during the first 24 hours. Unless rapidly recognized and corrected, this can threaten the life of an infant in whom the prognosis is otherwise good.

Upper urinary tract complications

Very severe degrees of hydronephrosis and hydroureter are found in infantile cases of urethral valves and an early return to normal function cannot be expected. In those with an acute exacerbation there is sometimes a surprising recovery but in more chronic cases any improvement takes place over a prolonged period of months or even years (*Figures 21.10 and 21.11*). Careful monitoring of renal function and of the efficiency of upper tract drainage is an essential part of the postoperative management of urethral valves and the difficulty lies in deciding when further operative intervention is required.

It has already been mentioned that reflux is a relatively common complication of urethral valves. In 100 cases with hydronephrosis reviewed by the author unilateral reflux was present in 21 per cent and bilateral reflux in 27 per cent. There is a considerable trend towards spontaneous cessation following valve resection which was well exemplified by Johnston's 1979 series. However, reflux is always associated with poorly functioning kidneys and consideration must be given to an operative approach. In unilateral examples the refluxing kidney may be functionless or nearly so, and very great benefit is then obtained from nephrectomy and removal of the hugely dilated ureter, which was undertaken in 9 per cent of the author's 100 cases (*Figure 21.12*). Radioisotopic scanning satisfactorily identifies functionless organs.

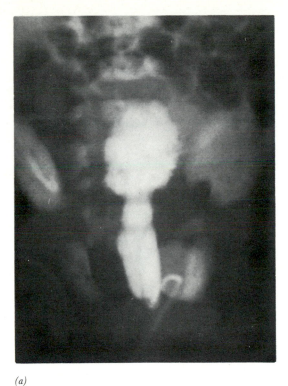

(a)

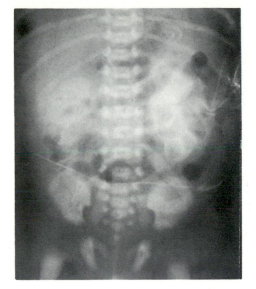

(b)

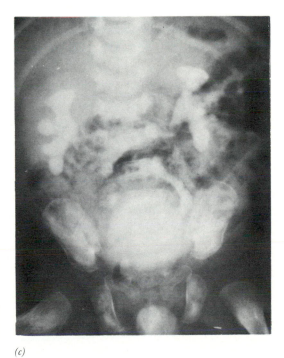

(c)

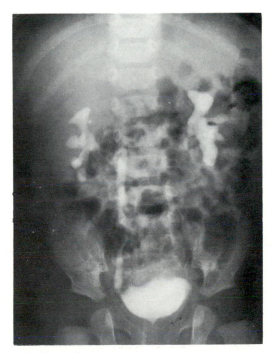

(d)

Figure 21.10. Urethral valves in a neonate. (*a*) Cystourethrogram. (*b*) Intravenous urogram on admission. (*c*) Intravenous urogram 2 months after valve ablation. (*d*) Intravenous urogram 12 months after valve ablation.

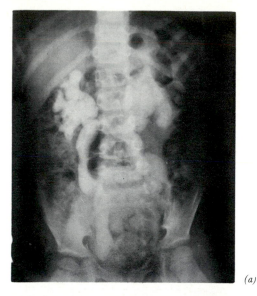

(a)

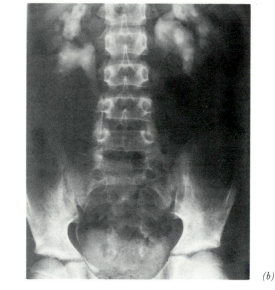

(b)

Figure 21.11. Urethral valves showing slow recovery of ureters. (*a*) Intravenous urogram 2 months after valve ablation at 5 years of age. (*b*) Intravenous urogram 8 years later.

Where reflux takes place into functioning kidneys there should still be hesitation in undertaking reimplantation, which in the circumstances of the grossly dilated ureter and the hypertrophied sacculated bladder is never a simple operation and is liable to a number of complications. Therefore, when the urine remains sterile and renal function is steady or improving an expectant attitude may be maintained in the hope that spontaneous cessation

will ultimately occur. If infections are troublesome, it must first be ensured that bladder outflow obstruction has been satisfactorily eliminated and only then should reimplantation be considered. The operation is inevitably accompanied by a considerable shortening and remodelling of the dilated tortuous ureter and great care must be taken to preserve the longitudinal blood supply. The entry point for the reimplantation should be selected posteriorly and not laterally on the bladder wall and the tunnel must not be so tight as to risk any constriction of the ureter. Indwelling ureteric catheter drainage is obligatory postoperatively.

There are some infants with reflux and renal failure so severe that reimplantation is too dangerous to attempt. In these cases a temporary diversionary procedure may be considered.

Secondary ureterovesical obstruction is another possible complication and should be revealed by careful monitoring of postoperative progress. It becomes evident if there is no improvement in the hydronephrosis despite the restoration of normal bladder emptying and the absence of reflux (*Figure 21.13*). Operative intervention should not be delayed and early reimplantation is required to save the kidney.

Diversionary procedures

At times urologists have resorted to urinary diversion too early and too often in cases of urethral valves with gross upper tract dilatation. Nevertheless these procedures have a small but important place in treatment. Nephrostomy is the simplest form and should be undertaken preoperatively or postoperatively if there is evidence that simple bladder drainage is not deflating an infected hydronephrosis. The operation, which is usually bilateral, should be undertaken through a short oblique incision in the loin. The kidney and the renal pelvis are exposed with the minimum mobilization, the renal pelvis is incised and a haemostat is passed through to protrude at one of the thin dilated calyces. The parenchyma is punctured at this site and a Malecot catheter of about 14 F is drawn in. The renal pelvic incision is then sutured and the tissues of the loin are closed around the catheter. Only where the hydronephrosis is extremely tense and infected should a direct puncture be

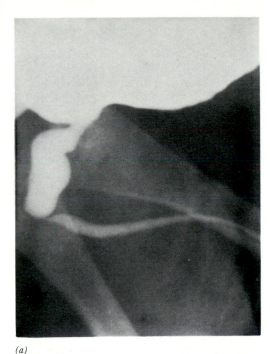

(a)

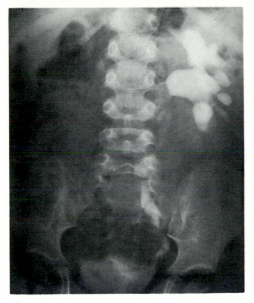

(c)

Figure 21.12. Urethral valves in a neonate. (*a*) Cystourethrogram. Right-sided reflux is present. (*b*) Intravenous urogram before treatment showing no opacification on the right and gross hydronephrosis on the left. (*c*) Intravenous urogram 3 years after valve ablation and right nephrectomy showing good recovery of the left kidney.

(b)

made in the outer surface of the kidney. Postoperatively the catheter should drain satisfactorily if it is firmly secured to the skin. Nephrostomies can be employed on a long-term basis of some months but accidents to the tube are not uncommon and it is preferable to treat this method as a relatively short-term (3–4 weeks) temporary diversion. The technique has no use

where the renal pelvis is too small and intrarenal to accommodate the mushroom end of the catheter.

Cutaneous ureterostomy had a considerable vogue in the treatment of urethral valves because the elongated tortuous ureter was easy to bring up as a loop on to the surface (Johnston, 1963). The method has considerable disadvantages in relation to ultimate reconstruction and should only be employed in uraemic infants whose renal function and ureteric tissues threaten to make remodelling and reimplantation a hazardous procedure. It then has the advantage that satisfactory upper tract drainage can be established without an indwelling catheter for a year or more during which time both renal and ureteric function may improve considerably. In performing a cutaneous ureterostomy a high loop a little below the renal pelvis should be chosen, mobilized and drawn up through the abdominal wall. The abdominal muscles may then be approximated behind the loop, which is opened longitudinally so that the cut edges of the ureter can be stitched to the skin edges. A well placed cutaneous ureterostomy of

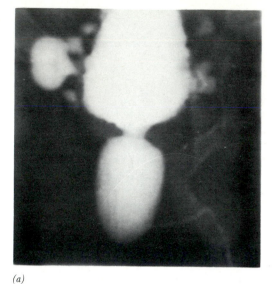

(a)

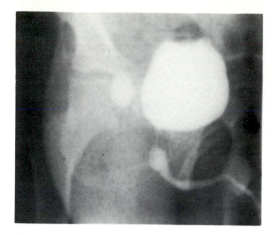

(b)

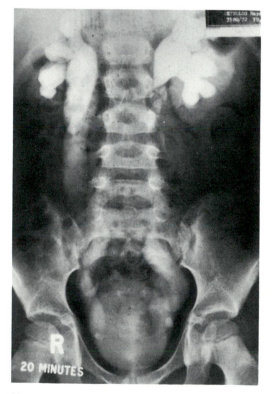

(c)

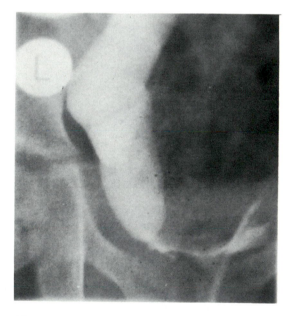

(d)

Figure 21.13. Urethral valves in 6-year-old boy. (a) Micturating cystourethrogram showing a sacculated bladder and a dilated posterior urethra. (b) Postoperative cystourethrogram showing normal bladder emptying. (c) Postoperative intravenous urogram showing persistent dilatation. (d) Antegrade ureterogram showing ureterovesical obstruction.

this type can secure a dramatic general improvement in the infant's condition and is not subject to local stenosis as is the terminal ureterostomy.

There are two major complications. First, the nonfunctioning bladder may contract down, particularly if it is sacculated and infected. In the series analysed by Lome and Williams (1972) six out of 21 patients suffered this change. However, most bladders if reconnected gradually distend to resume normal function and capacity. Secondly, the ureter may require reimplantation either for the prevention of reflux or for the correction of obstruction, and the presence of the ureterostomy especially if it is too low can interfere with this operation making mobilization difficult and hazarding the blood supply of the reimplanted segment. A reimplantation done dry below a cutaneous ureterostomy is at risk from immediate stenosis and should always be protected by an indwelling catheter.

To avoid the total defunctioning of the bladder alternative methods of ureterostomy have

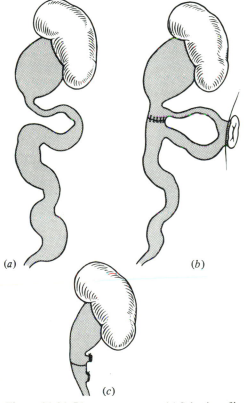

(a)   (b)

(c)

Figure 21.14. Ring ureterostomy. (*a*) Selection of loop of ureter. (*b*) Formation of ring. (*c*) Excision of superficial arc for closure.

been suggested, the simplest being the ring operation described by Williams and Cromie (1976) in which an anastomosis is made between the afferent and efferent arcs of the loop (*Figure 21.14*). Thus although the superficial appearance of the cutaneous ureterostomy is similar to that with a simple loop and is as little liable to stenosis, there is in addition a patent channel from the kidney to the bladder down which some urine flows. Moreover closure of the ring ureterostomy is accomplished by simple excision of the superficial arc, while in the classic loop ureterostomy excision and reanastomosis are ordinarily required.

In most series where cutaneous ureterostomy is confined to children with very severe failure there are a number in whom reconstitution is never possible. The mortality rate in this group is high, so that the need for rediversion to a stoma that can more easily accept a collecting bag is very seldom required.

Vesicostomy was suggested by Duckett (1974) as an easily reversible form of long-term temporary diversion for uraemic infants. This operation is appropriate for those with a large bladder capacity and care should be taken to use the apex of the bladder rather than the anterior wall. The technique of the procedure is described in Chapter 28. It may be appropriate where free reflux is present but is of no value if the upper tract dilatation results from ureterovesical obstruction, and there is some danger that the contraction of the bladder following vesicostomy may itself accentuate such an effect. There is the great advantage that closure is simple and may be accompanied by remodelling and reimplantation of the ureters in a virgin field.

Long-term consequences

The long-term prognosis in the majority of patients with urethral valves is satisfactory. Even among those with hydronephrosis in the author's series 61 per cent ultimately showed normal renal function. The mortality rate should be small with intensive nephrological care. In the above series it was 5 per cent, the fatal cases being infants whose renal function failed to improve following valve ablation and upper tract drainage. Some long-term problems of renal failure will undoubtedly be encountered, perhaps on a more extensive scale following the improved survival rate in infancy. In general it has been found that when the serum creatinine level returns to normal within 2 years the prognosis is good. When it remains moderately raised there is a risk that in adolescence or early adult life there will be a deterioration not easily accounted for by urinary tract changes. This may be accompanied by the onset of proteinuria and hypertension, and after another 2–3 years dialysis or transplantation may be required. Usually a bladder that was obstructed in infancy has recovered sufficiently by adolescence to accept a transplanted ureter without difficulty.

The possible complications of incontinence have already been mentioned. Potency is not affected although some of these young men are sterile because of reflux of semen through the dilated bladder neck. However, bladder neck tightening for the cure of either incontinence or sterility is a hazardous procedure and risks reconstituting the obstruction.

Posterior urethral polyp

A pedunculated fibrous polyp is an occasional cause of obstruction of bladder outflow. The lesion is quite distinct from the small mucosal polyps seen in adults at the bladder neck or in the urethra. The obstructive polyp is single, often 1–3 cm across and usually has a long stalk arising in the neighbourhood of the verumontanum. Histological examination of the author's cases has shown only loose fibrous tissue in the stroma.

The symptoms are those of mild obstruction with urinary tract infection or acute retention. Large polyps are just palpable on rectal examination and all sizes may be seen on urethroscopy. On good cystourethrograms the polyp appears as a filling defect (*Figure 21.15*) either up at the bladder neck or down below the verumontanum and the variation in its position can sometimes be demonstrated. Three of the author's cases (Williams and Abbassian, 1966; Stadaas, 1973) were associated with reflux, but it was not clear whether the polyp was the cause or whether the chronic infective process accompanying the reflux set up the inflammatory process that produced the polyp.

Endoscopic resection is suitable for small polyps and large ones may be excised through the open bladder. They do not recur.

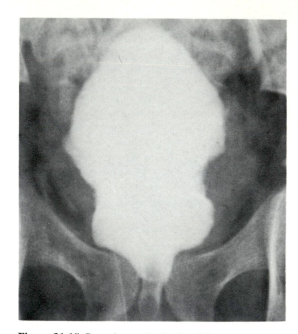

Figure 21.15. Posterior urethral polyp. Micturating cystourethrogram in a 4-year-old boy with episodes of retention. The polyp is seen as a filling defect extending upwards from the verumontanum to which it was connected by a narrow stalk.

Urethral stricture

Meatal stenosis

When it affects the normally situated meatus, stenosis is essentially an acquired disorder of circumcised boys resulting from meatal ulceration as part of a more generalized ammoniacal dermatitis in the infant. Simple meatotomy ordinarily suffices to cure it. A haemostat is applied with one blade within the urethra and one outside, crushing the tissue between the meatus and the coronal sulcus. A simple incision is then made through the avascular area. No stitches are required. While some postoperative instrumentation may be necessary to prevent adherence of the cut edges most children have an adequate meatus without this additional treatment, although it is not as big as in the immediate postoperative period. Rare cases of balanitis xerotica obliterans are seen in childhood. The prepuce is white and thickened and the glandular epithelium and the meatus are sometimes similarly affected. Circumcision is always required but a few boys also need a formal flap meatoplasty.

Stenosis of the hypospadiac meatus is common in the coronal situation and is almost always accompanied by a short blind sinus lying dorsal to the urethra and opening somewhat distal to it. A meatotomy that cuts the septum between this sinus and the urethra relieves the stenosis without accentuating the deformity. Again no stitches are required.

Although meatal stenosis often allows the passage of only a very thin stream of urine, retention of urine is rarely a complication and hydronephrosis is very uncommon. This suggests that the cushioning effects of the proximal urethra protect the upper urinary tract. Nevertheless great symptomatic improvement follows meatotomy in an appropriate case.

Anterior urethral stricture

Stricture in boys is occasionally congenital but most often traumatic in origin. Not infrequently it results from the instrumental treatment of congenital disorders.

Cases due to external trauma or to a lacerating wound present no problem of diagnosis. Children over 5 years are usually involved. Most have suffered a rupture following a fall astride a sharp object or have had a penetrating injury. The stricture is in the bulb and is short and tight with fibrosis affecting the corpus spongiosum as well as the urethra itself while behind and beyond the stricture the urethra is healthy and elastic. Cases due to instrumental trauma or of unknown or possibly congenital origin are not so apparent and many patients are referred after a variety of misdirected procedures have been undertaken. In postinstrumentation cases the stricture is most often at the penoscrotal junction (*Figure 21.16*) but sometimes affects the bulb. The area concerned may be 2–3 cm long and is not very clearly defined from the healthy urethra. The fibrosis does not spread deeply and affects mainly the epithelial and muscular layers of the urethra leaving the corpus spongiosum normal. Damage sometimes occurs after a single catheterization that was not recognized at the time as being particularly traumatic. It has also resulted from the passage of larger instruments for resection of the bladder neck or urethral valves.

Children with stricture due to instrumentation are in general much younger than those in whom it is due to external trauma since it is the

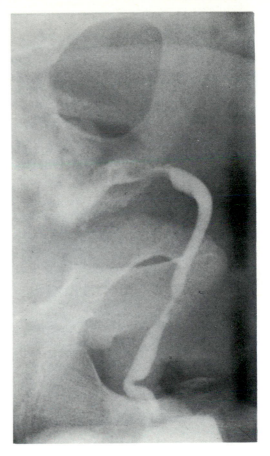

Figure 21.16. Anterior urethral stricture. Injection urethrogram in a 9-year-old boy presenting with episodes of retention. There was a history of catheterization during hernia repair in infancy. A soft stricture is visible at the penoscrotal junction.

infant's urethra that is so easily damaged. The young child himself seldom complains of a slowing of the stream and the disease is therefore not recognized early. Often the diagnosis is not even considered until an attack of retention has occurred. Such retention does not necessarily mean an exceptionally tight stricture or one that will resist catheterization. The passage of the catheter may itself dilate the stricture which is then easily missed in the subsequent cystourethrogram, particularly since interest in reflux and in the posterior urethra frequently diverts attention from the penoscrotal area.

It must therefore be emphasized that the diagnosis of anterior urethral stricture is best reached by performing a viscous medium injection urethrogram before any other instrumentation is undertaken. This clearly delineates the site and the length of the stricture although it does not give any information about the area above the external sphincter. Where the suspicion of a stricture arises only after instruments have been passed the child should be left untreated and reinvestigated 3–4 weeks later when the stricture, if present, will have tightened up.

Strictures of unknown origin have in the author's experience fallen into three groups. Some resemble those due to instrumental trauma, being in the penoscrotal area with a relatively long and ill defined narrowing; some

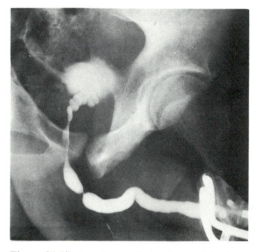

Figure 21.17. Anterior urethral stricture. Injection urethrogram in a 13-year-old boy presenting with difficult micturition. There is a ring stricture in the bulb; the appearance strongly suggests previous external trauma but no history could be obtained.

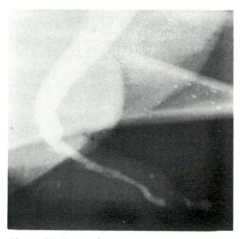

Figure 21.18. Anterior urethral stricture. Injection urethrogram in a 10-year-old boy without history of injury. Histologically there were features suggestive of balanitis xerotica obliterans.

simulate cases due to external trauma (*Figure 21.17*); and some are long lesions with a pathological epithelium, fibrosis and small saccules. The majority are therefore indicative of some trauma, either external and unrecorded or internal resulting from some instrumentation by a doctor, the patient or his friends. A very short bulbar stricture suggesting external trauma is commonly seen in adolescence. The origin of the very long stricture is quite obscure but a possible extension of balanitis xerotica obliterans may be involved (*Figure 21.18*). Urethritis has been considered as a cause but never definitely incriminated. Complete atresia of the urethra occurs in some duplications (*see* Chapter 20).

Treatment of urethral stricture in boys is surgical and intermittent dilatation has no place in long-term management. For a full discussion of the operative techniques of urethroplasty see Turner-Warwick (1977). Most of the author's cases have been satisfactorily treated by island implants of penile skin to enlarge the urethral calibre.

Posterior urethral stricture

Posterior urethral stricture almost always results from fracture of the pelvis and this is discussed in Chapter 31. Rare cases are seen following diathermy treatment of urethral valves. Such damage is almost always distally placed and can be treated in the same way as anterior strictures by insertion of a scrotal pedicle or free skin graft to enlarge the calibre. Techniques of operative reconstruction are discussed by Waterhouse (1977).

Dyssynergia

There remain a few boys with periodic urethral obstruction for whom pathological categorization still presents difficulties. The possibilities of occult neuropathic bladder and incomplete prune belly syndrome may be explored if there is no evidence of an organic obstructive lesion, but even these rather unsatisfactory diagnoses cannot be applied to all cases of retention. For the present it seems that we should accept that there are cases of unexplained detrusor-sphincter dyssynergia, as in the example illustrated in *Figure 21.19*. In these boys urethrotomy appears to be remarkably effective.

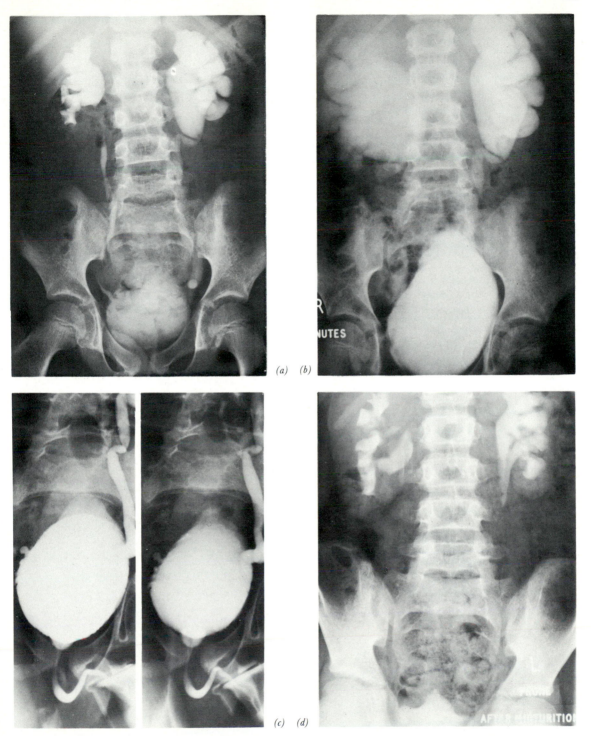

(a) *(b)*

(c) *(d)*

Figure 21.19. Detrusor-sphincter dyssynergia. Serial X-rays in a boy presenting with mild dysuria. (*a*) Intravenous urogram at 8 years. No treatment had been given. (*b*) Intravenous urogram 2 years later at the time of referral following an episode of retention. (*c*) Micturating cystourethrogram showing dilated posterior urethra. There was no detectable CNS abnormality and cystourethroscopy did not reveal any evidence of urethral valves. An Otis urethrotomy was performed. (*d*) Intravenous urogram 18 months later showing normal micturition and normal control.

References

Bazy, P. (1903) Retrecissements congenital de l'uretre chez l'homme. *Presse Medicale*, **11**, 215

Bodian, M. (1957) Some observations on the pathology of congenital idiopathic bladder neck obstruction. *British Journal of Urology*, **29**, 393

Cendron, J., Deburge, J.P. and Karlaftis, C. (1969) Valvulae of the posterior urethra. *Journal d'Urologie et Nephrologie*, **75**, 15

Duckett, J.W. (1974) Current management of posterior urethral valves. *Urological Clinics of North America*, **1**, 471

Field, P.L. and Stephens, F.D. (1974) Congenital urethral membranes causing urethral obstruction. *Journal of Urology*, **111**, 250

Hendren, W.H. (1970) A new approach to infants with severe obstructive uropathy: early complete reconstruction. *Journal of Paediatric Surgery*, **5**, 184

Hendren, W.H. (1971) Posterior urethral valves in boys: a broad clinical spectrum. *Journal of Urology*, **106**, 298

Henneberry, M.O. and Stephens, F.D. (1980) Renal hypoplasia and dysplasia in infants with posterior urethral valves. *Journal of Urology*, **123**, 912

Johnston, J.H. (1963) Temporary cutaneous ureterostomy in the management of advanced congenital urinary obstruction. *Archives of Disease in Childhood*, **38**, 161

Johnston, J.H. (1979) Vesico-ureteric reflux with urethral valves. *British Journal of Urology*, **51**, 100

Kaplan, G. (1976) in Clinical Pediatric Urology (edited by Kelalis, P.P., King, L.R. and Belman, A.B.). Saunders, Philadelphia. p.301

Kjellberg, S.R., Ericsson, N.O. and Rudhe, U. (1957) The Lower Urinary Tract in Childhood. Livingstone, London

Lome, L.G. and Williams, D.I. (1972) Urinary reconstruction following temporary cutaneous diversion in children. *Journal of Urology*, **108**, 162

Moorman, J.G. (1973) Zur Problematik der Harnröhrenklappen. *Urologe*, **12**, 219

Rattner, W.H., Meyer, R. and Bernstein, J. (1963) Congenital abnormalities of the urinary system: valvular obstruction of the posterior urethra. *Journal of Paediatrics*, **63**, 84

Robertson, W.B. and Hayes, J.A. (1969) Congenital diaphragmatic obstruction of the male posterior urethra. *British Journal of Urology*, **41**, 592

Stadaas, J.O. (1973) Pedunculated polyps of the posterior urethra in children causing reflux and hydronephrosis. *Journal of Pediatric Surgery*, **8**, 517

Turner-Warwick, R.T. (1977) Repair of urinary vaginal fistulae. *In* Operative Surgery: Urology (edited by Rob, C. and Smith, R.). Butterworths, London. p.206

Waterhouse, K. (1977) The surgical repair of membranous urethral stricture in children. *Transactions of the American Association of Genito-Urinary Surgeons*, **67**, 81

Whitaker, R.H., Keeton, J.E. and Williams, D.I. (1972) Posterior urethral valves: a study of urinary control after operation. *Journal of Urology*, **108**, 167

Williams, D.I. and Abbassian, A. (1966) Solitary pedunculated polyp of the posterior urethra in children. *Journal of Urology*, **96**, 483

Williams, D.I. and Cromie, W.J. (1976) Ring ureterostomy. *British Journal of Urology*, **47**, 789

Young, H.H., Frontz, W.A. and Baldwin, J.C. (1919) Congenital obstruction of the posterior urethra. *Journal of Urology*, **3**, 289

22 Urinary Tract Complications of Imperforate Anus

D. Innes Williams

Anatomy of the malformations

The common embryological origin from the cloaca of the rectum and the lower urinary tract makes it inevitable that malformations of the former affect the latter while at the same time surgical procedures on the bowel endanger the integrity and the nerve supply of the bladder and the urethra. The imperforate anus malformations form a distinct group in which urinary tract complications are relatively common. The anatomy of the primary anomaly requires a preliminary description, even though the urologist is likely to be concerned only after initial treatment has been undertaken by the paediatric surgeon. These malformations appear to arise from agenesis of the terminal bowel with or without incomplete separation of the rectum from the urogenital sinus. High or supralevator lesions can be regarded as examples of rectal agenesis and low or infralevator lesions as anal agenesis. A high lesion in the male is almost always accompanied by a rectourethral fistula opening immediately below the verumontanum (*Figure 22.1*). The rectovesical fistula so commonly referred to in the older literature is in fact very rare. The fistulous track may vary greatly in calibre and may even be atretic. Its presence deforms the urethra a little but does not interfere with the sphincteral system.

In the female rectal agenesis can occur with or without a fistula into the posterior wall of the vagina. Sometimes there is a common cloacal track into which drain the bladder or the urethra, the vagina (which is often duplicated) and the rectum (*Figures 22.2, 22.3, 22.4 and 22.5*).

Low lesions in the male may present with simple anal stenosis or prolongation of the anal canal into a sinus along the perineal raphe. At times the bowel joins the distal urethra as an anobulbar fistula. Very rarely the fistula lies further forward at the penoscrotal junction. Low

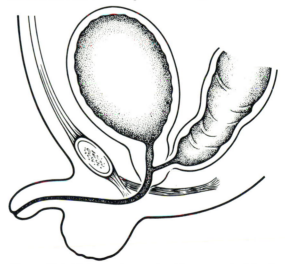

Figure 22.1. Male rectal agenesis with rectourethral fistula. (Reproduced by permission of the editor, *British Journal of Urology*.)

lesions in the female usually have a stenotic anal ectopic opening at the vestibule. A few have a covered anus in which a thick bar of perineal skin appears to have grown forward to cover the anal opening and the posterior vulva.

In general the immediate treatment for low lesions is a perineal operation opening up the

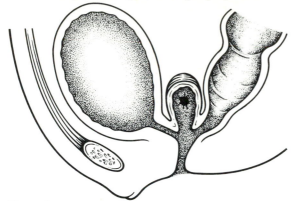

Figure 22.2. Female rectal agenesis with cloaca. (Reproduced by permission of the editor, *British Journal of Urology*.)

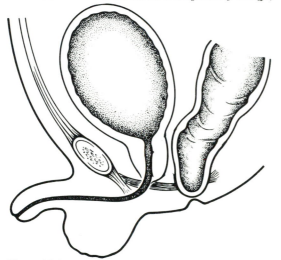

Figure 22.3. Male anal agenesis with anal stenosis. (Reproduced by permission of the editor, *British Journal of Urology*.)

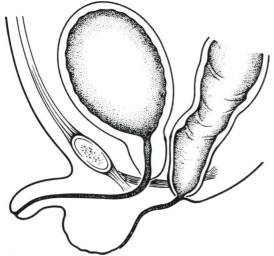

Figure 22.4. Male anal agenesis with perineal sinus. (Reproduced by permission of the editor, *British Journal of Urology*.)

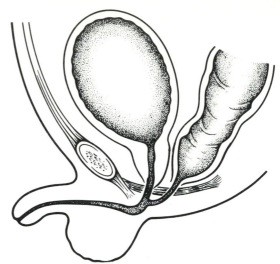

Figure 22.5. Male anal agenesis with anobulbar fistula. (Reproduced by permission of the editor, *British Journal of Urology*.)

stenotic anus, following back the track of the perineal sinus or cutting back the vestibular ectopic anus. High lesions almost certainly necessitate a preliminary colostomy and a subsequent reconstructive operation aiming to sever the rectourethral or rectovaginal fistula and to pull the rectum down to the perineum, making a channel within the puborectalis sling to give the child continence. Various techniques of operation have been described (Kieswetter, 1979).

Urinary tract involvement

When the urinary tract is considered in relation to imperforate anus there are five groups of disorder as follows:

1. Concomitant urinary tract anomalies
2. Concomitant spinal cord anomalies
3. Complications of the primary fistula
4. Complications of pelvic surgery in the male
5. Complications of cloaca in the female.

Some symptoms such as urinary incontinence may be due to factors in any one of these groups and it is sometimes difficult to make an accurate diagnosis, yet the prognosis differs widely according to the cause.

Concomitant urinary tract anomalies

Quite apart from rectourethral fistula or cloaca, congenital anomalies of the urinary tract frequently accompany imperforate anus. The exact incidence is hard to determine since intravenous pyelograms have been performed routinely in very few large series. Garrett and Yurdin (1958) found a rate of 19 per cent of anomalies unconnected with the actual fistula. Scott, Swenson and Fisher (1960) analysed 63 cases according to the level of the obstruction and found 17 per cent had urinary tract anomalies which were evenly distributed between the high and low groups. Smith (1968) reported urinary tract anomalies in 24 per cent of low bowel deformities and in 38 per cent of patients with rectal atresia. Wiener and Kieswetter (1973) reviewed 200 cases and found major urinary tract anomalies in 28 per cent, 15 per cent of which were incompatible with survival.

The type of anomaly varies considerably. There may be absence, malrotation or ectopia of a kidney, or ureteric duplication, megaureter, ureterocele or ectopic ureter. Exstrophy of the bladder, urethral valves and hypospadias are all seen from time to time. Most of these anomalies require treatment on their own account. It is important to recognize that if a dilated ureter is found after treatment of imperforate anus this can be a concomitant anomaly rather than the result of treatment.

Concomitant spinal cord anomalies

Partial sacral agenesis is a common finding in severe cases of rectal anomaly and it can occur in less severe cases as well. Sometimes the appearance is misleading in that there is a long lumbar spine and a relatively short sacral one, and Smith (1968) reported some sacral anomaly in 45 per cent of cases of high rectal atresia. Nevertheless absence of the coccyx and the last two or three segments of the sacrum is important, since if three segments are missing the nerve supply to the bladder is virtually certain to be involved (Williams and Nixon, 1957). It is not necessary for the conus of the spinal cord to be tethered to the vertebral anomaly as it is in spina bifida occulta and other vertebral defects, and consequently there is little chance of improving the condition by surgical interference with the spinal cord. There appears to be a simple deficiency of the spinal nerve roots rather than any more complex lesion. The paralysis of the bladder that results is a lower motor neurone lesion and closely simulates the disorder resulting from pelvic nerve damage discussed later.

Because of the importance of this condition it is essential to obtain good X-rays of the sacrum in every case of imperforate anus.

Complications of the primary fistula

Shortly after birth the presence of a rectourethral fistula may be recognized from the passage of meconium per urethram and sometimes by the distension of the bladder with flatus. In these circumstances immediate diversionary colostomy is likely to be performed, if not definitive closure of the fistula itself. The complications of the primary fistula seen by the urologist, therefore, are usually in children with a colostomy who have leakage of urine into the bowel or of bowel contents into the urethra. While the fistula is present there is a liability to urinary tract infection and, since the urine not infrequently fills the distal segment of the bowel beyond the colostomy, calcification may occur in faecal masses giving the appearance of rectal calculi. These can be removed by washout of the distal loop of the colostomy or at surgical operation, but it is important to realize that they are present in the bowel and not the urinary tract. In one observed case the absorption of urine from the bowel was sufficient to cause an acidosis similar to that seen after ureterocolic transplantation.

Complications of pelvic surgery in the male

Whereas concomitant urinary anomalies and spinal cord disorders are more or less evenly distributed between the sexes and between high and low rectal anomalies the complications of pelvic surgery are much more common in the male and in high anomalies. The majority of problems arise from attempts to sever the rectourethral fistula and pull through the rectum so that it lies within the sling of puborectalis in order to obtain rectal control. In the female there is no rectourethral fistula to sever and the nerve supply to the bladder, being displaced laterally around the vagina, is less liable to damage at pull-through. If the low fistula is recognized for what it is, in either the male or the female, it can be approached from below and there is therefore small risk of interfering with the nervi erigentes.

It is difficult to give any precise estimate of the frequency with which complications occur, because much depends upon the skill of the surgeon concerned. Cozzi and Wilkinson (1968) found some urinary incontinence in 12 out of 76 cases of imperforate anus, although in seven this could be attributed to sacral agenesis or anatomical lesions and two patients were probably enuretic, leaving only three that could reasonably be put down as surgical complications. However, the urologist is not likely to see the straightforward case in which all has gone well but is presented with the mishaps, first of all with prolonged retention after operation and later with incontinence, persistent fistula or recurrent infection. Analysis of cases that have come under the author's care shows them to fall into seven groups.

Pelvic nerve injury

This is the adult complication most familiar to urologists and it does not differ greatly in children. In the immediate postoperative period there is retention of urine which is treated by prolonged catheterization. After a time the urine can be expelled by straining but a large residue remains. Over the course of some months the residue probably diminishes while incontinence continues. At this late stage it is found that the child has no sensation of fullness of the bladder, that the bladder neck is somewhat relaxed and that the urine can be expelled by manual compression. Intelligent and less severely affected children can develop the habit of straining to pass urine and may be able to remain dry for reasonable periods between these acts of micturition. A few develop serious upper tract dilatation and a larger number have recurrent urinary tract infections. Impotence is to be expected in adult life. Treatment for the most part has been directed towards the management of incontinence by training or appliances. Since the external sphincteral complex is probably intact there may be a place for the implanted electronic stimulator.

The pulled-up bladder

Some cases of retention following operation have proved to be due to a curious lip formation at the anterior bladder neck. This has been satisfactorily corrected by anterior bladder neck Y-V plasty. It appears that the deformity arises from excessive mobilization of the bladder and the urethra posteriorly in the attempt to cut the rectourethral fistula flush and to ensure that the rectum is brought down close to the urethra through the puborectalis sling. Thus the posterior bladder wall is pulled up while the anterior wall remains fixed. This is the only type of bladder neck obstruction the author has been able to diagnose with certainty in this group.

The rectal stump

If a considerable length of rectum is left attached to the urethra as a blind diverticulum the child may be liable to recurrent urinary tract infection, haematuria and stone formation. In fact complications are usually seen only when a stone is present; this appears to form on retained meconium within the stump or on an non-absorbable suture. The opacity that the calculus causes may be mistaken for a vesical or ureteric calculus, or when it does not appear to be in either of these viscera it may be dismissed as a phlebolith. The stump itself does not necessarily fill either on a micturating cystourethrogram or an injection urethrogram, so that urethroscopy and catheterization of the fistula are required for diagnosis (*Figure 22.6*). Treatment is largely concerned with the removal of the calculus but an attempt should be made to remove the stump completely. Operative approach to this area is never easy after the previous surgery and attempts to obtain anatomical perfection are likely to damage the nerve supply. A laparotomy approach has been used, either in the midline or from one side, aiming to palpate the stone and to dissect down to it. Results have on the whole been satisfactory. Rarely a large stump is left which fills with urine during micturition and subsequently empties, causing dribbling incontinence as in some cases of 'vaginal' diverticulum of the posterior urethra. Excision is then required.

High rectourethral fistula

The persistence of a rectourethral fistula (*Figure 22.1*) after an anus has been formed may be due either to failure to recognize the presence of the primary fistula so that the perineal opening of

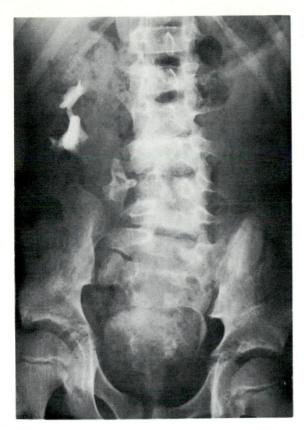

(a)

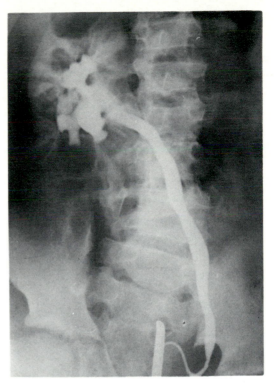

(b)

Figure 22.6. Imperforate anus with urinary tract anomalies and late complications of pull-through operation in infancy. This boy presented with continuous dribbling incontinence. *(a)* Intravenous urogram showing vertebral anomalies and right renal opacification only. *(b)* Retrograde ureterogram showing solitary crossed ectopic kidney. *(c)* Micturating cystourethrogram showing distended bladder with large posterior urethral diverticulum, that is the rectal stump. Excision of the diverticulum restored normal urinary control.

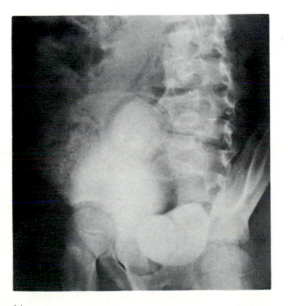

(c)

the bowel is basically into the side of the rectum or to a breakdown following infection and trauma. In the latter case it may be associated with nerve damage to the bladder. Where bladder function is normal the child expels his urine partly per urethram and partly per rectum but does not wet himself between the acts of micturition. If concomitant pelvic nerve damage is present there is likely to be continual urinary incontinence per rectum. Diagnosis presents no great difficulty since a sound passed per urethram emerges into the rectum and the level of the lesion can be estimated. The fistula can also be visualized by micturating cysto-urethrography. Treatment, however, is frequently a matter of great difficulty and it is not uncommon for the case to be referred to the urologist after two or three attempts have been made to close the opening.

In such circumstances it is very unlikely that closure will be effected simply by exposing the area from the perineum and suturing the two viscera separately, and some more radical approach is required. Many paediatric surgeons favour a repetition of the pull-through procedure as in the primary operation so that healthy bowel is placed in contact with the urethra and the fistula then closes. This is certainly appropriate if the terminal bowel has been largely destroyed by sepsis and retraction. Where a healthy rectum reaches the perineum the author's preference is for an omental interposition.

A synchronous combined approach is made from above and below and a plane established between the urinary tract and the bowel. This plane when opened up inevitably severs the fistula, but it need not be dissected widely on either side, indeed to do so would endanger the nerve supply to the bladder. The urethra is usually found to be scarred and impossible to close by a simple suture line. The rectum, on the other hand, being capacious can generally be closed by a double layer of sutures. Once this is done a leaf of omentum that has been completely mobilized from the greater curvature of the stomach and brought down to the right lateral paracolic gutter, as described by Turner-Warwick (1967), is brought through the plane separating the two viscera, the urethra being left unsutured. A diversionary colostomy should previously have been performed and the bladder drained either suprapubically or by a urethral catheter. Where there is concomitant nerve damage no reconstruction may be feasible and urinary diversion is preferable.

Low rectourethral fistula

This usually results from failure to recognize the presence of an anobulbar fistula as the primary condition. It is associated with urine loss per rectum or faecal contamination of the urine and is much less likely to be complicated by nerve damage than the high lesion. Being close to the perineum it is readily accessible and can often be closed by simple excision and suture.

Urethral stricture or diverticulum

Stricture of the posterior urethra can result from an overextended excision of the fistula, but most anterior strictures are due to infection and trauma or the effects of long-term catheterization in children with pelvic nerve damage or fistula formation. An acquired urethral diverticulum in the region of the penoscrotal junction may also result from the use of catheters. At times perineal surgery produces complete ablation of a section of the urethra so that fistula and stricture coexist. Following a preliminary colostomy these cases may be treated by dissecting the bowel off the urethra and closing it and then laying a scrotal flap (Blandy) into the posterior urethral wall above the fistula level. At a second stage the scrotal flap can be freed from the surrounding skin and used to complete the urethral closure.

Epididymitis

Recurrent and severe epididymitis is a secondary complication, particularly where a neurogenic bladder, a fistula or a stricture is present. Attacks may continue after satisfactory closure of a fistula and are probably due to local trauma to the vesicles or the ejaculatory ducts. In several cases a vasectomy has been required to relieve the attacks which had already rendered the epididymis severely and permanently scarred.

Complications of cloaca in the female

Girls presenting with this malformation have, behind a somewhat enlarged clitoris, a single opening only on the perineum. It leads into a channel of variable length and calibre which can be called a cloaca by analogy with the functional passage found in lower forms of life but bears little relation to the human embryological organ. Joining with this cloaca anteriorly is the bladder or the urethra. The bladder neck may be well formed and potentially continent or it may be seriously deficient. Ureteric anomalies are common and reflux is to be expected. The upper end of the cloaca communicates with the female genital tract which is usually duplicated and sometimes enormously distended with viscid fluid. The rectum is short and may or may not have a permeable track into the posterior wall of the cloaca immediately below the septum dividing the vagina.

At birth a colostomy is urgent and obligatory. Subsequent investigation reveals the precise anatomy. If the cloaca is narrowed it may be necessary to dilate it widely to drain the urine and to prevent its accumulation in the genital passages which can become seriously infected. In other cases it is preferable to postpone definitive treatment for some years. A pull-through procedure for the rectum is undertaken if there is sufficient pelvic musculature to give any hope of continence. Separation of the urethra and the vagina may be attempted and Hendren (1977) has given details of appropriate surgery. If the bladder neck is competent it may be sufficient to leave the urethral opening high in the vagina rather than to risk damage during the major surgery required for anatomical correction. Reflux prevention and other ureteric procedures may be required. The prognosis in regard to uterine function is not necessarily hopeless even when initially there has been a degree of hydrocolopos or hydrometra, but complications of the duplicated tract are to be anticipated. The management of the bladder and the urethra is further discussed in Chapter 23 in the section on the urogenital sinus.

References

Cozzi, F. and Wilkinson, A.W. (1968) Congenital abnormalities of the anus and rectum: mortality and function. *British Medical Journal*, i, 144

Garrett, R.A. and Yurdin, D. (1958) Urologic complications of imperforate anus. *Journal of Urology*, **79**, 514

Hendren, W.H. (1977) Surgical management of urogenital sinus anomalies. *Journal of Paediatric Surgery*, **12**, 339

Kieswetter, W.B. (1979) Rectum and Anus. *In* Pediatric Surgery, 3rd edn (edited by Ravitch, M.M.). Year Book Publications, Chicago. p.1059

Scott, J.E.S., Swenson, O. and Fisher, J.H. (1960) Surgical treatment of imperforate anus. *American Journal of Surgery*, **99**, 137

Smith, E.D. (1968) Urinary anomalies and complications in imperforate anus and rectum. *Journal of Paediatric Surgery*, **3**, 337

Turner-Warwick, R.T. (1967) The use of the omental pedicle graft in the repair and reconstruction of the urinary tract. *British Journal of Surgery*, **54**, 849

Wiener, E.S. and Kieswetter, W.B. (1973) Urological abnormalities associated with imperforate anus. *Journal of Paediatric Surgery*, **8**, 151

Williams, D.I. and Nixon, H.H. (1957) Agenesis of the sacrum. *Surgery, Gynecology and Obstretrics*, **105**, 84

23 Female Urethral Anomalies and Obstructions

D. Innes Williams

Although minor disorders of the female urethra are very commonly diagnosed and thought by many to account for a high proportion of cases of recurrent urinary tract infection, major congenital abnormalities are very rare and almost always involve some other organ. Thus in congenital absence of the urethra the bladder opens directly into a common channel with the vagina and this disorder is best considered under the heading of Urogenital sinus, as is a short urethra with a termination in the anterior vaginal wall (hypospadias), since externally there is only a single opening for both the urinary and the genital tracts. A short urethra with a normal external meatus and no proper formation of the bladder neck is better described as bilateral single ectopic ureters (*see* Chapter 16). Urethral valves in the female have nothing in common with the male disorder and the only truly valvular flap ordinarily observed is formed by the lower lip of a ruptured ectopic ureterocele (*see* Chapter 16). Epispadias in the female with an incomplete bladder neck is an important anomaly discussed in Chapter 25.

anlage and there may be two vulvas and duplication of the genital tract. In Boissonnat's (1961) case the urethras lay in the coronal plane and were associated with a bifid clitoris and pubic diastasis, suggesting an embryogenic relationship with epispadias.

The occurrence of two urethras draining a single bladder is exceptionally rare and the usual finding is that a narrow accessory channel lies posterior to a normal urethra. In the case seen by the author the supernumerary urethra opened into the vagina and led to urine leakage. Both urethras may, however, open on the vestibule and in such cases the patient may be continent. The vesical orifice of the accessory urethra is often situated some distance from the normal bladder outlet.

If an accessory urethra causes urinary incontinence or dysuria, its excision or its obliteration by diathermy coagulation or by the injection of a sclerosant may be necessary. When the two urethras are closely apposed surgery to the supernumerary structure carries a considerable risk to the normal one.

Urethral duplication

The rare condition of urethral duplication is most often encountered in association with complete duplication of the bladder. The urethras lie side by side in the coronal plane. This anomaly results from splitting of the vesicourethral

Urethral diverticulum

Urethral diverticula involve the posterior wall of the urethra and are mainly encountered as acquired lesions in parous women. Nevertheless, Johnson (1938) described a diverticulum in the urethra of a newborn infant.

In the author's experience an apparent urethral diverticulum in a girl may be the lower end of an ectopic ureter, the upper end of which is narrow or actually obliterated. The cavity fills by reflux during micturition and causes incontinence by its emptying afterwards. It is demonstrated on micturating cystourethrograms but a full investigation is required in view of its likely ureteric origin.

Excision of the diverticulum may occasionally be necessary. If the opening is very low down in the urethra then it is usually sufficient simply to perform a meatotomy up to the opening so that the diverticulum does not distend during micturition and does not, therefore, produce any symptoms.

Urogenital sinus

There is an important yet uncommon group of disorders that involves both the urethra and the vagina with a single shared opening at the vulva and so may be categorized as urogenital sinus anomalies. They have been analysed by Williams and Bloomberg (1976).

Since a terminal common channel for the urinary and genital tracts is a normal feature of the male it is inevitable that any virilization of the female fetus produces a urogenital sinus, and

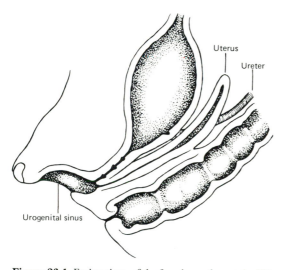

Figure 23.1. Embryology of the female urethra at the 100 mm stage, showing the downgrowth of the vagina and the widening out of the urogenital sinus.

this is commonly encountered in congenital adrenocortical hyperplasia. However, the process by which the normal female comes to have separate urinary and genital openings involves more than the absence of virilization and is also due to the caudal movement of the vaginal opening, taking place late in the course of fetal life (*Figure 23.1*). There is a variety of anomalies in which this process fails without any virilization and these present as urinary tract problems in childhood or as genital problems at puberty.

Urogenital sinus due to virilization of the female fetus

This well known condition is described in Chapter 44, but the anatomical deformity merits some discussion here and is demonstrated diagrammatically in *Figure 23.2a*.

Most of these children require clitoridectomy or clitoral reduction as well as vaginoplasty. A general discussion of these operations is outside the scope of this chapter, although it may be noted that only in a few cases is the vagina low enough to enable it to be stitched directly to the perineal skin. The method of vaginoplasty commonly employed by the author involves the raising of a posteriorly based perineal skin flap which is turned upward, as in the scrotal flap urethroplasty for male stricture, to meet the opened-out terminal vagina.

There is a considerable variation in the degree of virilization; sometimes the urogenital sinus is short and opens on the perineum and occasionally it is long and resembles a complete normal urethra opening on the glans of what appears to be a normal penis.

In general the greater the degree of virilization the higher is the vaginal orifice, and there are a few examples in which this lies above the external sphincteral mechanism corresponding in position to the male verumontanum. These cases present a difficult problem in treatment and it seems best to delay complete correction. An operation that excises the corpora cavernosa of the clitoris and preserves an opened-out urethral strip produces an acceptable female appearance in infancy, and vaginoplasty can be postponed until the approach of puberty when the vagina becomes much more accessible.

However, in some children the high position

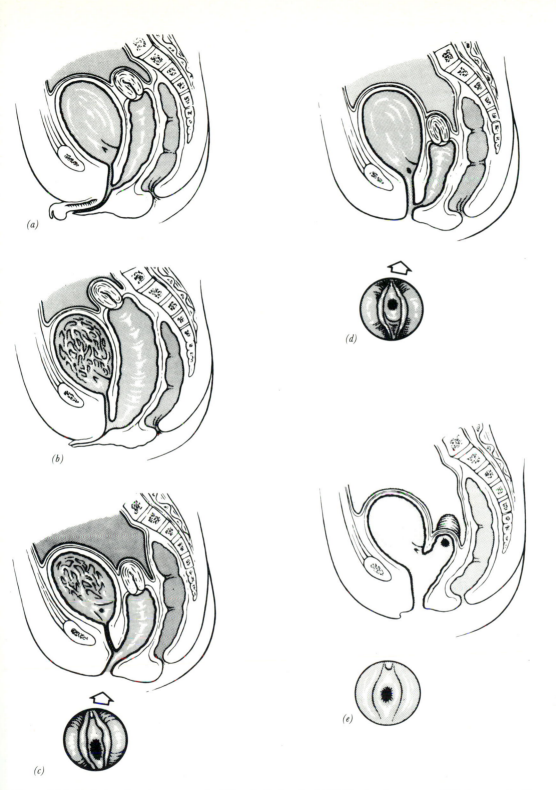

Figure 23.2. Varieties of persistent urogenital sinus in the female. *(a)* Virilization due to congenital adrenocortical hyperplasia. *(b)* Vulval obstruction with pseudopenis. *(c)* Female hypospadias. *(d)* Vaginal atresia with wide urethra. *(e)* Urovaginal confluence. (Reproduced by permission of the editor, *Journal of Pediatric Surgery*.)

of the vaginal opening is associated with reflux of urine, producing a huge hydrocolpos and complicating urinary tract infection. Such cases may demand early vaginoplasty to secure adequate drainage and one girl was treated by a combination of a parasacral and a perineal operation. The child was placed in the left lateral position and a parasacral incision was made, mobilizing the coccyx. The levator ani fibres were parted and the pelvic viscera displaced. The rectum was then gently retracted posteriorly so that the termination of the vagina in the urethra was easily exposed. The vagina was cut across at this point and the urethral wall repaired. The proximal cut end of the vagina was then anastomosed to a flap of perineal skin. Subsequently a stricture formed at this skin anastomosis, and it is planned on a future occasion to raise a more generous labial flap to effect the anastomosis to the vagina.

Vulval obstruction with pseudopenis

Although in this condition (*Figure 23.2b*) there is a suggestion of pseudohermaphroditism, there is no evident hormonal basis for the disorder and no chromosomal abnormality. Complete fusion of the labial folds produces anteriorly a small lax penis-like structure containing a narrow outlet for the urethra. The vagina and the urethra communicate beneath the labial folds and both are obstructed by the narrow urogenital sinus. This obstruction produces an enormous hydrocolpos as well as a trabeculated bladder, often with reflux, dilated ureters and somewhat dysplastic kidneys. The vulval fusion is not therefore an isolated abnormality. There may be a degree of fibrosis both of the terminal urethra and of the high vaginal opening, as well as upper urinary tract anomalies.

The majority of cases present at birth with an abdominal swelling that may be either the distended bladder or the distended hydrocolpos. On superficial examination these infants appear to be male, but the pseudopenis is found to be a flabby organ consisting of folds of skin without palpable corpora cavernosa. The scrotum is absent and no testicles are palpable. The urethra is too small to accept any catheter although cystourethrograms may be obtained by suprapubic puncture. A buccal smear reveals a positive sex chromatin and a karyotype of 46 XX constitution.

Once the diagnosis has been made a simple cut back opening up the labial folds relieves the urgent retention. Because the urethral and vaginal openings may also be stenosed more extensive surgery is likely to be required. Enlargement of the vaginal introitus by the rotation of a labial flap together with repeated urethral dilatation should suffice. Ureteric reimplantation for reflux prevention may be needed later.

Female hypospadias

In this anomaly the urethra enters the anterior wall of the vagina a centimetre or two above the introitus (*Figure 23.2c*). The condition has little in common with true hypospadias in the male but the term is convenient and has been generally accepted. On superficial examination the vulva appears to be normal with the usual vaginal introitus. On closer inspection it becomes evident that the urethral meatus cannot be seen, while a curved sound passed up the anterior vaginal wall ordinarily enters the urethra without difficulty. Minor degrees of this condition may be found in symptomless and otherwise normal children. Two important complications may be encountered, namely urethral stenosis and vaginal obstruction.

Most cases present early in life with urinary tract infection or straining on micturition. Repeated wide dilatation of the urethra is usually effective in securing normal bladder evacuation but anterior urethral myotomy and reimplantation of the ureters may also be required. Curiously, although the urethra is short and has been widely dilated, incontinence is not a major feature except in those cases where some other abnormality such as an ectopic ureter is present. Urinary hydrocolpos due to vaginal atresia can lead to postmicturition incontinence and persistent urinary tract infection. Episiotomy with inward rotation of a labial flap to open up the introitus is then required.

Vaginal atresia with wide urethra

In this condition the vulva is normal to superficial inspection, but on parting the labia only a single opening is found. This is rather wider than the normal urethra and leads directly into the bladder through a relaxed bladder neck (*Figure 23.2d*). The bladder itself is normal although stress incontinence of a severe degree results from the bladder neck incompetence. The vagina is atretic at its lower end and joins the urethra at some point above the meatus. This vaginal opening may be low and easily found or high and obstructed; at times it appears to be completely sealed off. Such cases may be mistaken for simple hydrocolpos. It is important to recognize that in this group not only is the urinary tract abnormal but also the vagina is short and atretic rather than simply obstructed by a membrane.

These children contrast with cases of female hypospadias in that they present much later in childhood with incontinence as the major complaint. Vaginoplasty should secure the external opening and continence may improve on imipramine treatment. If not, some operation to support the bladder neck is necessary.

Urovaginal confluence with absent bladder neck

These patients have a major abnormality of both the urinary and the genital system with complete confluence of the vagina, the urethra and the bladder neck (*Figure 23.2e*). No micturition is possible and such girls present at about 3 years of age when it is evident that there is no vestige of urinary control. Externally the condition resembles vaginal atresia with a wide urethra, having a single opening at the vulva that leads directly into the urinary tract, but there is no possibility of retention of secretion within the vagina. The bladder is of variable size and wide open caudally. Unilateral renal agenesis is common, as is reflux into the solitary ureter. The upper vagina and the uterus are likely to be bifid or asymmetrical.

In some cases the bladder is so small that primary diversion should be performed. In others an attempt should be made to construct a bladder neck using an anterior detrusor tube (Williams and Snyder, 1976). The creation of a sphincteral zone is more important than the separation of the whole length of the urethra from the vagina. Techniques for the latter procedure together with the management of related cases of 'cloaca' were discussed by Hendren (1977, 1980).

Distal urethral obstruction

It has long been recognized that instrumental urethral dilatation can lead to symptomatic improvement in females of all ages with a variety of minor urinary complaints, and this happy result has been ascribed at various times to the effects of dilatation upon the bladder neck, the inflamed mucosa or the external meatus. At present attention centres upon the distal urethra and obstruction due to either a collagenous ring of tissue (Lyon and Smith, 1963) surrounding the membranous urethra in girls or to a spastic condition of the external sphincter. Symptoms attributed to this obstruction are frequency, urgency, enuresis and recurrent infection. The condition may be recognized by urethral calibration, radiology or urodynamic methods.

Urethral calibration is a simple procedure that has become a routine part of endoscopic investigation in many centres. Bougies à boule are often employed although they are not essential for measurement. The calibre at which withdrawal of the expanded end produces whitening of the mucosa around the external meatus is noted. All urologists have observed on occasions definite stenosis of the external meatus, while this never approaches the degree characteristic of the male equivalent, and there is no doubt that in such cases symptoms are alleviated by instrumental dilatation or meatotomy. Doubt arises, however, in relation to the large number of girls with recurrent infection and without obvious abnormality in whom some investigators find distal urethral obstruction of lesser degree. Immergut, Culp and Flocks (1967) have shown from a study of urologically normal children undergoing otorhinolaryngological procedures that between 0–4 years the mean calibre of the external meatus is 15 F, between 5–9 years 17 F, between 10–14 years 21.4 F and between 15–20 years 26.2 F. They did not find any significant difference in calibre between the meatus itself and the distal urethral ring. In a further study Immergut and Notman(1965) investigated girls with recurrent infection and found they had slightly larger urethral calibres, the difference being small but statistically significant. It does not appear, therefore, that a fixed stenotic ring can account for the common problem of recurrent infection although obstruction may still be due to a spastic external sphincter.

Radiologically the female urethra has proved to be a difficult organ to study, with rapid changes of form during normal and interrupted micturition. The normal appearance may be of a simple tube with slight tapering from the bladder neck to the external meatus (*Figure 23.3*).

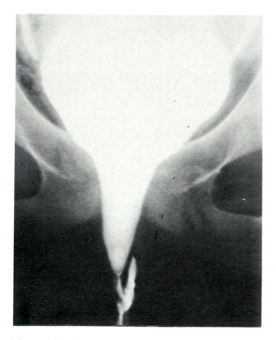

Figure 23.3. Normal cystourethrogram in a female showing the tapering outline of the urethra with no evidence of meatal stenosis.

Many girls show a distinct collar at the upper end with a widened area below, and any attempt at voluntary restraint of micturition produces a ballooning of the mid-section of the urethra which disappears with restoration of free flow (*Figure 23.4*). Where the widening appears to persist through all phases of micturition it has been suggested that there is a distal urethral obstruction, and unquestionably repeat studies after wide meatotomy show a simple tubular urethra. However, Schopfner (1967) in a very extensive study found no relationship between radiological appearance and urethral calibre, or between the urethral outline and the presence of reflux or residual urine. Allen (1970) also concluded that it was impossible to diagnose distal urethral obstruction radiologically. Harrow *et al.* (1960) regarded the very wide urethra found in some girls as evidence of congenital dilatation rather than obstruction.

Urodynamic pressure-flow measurements can give satisfactory evidence of obstruction in boys old enough to cooperate. Young girls have proved difficult to investigate and most authors examining cases with simple recurrent infection (for example Nunn, 1965; Whitaker, Johnson and Lawson, 1969) failed to identify distal urethral obstruction. The urethral pressure profile (*see* Chapter 18), which measures the lateral pressure upon the urethra in the resting state, has been considered an appropriate investigation for these cases and all observers agree that the peak of the normal profile is found well below the bladder neck and a little above the external meatus at a level corresponding to the external sphincter. Tanagho *et al.* (1971) showed that this peak can be lowered by general anaesthesia and abolished by curare. They postulated that inappropriate contraction of the sphincter during micturition can interrupt the stream and

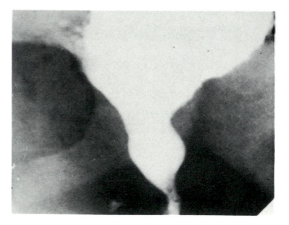

Figure 23.4. Normal cystourethrogram in a female showing transient proximal dilatation of the urethra.

cause proximal urethral dilatation. Lyon and Smith (1963) also noted intermittent flow in girls with recurrent urinary tract infection as evidenced by a sound recording of the process of micturition. They believed that local inflammation can cause tenderness in the urethra and spasm of the external sphincter, leading in turn to an interrupted stream and turbulence which carries bacteria back from the meatus to the bladder and thus perpetuates a vicious circle of infection.

However difficult and insecure the diagnosis of distal urethral obstruction is, very good results have been claimed from treatment both with forcible dilatation and with urethrotomy. Lyon, one of the original protagonists, repeated the excellent published results and emphasized the need for stretching the collagenous ring in the distal urethra beyond the point of rupture. Ordinarily bougies meet increasing resistance from the bladder wall up to about 24 F and then the ring appears to give way and dilatation becomes easier. It may be continued to 32–40 F. Lyon and Marshall (1971) reviewed 864 children. Of 283 with symptoms of cystitis 65 per cent had an immediate and sustained cure and in the long term 86 per cent were improved. Of 297 children with feverish attacks 82 per cent had an immediate cure and the failures were mostly in children with reflux. Kerr, Leadbetter and Donaghue (1966) advocated the use of the Otis urethrotome and recorded 72 per cent of improvements in 44 children, many of whom had previously required continuous chemotherapy. The disappearance of minor degrees of reflux was common in these cases but major degrees remained unchanged. Vermillion, Halverstadt and Leadbetter (1971) reported a group of 106 girls also treated by urethrotomy and recorded a cure rate of 78 per cent.

Controlled trials have not given such clear-cut answers. Kaplan, Sammons and King (1973) made a blind comparison between dilatation, urethrotomy and medication alone and found no difference in the cure rates. There could possibly have been a slight disadvantage to urethrotomy, and there was some suggestion that very long-standing recurrent infection was improved by dilatation techniques. Hendry, Stanton and Williams (1973) found no overall difference between children treated with medication alone and those treated by urethral dilatation plus medication. There were occasional examples of apparent benefit in children with uninhibited bladder contractions.

In conclusion there seems every reason to undertake either urethral dilatation or urethrotomy on any child found to have a urethral calibre less than normal and in others where recurrent infection is associated with small volumes of residual urine or evidence of an interrupted urine stream. The wholesale treatment of girls with minor symptoms cannot, however, be justified.

Covered meatus

In a few girls without other abnormalities partial closure of the urethral folds carries the urethra towards the clitoris and the meatus is then directed forwards by a posterior mucosal fold. Meatotomy is required if the urine stream is diverted anteriorly to such a degree that micturition in the sitting position is difficult.

Paraurethral cyst

Cystic dilatation of an obstructed paraurethral gland or duct usually presents clinically in infancy or early childhood. The swelling protrudes through, or bulges immediately below or lateral

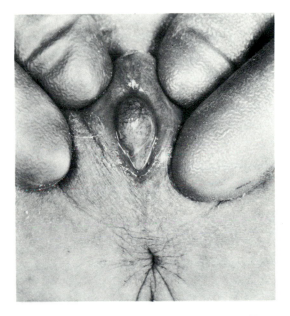

Figure 23.5. Simple paraurethral cyst closely resembling hydrocolpos or prolapsed ectopic ureterocele.

to, the meatus (*Figure 23.5*) and may simulate a prolapsed ectopic ureterocele. Excision or marsupialization of the cyst is required.

Urethral prolapse

Prolapse of the urethral mucosa is commoner during childhood than in adult life. The condition may occur in an otherwise healthy child or may follow a period of severe coughing or straining at stool. The prolapse involves the entire circumference of the urethra so that the meatus is hidden by a rosette of mucosa which becomes engorged, haemorrhagic (*Figure 23.6*) and possibly gangrenous. The swelling gives the appearance of having a pedicle and may be misdiagnosed as of neoplastic nature.

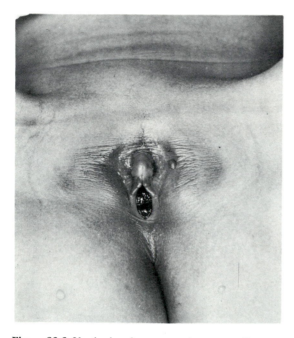

Figure 23.6. Urethral prolapse appearing as a small haemorrhagic protrusion.

The presenting complaint is bleeding. Dysuria may also be present but this is not invariable. Following preliminary cleansing by sitz bathing the redundant mucosa may be circumcised and the urethral meatus resutured to the meatus. A period of postoperative catheter drainage is required. Alternatively a ligature may be tied around the base of the prolapse over an indwelling catheter so that the mucosa sloughs off. There is little or no tendency to stricture formation after either procedure.

Traumatic stricture and fistula

As in the male, although much less commonly, stricture of the urethra results from rupture associated with fractures of the pelvis. The injury almost always includes either the anterior wall or the circumference of the vagina, and when healing occurs a urethrovaginal fistula develops. Trauma can occur at various levels up to and including the bladder neck.

In low strictures with urethrovaginal fistula continence is preserved and only dilatation of the fistula may be required unless the vaginal outlet itself is stenosed, producing a hydrocolpos. In mid-section fistulas it is desirable to restore the continuity of the urethra and to separate the vagina from it. The two viscera can be divided by an abdominoperineal approach and the vagina, which is capacious, is easily closed. Often the urethra must be left as a simple strip of anterior wall backed by a leaf of omentum. In high injuries incontinence can result from encroachment upon the bladder neck and paradoxically the stricture may be present above the fistula. Anterior bladder neck Y-V plasty may sometimes overcome the stricture problem and allow concomitant closure of the fistula, but frequently incontinence remains and further reconstructive operations are required (Williams, 1975).

References

Allen, P.R. (1970) The lower urinary tract. *Progress in Pediatric Radiology*, **3**, 139

Boissonnat, P. (1961) Complete double functional urethra with a single bladder. *British Journal of Urology*, **33**, 453

Hendren, W.H. (1977) Surgical Management of Urogenital sinus abnormalities. *Journal of Pediatric Surgery*, **12**, 339

Hendren, W.H. (1980) Construction of female urethra from vaginal wall and perineal flap. *Journal of Urology*, **123**, 657

Hendry, W., Stanton, S. and Williams, D.I. (1973) *British Journal of Urology*, **45**, 72

Immergut, M. and Notman, G.E. (1965) The urethral calibre of female children with recurrent urinary tract infection. *Journal of Urology*, **99**, 189

Immergut, M., Culp, D. and Flocks, R.H. (1967) The urethral calibre in normal female children. *Journal of Urology*, **97**, 693

Johnson, C.M. (1938) Diverticulum of the female urethra. *Journal of Urology*, **39**, 506

Kaplan, C.G.W., Sammons, P.A. and King, L.R. (1973) Blind comparison of dilatation urethrotomy and medication alone in the treatment of urinary tract infection in girls. *Journal of Urology*, **109**, 917

Kerr, W.S., Leadbetter, G.W. and Donahue, J. (1966) An evaluation of internal urethrotomy in female patients with urethral obstruction. *Journal of Urology*, **95**, 218

Lyon, R.P. and Marshall, S. (1971) Urinary tract infection and difficult micturition in girls: long term follow-up. *Journal of Urology*, **105**, 314

Lyon, R.P. and Smith, D.R. (1963) Distal urethral stenosis. *Journal of Urology*, **89**, 414

Nunn, I.N. (1965) Bladder neck obstruction in children. *Journal of Urology*, **93**, 693

Schopfner, C.E. (1967) Roentgen evaluation of distal urethral obstruction. *Radiology*, **99**, 222

Tanagho, E.A., Miller, P.R., Lyon, R.P. and Fisher, R. (1971) Spastic striated external sphincters and urinary tract infection in girls. *British Journal of Urology*, **43**. 69

Vermillion, C.D., Halverstadt, D.R. and Leadbetter, G.W. (1971) Internal urethrotomy and urinary tract infection in girls. *Journal of Urology*, **106**, 154

Whitaker, J., Johnson, T.S. and Lawson, J.D. (1969) Urinary outlfow resistance estimation in children. *Investigative Urology*, **7**,\127

Williams, D.I. (1975) Rupture of the female urethra in childhood. *European Urology*, **1**, 129

Williams, D.I. and Bloomberg, S. (1976) Urogenital sinus in the female child. *Journal of Pediatric Surgery*, **11**, 51

Williams, D.I. and Snyder, H. (1976) Anterior detrusor tube repair for urinary incontinence in children. *British Journal of Urology*, **48**, 671

24 Prune Belly Syndrome

D. Innes Williams

The prune belly syndrome has attracted a great deal of attention in the paediatric literature under a variety of names and a full bibliography was provided by Wigger and Blanc (1977). Earlier papers sometimes refer to the Eagle-Barrett syndrome. Stephens (1963) used the term triad syndrome because of the three characteristic anomalies, namely the absence of abdominal muscles, cryptorchidism and urinary tract deformities. The prune-like appearance of the neonatal abdominal wall determined the titles of papers by Burke, Shin and Kelalis (1969) and Waldbaum and Marshall (1970). Many systems of the body are affected and it is not possible to say that any one abnormality is primary.

There is very little information as to the overall incidence of the syndrome. Perhaps the long-term nature of the complaint and repeated attendances at clinics over many years have given urologists an exaggerated idea of its frequency. The author saw just 46 cases in 30 years of practice. The fully developed syndrome is seen only in males although on rare occasions abdominal muscular defects occur in both sexes in a variety of circumstances (for example arthrogryposis and pterygium syndrome) unconnected with the typical prune belly changes in the urinary tract. In most patients the chromosomes are normal, but a defect was reported in one case by Harley, Chen and Rattner (1972). There is no record of a familial incidence.

Pathology

The abnormalities of structure and function in the various systems affected require separate consideration since it is difficult to discern any causative relationship between one and another.

Abdominal musculature

The essential defect is the absence of muscles in the lower and medial parts of the abdominal wall, although the upper rectus and outer oblique muscles are developed. The severity of the condition is variable and it is often asymmetrical. Welch and Kearney (1974) claimed that the muscles are hypoplastic rather than absent. Wigger and Blanc (1977) found individual muscle fibres sometimes had an appearance of secondary atrophy while surviving bundles were sometimes hypertrophied. The abdominal wall in the affected area consists of skin, fat and a condensation of fibrous tissue lying on the peritoneum. In the relaxed state it takes on the characteristic wrinkled prune-like appearance (*Figures 24.1 and 24.2*). It is readily stretched and with the passage of time the wrinkles flatten out, leaving a protuberant lower abdomen. The intact upper rectus muscles may pull the umbilicus upwards.

The disability resulting from this absence of muscles is less than might be suspected. The

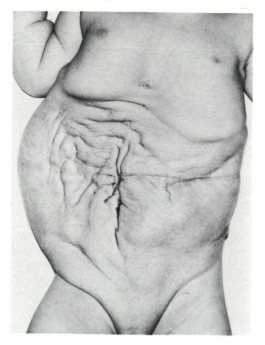

Figure 24.1. Prune belly syndrome. The appearance of the abdominal wall in the infant.

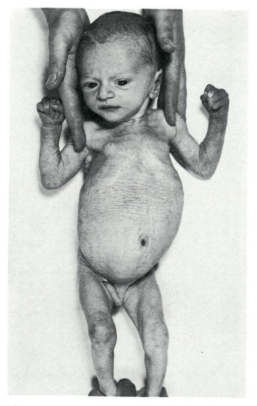

Figure 24.2. Prune belly syndrome in the infant. Note the long flabby penis.

child may have some difficulty in rising from the supine position and in very severe cases the lower chest is flared outwards with a central depression. Because the ability to cough effectively is impaired infants are liable to respiratory infection.

Healing of abdominal wall wounds after incision proceeds satisfactorily even though the suturing procedure may seem inadequate because of the lack of well defined layers. The absence of muscle tension seems to eliminate any tendency to dehiscence.

Urinary tract

The whole length of the urinary tract is involved to a greater or lesser extent in the anomaly. Ordinarily secondary changes following infection and obstruction complicate the picture so that it may be difficult to distinguish primary from consequent pathology. The characteristic gross dilatation of the upper urinary tract results from the effect of lower tract dysfunction upon the abnormally muscularized ureters and dysplastic kidneys. Elimination of outflow obstruction or reflux can lead to improvement of function but seldom to normality. Severe urethral obstruction in fetal life produces renal dysplasia of a degree that badly impairs function. Often the dysplasia in prune belly syndrome occurs without obstruction and appears to be part of the primary pathology.

The kidneys may be normal although the majority are dysmorphic or dysplastic to some degree and most are complicated by hydronephrosis. A typical picture of mild dysmorphism shows a kidney of normal size with a thick parenchyma but elongated infundibula terminating in clubbed calyces, yet without any evidence of parenchymal scarring (*Figure 24.3*). Cystic spaces in the pyramids are seen from time to time. In more severely affected kidneys there may be gross distortion of form accompanied by deterioration of function and histologically dysplastic changes. In the most extreme cases there is a multicystic kidney with an atretic upper ureter (*see* Chapter 14). The hydronephrosis is seldom associated with pelviureteric obstruction and more often coincides with gross ureteric dilatation (*Figure 24.4*). Often renal function is surprisingly well preserved in spite of the hydronephrosis and rapid deterioration is quite unusual

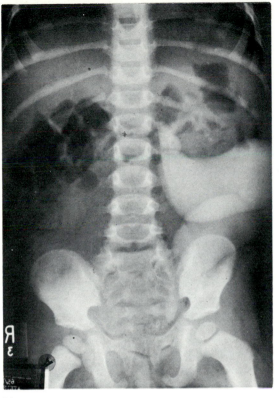 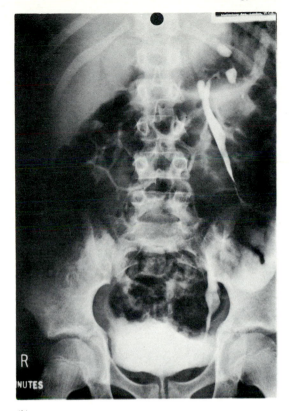

(a) *(b)*

Figure 24.3. Prune belly syndrome. *(a)* Intravenous urogram at 5 years. There is no opacification of the right side and a grossly dilated tortuous ureter on the left, but good renal function. *(b)* Intravenous urogram at 10 years, following urethrotomy. Ureteric dilatation is much improved and there is a thick renal parenchyma with globular calyces.

except where there has been chronic infection or very severe dysplasia.

The extreme tortuosity of the ureters produces a radiological appearance that is often immediately recognizable as associated with absent abdominal muscles, although of course the degree of dilatation varies. The lower end of the ureter is more severely affected than the upper one, and there are occasional saccular dilatations of the middle segment. Histological examination of the ureteric muscle (Palmer and Tesluk, 1974) reveals fibrosis and scarcity of muscle bundles. Ehrlich and Brown (1977) studied the structure by electron microscopy and found a marked decrease in nerve plexuses with evidence of irregularity and degeneration of the nerve trunks. These findings are in keeping with the poor propulsive power of the ureters, and the unusual form of the dilatation results from lower tract dysfunction. Reflux is present in many but not all cases. It can be re-emphasized that renal

function is often surprisingly well preserved in the face of apparently severe ureteric pathology.

The bladder has a large capacity and an irregular outline. It is generally attached to the umbilicus where there may be an apical diverticulum. While the bladder wall is thickened it is often not trabeculated in the ordinary form of prune belly syndrome, there being a rather more homogeneous enlargement of the muscle bundles. The trigone is very wide with, as a rule, dilated ureteric orifices that allow reflux. The bladder neck itself is relaxed and below it there is a tapering dilatation of the posterior urethra which narrows down to a point at approximately the membranous level. Occasionally a true urethral valve is found in this situation but in general there is no more than a smooth constriction. In very severe cases the membranous urethra is the site of complete obliteration which leads to enormous dilatation of the posterior urethra (*Figure 24.5*) so that it cannot be defined from the bladder itself. In

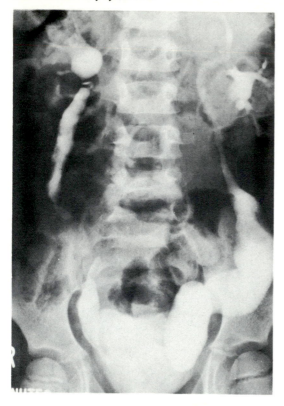

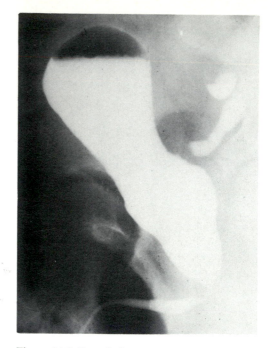

Figure 24.5. Prune belly syndrome. Micturating cystourethrogram showing dilated posterior urethra and reflux.

Figure 24.4. Prune belly syndrome. Intravenous urogram in a symptomless boy. During orchidopexy a pressure-perfusion study showed no evidence of obstruction at the left ureterovesical junction.

many cases there is a tubular diverticulum at the site of the utricle (*Figure 24.6*) and this appears to be a developmental anomaly rather than simply the result of obstruction.

The function of the bladder in mild prune belly syndrome is often normal. There are some clear-cut examples of obstruction to the urethra while in other children there appears to be a progressive failure of efficient bladder emptying, perhaps due to imbalance between the force of bladder contraction and the urethral resistance. Clinical evidence clearly demonstrates that the resistance lies in the membranous zone even though there is no evident pathological change. Urethrotomy at this point can restore surprisingly normal bladder function.

The anterior urethra is usually normal although megalourethra may occur with gross dilatation of the penile segment (*see* Chapter 20). This is associated with enlargement of the penis but seldom with definite obstruction to the distal urethra.

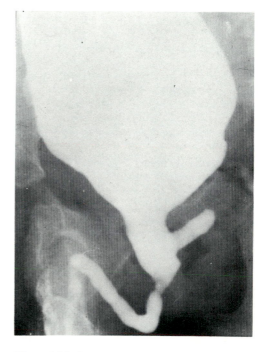

Figure 24.6. Prune belly syndrome. Micturating cystourethrogram showing utricular diverticulum.

Testicles

Bilateral cryptorchidism is an essential feature of prune belly syndrome, the testicles being placed high on the posterior abdominal wall. It is reasonable to link the failure of descent with the absence of the abdominal muscles and of the gubernaculum. However, the latter is usually regarded as important only in the final phases of descent and its absence should leave the testicle immediately above the internal inguinal ring, whereas a much higher situation is characteristic of prune belly syndrome. The testes themselves are often well developed, better for instance than those in male intersex children, although the epididymis may be elongated and drawn away from the gonad itself. After puberty, atrophy of the testicular tubules occurs but normal virilization can be expected. As yet there has been no report of tumour complicating this type of cryptorchidism.

Intestinal tract

Imperforate anus is a common association of the most major degrees of prune belly syndrome in the newborn. Usually in these cases there is complete destruction of the kidney with urethral atresia, and rectal deformity is not therefore a clinical problem. Almost all the children have a universal mesentery with an unattached caecum which can result in intestinal malrotation.

Limb deformities

In very severe prune belly syndrome when there is obliteration of the membranous urethra and failure of urine excretion oligohydramnios results. Major compression deformities of the limbs are then seen; even in less extreme cases talipes equinovarus occurs quite frequently and bilateral congenital dislocation of the hips occasionally. Most patients exhibit a dimple on the outer aspect of the knee and the elbow where the skin is bound down to the underlying joint tissues. While this deformity has no obvious clinical significance its regular appearance emphasizes the generalized nature of the disorder.

Presentation and natural history

Although all patients with the diagnosis of prune belly syndrome have major anomalies of the urinary tract, the severity varies considerably and with it the prognosis. It can be said that there is a continuous spectrum of variability, but there are certain characteristic presentations that simplify description. The diagnosis of absent abdominal muscles should present no difficulty whatever the complaint that brings the child to hospital. Agenesis is most obvious at birth and the only confusion that can arise is with attenuated and atonic musculature of the abdominal wall in a uraemic infant with obstruction due, for instance, to urethral valves. Another conceivable source of error is the huge ventral hernia found in association with the split symphysis in variants of bladder exstrophy. Partial agenesis is not quite so easily recognized and, as will be seen, there are examples of incomplete prune belly syndrome in which the characteristic urinary tract changes occur without abnormality of the abdominal wall.

Neonates with complete urethral obstruction may be stillborn but are in any case easily recognized to have anuria and the signs of oligohydramnios, that is the Potter facies, compression signs in the limbs and pulmonary hypoplasia. Many of these children die of respiratory failure soon after birth and a few develop spontaneous pneumothorax during the first 48 hours; if they survive the pulmonary lesions they succumb to renal failure within 10 days. The obliterated urethra prevents catheterization but the urinary tract may be outlined radiologically by percutaneous puncture of the bladder. Once the nature of the syndrome is recognized there is no merit in attempting drainage procedures which release only a scanty flow of dilute urine and do not affect the outcome.

A few infants with complete urethral atresia have a patent urachal fistula allowing some urine flow. Although renal function is likely to be poor, the situation is not so desperate and treatment is therefore justifiable. A simple method is enlargement of the fistula to form a vesicostomy, allowing free drainage until such time as it becomes apparent whether there is sufficient renal tissue to support life.

There is a relatively large group of infants

diagnosed at birth as suffering from the prune belly syndrome who have a patent urethra and a good urine stream but such advanced urinary tract disorders with complicating uraemia and infection that treatment is demanded during the first days or weeks of life. The general problem of dehydration and electrolyte disorders parallels that found in neonates with urethral valves. Intravenous urograms show dysplasia and gross hydronephrosis, often with failure of function on one side. A voiding cystogram reveals an enormous bladder displaced upwards out of the pelvis and distending the lower abdomen to such an extent that its ventral wall lies almost parallel to the anterior urethra. The bladder neck is ill defined and the urethra tapers to a relative narrowing below the verumontanum. Any instrumentation in these infants can be hazardous since the introduction of infection may well lead to septicaemia with a disastrous outcome. Nevertheless well managed urethral catheter drainage is the simplest emergency treatment pending the restoration of biochemical equilibrium, and in a few cases this alone suffices to get the infant through the immediate difficulties so that the prognosis even without major surgery may be good. In others failure of bladder emptying and reflux produce progressive renal damage.

Most neonates recognized as suffering from agenesis of the abdominal muscles have no complaints relating to the urinary tract in spite of major abnormalities shown by urography. In the past many of these infants were not referred to the urologist until later in childhood. This group was the subject of a study by Woodhouse, Williams and Kellett (1979). Of 11 patients seen in infancy nine remained well for periods up to 24 years with normal micturition, normal renal function and few, if any, episodes of urinary tract infection. One was lost to follow-up after 15 years of satisfactory progress and one developed chronic retention with renal failure. Of 16 additional patients in whom initial treatment elsewhere had been conservative and who were referred because of increasing retention and hydronephrosis and treated by urethrotomy 11 showed an improved and stabilized condition, four developed progressive failure and one suffered brain damage after respiratory arrest. It seems clear that the major hazard in these boys is the relative obstruction at the membranous urethral level, although as already remarked the pathology of this obstruction remains obscure.

Treatment

The prune belly syndrome should be recognized by the paediatrician at routine postnatal examination or on presentation with signs of urinary tract infection or renal failure. The paediatrician or nephrologist is rightly involved in the treatment of neonatal emergencies but the main responsibility for overall management lies with the urologist. The author's preference has been for a conservative approach with minimal surgical interference, concentrating first upon securing adequate bladder function by urethrotomy and reserving bladder or upper tract surgery for complicated cases. Other urologists have taken a different approach (Hendren, 1973; Jeffs, 1975) and advocate major reconstruction of the upper and lower urinary tracts at the earliest opportunity.

Relief of outflow obstruction

Any child with a bladder residue, major reflux and a dilated posterior urethra should be regarded as suffering from obstruction at the level of the membranous urethra and a urethrotomy should be performed. In older boys the Otis urethrotome can be employed, making two cuts anterolaterally at 24 F and 30 F (*Figure 24.7*). In infants an endoscopic incision should be made in a similar situation, using either a cold knife or a pointed electrode. Loop resection of tissue is not required. Catheter drainage for 5–7 days should follow and subsequently the efficiency of voiding should be checked. The procedure can be repeated if the first attempt has been overcautious. A minor degree of incontinence is not unusual but does not last more than a few weeks. Following successful urethrotomy a major improvement in upper tract dilatation can be anticipated. Regular monitoring of progress is essential.

Reduction cystoplasty

A very large bladder may fail to empty because of detrusor incompetence, even when urethral obstruction has been eliminated. A reduction cystoplasty should then be considered and successful results were recorded by Perlmutter (1975).

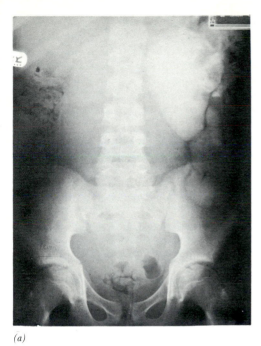
(a)

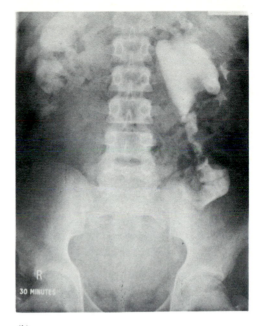
(b)

Figure 24.7. Prune belly syndrome. *(a)* Intravenous urogram before treatment showing gross left hydronephrosis, no opacification on the right and an enormously distended bladder. *(b)* Intravenous urogram following urethrotomy showing considerable improvement on both sides.

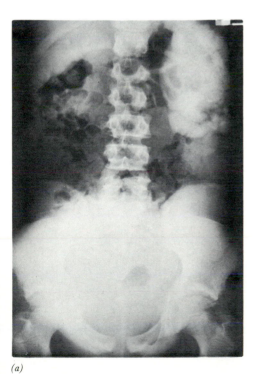
(a)

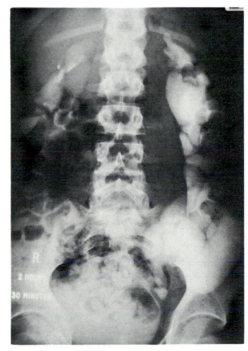
(b)

Figure 24.8. Prune belly syndrome. *(a)* Intravenous urogram before treatment. *(b)* Intravenous urogram following urethrotomy and bilateral ureteric reimplantation.

Ureteric reconstruction

The refluxing, dilated, tortuous and poorly propulsive ureters of the prune belly syndrome are obvious predisposing causes of urinary tract infection. It has already been remarked that they are associated with progressive damage less often than might be expected and it is evident that operative correction is always difficult and even hazardous. Nevertheless, as with urethral valves correction of bladder outflow obstruction may fail to improve the situation so that recurrent infection or increasing dilatation may demand treatment. The infant's ureter is more likely to have functioning muscle and the adolescent's is more likely to be atonic and fibrotic. Operation should not therefore be unduly postponed.

Simple reimplantation for reflux prevention is inappropriate and major remodelling is required, with excision of a considerable length of the lower end which is the most seriously affected portion of the ureter. When straightening the tortuous curves the greatest care must be taken to preserve the longitudinal blood supply (*Figure 24.8*). A second operation for upper end reconstruction to relieve pelviureteric dysfunction may be required. Total remodelling of the entire length of the ureter, although possible, is risky.

Nephroureterectomy

Asymmetrical upper tract damage is common and one kidney may be functionless due to either hydronephrosis or dysplasia. When total failure is confirmed by radioisotopic renography, nephroureterectomy should be performed.

Urinary diversion

As in cases of urethral valves, urinary diversion may be required as a temporary measure in the infant with severe dilatation when the ureters are enormous and aperistaltic so that reconstruction, although indicated by the progressive deterioration, seems to constitute too severe a hazard. These are exceptional circumstances and diversion should be employed very seldom. Bilateral nephrostomy is a possible method but the simplest and perhaps safest technique for infants with prune belly syndrome is a vesicostomy since the bladder is of large capacity and attached to the umbilicus, and occasionally has a fistula. The technique is discussed in Chapter 28. Cutaneous ureterostomy can also provide a satisfactory long-term temporary diversion, preferably employing the high ring technique (*see* Chapter 24). Permanent diversion is very rarely necessary, although patients with major deformities approaching terminal renal failure can sometimes be managed for a period by this expedient. If an ileal loop is employed it should be very short and anastomosed directly to the renal pelvis, which should itself be reduced in size to eliminate the atonic wall. Perhaps the best conduit is a short segment of transverse colon anastomosed at either end to the renal pelvis and opened in the middle.

Orchidopexy

The abdominal testis is found in close relationship to the dilated ureter and if ureteric surgery is planned then orchidopexy should be undertaken at the same time. Either operation performed alone produces fibrosis which renders the subsequent one more difficult. Except in neonates, the testicular vessels are too short to allow standard orchidopexy even if staged. However, the artery to the vas is usually well developed and can provide an adequate blood supply to the testis, particularly if it is carefully preserved by not disturbing the adherence of the vas to the peritoneum. The author's practice is therefore to perform orchidopexy through a laparotomy approach by cutting the testicular vessels and isolating the testicle and the vas with a continuous flap of peritoneum which is turned down, brought out through an inguinal incision and placed in the scrotum.

Very rarely orchidopexy is altogether impossible. The testicles should then be left in the abdomen until after puberty and prostheses placed in the scrotum.

Plication of the abdominal wall

Abdominal wall surgery has been advocated as a method of improving respiratory function (De Bord, 1955), although there is little evidence that it works in this way. There may be a demand for cosmetic improvement of the child's appearance, which is better met by surgery than by a corset. The redundant skin and subcutaneous tissue can be excised, preferably leaving the umbilicus and the midline intact, and the deeper tissues can be plicated to give some semblance of a normal abdominal contour.

Anaesthetic problems

A number of reports, for instance Karamanian *et al.* (1974), refer to unexpected anaesthetic difficulties and death due to respiratory depression in the early postoperative phase. It is not clear whether this disaster specifically relates to the muscular deficiency or to a particular drug, but the anaesthetist should be warned of the possible dangers.

Incomplete prune belly syndrome

Partial and unilateral absence of abdominal muscles may be accompanied by all the urinary tract changes already described. In other children a wrinkled prune-like skin is found although some active muscle is present in all areas. In a few the abdominal wall is entirely normal but the urinary tract exhibits all the features of the visceral syndrome in its less severe form. Cryptorchidism appears to follow the condition of the abdominal wall rather than the state of the urinary tract. It seems improper to label children with localized abnormalities in the urinary tract alone as incomplete prune

belly syndrome. However, when the entire urinary system is involved recognition of the affinity to prune belly syndrome is helpful in deciding treatment and prognosis.

References

Burke, E.C., Shin, M.H. and Kelalis, P.P. (1969) Prune belly syndrome: clinical findings and survival. *American Journal of Diseases of Children*, **117**, 668

De Bord, R.A. (1955) Congenital deficiency of abdominal musculature: case report with new method of surgical repair. *Annals of Surgery*, **142**, 863

Ehrlich, R.M. and Brown, W.J. (1977) Ultrastructural anatomic observations of the ureter in the prune belly syndrome. *In* Birth Defects Original Article Series, Vol 13. (edited by Bergsma, D. and Duckett, J.W.). Liss, New York. p.101

Harley, L.M., Chen, Y. and Rattner, W.H. (1972) Prune belly syndrome. *Journal of Urology*, **108**, 174

Hendren, W.H. (1973) *In* Problems in Paediatric Urology (edited by Johnston, J.H. and Scholtmeijer, R.J.). Excerpta Medica, Amsterdam. p.1

Jeffs, R.D. (1975) Paper presented at Northeastern Section Meeting of the American Urological Association, Sept. 21–24.

Karamanian, A., Kravath, B., Nagashima, H. and Gentsch, H.H. (1974) Anaesthetic management of "prune belly" syndrome: case report. *British Journal of Anaesthesia*, **46**, 897

Palmer, J.M. and Tesluk, H. (1974) Ureteral pathology in the prune belly syndrome. *Journal of Urology*, **111**, 701

Perlmutter, A.D. (1975) Reduction cystoplasty in prune belly syndrome. *Transactions of the American Association of Genito-Urinary Surgeons*, **67**, 87

Stephens, F.D. (1963) Congenital Malformation of Rectum, Anus and Genito-Urinary Tracts. Livingstone, London

Waldbaum, R.S. and Marshall, V.F. (1970) The prune belly syndrome: a diagnostic therapeutic plan. *Journal of Urology*, **103**, 668

Welch, K.J. and Kearney, G.P. (1974) Abdominal musculature deficiency syndrome: prune belly. *Journal of Urology*, **111**, 693

Wigger, H.J. and Blanc, W.A. (1977) *In* Pathological Annual, Part II, Vol. 12 (edited by Sonners, S.C. and Rosin, P.G.). Appleton-Century-Crofts, New York

Woodhouse, C.R.J., Williams, D.I. and Kellett, M.J. (1979) Minimal surgical interference in the prune belly syndrome. *British Journal of Urology*, **51**, 475

25   The Exstrophic Anomalies

J.H. Johnston

The exstrophic lesions are represented by a range of developmental anomalies. The commonest is bladder exstrophy, which occupies a central position as regards severity. Lesser degrees of the same basic embryological defect produce epispadias and superior vesical fissure. The most extreme form is exstrophy of the cloaca.

Embryology

Since the normal embryo does not pass through such a phase the exstrophic lesions are due to abnormal embryogenesis and not simply to an arrest in development. The fundamental developmental abnormality in all forms of exstrophy is a failure of primitive streak mesoderm to invade the allantoic extension of the cloacal membrane (the infraumbilical membrane). As a result the ectoderm and the endoderm are in contact abnormally in the developing lower abdominal wall in the same way as they normally are in the cloacal membrane. The absence of mesoderm constitutes an unstable state so that the infraumbilical membrane disintegrates with the cloacal membrane and the pelvic viscera are laid open on the abdominal surface. The abdominal musculature derived from the thoracic somatic mesoderm is normal on each side of the ventral defect.

The abnormally extensive cloacal membrane produces a wedge effect which holds apart the developing structures in the abdominal wall and is responsible for the separation of the pubic bones and the existence above the exstrophy of a wide linea alba or, in more severe degrees, of an exomphalos. The same effect may cause duplication of the penis or the female genital tract due to a failure of fusion of the paired genital tubercles or the müllerian ducts (Marshall and Muecke, 1968).

The precise form an exstrophic lesion takes is dependent upon the extent of the allantoic extension of the cloacal membrane onto the abdominal wall and upon the time in embryonic life at which dehiscence of the membrane occurs. The commonest anomaly, which is vesical exstrophy with epispadias, is due to the breakdown of an extensive membrane after the completion of the urorectal septum at the 16 mm stage so that the primitive urogenital sinus is exteriorized. A less extensive infraumbilical membrane leads to the occurrence of epispadias without exstrophy. If only the cranial portion of the membrane is uninvaded by mesoderm, its dehiscence produces superior vesical fissure.

Cloacal exstrophy probably represents the same basic anomaly as bladder exstrophy with earlier dehiscence of the infraumbilical and cloacal membranes at about the 5 mm stage, before the formation of the urorectal septum. Exstrophy developing at this stage would explain the occurrence of a central bowel field between two bladder fields (*Figure 25.1*). A possible objection to this hypothesis is that the exstrophic bowel does not involve the termination of the gut but the ileocaecal region, which

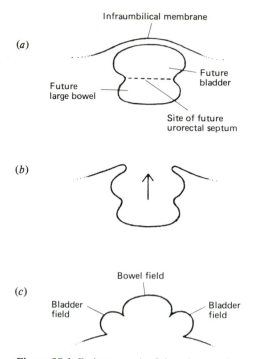

Figure 25.1. Embryogenesis of cloacal exstrophy. Following dehiscence of the infraumbilical membrane, eversion of the exstrophied cloaca leads to the occurrence of a central bowel field between two bladder fields.

does not normally enter into the formation of the cloaca. However, Johnston (1913) pointed out that the hindgut, which he believed to begin at the usual site of a Meckel's diverticulum, would be greatly restricted in growth by its involvement in exstrophy. He suggested that the exposed bowel represents an extremely short hindgut and that the distal blind length of intestine is the persistent postanal or tail gut.

Johnston and Penn (1966) reported cases supporting Johnston's (1913) theory in that they represented the occurrence of exstrophy at a phase of development between those leading to the typical vesical and cloacal forms. The exstrophic bowel lay entirely caudal to the bladder, indicating a breakdown in the cloacal and infraumbilical membranes at about the 8 mm stage, after the formation of the urorectal septum and before its fusion with the endoderm lining the cloacal membrane.

The embryogenesis of the exstrophy complex is further complicated by the fact that mesodermal invasion of the infraumbilical membrane may be merely delayed rather than entirely absent, so that secondary closure of the

parietes occurs after the formation of an exstrophy. Such a development produces covered bladder or cloacal exstrophy. On occasions delayed parietal closure leads to portions of the exstrophied organs becoming sequestrated on the abdominal surface without communication with the underlying structures. Rarely sequestration includes portions of viscera not ordinarily involved in exstrophy.

Bladder exstrophy

Bladder exstrophy has an incidence in different communities of between one in 10000 (Rickham, 1961) and one in 40000 (Marshall and Muecke, 1968) live births. It is twice as common in the male. The abnormality has been reported in twins (Higgins, 1962) and in siblings (Cendron and Petit, 1971) but a familial incidence is rare and parents of an affected child can be reassured on this point.

The size of the exstrophic bladder varies considerably. In some cases its surface area approaches that of a normal bladder while in others little more than the trigone is represented. At birth the exposed mucosa is thin and

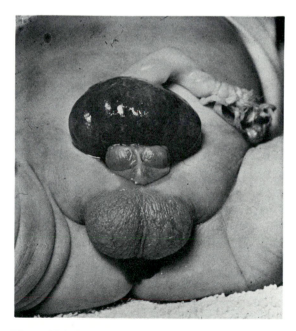

Figure 25.2. Bladder exstrophy in a newborn boy. The thin-walled bladder is everted by intra-abdominal pressure.

smooth and the muscular coat is soft and pliable; the organ is bulged outwards by intra-abdominal pressure (*Figure 25.2*) and can be inverted by digital compression. With exposure and unavoidable infection the mucosa becomes thickened and a polypoid and squamous metaplasia occurs, especially towards the bladder apex. Eventually the detrusor musculature becomes fibrotic so that the bladder forms a thick rigid plaque that can no longer be inverted. In the neonate the umbilical cord is inserted immediately above the bladder and later the umbilical scar is barely detectable. In the great majority of cases the upper urinary tract is normal at birth and, although the ureters have to curve upwards to reach the bladder, ureteric peristalsis is normal. With the development of mucosal changes the ureteric orifices may later become obstructed, leading to hydro-ureteronephrosis.

In boys complete epispadias is almost always present. The glans is wide with a dorsal groove and the urethra is represented by a mucosal strip on the dorsum of the short upturned penis. The scrotum is wide and shallow and undescended testes are common. Inguinal hernias are frequent associated lesions. In girls, too, there is total epispadias in which the clitoris is duplicated and the labia are wide apart anteriorly. In both sexes the anus lies in an unusually anterior position.

As with all forms of exstrophy the pubic bones are separated, although the width of the gap varies in different cases. A narrow interpubic space is associated with a small bladder but in the male the penis is well developed; the converse also holds true. As a result of the bony anomaly the gait is broad-based, but there is no serious orthopaedic disability. However, the consequent separation of the two halves of the pelvic diaphragm causes a lack of suspensory support for the rectum so that complete rectal prolapse may occur. Usually the liability to prolapse corrects itself with time and this complication rarely requires more than a temporary Thiersch operation, using a subcutaneous perianal nylon suture.

Although individuals with untreated bladder exstrophy can survive in good health to middle age or older, their total uncontrollable urinary incontinence is socially unacceptable in a civilized environment. Two basic methods of management are possible, namely bladder reconstruction and urinary diversion.

Bladder reconstruction

Among the earliest reconstruction operations for bladder exstrophy aimed at producing urinary continence were those performed by Trendelenberg who reported the results of surgery in two men and one boy in 1906. The adult operations were failures from the outset and the boy obtained only a temporary period of urinary control. Following Trendelenberg's report, bladder reconstruction was largely abandoned in favour of ureterosigmoidostomy. In the 1950s there was a revival of interest in the procedure, partly because of recognition of the then often unsatisfactory late results of colonic urinary diversion and partly because of the introduction of posterior iliac osteotomies to allow closure of the pubic gap and the abdominal wall defect. There is general agreement as regards the basic principles of bladder reconstruction but opinions differ as to timing, staging and details of technique (see below). The following outline is descriptive of the method used by the author in most cases (Johnston, 1977).

With the child prone, bilateral iliac osteotomies are performed through vertical incisions just lateral to the sacroiliac joints. The two halves of the pelvis are then forcibly compressed together so as to stretch the ligamentous and muscular attachments that still tend to hold them apart.

Bladder reconstruction is performed at the same session. Through a circumferential incision around its margins the bladder is mobilized from the skin, the rectus muscles and, superiorly, the peritoneum (*Figure 25.3*). At the bladder neck the incision is continued on each side of the urethral mucosa and the epispadial urethra is mobilized sufficiently to allow it to be closed into a tube. In the female the entire urethra is constructed but in the male closure is limited to the posterior urethra so that penile lengthening and chordee correction can be carried out before the formation of a penile urethra. The bladder neck is narrowed and the posterior urethra is lengthened by excising a wedge of bladder wall on each side of the vesicourethral junction.

After closure of the bladder and the urethra with apical bladder drainage the interpubic fibromuscular band representing the splayed-open external urethral sphincter is detached from the bone on each side and sutured around the bladder outlet. It is doubtful if the sphincteral reconstruction makes any useful contribution

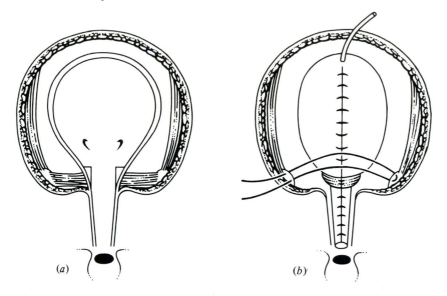

Figure 25.3. Closure of exstrophic bladder in female. *(a)* The bladder is freed from the skin, the recti abdominis and the peritoneum, a wedge of tissue is excised from each side of the bladder neck and a urethral strip is mobilized. *(b)* The bladder and the urethra are closed with bladder drainage. The interpubic band is detached from the bone on each side and sutured around the bladder neck. Strong catgut suture is passed through the pubic bones. (Reproduced by permission of Year Book Medical Publishers.)

to subsequent continence, but the procedure serves to protect the constructed urethra. The two halves of the pelvis are then compressed together and the pubes are sutured in apposition using strong catgut sutures passed through the bone. Closure of the pubic gap approximates the recti and the skin and allows easy wound closure. Following operation the child's legs are bandaged together to lessen tension on the pubic sutures and he is subsequently nursed with his legs elevated on a gallows frame.

In children over the age of 9 months or so it is commonly found that even with iliac osteotomies closure of the pubic gap can be obtained only with excessive tension so that there is an increased risk of wound dehiscence. Closure of the abdominal defect in these cases is preferably obtained by the raising of musculofascial and skin flaps.

Although vesicoureteric reflux is generally present following exstrophy reconstruction, at the initial operation the author does not attempt to prevent it. Ureteric reimplantation is less certain of success with an open exstrophic bladder, and during the early postoperative months the reconstructed bladder behaves more like a conduit than a reservoir so that reflux at this time is not harmful provided that there is no infravesical obstruction or uncontrollable infection. Antireflux surgery is performed later in the child who achieves useful control or else during secondary operations at the bladder neck aimed at improving continence.

Variations in methodology

The author's preference is to reconstruct the exstrophic bladder during the neonatal period because the organ at that time is thin and pliable and easily inverted, and because closure of the pubic gap is easily achieved. Fisher and Retik (1969) and Jeffs *et al.* (1972) also favoured early reconstruction but Chisholm (1969) advised deferring operation until the pubic bones are sufficiently mineralized to hold wire sutures. During the first day or two of life the pubes may be approximated without iliac osteotomies, possibly because of the influence of the maternal hormone relaxin. After this period division of the bony pelvic ring is necessary to relieve tension at the pubic connection.

The pubic bones later reseparate even when nonabsorbable sutures are employed, and most authors have considered that approximation of the pelvis is of value solely as a means of securing easy wound closure. However, Chisholm (1969) suggested that maintaining correction of the pelvic anomaly is important as regards urinary control and he advocated wiring the pubes and keeping the child in a plaster cast for 4–6 months after operation. Williams and Keeton (1973) and Marshall and Muecke (1970) advised the employment of osteotomies only when the pubic gap is unusually wide and otherwise the use of mobilized aponeurotic and skin flaps to close the defect. In boys Duckett (1977) reported the use of the strips of epithelium between the skin and the mucosa on each side of the exstrophy to fashion a neourethra and so allow penile and urethral lengthening.

Williams and Keeton (1973) stated that they prefer to perform bladder reconstruction at the age of 2–3 years. In boys the penile abnormality is corrected first and at the initial reconstruction no attempt is made to produce a continent bladder neck. One year later tightening of the vesical outlet by the Young-Dees (Young, 1922; Dees, 1949) or Leadbetter (1964) technique is performed and at the same time the ureters are reimplanted higher in the bladder using an antireflux technique. This two-stage approach to obtaining continence has also been employed by Jeffs *et al.* (1972), Megalli and Lattimer (1973) and Cendron and Petit (1971). Megalli and Lattimer (1973) advised that detrusor function should be assessed and shown to be adequate before bladder neck tightening is performed. They found that in 29 of 37 patients with a reconstructed exstrophy the bladder musculature had ineffective contractility. Toguri *et al.* (1978) defined continence length as the distance on the urethral pressure profile between the first pressure rise in the urethra and the highest point on the tracing. These authors noted that the minimum length needed for continence was 0.6 cm and considered that a measurement of at least 1.5 cm should be aimed at during bladder outlet construction.

Results

In 1974 Johnston and Kogan reviewed the recorded results of bladder exstrophy reconstruction and reported that 91 (21.9 per cent) of 415 patients were stated to have achieved continence. They considered that the percentage probably overestimated the effectiveness of surgery since some authors were rather vague as to the degree of control their patients actually achieved. The overall success rate was reduced further by the fact that a considerable proportion of children who did acquire control had to have urinary diversion because of upper tract deterioration. In 1978 Jeffs reported much more satisfactory results. Of 39 children with completed two-stage correction 60 per cent were continent, 20 per cent were partly continent and expected to improve further and 20 per cent were failures. Chisholm (1979), also employing a two-stage procedure, reported that 31 (42 per cent) of his 74 patients were continent, 19 (26 per cent) had some control and 24 (32 per cent) had none.

Complications

WOUND BREAKDOWN

Some degree of postoperative wound dehiscence is not uncommon, especially at the lower extremity of the reconstruction involving the bladder outlet in boys and the urethra in girls. Following closure of the pelvic ring, if there is excessive tension on the pubic sutures and especially if the child is restless and intolerant or there are difficulties with urinary drainage then complete breakdown of the repair with reformation of the exstrophy may occur. This complication does not preclude the possibility of success at a second attempt.

UPPER URINARY TRACT DETERIORATION AND CALCULI

The main late complication of bladder reconstruction is upper tract and renal deterioration resulting from obstruction, defective detrusor function, reflux and infection. It is difficult to determine from the literature the precise incidence of such changes, particularly since their onset may be considerably delayed. The author's experience from 32 bladder reconstructions is similar to that of Williams and Keeton (1973) who reported significant upper tract dilatation in about one case in five. Renal calculi formed in three of the author's cases. Eight of the 26 continent patients described by Jeffs *et al.* (1972) showed only minor upper tract changes. King and Wendell (1972) reported that 10 of their 11 patients developed hydroureteronephrosis whether or not they were continent. Three of the 12 patients of Stagner and Hodges (1963) developed renal stones and others showed pyelonephritic changes on pyelography. Megalli and Lattimer (1973) stated that in their series 12 of 40 initially normal ureters became dilated after operation but 17 of 23 previously dilated ureters improved. Bladder stones formed in four of the author's cases and have been reported by other workers. In the absence of upper tract deterioration these are not an indication for diversion. Vesical stones are most easily removed by transperitoneal cystotomy.

NEOPLASIA

The predisposition of an untreated exstrophic bladder to malignant tumour, most commonly adenocarcinoma, has long been recognized. In most cases neoplastic change occurs in adult life although it has been reported in a 14-year-old boy (Raghavaiah and Reddy, 1976). This complication has generally been assumed to result from chronic irritation of the exposed mucosa, but there is now evidence that a reconstructed exstrophic bladder may similarly be liable to malignant change. Two epithelial carcinomas and two rhabdomyosarcomas developing after bladder closure have been reported (Jacobsen and Olesen, 1968; Semerdjian, Texter and Yawn, 1972; Engel, 1973).

Microscopy of the mucosa of an exstrophic bladder has shown that inflammatory changes and squamous metaplasia can develop before the age of 2 weeks, and even at birth cystitis cystica and cystitis glandularis may be present (Culp, 1964; Engel, 1973). From electron microscopic studies Clark and O'Connell (1973) reported that the mucosal cells lacked the normal surface ridges and showed microvilli, features that occur in transitional cell carcinoma. Histological mucosal changes present before bladder closure generally persist afterwards (Ruden, Tannenbaum and Lattimer, 1972) and on occasions extensive metaplasia of the transitional epithelium to a colonic type of mucosa may occur *de novo* following reconstruction (Johnston and Kogan, 1974).

According to present knowledge the risk of malignancy is not sufficiently great to contraindicate bladder reconstruction when the patient is otherwise suitable. Nevertheless, regular postoperative urinary cytology and cystoscopy are advisable and if or when secondary urinary diversion is needed cystectomy should be performed.

Comment

The ideal result of bladder reconstruction for exstrophy, namely a fully continent patient with a persistently normal upper urinary tract, is achieved in only a minority of cases. Although the operation carries some risk to the kidneys from obstruction, reflux and infection, this exists also (and probably to no less degree) when the child is treated from the outset by urinary diversion. Turner, Ransley and Williams (1980) recorded that the risk of renal damage was 27 per cent with initial diversion, 15 per cent with exstrophy closure and 33 per cent if closure was followed by diversion. It is now generally accepted that the two-stage approach offers a better chance of obtaining continence with less hazard to the upper tracts than the original one-stage procedure. When the exstrophic bladder is large and pliable early reconstruction offers the child a reasonable chance of being normal or nearly normal, and even if control is not achieved the patient is spared the discomfort of the exposed sensitive bladder. Also, parental morale improves greatly when the unsightly deformity no longer exists. It is always necessary to carry out careful postoperative supervision indefinitely to ensure that irreversible upper tract pathology does not occur. In the patient who has had a successful reconstruction the possibility of neoplastic change must be remembered.

Urinary diversion

Indications

Some authorities (notably Spence, 1966) have opposed bladder reconstruction for exstrophy on the grounds that the likelihood of complete success is small, multiple operations may be needed and the risk of complications is considerable, and have advocated urinary diversion as the primary method of management. The proponents of bladder reconstruction resort to diversion only as a second choice in the patient whose bladder is unsuitable for reconstruction or when reconstruction fails to achieve continence or is followed by upper tract complications.

In the child whose upper tracts remain normal but who shows little or no sign of obtaining urinary control following bladder and bladder neck reconstruction it can often be difficult to decide when to abandon hope of success and advise diversion. In the author's series diversion is generally performed in such cases before school age so as to spare the child the discomfort and the embarrassment of being continually wet. However, Fisher and Retik (1969) stated that they favour waiting until the patient is postpubertal because they have found that late improvement in control is possible. Lattimer *et al.* (1978) similarly noted that continence improves with age and they advised that the patient, particularly the male in whom a urine collecting appliance can be used, should be encouraged to tolerate incontinence until 20 years of age.

When there is adequate anal control and when the ureters are undilated and kidney structure and function are normal the author's practice, like that of Spence (1966), is to perform ureterosigmoidostomy when diversion is needed. If the anal sphincters are defective or there is upper tract dilatation then external diversion by intestinal conduit, or preferably by cutaneous ureterostomy with transureteroureterostomy, is necessary. The various methods of urinary diversion are discussed in Chapter 28.

Cystectomy

When urinary diversion is performed as the primary method of treatment, removal of the exstrophy and closure of the abdominal defect are needed. It is not necessary to excise the bladder entirely. The mucosa is stripped off the musculature as far as the bladder neck, carefully preserving the posterior urethra in the male. The bladder muscle is then plicated with catgut sutures to produce a thick firm plaque and the skin defect is closed by flaps rotated from each side (Allen, Spence and Salver, 1974). When urinary diversion is needed following bladder reconstruction, cystectomy should be performed because of the possibility of neoplastic change.

Replacement of the bladder by colon

Arap (1980) devised an alternative method of exstrophy closure whereby a sigmoid conduit is fashioned with antireflux ureteric implants and, at the same operation, the exstrophic bladder is tubularized to constitute a urinary sphincter. The abdominal wall is reconstructed. Three months later the conduit is detached from the skin and anastomosed to the bladder. Of 20 cases followed for 5 years or more 15 are reported to be continent by day and to have normal upper urinary tracts.

Epispadias

Epispadias in the absence of exstrophy varies in degree. In boys balanic, penile and penopubic

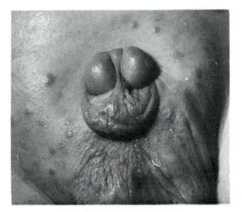
(a)

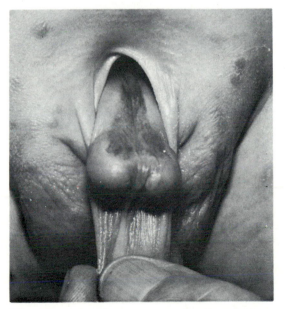
(b)

Figure 25.4. Epispadias in a boy. *(a)* The short upturned penis. *(b)* This shows the meatus at the penile base, the splayed open glans and the prepuce confined to the ventrum.

types can be recognized according to the position of the urethral meatus. The penis is short and broad with a splayed-open glans and there is marked dorsal chordee so that it curves upwards to lie in contact with the pubic skin (*Figure 25.4*). The prepuce is usually represented by a ventral hood of skin but rarely there is a complete and possibly unretractable foreskin

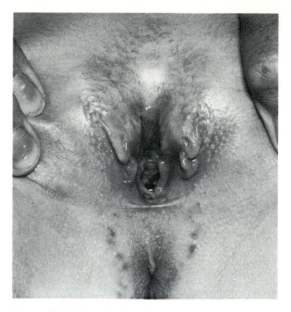

Figure 25.6. Epispadias in a girl showing the urethra which is deficient dorsally and the double clitoris.

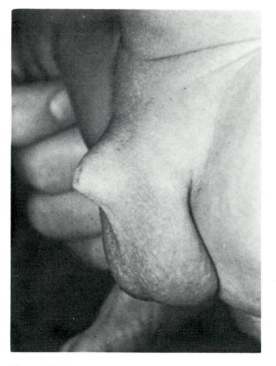

Figure 25.5. Epispadias with a complete phimotic prepuce.

(*Figure 25.5*). In the female, also, the urethra is defective dorsally to a variable extent and the clitoris is duplicated (*Figure 25.6*). The degree of urinary control possessed by the patient ranges from normal continence to total incontinence. In the incontinent child the urethra above the urogenital diaphragm is short and wide and the inadequate sphincter is incapable of maintaining a closed lumen. In boys the grade of sphincteral deficiency is generally proportionate to the severity of the penile defect. The bladder mucosa may prolapse through the wide urethral meatus in either sex.

The totally incontinent patient with epispadias has an almost constant dribble of urine when he is upright and active. On recumbency there are often periods of dryness, and on rising passive voiding of an appreciable volume of urine can occur. Cystography shows involuntary leakage from the bladder to the urethra. Urethral pressure profilometry demonstrates an extremely low or totally absent urethral resistance. Electrical stimulation of the pelvic diaphragm generally produces no rise in urethral pressure, indicating that the voluntary as well as the involuntary sphincter is ineffective, presumably because the same anatomical abnormality occurs as with bladder exstrophy. Often the bladder is extremely small and thin-walled since it has never been called upon to retain and expel urine.

Bladder outlet reconstruction

Surgery for incontinence in epispadiac patients may be directed at narrowing and tightening the existing bladder neck or lengthening the posterior urethra by the formation of a tubular neourethra from the vesical wall. Some authors (Klauber and Williams, 1974; Jeffs, 1978) have combined the reconstruction with a suspension operation of the Marshall-Marchetti-Krantz or Millin type.

In the Young-Dees (Young, 1922; Dees, 1949) operation the bladder neck and the proximal urethra are opened anteriorly and narrowed by the excision of a wedge of tissue from each side. Resuturing then converts the funnelled outlet into a tubular shape. The technique may be modified by excising mucosa only, when the excess of muscle is overlapped to produce a stronger sphincteral effect.

Lengthening of the posterior urethra using bladder wall is based on the concept that continence depends less on the activity of anatomically well defined sphincters than on the muscular and elastic tone of the entire urethra above the urogenital diaphragm. A tube formed from the bladder should therefore provide urinary control so long as it contains enough musculoelastic tissue and has sufficient length. In the Leadbetter (1964) technique a strip of trigone is tubularized after reimplantation of the ureters higher

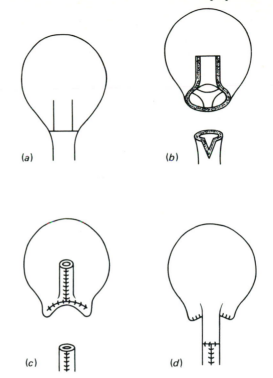

Figure 25.8. The Tanagho-Smith bladder outlet reconstruction. *(a and b)* The bladder neck is divided, an anterior flap is fashioned and a wedge is excised from the proximal end of the urethra. *(c and d)* The flap is tubularized, the bladder closed and the neourethra anastomosed to the narrowed urethra. (Reproduced by permission of Year Book Medical Publishers.)

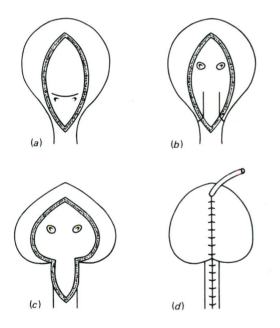

Figure 25.7. Leadbetter procedure for bladder outlet reconstruction. *(a)* The bladder is opened anteriorly. *(b)* The ureters are reimplanted higher in the bladder and the trigonal strip is outlined. *(c and d)* The trigonal strip is tubularized to form a neourethra. (Reproduced by permission of Year Book Medical Publishers.)

in the bladder (*Figure 25.7*). With the Tanagho-Smith (Tanagho and Smith, 1972) method a flap, which is based upwards, of the anterior bladder wall is tubularized. After the bladder outlet is divided and the proximal urethra is narrowed the neourethra is inserted between the two (*Figure 25.8*). The length of the tube is

maintained by suturing its upper end to the pubic region of the abdominal wall. Williams and Snyder (1976) modified the operation by using an anterior bladder strip instead of a flap. Retaining continuity between the bladder wall and the urethra lessens the risk of tissue devascularization.

The Leadbetter (1964) method has the advantage that as a rule the trigone provides better musculature for the neourethra than does the anterior wall of the bladder. However, following the construction of a posterior neourethra the bladder falls into the preurethral dead space so that a retort shape develops with the new urethral meatus lying high on the posterior vesical wall. As a result some patients have difficulty in initiating micturition and sustaining a normal urine flow. This complication can be prevented by using an omental graft to fill the dead space and so maintain a dependent

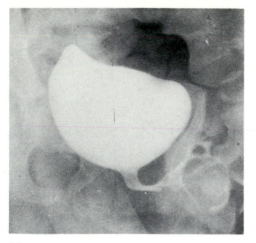

(a)

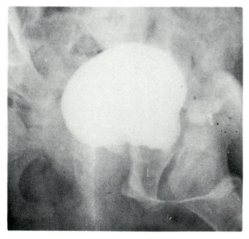

(b)

Figure 25.9. Micturating cystourethrograms in an incontinent boy with epispadias. *(a)* Before surgery. There is a short wide incompetent posterior urethra. *(b)* Following a successful Tanagho-Smith operation. The neourethra opens at the dependent part of the bladder.

bladder outlet (Johnston, 1977). With the anterior flap or strip procedures the bladder has less tendency to angulate on the neourethra (*Figure 25.9*) and since the divided trigonal apex is resutured to the posterior margin of the new bladder neck the trigone may retain its normal opening effect when the detrusor contracts.

Results

It is not possible from a study of the literature to compare the effectiveness of the different techniques of bladder neck reconstruction because

they are often modified by individual surgeons and applied to differing degrees of incontinence and bladder development. The Young-Dees operation has been widely employed. Young (1922) reported 10 good results and one fair result in 12 boys. Dees (1949) had three good and two poor results in five boys. Eighteen of Welch's (1969) 27 patients and 28 of Culp's (1964) 30 patients became continent. Klauber and Williams (1974) achieved continence in nine of 17 girls and 13 of 27 boys while five patients required a second operation. The Leadbetter (1964) technique was reported by Leadbetter and Fraley (1967) and Cibert and Cibert (1965) to be successful in respectively two of three and three of 17 patients with epispadias. Tanagho and Smith (1972) performed their procedure effectively in one boy with epispadias.

The efficacy of any of the techniques designed to cure epispadial incontinence depends mainly on the size of the bladder and the muscularity of its wall. When the bladder is very small and very thin-walled, as is often the case in the totally incontinent child, it may be possible neither to provide enough muscular tissue at the bladder outlet nor to construct a sufficiently muscularized neourethra of adequate length to allow any real prospect of success. The child who has some natural control generally has a better developed bladder and the prognosis after surgery is correspondingly improved.

The achievement of full control following operation is often delayed for months or even years. In some instances a striking spontaneous improvement occurs at puberty. Culp (1973) reported that in his series maturity contributed as much to continence as did the surgeon and Welch (1969) found that control developed at puberty in six of 12 boys with epispadias who had been considered operative failures until that time. In the male growth of the prostate is probably important in promoting control, and in both sexes increased awareness of the social advantages of being dry undoubtedly provides a strong stimulus.

Complications

The main complication of surgery for incontinence due to epispadias is a relative vesical outlet obstruction which results from a defective detrusor being unable to overcome the increased, but not necessarily abnormal, resistance at the reconstructed bladder exit. Incomplete emptying, infection, stone formation and upper tract dilatation may follow. Vesicoureteric reflux is often present with epispadias so that ureteric reimplantation may be indicated even when resiting of the ureters is not needed as part of the bladder neck reconstruction.

Superior vesical fissure

In this rare condition the exstrophy is restricted to the apical part of the bladder, and the rest of the viscus, the urethra and the abdominal wall are normal except for the typical skeletal abnormality and the consequent separation of the recti abdominis (*Figure 25.10*). Treatment involves operative closure of the open portion of the bladder. As a rule the child subsequently has normal urinary control.

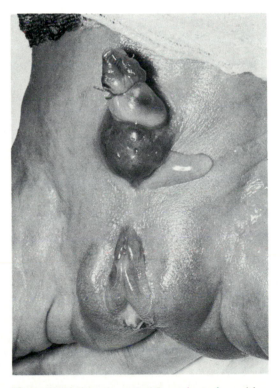

Figure 25.10. Superior vesical fissure in newborn girl. (Reproduced by permission of Year Book Medical Publishers.)

Cloacal exstrophy

Exstrophy of the cloaca represents the most extreme degree of the disorder. It is the result of dehiscence of the cloacal infraumbilical membranes at the 5 mm stage and before the formation of the urorectal septum. Anatomical details differ although most patients show the same basic deformities. An exstrophic hemibladder with its ureteric orifice lies on each side and between them is a zone of exposed intestinal mucosa with an upper and a lower orifice (*Figure 25.11*). The exstrophic bowel is the ileocaecal

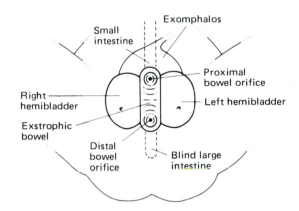

Figure 25.11. Anatomy of classic cloacal exstrophy.

region, the upper orifice being the terminal ileum which commonly prolapses. The lower orifice leads to a short length of colon that ends blindly in front of the sacrum. Sometimes the orifice of the appendix is visible and on occasions there are two appendices. Above the area of exstrophy is a large exomphalos containing bowel and often liver. The anus is imperforate (*Figure 25.12*).

Other congenital abnormalities are very commonly present. Soper and Kilger (1964) reviewed 57 cases of cloacal exstrophy. Of 30 in which the urinary tract was described 15 had gross unilateral or bilateral lesions such as multicystic kidney, renal aplasia or severe dysplasia and ureteric atresia or stricture. In the series of Johnston and Kogan (1974) seven of 16 cases showed similar renal and ureteric pathology. One boy had union between the ureters and the vasa deferentia bilaterally.

In boys the phallus is generally duplicated and each moiety is rudimentary. The penes were epispadial in all recorded cases except that of

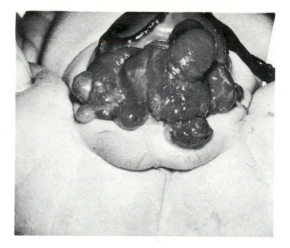

Figure 25.12. Cloacal exstrophy in a newborn boy showing a central bowel field between two bladder fields, a large exomphalos and no anus

Hall, McCandless and Rickham (1953) where each organ had a small central urethra. Bilateral cryptorchidism is almost invariable. Duplication of the genital tract of varying degree occurred in each of the four female cases of Johnston and Kogan (1974) and in 22 of 24 girls in Soper and Kilger's (1964) series. Some children with cloacal exstrophy have no external genitalia. Spina bifida of various grades of severity existed in six of Johnston and Kogan's (1974) 16 cases and in 32 of the 57 reviewed by Soper and Kilger (1964). The small intestine is often congenitally abnormally short and its effective length becomes even less when there is ileal prolapse.

Management

Although an untreated long-term survivor has been reported (Remigailo *et al.*, 1976), the child with cloacal exstrophy is generally born prematurely and unless corrective measures are undertaken promptly the profuse fluid losses from the short alimentary tract often quickly prove fatal. Whether or not intervention is warranted is a difficult ethical and moral problem. The most successful result of treatment is exemplified by an individual with both faecal and urinary stomas and, especially in the male, severe genital deformities. Frequently there are other problems arising from renal lesions and from spina bifida.

When treatment is considered to be justified, early intervention is needed. The exomphalos is

excised and the exposed bowel is separated from the hemibladder on each side. It may be necessary to resect the exstrophic bowel and fashion a terminal ileostomy, but often the open intestine can be tubularized and the extremity of the colon brought to the abdominal surface and opened so as to preserve a larger absorptive surface. The two hemibladders are sutured to each other and to the abdominal wall above. The child is thus left with a bladder exstrophy that later requires cutaneous urinary diversion and cystectomy.

Covered exstrophy and visceral sequestration

Embryologically, covered exstrophy is the result of delayed closure of the defect in the abdominal parietes following the formation of an exstrophy. Affected patients show the typical separation of the pubes and a wide linea alba and in some instances these are the only obvious abnormalities. Most cases of covered exstrophy represent late embryological closure of exstrophy of the bladder. The umbilicus is sited low and abuts on a paper-thin scar composed essentially of cutaneous epithelium and the anterior bladder wall. Often the child has epispadias although urinary control may be normal.

Johnston and Koff (1977) reported two boys with covered exstrophy of the cloaca. In each the lower abdominal wall was extremely thin. The bladder was bilobed in the sagittal plane and a short colon or the caecum opened into its posterior aspect. The upper urinary tract was normal apart from unilateral renal ectopia. The anus was imperforate. The penis and the urethra were normally formed but each child had incomplete urinary control as a result of sacral dysgenesis. The authors suggested that dehiscence of the upper portion of the infra-umbilical membrane occurred at the 5 mm stage to produce cloacal exstrophy and that later mesodermal and ectodermal infiltration closed the defect secondarily while further visceral development did not occur.

Variations on the same theme have been recorded. In the patient of Koontz, Joshi and Ownby (1974) there was a partially covered exstrophy of the cloaca in which the exstrophied zone was confined to the umbilical region. Williams (1974) and Emery, Campbell and Hodges (1974) described examples of unilateral exstrophy with a contralateral normally formed hemibladder. Duplication of the hindgut and imperforate anus may coexist in such cases.

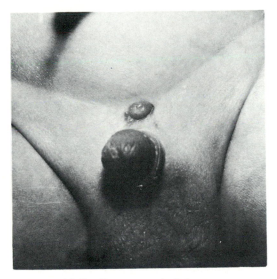

Figure 25.13. Duplicate exstrophy in boy.

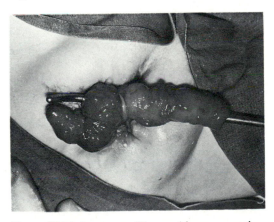

Figure 25.14. A segment of ileum, with mucosa on the exterior, sequestrated on the abdominal surface in a girl with epispadias. The alimentary tract was intact.

Some instances of covered exstrophy show secondary parietal closure leading to the sequestration of portions of viscera on the body surface. In duplicate exstrophy a small area of bladder wall is situated on the abdominal skin; the underlying bladder is intact and as a rule the urethra is normal (*Figure 25.13*). In Johnston and Penn's (1966) case of incomplete cloacal exstrophy the proctodaeum and part of the rectum were completely exteriorized on the perineum. In the girl shown in *Figure 25.14* a T-shaped segment of small intestine with its mucosal surface on the exterior was attached just posterior to the vaginal introitus. The exteriorized bowel had no communication with the intact alimentary tract. The child had a double clitoris and an epispadial urethra; total urinary incontinence necessitated diversion. A very similar lesion in a boy was recorded by Williams (1974). In his case the extra-abdominal bowel was attached to the pubic region above the penis.

Associated genital abnormalities

In some cases of exstrophy there are genital anomalies that appear to be coincidental and unrelated to the basic embryological fault. Johnston and Kogan (1974) recorded vaginal atresia with hydrocolpos in a girl with bladder exstrophy, and also total absence of the external genitalia in a baby of undetermined sex with exstrophy of the cloaca. Vaginal aplasia with bladder exstrophy was reported by Ezell and Carlson (1970). As a rule the genital lesions seen with exstrophy can be attributed to the wedge effect of the infraumbilical membrane which holds apart and prevents normal union of the originally paired genital tubercles and of the müllerian ducts.

In the female duplication of the clitoris is almost invariable, even with mild degrees of epispadias, and the labia majora are wide apart anteriorly. Various degrees of duplication of the uterus and the vagina are nearly always present with exstrophy of the cloaca. They occurred in 22 of the 24 female cases reported by Soper and Kilger (1964). In Johnston and Kogan's (1974) series three of four girls with cloacal exstrophy had vaginal duplication and the fourth had a double uterus. In cases of bladder exstrophy the female genital tract is usually single although double vagina has been recorded (Johnston and Kogan, 1974). Duplex vaginas often lie in the sagittal rather than the expected coronal plane or may be obliquely arranged.

Management of the female genital anomalies depends on their degree. Double uterus generally needs no interference. With vaginal duplication, division of an intervening septum may be all that is required. When the vaginas are widely separated excision of one vagina and hemiuterus may be needed. Because of the pelvic bony abnormality and the resulting gap in the pelvic diaphragm, pregnancy in women who have had bladder exstrophy carries the strong possibility of fetal malpresentation and of prepartum, intrapartum or postpartum uterine prolapse (Krisiloff *et al.*, 1978).

Allen, Spence and Salver (1974) described techniques for improving the appearance of the external genitalia in women who have epispadias or have undergone excision of an exstrophic bladder. Resection of the skin over the pubic gap and approximation of flaps raised from each side produces a normal pubic hair distribution. The two clitorides are mobilized and joined to form a single midline organ.

In the boy with bladder exstrophy or with epispadias alone the penis is abnormally short and is tilted and curved upwards. The chordee is due partly to fibrous bands on the penile dorsum and partly to the shortness of the

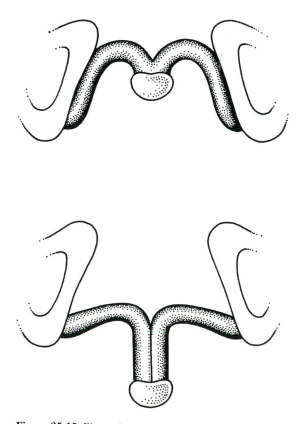

Figure 25.15. Elongation of the penis by partial separation of the crura from the puboischial rami.

urethra which produces a bow-string effect. Its elimination requires the fibrosis to be excised and the urethra to be mobilized from the corpora cavernosa and allowed to retract proximally. Any residual intrinsic corporal curvature can be corrected by the excision of one or more transverse ellipses of tunica albuginea from the ventrum of the penis. Resuture of the edges straightens the shaft.

The shortness of the penis is caused mainly by the separation of the pubic bones. The length of each corpus cavernosum is essentially normal but much of it is wasted between the shaft and the bony attachment. In order to lengthen the penis the extrapenile parts of the corpora cavernosa must be advanced into the penile body. Approximation of the pubic bones does not help in this regard since correction of the bony deformity leads to a forward tilting of the front of the pelvis and the penis retracts behind the pubis to become even less prominent than before. The most effective technique is to detach the penile crura partially from their puboischial insertions (*Figure 25.15*; Johnston, 1975) Complete separation of the crura from the bone as described by Kelley and Eraklis (1971) appears to carry an appreciable risk of injuring the neurovascular bundle that enters the extremity of the crus and causing penile devascularization or denervation.

Skin cover for the denuded penis is best obtained by using the redundant ventral foreskin. Separation of the two layers of the prepuce produces a large skin surface which is then incised longitudinally before each half is brought to the penile dorsum. Alternatively when sufficient preputial skin is not available a split-skin graft may be applied (*Figure 25.16*) or the penile shaft may be buried temporarily under the skin on the front of the scrotum and then freed some 3 months later at which time the ventrum is covered with scrotal flaps. With the latter method it is difficult to achieve a close skin fit for the penis and the appearance is often unsatisfactory.

Penile lengthening and chordee correction are carried out at the same operative session. About 6 months later a penile urethra may be constructed from a dorsal skin strip and a glandular urethra fashioned by suturing in apposition de-epithelialized triangles from each side of the splayed-open glans. The formation of a penoglandular urethra is essential in the continent patient. However, if urinary diversion has been

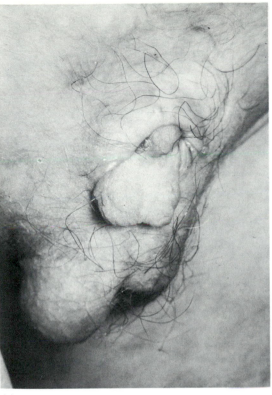

(a)

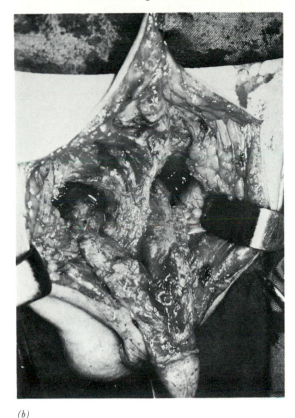

(b)

Figure 25.16. Penile lengthening in a 12-year-old boy who had had reconstruction of an exstrophic bladder and later a urinary diversion. *(a)* Before surgery. Only the tip of the glans is visible. *(b)* During operation. The penile crura are mobilized from the bone. A free skin graft is applied because of insufficient local skin. *(c)* Appearance 2 years after surgery.

performed then a neourethra that is not transporting urine is very prone to stricture. In these circumstances, although the glandular deformity may be corrected early for cosmetic reasons, it is preferable to defer full urethral construction until seminal emissions begin after puberty. When a split-skin graft has been employed to cover a denuded penile shaft the formation of a penile urethra may not be possible. Nevertheless, in circumstances in which grafting is necessary the penis before operation is generally extremely short and the patient is usually perfectly satisfied with a serviceable phallus and is not overconcerned about the site of emergence of seminal fluid.

The late results of male genital reconstruction for epispadias and bladder exstrophy have been reviewed by Hanna and Williams (1972). All patients reported good erections and most were capable of satisfactory copulation. A normal

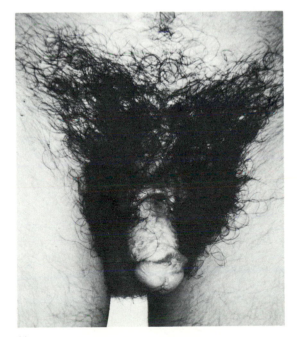

(c)

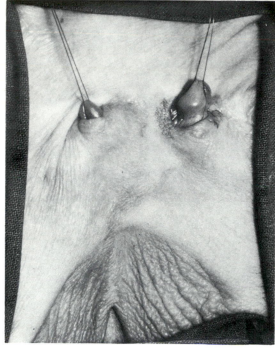

(a)

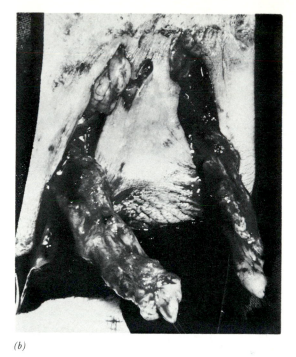

(b)

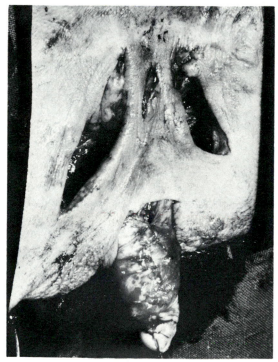

(c)

seminal analysis was found in most patients with epispadias but in only one of eight men who had had bladder exstrophy. Lattimer (1978) had three male exstrophy patients who fathered children. Retrograde ejaculation may occur through an incompetent bladder neck but an important danger to future fertility is iatrogenic damage to the verumontanum and ejaculatory apparatus caused by surgery aimed at producing a continent bladder outlet.

During early childhood the surgeon tends to concentrate on the purely urological aspects of bladder exstrophy and epispadias. However, it is important that bladder and urethral surgery should not jeopardize the boy's chances of becoming a sexually active man. Lattimer (1973) has shown from patient questionnaires that the boy and his parents are often concerned mainly with the possibility of his possessing a penis of normal appearance and adequate function and less with where his urine emerges.

The boy with cloacal exstrophy generally has two very rudimentary widely separated penes and Tank and Lindenauer (1970) recommended that such patients be demasculinized and raised as girls. When a male role has already been

Figure 25.17. Minute double hemiphalli in a 6-year-old boy born with cloacal exstrophy. *(a)* Before treatment. *(b)* The hemiphalli are mobilized from their bony attachments. *(c)* The hemiphalli are joined to form a single organ emerging just above the scrotum and a free skin graft is applied.

allocated it is possible by freeing and lengthening each penis from its bony attachments to unite them, apply a skin graft and fashion an acceptable, if not normal, organ (*Figure 25.17*).

References

Allen, T.D., Spence, H.M. and Salver, K.E. (1974) Reconstruction of the external genitalia in exstrophy of the bladder. *Journal of Urology*, **111**, 830

Arap, S. (1980) Personal communication

Cendron, J. and Petit, P. (1971) Symposium on treatment of complete exstrophy of the urinary bladder. *Annales Chirurgie Infantiles*, **6**, 359

Chisholm, T.C. (1969) Exstrophy of the bladder. *In* Pediatric Surgery (edited by Mustard, W.T., Ravitch, M.M., Snyder, W.H., Welch, K.J. and Benson, C.D.). Year Book Medical Publishers, Chicago.p.1213

Chisholm, T.C. (1979) Exstrophy of the urinary bladder. *In* Pediatric Surgery, 3rd edn (edited by Ravitch, M.M., Welch, K.J., Benson, C.D., Aberdeen, E. and Randolph, J.G.). Year Book Medical Publishers, Chicago. p.1239

Cibert, J. and Cibert, J. (1965) Traitement de l'incontinence urinaire feminine avant 15 ans. *Annales Chirurgie Infantiles*, **6**, 255

Clark, M.A. and O'Connell, K.V. (1973) Scanning and transmission electron microscopic studies of an exstrophic human bladder. *Journal of Urology*, **110**, 481

Culp, D.A. (1964) Histology of the exstrophied bladder. *Journal of Urology*, **91**, 538

Culp, O.S. (1973) Treatment of epispadias with and without urinary incontinence: experience with 48 patients. *Journal of Urology*, **109**, 120

Dees, J.E. (1949) Congenital epispadias with incontinence. *Journal of Urology*, **62**, 513

Duckett, J.W. (1977) The use of paraexstrophy skin pedicle grafts for correction of exstrophy and epispadias repair. Birth Defects Original Article Series, Vol. 13, No.5 (edited by Bergsma, D. and Duckett, J.W.). Liss, New York. p.175

Emery, J.A., Campbell, J.R. and Hodges, C.V. (1974) Duplication of the hindgut: low male imperforate anus and unilateral exstrophy of the bladder. *Journal of Urology*, **112**, 532

Engel, R.M.E. (1973) Bladder exstrophy: vesicoplasty or urinary diversion. *Urology*, **2**, 20

Ezell, W.W. and Carlson, H.E. (1970) A realistic look at exstrophy of the bladder. *British Journal of Urology*, **42**, 197

Fisher, J.H. and Retik, A.B. (1969) Exstrophy of the bladder. *Journal of Pediatric Surgery*, **4**, 620

Hall, E.G., McCandless, A.E. and Rickham, P.P. (1953) Vesicointestinal fissure with diphallus. *British Journal of Urology*, **25**, 219

Hanna, M.K. and Williams, D.I. (1972) Genital function in males with vesical exstrophy and epispadias. *British Journal of Urology*, **44**, 169

Higgins, C.C. (1962) Exstrophy of the bladder: report of 158 cases. *Annals of Surgery*, **28**, 99

Jacobsen, B.E. and Olesen, S. (1968) Bladder exstrophy complicated by adenocarcinoma. *Danish Medical Bulletin*, **15**, 253

Jeffs, R.D. (1978) Exstrophy and cloacal exstrophy. *In* Urologic Clinics of North America, Vol. 5, No. 1 (edited by McNally, K.S.), Saunders, Philadelphia. p.127

Jeffs, R.D., Charrois, R., Many, M. and Juriansz, A.R. (1972) Primary closure of the exstrophied bladder. *In* Current Controversies in Urologic Management (edited by Scott, R., Gordon, H.L., Scott, F.B., Carlton, C.E. and Beach, P.D.). Saunders, Philadelphia. p.235

Johnston, J.H. (1975) The genital aspects of exstrophy. *Journal of Urology*, **113**, 701

Johnston, J.H. (1977) Exstrophy of the bladder and epispadias. *In* Operative Surgery: Urology, 3rd edn (edited by Williams, D.I.). Butterworths, London. p.228

Johnston, J.H. and Koff, S.A. (1977) Covered cloacal exstrophy: another variation on the theme. *Journal of Urology*, **118**, 666

Johnston, J.H. and Kogan, S.J. (1974) The exstrophic anomalies and their surgical reconstruction. Current Problems in Surgery. Year Book Medical Publishers, Chicago

Johnston, J.H. and Penn, I.A. (1966) Exstrophy of the cloaca. *British Journal of Urology*, **38**, 302

Johnston, T.B. (1913) Extroversion of the bladder complicated by the presence of intestinal openings on the surface of the extroverted area. *Journal of Anatomy*, **48**, 89

Kelley, J.H. and Eraklis, A.J. (1971) A procedure for lengthening of the phallus in boys with exstrophy of the bladder. *Journal of Pediatric Surgery*, **6**, 645

King, L.R. and Wendell, E.F. (1972) Primary cystectomy and permanent urinary diversion in the treatment of exstrophy of the urinary bladder. *In* Current Controversies in Urologic Management (edited by Scott, R., Gordon, H.L., Scott, F.B., Carlton, C.E. and Beach, P.D.). Saunders, Philadelphia. p.244

Klauber, G.T. and Williams, D.I. (1974) Epispadias with incontinence. *Journal of Urology*, **111**, 110

Koontz, W.W., Joshi, V.V. and Ownby, R. (1974) Cloacal exstrophy with the potential for urinary control: an unusual presentation. *Journal of Urology*, **112**, 828

Krisiloff, M., Puckner, P.J., Tretter, W., McFarlane, M.T. and Lattimer, J.K. (1978) Pregnancy in women with bladder exstrophy. *Journal of Urology*, **119**, 478

Lattimer, J.K. (1973) Communication to the International Society of Urology, Amsterdam

Lattimer, J.K. (1978) Fertility in exstrophy of the bladder. Society for Pediatric Urology Newsletter, July 19

Lattimer, J.K., Beck, L., Yeaw, S., Puckner, P.J., McFarlane, M.T. and Krisiloff, M. (1978) Long-term follow-up after exstrophy closure: late improvement and good quality of life. *Journal of Urology*, **119**, 664

Leadbetter, G.W. (1964) Surgical correction of total urinary incontinence. *Journal of Urology*, **91**, 261

Leadbetter, G.W. and Fraley, E.E. (1967) Surgical correction of total urinary incontinence: 5 years later. *Journal of Urology*, **97**, 869

Marshall, V.F. and Muecke, E.C. (1968) Malformations. *In* Encyclopedia of Urology, Vo.7, Part 1 (edited by Alken, C.E., Dix, V.W., Goodain, W.E., Weyrauch, W.M. and Wildbolz, E.). Springer-Verlag, New York.p.191

Marshall, V.F. and Muecke, E.C. (1970) Functional closure of typical exstrophy of the bladder. *Journal of Urology*, **104**, 205

Megalli, M. and Lattimer, J.K. (1973) Review of the management of 140 cases of exstrophy of the bladder. *Journal of Urology*, **109**, 246

Raghavaiah, N.V. and Reddy, C.R.R.M. (1976) Adenocarcinoma of the bladder in a boy. *Journal of Urology*, **116**, 526

Remigailo, R.V., Woodard, J.R., Andrews, H.G. and Patterson, J.H. (1976) Cloacal exstrophy: 18 year survival of untreated case. *Journal of Urology*, **116**,811

Rickham, P.P. (1961) The incidence and treatment of ectopia vesicae. *Proceedings of the Royal Society of Medicine*, **54**,389

Ruden, L., Tannenbaum, M. and Lattimer, J.K. (1972) Histologic analysis of the exstrophic bladder after anatomic closure. *Journal of Urology*, **108**,802

Semerdjian, H.S., Texter, J.H. and Yawn, D.H. (1972) Rhabdomyosarcoma occuring in repaired exstrophic bladder: case report. *Journal of Urology*, **108**,354

Soper, R.T. and Kilger, K. (1964) Vesico-intestinal fissure. *Journal of Urology*, **92**,496

Spence, H.M. (1966) Ureterosigmoidostomy for exstrophy of the bladder. *British Journal of Urology*, **38**,36

Stagner, R.V. and Hodges, C.V. (1963) Experiences with exstrophy of the bladder. *Journal of Urology*, **89**,53

Tanagho, E.A. and Smith, D.R. (1972) Clinical evaluation of a surgical technique for the correction of complete urinary incontinence. *Journal of Urology*, **107**, 402

Tank, E.S. and Lindenauer, S.M. (1970) Principles of management of exstrophy of the cloaca. *American Journal of Surgery*, **119**,95

Toguri, A.G., Churchill, B.M., Schillinger, J.F. and Jeffs,

R.D. (1978) Continence in cases of bladder exstrophy. *Journal of Urology*, **119**,538

Trendelenberg, F. (1906) Treatment of ectopia vesicae. *Annals of Surgery*, **44**,281

Turner, W.R., Ransley, P.G. and Williams, D.I. (1980) Patterns of renal damage in the management of vesical exstrophy. *Journal of Urology*, **124**,412

Welch, K.J. (1969) Epispadias. *In* Pediatric Surgery (edited by Mustard, W.T., Ravitch, M.M., Snyder, W.H., Welch, K.J. and Benson, C.D.). Year Book Medical Publishers, Chicago. p.1333

Williams, D.I. (1974) Epispadias and exstrophy. *In* Encyclopedia of Urology, Vol. 15, Suppl. (edited by Andersson, L., Gittes, R.F., Goodwin, W.E., Lutzeyer, W. and Zingg, E.). Springer-Verlag, New York. p.266

Williams, D.I. and Keeton, J.E. (1973) Further progress with reconstruction of the exstrophied bladder. *British Journal of Surgery*, **60**,203

Williams, D.I. and Snyder, H.N. (1976) Anterior detrusor tube repair for urinary incontinence in children. *British Journal of Urology*, **48**,671

Young, H.H. (1922) An operation for the cure of incontinence associated with epispadias. *Journal of Urology*, **7**,1

26   Enuresis

W. Keith Yeates

The term enuresis should be used to refer only to the condition of repeated involuntary acts of micturition in childhood without detectable urological or neurological cause. It should not be used synonymously with urinary incontinence of which enuresis is just one type.

Mature bladder function

The final objective in the development of bladder function is the degree of bladder control of the normal adult. The features of normal micturition in the adult during the day can be summarized on a diagrammatic filling and

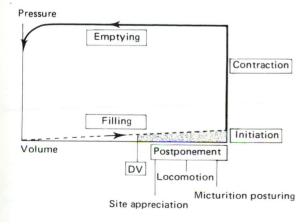

Figure 26.1. The micturition cycle showing the main features of mature bladder function. DV = the sensation of bladder distension

emptying cystometrogram (*Figure 26.1*). During filling at physiological rates the intravesical pressure remains low. The sensation of bladder distension is felt when the bladder is about two thirds full. Bladder contraction does not occur until the premicturition requirements of reaching a socially acceptable micturition site, adjusting the clothing and adopting a micturition posture have been completed. Therefore in addition to the possession of a water-tight outlet during filling, bladder control during the day depends on two basic factors, namely the appreciation of a moderate degree of bladder distension and the ability to inhibit bladder contraction. To these should be added the ability to initiate micturition at any convenient time.

Bladder function in the adult during the night is represented by bladder filling short of the desire to micturate. The functional capacity of the normal bladder easily accommodates the output of urine during the night on a fluid intake dictated by thirst rather than by social habits. If greater bladder distension occurs during sleep, the sensation awakens the individual. Bladder control during sleep therefore depends on both the adequacy of the bladder capacity and the ability to be wakened by bladder distension. Deficiency of only one of these factors does not produce nocturnal incontinence.

In summary, mature bladder function is characterized by such great powers of voluntary postponement and initiation that micturition interferes minimally with the day's activities and allows a full night's sleep. At no time should there be inappropriate cerebral stimulation of micturition.

Bladder function in childhood

For about the first 6 months of life the bladder responds to distension by immediate evacuation. The stream is forceful and emptying is complete, and the child is dry until the next act 1 or 2 hours later. During the following 2 years there is a progressive decrease of frequency, fluctuating as the child acquires other new skills. At some time during this period the infant begins to convey to its mother that it is about to micturate and unconsciously inhibits micturition for increasing lengths of time. The decrease in frequency naturally allows longer periods of dry sleep, and finally wakening can be caused by the sensation of bladder distension.

The order of development of bladder control varies. In some infants the frequency of micturition decreases first, in others wakening from sleep by bladder distension occurs first and in some both signs of control appear together. Involuntary stimulation of micturition is not recognizable as an entity but, if it is occurring, maturation brings about its cessation.

Enuresis

The reported incidence of enuresis varies somewhat with different authors' definitions. This is so particularly in the frequency required for it to be included in a series of cases, for example wetting more than one night a month. In the UK mature bladder function is achieved in about 77 per cent of children aged 3 and in 90 per cent by the age of 5 (Miller *et al.*, 1960). In other countries such as the USA, Australia and Sweden the average age of attaining bladder control is different (Oppel, Harper and Rider, 1968).

Delayed development of one or both of the two main factors in bladder control, that is sensation and inhibition, results in the production of different clinical pictures. In 50 per cent of cases there is both nocturnal incontinence and diurnal urgency and frequency. There may also be incontinence during the day, particularly if the child is preoccupied, and this is presumably a manifestation of deficiency in sensation. In 10 per cent of patients there are only the diurnal symptoms of frequency and urgency. In the remaining 40 per cent the obvious dysfunction is nocturnal incontinence, although sometimes detailed enquiry elicits a history of a minor degree of frequency and urgency also during the day in contrast to children who have complete bladder control at night. The nocturnal incontinence may occur one or more times during the night, every night or nearly every night, or at irregular intervals. Often a child is wet for a few nights in succession followed by some days or weeks of dry nights. The exacerbation may be clearly related to emotional situations or to changes in the weather or environment, but frequently there is no obvious or admitted cause. Although there is clearly a hereditary factor in many cases of enuresis the effect of a similar environment makes the importance of heredity among the children of one family difficult to assess.

The majority of cases of enuresis, at least under the age of 5, appear to be due to failure to develop bladder control. However, in about 15 per cent the symptoms appear in children who had gained satisfactory bladder control at least a year previously. This is often referred to as onset enuresis and clearly cannot be attributed simply to delay in maturation. These patients can be regarded as having latent enuresis that has been made manifest by some often unknown change of circumstances (Yeates, 1973).

Enuresis naturally tends to disappear progressively as the child gets older, girls gaining control much faster than boys. In many the cessation of enuresis occurs at puberty, leaving about 2 per cent still enuretic at the age of 15 (Miller *et al.*, 1960). About half of this small remainder continue to have enuresis into adult life. Where there is a strong family history of enuresis the age of acquiring control is often very similar in members of the same family. It is fortunately rare for nocturnal enuresis to persist into adult life, but it is very common for individuals who have had enuresis with diurnal urgency and frequency to continue to have a reduced functional bladder capacity with urgency during the day and sometimes with nocturnal frequency which wakens them. A common syndrome is the youth or young adult whose nocturnal enuresis ceases about puberty yet constantly recurs after drinking a few pints of beer late in the evening.

Mechanism

Many aspects of bladder function continue to be very imperfectly understood, but it is useful to

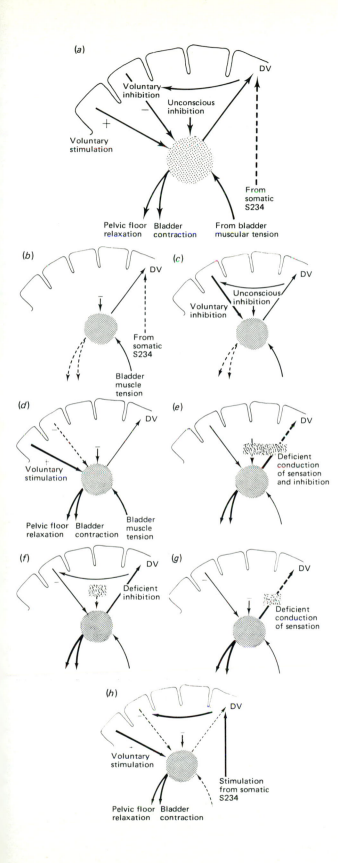

Figure 26.2. Working hypotheses of bladder control. *(a)* The functional micturition centre and its connections. *(b)* The desire to micturate. *(c)* Normal inhibition of bladder contraction. *(d)* Micturition. *(e)* Deficiency of both unconscious inhibition and conduction of sensation. *(f)* Deficient unconscious inhibition. *(g)* Deficient conduction of bladder sensation. *(h)* Bladder irritability induced by somatic afferents from cystitis.

have a working hypothesis. Coordinated micturition (that is a sustained bladder contraction combined with reciprocal relaxation of the pelvic floor) requires reflex arcs about as high as the upper part of the brainstem and the hypothalamus, and it is useful to conceive of there being a functional micturition centre at this site (*Figure 26.2a*). Even in infancy micturition is a coordinated act so that it occurs through the same centre. This centre is charged by impulses from the distending bladder. When a sufficient number have accumulated the tension in the centre is transmitted to the cerebral cortex producing an early warning of bladder distension (*Figure 26.2b*). The tendency for the centre to fire down the efferent tract to stimulate bladder contraction is suppressed by unconscious inhibitory impulses from the basal ganglia and the cerebral cortex (*Figure 26.2c*). Later these are reinforced by inhibitory impulses from the cortex. When micturition is desired the excitatory state in the centre is supplemented by stimulation from the cerebral cortex combined with removal of the inhibition (*Figure 26.2d*). Micturition then occurs by the combination of a sustained bladder contraction with reciprocal relaxation of the pelvic floor.

The first part of maturation, namely an increase in the functional bladder capacity, can be thought of as due to the development of involuntary inhibition later supplemented by voluntary inhibition from the frontal cortex. One cause of frequency and one aspect of urgency are due to delay in the development of unconscious inhibition (*Figure 26.2f*). The frequency is owing to the relative reduction in bladder capacity so that the bladder reaches its functional capacity during the night. Delay in the development of the sensory tracts from the centre to the sensory cortex (*Figure 26.2g*) results in the other mechanism of urgency such that impulses break through from the centre to the sensory cortex only when the centre is fully charged at the onset of the bladder contraction. This deficiency of sensory transmission also accounts for unawareness of bladder distension and for micturition during sleep when the functional bladder capacity has been reduced by a concomitant delay in the development of inhibition (*Figure 26.2e*). In addition deficiency in bladder sensation explains associated occasions of unconscious incontinence during the day, especially when the child is preoccupied with other interests.

Maturation appears to be due to the progressive development of function in these tracts, the variable pattern of enuresis depending on their different rate or order of development. As previously mentioned the rate and the pattern of maturation often seem to have a genetic basis.

It is not easy to explain nocturnal incontinence in the complete absence of diurnal symptoms without invoking the mechanism of unconscious active stimulation of the centre by the frontal cortex during sleep (*Figure 26.2d*). This could well be the important factor in episodes of incontinence during the day associated with behaviour disorders.

Clinical aspects

Children with enuresis may be referred to hospital on account of the delay in the development of bladder control itself or due to other conditions, the enuresis coming to light on routine enquiry. Although, as the corollary of the definition of enuresis, there are no detectable organic causative factors in the great majority of cases, in some there are associated abnormalities of the CNS or the urinary tract which merit discussion.

Abnormalities of the CNS

Mental deficiency

Mental deficiency is commonly associated with urinary incontinence of enuretic type which is presumably the result of general delayed cerebral development.

Minor habit disorders

It is frequently stated that there is an association between enuresis and deviant behaviours such as nail biting, tics, temper tantrums, thumb sucking and so on. However, such assessments were carried out before the use of sophisticated statistical methods, and their significance is difficult to judge.

Psychological disorders

Repeated careful studies by many workers have failed to show any consistent psychological disorder with enuresis. However, there is a high incidence of enuresis in deprived children in institutions which often ceases dramatically when the child is brought into hospital. It is also a common clinical observation that enuresis stops when any child is away from home, on holiday, or admitted to hospital. In summary, deficient bladder control of enuretic type is common in a number of abnormal mental states (when involuntary stimulation of micturition may be an important factor) while there is no evidence that an abnormal mental state is a causative factor in the ordinary case of enuresis. Similarly, electroencephalography may show abnormalities in epileptic children with nocturnal incontinence, but there are no characteristic findings in enuretic patients when fits have not actually been observed.

Abnormalities in the urinary tract

Infection

Urinary tract infection is related to enuresis in the following ways:

1. In the vast majority of cases there is no urinary tract infection.
2. Urinary tract infection may appear to be purely coincidental as shown by enuresis having been present beforehand and continuing after treatment has removed the infection.
3. Urinary tract infection may appear to have precipitated the enuresis and when the infection clears up the enuresis ceases. It is easiest to think of these cases as latent enuresis which becomes manifest when the bladder capacity is decreased and urgency is increased by mucosal irritation (*Figure 26.2h*).

Anatomical abnormalities

Enuresis has been attributed to apparent radiological abnormalities such as a wide bladder neck or mucosal folds in the posterior urethra, which have subsequently been found to be just variations of the normal, or to phimosis or meatal stenosis. Ureteric reflux may be found in the course of investigation of enuresis. Although it is true that enuresis sometimes ceases following corrective surgery of genitourinary abnormalities (as it sometimes does following appendicectomy), it is very difficult

either theoretically to imagine or statistically to show that there is any true causal relationship.

Investigation of bladder function

Functional bladder capacity

This should be measured after the child has postponed micturition for as long as possible and it is very often reduced in enuresis. Patients with frequency and urgency have an average capacity of about half that of control cases. Those that manifest only nocturnal incontinence have on average a bladder capacity about two thirds that of normal controls (Zaleski, Gerrard and Shokeir, 1973).

Intravenous urography

No abnormality is present except that the bladder capacity sometimes looks reduced. This is also the only common finding on cystography.

Cystoscopy

The only abnormality is that often the bladder capacity is reduced, and under a light anaesthetic there is often deep respiration at a significantly smaller capacity than one would expect in normal children. In older enuretics there is sometimes a moderate degree of bladder trabeculation and the appearance of a posterior bar at the bladder neck on both micturation cystourethrography and cystourethroscopy.

Urodynamic studies

The history suggests that on filling uninhibited contractions will be readily demonstrable in all cases with frequency and urgency. It is true that such uninhibited contractions are much more frequently found in patients with frequency and urgency than in those with nocturnal incontinence alone, but the correlation is not nearly as close as one might expect.

The desire to micturate is often immediately followed by a contraction wave, although sometimes the sensation is delayed until the contraction wave has actually begun. In adults with enuresis the flow rate is often greatly increased. The urethral pressure profile is high and the patient can voluntarily squeeze the urethra particularly powerfully. Finally the bladder pressure, which is normal during free micturition, rises excessively when the patient voluntarily obstructs the urethra.

All these findings seem to be the result of the patient with long-standing frequency and urgency having to contract the pelvic floor a number of times a day to prevent leakage. It is easy to postulate that this voluntary obstruction at external sphincteral level will cause a blow-out of the prostatic urethra below the bladder neck giving the appearance of a posterior bar, exercise the bladder muscle against resistance and so produce bladder hypertrophy and a high rise of pressure on voluntarily obstructing the urethra during micturition (Yeates, 1973), and also explain the raised urethral pressure profile and the increased voluntary power to compress the urethra.

Differential diagnosis

As has been indicated organic findings in enuresis are coincidental. Nevertheless enuresis may mimic, in the vast majority of cases only superficially, important organic diseases that cause incontinence of urine. These include abnormalities of the CNS, particularly spina bifida, and local bladder abnormalities such as cystitis, bladder diverticula and true posterior urethral valves. However, in any of these conditions it is extremely rare for micturition itself to appear normal, the bladder to feel empty, the urine to be uninfected, and the child to be thriving. Persistent and doubtful cases warrant a thorough urological investigation, but positive organic findings are rare when the history is not suspicious of organic disease and the ordinary clinical examination is entirely negative.

Treatment

In exceptional cases where there is incidental urinary tract infection this should be treated as a priority.

Drugs

It is generally agreed that the most useful group of drugs are the tricyclic antidepressants. Although imipramine is probably the most widely used, clinical trials have not convincingly demonstrated that any one of this group is better than the others (Blackwell *et al.*, 1972). Their mechanism of action is not clearly understood. Unlike their effect on depression there is nearly always a response in the first week. These drugs appear to have a specific effect on bladder activity: whether centrally or peripherally is not know.

The effective dose varies from 25–75 mg at bed-time. All clinical trials do not report the same results, but on average the effects seem to relate more to the individual than to the dosage. Treatment should commence with 25 mg for a week and if this is not effective then the dose should be increased to 50 mg and then 75 mg the following 2 weeks. If there is no very obvious benefit by the end of the third week, the drug should be discontinued. Effective therapy should be maintained for 3 months in the first instance. Recurrence rates following withdrawal of the drug vary between 5–40 per cent. The results compare unfavourably with the much lower recurrence rate following withdrawal of the pad and bell (Dische, 1971) which should therefore take precedence in older children.

Pad-and-Bell therapy

The pad-and-bell alarm apparatus should be tried as a first line of treatment in children old enough to be enthusiastic about being dry and to cooperate in the use of the apparatus, which usually means aged 7 and over. Most children show a noticeable improvement after 1–4 weeks of therapy, but the results progressively improve up to 4 months when about 80 per cent are dry. Approximately 30 per cent subsequently relapse and they usually respond to a second course (Dische, 1971).

Operative procedures

Surgery has no part to play in enuresis in childhood. Overdistension of the bladder is difficult and unsatisfactory in children as it requires an epidural anaesthetic lasting for at least 2 hours to be successful.

The adult with enuresis

The few cases of enuresis with incapacitating urgency and/or nocturnal incontinence that persist into adult life should be seriously considered for surgical procedures. They rarely respond to drugs, which in any case it would be undesirable to continue indefinitely. The principle of treatment is to increase the functional bladder capacity by some means affecting only the bladder itself so that a night's output of urine can be accommodated and the contractile responses of the bladder to stretch are reduced. The nearer to the bladder muscle the treatment is applied the more likely are these objectives to be achieved.

Overdistension under epidural anaesthesia at systolic pressure for four periods of half an hour with 5 minutes rest has about a 30 per cent chance of producing considerable lasting improvement (Ramsden *et al.*, 1976). In persistent cases complete transection and resuture of the bladder wall about 2 cm above the bladder neck and interureteric bar with the theoretical object of dividing the nervous supply to the detrusor has given lasting excellent results in about 70 per cent of cases (Hindmarsh, Essenhigh and Yeates, 1977). Transection has much more beneficial effects than might be expected from postoperative cystometric investigations which demonstrate only partial denervation at most.

Fortunately there is quite a high incidence of spontaneous cessation of enuresis even as late as the early 30s. In very few cases indeed is enuresis in the otherwise normal individual a lifelong state.

References

Blackwell, B., Lipkin, J.O., Meyer, J.H., Kzma, R. and Boulter, W.V. (1972) Dose responses and relationships between anticholinergic activity and mood with tricyclic antidepressants. *Psychopharmacologia*, **25**, 205

Dische, S. (1971) Management of enuresis. *British Medical Journal*, ii, 33

Hindmarsh, J.R., Essenhigh, D.M. and Yeates, W.K. (1977) Bladder transection for adult enuresis. *British Journal of Urology*, **49**, 515

Miller, F.J.W., Court, S.D.M., Walton, W.S. and Knox, E.G. (1960) *In* Growing up in Newcastle upon Tyne. Oxford University Press, London. p.150

Oppel, W.C., Harper, P.A. and Rider, R.V. (1968) The age of attaining bladder control. *Pediatrics*, **42**, 614

Ramsden, P.D., Smith, J.C., Dunn, M. and Ardran, G.M. (1976) Distension therapy for the unstable bladder; later results including an assessment of repeat distensions. *British Journal of Urology*, **48**, 623

Yeates, W.K. (1973) Bladder function: increased frequency and nocturnal incontinence. *In* Bladder Control and Enuresis (edited by Kolvin, I., MacKeith, R.C. and Meadow, S.R.). Heinemann, London. p.155

Zaleski, A., Gerrard, J.W. and Shokeir, M.H.K. (1973) Nocturnal enuresis: the importance of a small bladder capacity. *In* Bladder Control and Enuresis (edited by Kolvin, I., MacKeith, R.C. and Meadow, S.R.). Heinemann, London. p.95

27 The Neuropathic Bladder

Herbert B. Eckstein and D. Innes Williams

Introduction

Normal micturition, or the ability to empty the bladder at will, is a complicated process that usually develops between the first and third years of life. Cortical and subcortical centres for micturition, spinal pathways and a special centre in the sacral part of the spinal cord all affect the bladder through peripheral, sympathetic and parasympathetic nerves, and must all be intact to ensure normal micturition. The normal anatomy (Donker, Dvoes and Van Ulden, 1976) and central nervous connections (Nathan, 1976) are described in detail in standard textbooks, while the various theories relating to the development of normal micturition and of the neuropathic bladder were discussed in detail in the previous edition of this volume (Eckstein, 1968). Recent work has centred mainly on the intrinsic nervous mechanisms and the role of cholinergic, alpha-adrenergic and beta-adrenergic receptors (El Badawi and Shenk, 1974; Caine and Raz, 1975; Sundin *et al.*, 1977). These developments are of interest in connection with the possible treatment of bladder dysfunction by pharmacological agents.

Causes

Damage to any of the nervous pathways to the bladder can result in neuropathic dysfunction. It is important to realize at the outset that in paediatric practice such interruption is ordinarily partial rather than complete, so that the clinical and pathological picture may be unexpected, confused and unpredictable and may not conform to the patterns classically described in the adult patient with traumatic paraplegia.

Myelomeningocele

Undoubtedly myelomeningocele is at present still the commonest cause of a neuropathic bladder in childhood. The importance of this major spinal abnormality is altering because of the overall declining birth rate, the changing medical attitude towards the treatment of severely handicapped neonates with myelomeningocele, and above all the possibility of antenatal diagnosis by the alpha-fetoprotein test with subsequent termination of pregnancy when indicated. These factors have already reduced the number of cases of myelomeningocele requiring treatment and will no doubt continue to do so in the years to come.

However, the small and often skin-covered lesions of sacral myelomeningocele cannot be detected by alpha-fetoprotein estimations, either on blood or on amniotic fluid, or for that matter by ultrasound investigation of the mother. There will therefore always remain a hard core of children with myelomeningocele who have a neuropathic bladder and in whom urinary incontinence and other related problems are a major factor.

There is no real correlation between the level of the myelomeningocele and the type of neuropathic bladder that develops. In clinical practice lesions of the cervical and dorsal spine may be associated with normal micturition and normal leg movement. The reason is that extensive cervical and dorsal spinal lesions result in a significant paralysis of the respiratory muscles and babies with high lesions are virtually certain to die soon after birth, so that there is a certain amount of selection. Infants with relatively minor lesions of the cervical or dorsal spine are likely to survive without significant neurological deficit. The majority of myelomeningoceles are in the lumbar region and the bladder is usually affected but there is no clear correlation between the level of the lesion or the associated lower limb paralysis and the type of neuropathic bladder. Nevertheless it is of great importance to realize that children with sacral lesions and minimal additional handicaps tend to develop obstructive uropathy due to the neuropathic bladder and that an overactive external sphincter is the usual cause of upper tract dilatation in these patients. The same comment applies to children with so-called sacral lipoma, which is essentially a skin-covered neural tube defect, and here again the chances of progressive upper tract dilatation are high. Since children with sacral myelomeningocele or sacral lipoma tend to be otherwise physically and mentally normal, the control and the management of the urinary tract is particularly important.

Sacral agenesis

Agenesis of the sacrum is relatively uncommon and is frequently associated with other congenital abnormalities such as anorectal agenesis. Children with sacral agenesis are likely to have a deficient bladder innervation and therefore a neuropathic bladder (Williams and Nixon, 1957).

In general the absence of three or less sacral segments does not interfere with normal micturition, while that of four or more is associated with urinary incontinence. As in the case of very low myelomeningoceles, sacral agenesis tends to be related to obstructive uropathy in association with incontinence, and again overactivity of the external sphincter appears to be the cause of outflow obstruction. Investigation and treatment must be aimed accordingly. Anorectal agenesis is not infrequently associated with sacral agenesis and a significant number of infants with anorectal agenesis have a urinary tract abnormality in any event, even if the sacrum is normal. It is therefore imperative to perform adequate urological investigations in all children born with anorectal agenesis.

Spinal dysraphism and diastematomyelia

Other vertebral abnormalities capable of affecting the spinal cord are not exceptionally uncommon and cannot always be detected by clinical examination of the spine. Spina bifida occulta has a variable significance. For example simple failure to fuse of the laminae of the fourth and fifth lumbar vertebrae is unlikely to be important, but if the spinal canal is noticeably widened at the same level or there is a hairy patch on the back there may well be cord involvement. A bony or cartilaginous spur transfixing the cord in the midline (diastematomyelia) or an attenuated and shortened filum terminale may produce traction injury of the spinal cord. This results in a neuropathic bladder in children who appear to be neurologically normal in infancy but develop urinary incontinence around 3 years of age or more. The child who has normal micturition initially and then becomes incontinent must be suspected of having spina bifida occulta, diastematomyelia or a tumour of the spinal cord and accordingly has to be investigated from a neurological and neurosurgical point of view.

Tumours affecting the spinal cord

Primary tumours of the spinal cord are rare, although secondary tumours causing spinal cord compression, especially in relation to neuroblastoma, are not infrequently seen. While such lesions may produce peripheral paralysis and obvious physical signs it is not unusual for a disturbance of micturition to be the initial symptom in an infant or child. Again, myelography and other relevant investigations are essential.

Trauma

Accidental injury to the vertebral column and the spinal cord is surprisingly rare in childhood in contrast to adult life. Traumatic paraplegia with a neuropathic bladder is occasionally seen following major road traffic injuries and the diagnosis should present no problems. On the other hand, surgical trauma to the nerve supply of the bladder is unfortunately not so uncommon after procedures for correction of either anorectal abnormalities or Hirschsprung's disease. Such trauma can usually be avoided by meticulous and careful dissection keeping close to the bowel wall. In relation to Hirschsprung's disease the operative procedures described by Rehbein (1959), Soave (1966) and Duhamel (1956) have a greatly reduced incidence of neuropathic damage to the bladder compared to the original pull-through procedure described by Swenson (1950).

Viral infections

Transverse myelitis occasionally produces a neuropathic bladder with or without associated paraplegia. Radiological investigations are unrewarding and the diagnosis is made essentially by the exclusion of other processes. Encephalitis associated with measles is a very rare cause. While retention of urine may develop during an episode of poliomyelitis the majority of patients so affected recover spontaneously with conservative treatment.

Osteomyelitis of the vertebral column

Osteomyelitis of the vertebrae in infancy may lead to overall spinal cord compression or localized interference with spinal pathways so that bladder function may be affected. This diagnosis should be considered as a possibility in the ill child who presents with a neuropathic bladder without obvious cause. The bladder disturbance may become apparent before any radiological changes can be detected in the vertebrae. A radioisotopic bone scan may be useful for early diagnosis of a pathological process in a vertebral body.

Occult neuropathic bladder

There are a considerable number of children who have symptoms suggesting a neuropathic bladder, namely incontinence, inadequate emptying, retention and subsequent infection or upper tract damage, and in whom a full neurological examination shows no deficit whatever. Radiological investigations and myelography of the vertebral column give completely normal results and there are no obvious congenital abnormalities. Concomitant bowel disturbance, generally in the form of constipation with overflow incontinence, is not unusual. It must be assumed that in this group of patients there is isolated damage, either congenital or acquired, to the nerve supply or to the intrinsic nervous mechanism of the bladder and at present the term occult neuropathic bladder must be accepted as a clinical diagnosis (Allen, 1979). It need not be assumed that the prognosis for these cases is as certain as it is in true neuropathies, and recovery of function is not unknown (*see* Chapter 19).

Types of neuropathic bladder

A great deal has been written about the various types of neuropathic bladder but such studies were essentially based on adult patients with traumatic paraplegia (Bors and Comarr, 1971). Clearly in children with congenital lesions or lesions acquired soon after birth the situation is different, and it is difficult to define the various types in spite of the many attempts at classification using radiological or urodynamic findings.

In the congenital neuropathic bladder normal function is unlikely to be preserved in either the detrusor or the sphincter system, yet both may exhibit independent hyperactivity or inactivity which in various combinations determines the functional disorder. Thus it is possible, although rare, for a relaxed sphincter system with an atonic detrusor to produce a situation where urine dribbles from a bladder that is not significantly distended. Much more often the bladder is found to be of large capacity and flaccid, emptying by overflow from a large residue. The wall of such a bladder tends to be thin and untrabeculated, and because of detrusor distension vesicoureteric reflux is likely to follow and upper tract dilatation may result. Other patients have a small capacity hyperactive contractile bladder with dyssynergic contraction of the external sphincter resulting in detrusor hypertrophy. While reflux is usually no major problem in these patients, severe hydronephrosis can be consequent upon the obstructive factor.

No type of bladder dysfunction remains unchanged over the years and it is for this reason that categorization is difficult. At birth the intravenous pyelogram seldom reveals major abnormalities in cases of myelomeningocele but Devens, Pompino and Kubler (1978) have shown that in a group not subjected to active treatment of the urinary tract there was a very considerable incidence in later life of upper tract dilatation and renal scarring. The age and the speed at which these changes occur are somewhat unpredictable. The passage of time associated with recurrent or continuous infection may convert a large flabby bladder into a small contracted one, while the bladder outlet obstruction resulting from sphincteral spasm may enlarge a small hyperactive bladder and rapidly increase the upper tract dilatation. The onset of infection is always deleterious as regards both the symptoms and the radiological changes, but some reversal may be obtained by control of infection together with elimination of obstruction. In the paediatric age group there is no correlation between the various types of neuropathic bladder, the site of the spinal lesion and the degree of paraplegia. Nevertheless cases of spina bifida occulta with tethered conus and of diastematomyelia are those most likely to show deteriorating neurological signs as growth progresses and the tension within the cord increases. Such deterioration may be observed in late childhood or adolescence. By contrast it is also among the lesser forms of spinal dysraphism that an apparent improvement in vesical control is observed as a result of voluntary effort.

Diagnosis and investigation

Diagnosis is concerned with the identification of a neuropathy as the cause of urinary tract symptoms and with the assessment of the consequences of the bladder dysfunction. In the majority of cases the spinal cord lesion is a clinically obvious myelomeningocele and there can be no doubt that the urinary disorder is of CNS origin. However, many children presenting to the urologist with frequency, urgency, incontinence, urinary tract infection and vesical retention have no immediately recognizable local abnormality as the cause of their complaint and may therefore be suspected of suffering from some form of spinal dysraphism or an occult neuropathic bladder. Investigation of these children should include full clinical neurological examination with particular attention to the territory of the sacral nerves, and other studies are essential. The entire vertebral column must be X-rayed, since high thoracic anomalies may well accompany lower ones; the lumbosacral region requires special study and the lower part of the sacrum must not be omitted. If the spine is clearly demonstrated and normal, it can be assumed that there is no congenital spinal cord anomaly which could be responsible for a bladder disorder. However, if spina bifida occulta, a localized widening of the interpedicular distance, diastematomyelia or a more complex bony deformity is revealed then a neuroradiological opinion should be sought and myelography planned. Simple sacral agenesis, if clear-cut, is seldom worth further radiological investigation because although it may be associated with a neuropathic bladder there is very little chance of remediable tethering of the conus.

Investigations directed towards the urinary tract are essential for adequate assessment, but on their own they can seldom make a positive diagnosis of neuropathic bladder (*Figure 27.1*). Micturating cystourethrograms often reveal a sacculated bladder with a relaxed neck, an absence of coordinated detrusor contractions and a large residual volume. The addition of pressure-flow measurements to the video studies provides information on detrusor instability, flow rate and external sphincteral spasm. Together all this evidence builds up a picture of the neuropathic bladder which can vitally affect management but which in young children may not be easy to differentiate from that of obstructive uropathy. The bethanecol stimulation test (Lapides, 1962) identifies the greater response of denervated muscle to chemical stimulation and has been claimed to be diagnostic in doubtful cases; however, it has not proved reliable in practice. Although electromyography of the anal and external urethral sphincters may be helpful in diagnosis (Firlit, 1979) the results can be difficult to interpret. In summary most congenital neuropathic bladders are easily recognized by clinical examination and spinal radiol-

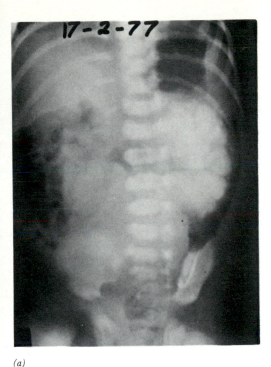
(a)

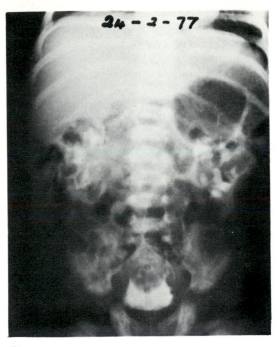
(b)

Figure 27.1. *(a)* Excretory urogram of an infant with a myelomeningocele showing large bladder and gross upper tract dilatation (routine postspinal-closure intravenous pyelogram). *(b)* Same patient. Excretory urogram after 1 week's drainage of bladder by urethral catheter. Note marked improvement in upper urinary tract.

ogy. Urinary tract investigations are concerned with monitoring the progress of the disease and occult neuropathies must always be subject to some doubt.

In cases of myelomeningocele the earliest investigations are simply urine analysis, plasma creatinine estimation and intravenous urography and are performed during the first month of life. The greatest danger in the first 2 years is from infection and urine culture should be undertaken monthly for this period with repeat intravenous urography at the end of it. Similar studies should be repeated at longer intervals throughout childhood. Cystograms are not necessary for the infant who has not had infection. Video studies together with cystometry may be required later when the choice of treatment regimen is to be made. Older children who have suffered from infection or show signs of upper tract dilatation may require the full gamut of tests. Mayo, Chapman and Shurtleff (1979) surveyed a series of fully investigated myelomeningocele cases and concluded that the amount of vesical residue and the fluoroscopic appearance of the bladder were the most valu-

able parameters for monitoring progress. Cystoscopy is seldom needed. Renal function studies may be necessary for follow-up in children with upper tract damage.

Management

The majority of children, and certainly of infants, with a neuropathic bladder suffer from spina bifida or myelomeningocele. In 1957 the development of shunt systems by Holter and Pudenz and others made the associated hydrocephalus a treatable condition, and from the early 1960s the majority of infants with myelomeningocele were treated as emergencies by primary back closure and subsequent shunt insertion. The review by Lorber (1971) suggested that the overall results of this approach were often unsatisfactory and since then a process of selection has been developed so that only those infants who have reasonable leg movement and a fair prognosis are treated.

In such infants the back is still closed within 24 hours and a shunt is inserted as soon as progressive hydrocephalus is evident. Since many of these children have paralysis and deformity of their lower limbs a team approach to the problem is necessary, and the urologist or paediatric surgeon must become involved in the care of the urinary tract. With all types of neuropathic bladder the child is incontinent with varying elements of sphincter weakness, outflow obstruction and detrusor hyperactivity. There is a risk of developing hydronephrosis with complicating infection, pyelonephritis and renal failure. Management must therefore take into account the relief of incontinence together with the preservation of the kidneys. Both these objectives demand that the bladder is regularly emptied by voluntary effort, expression, catheterization or even ultimately diversion. In the first 2–3 years of life a child with a normal upper urinary tract may continue untreated, although often regular expression can be helpful. More active management at this stage is only indicated by recurrent infection and increasing vesical residue.

As the child grows and approaches school age management decisions become increasingly important. Many of those with continuous incontinence and without serious retention can carry on wearing napkins for a much longer period. Children with lesser degrees of lower limb paralysis and less severe involvement of the bladder are most keen to attain some voluntary continence and in a few cases drug therapy may help them to do so. Increasingly in recent years intermittent catheterization has been employed, particularly for children of 7 years and over who can manage the instrument themselves. For the obese chair-bound paraplegic girl diversion still holds its place. Each of the common methods of management must be considered separately.

Bladder expression

Expression of the bladder or the so-called Credé manoeuvre is a well recognized procedure. It is certainly applicable to newborn infants with myelomeningocele once their backs have healed completely, but should on no account be employed until this has taken place because wound breakdown, infection and possibly meningitis could otherwise result. Early bladder expression reduces the residual urine to a minimum and leads to a reduction in urinary tract infection. Some older children can be managed perfectly well by regular 3-hourly bladder expression provided that they are cooperative and the mother and the school nurse are prepared to help. Such bladder expression can only work if the child has a large capacity bladder and sufficient outflow obstruction so as not to dribble continually, and does not suffer from massive reflux and hydronephrosis. This procedure should always be attempted since it is less invasive and interfering than any of the other methods. In clinical practice as a long-term technique of keeping the child dry it is probably successful in about 10 per cent of myelomeningocele patients with a neuropathic bladder.

Drug management

Chemotherapy, either intermittent or continuous, is frequently required for the control or prevention of infection in the neuropathic bladder, while drugs aimed specifically at the neuromuscular mechanisms have only a small place. Success can be claimed in selected cases, often when drugs are an adjuvant to other methods of management.

There are a few older children who can void by voluntary effort with only a small residue and yet are incontinent because of frequency and urgency. Cystometrograms in such cases show detrusor instability. In these children and in those on intermittent catheterization who are wet as a result of uninhibited contractions probanthine or emepronium can be helpful, although it should be remembered that the former also acts on the large bowel and may increase the problems of constipation which are in any case common in children with myelomeningocele. Imipramine has been used in this situation but the authors' experience with it has been disappointing. By contrast detrusor contraction can be stimulated by bethanechol, carbachol or other parasympathomimetic drugs. Their effect is short lived and they can only be appropriately used with the transient retention that sometimes follows spinal cord surgery.

Drugs may also be employed to influence the sphincteral system through stimulation or inhibition of the alpha-adrenergic receptors which are concentrated in the bladder base and the upper urethra. In children on intermittent catheterization bladder neck relaxation rather than detrusor instability may be the cause of wetting soon after the bladder has been emptied and ephedrine may be helpful. If, on the other hand, a child is voiding voluntarily while building up a vesical residue then the alpha blocker phenoxybenzamine may be used in a dosage of 0.3–0.5 mg/kg per day. The side effects of this drug include fatigue and orthostatic hypotension but these improve after a few days. Chronic constipation is, if anything, likely to lessen on this treatment.

The drugs at present available have no effect upon spasm of the external sphincter, for which urethrotomy may be required. However, by a combination of surgery and drug treatment a 'pseudocontinence' (Stockamp, 1977) may sometimes be acquired.

Intermittent catheterization

Intermittent catheterization of the urinary bladder in children with neuropathic incontinence was suggested by Lapides *et al.* (1972) and Lyon, Scott and Marshall (1975) and a further series was reported by Hunt, Whithycombe and Whitaker (1978). The authors' experience (Eckstein, 1979) showed that intermittent catheterization can be highly successful provided that the patients are selected carefully. A bladder of reasonably large capacity is essential and there must be no serious detrusor instability. The physical ability of the patient to catheterize herself or himself must be considered seriously. This type of treatment is unlikely to work in the child with multiple handicaps and gross physical deformity or with a markedly reduced intellect. A significant number of shunt-treated hydrocephalic children have some degree of spasticity involving their upper limbs which may interfere with fine finger movements. Such spasticity is a contraindication to intermittent catheterization. The success of the method is largely dependent upon the enthusiasm of the nursing staff who have to teach the child or mother the technique. Ideally catheterization should be performed at 4-hourly intervals, although the timing depends upon the bladder capacity. Many children can be kept dry for 3 hours but not for 4 hours and then more frequent catheterization is essential. In the long

term it is unrealistic and impractical to use this technique at less than 3-hourly intervals because it would interfere too much with schooling and other activities. On the other hand during the initial training process 2-hourly catheterization is acceptable to give the child confidence and the periods between catheterizations are then gradually increased.

While antireflux surgery in patients with a neuropathic bladder is not generally recommended and has a high failure rate, there may be a place for such surgery in children who are managed by intermittent catheterization and have vesicoureteric reflux (Jeffs, Jonas and Schillinger, 1976). Bladder neck tightening followed by intermittent catheterization has been successful in the authors' experience.

Continuous catheterization

Continuous catheterization of the neuropathic bladder by indwelling balloon catheters is advised by a number of people (Forrest, 1974) but in the authors' experience it has been singularly unsuccessful. There tends to be leakage around the catheter and increasingly larger instruments have to be employed to prevent this. In many patients even the larger indwelling catheter is unable to control persistent urine leakage. Another problem of continuous catheter drainage is the tendency to bladder infection, especially with organisms resistant to virtually all antibiotics.

Conversely continuous catheter drainage of the bladder is recommended in children with neuropathic bladder who are undergoing major orthopaedic or spinal surgery and are immobilized in hip spicas. The indwelling catheter reduces the contamination of the plaster and the wound by urine.

Endovesical electrostimulation

Endovesical electrostimulation was suggested by Katona (Katona and Eckstein, 1974). Although this method seemed successful initially, it has become apparent that any success can only be attributed partly to the effect of catheterization and partly to the whole-hearted attention to the urinary tract of children with myelomeningocele (Nicholas and Eckstein, 1975). The electrical stimulator is probably irrelevant to the successes reported.

Implanted pacemakers

Direct stimulation of the detrusor muscle by an implanted pacemaker has been successfully undertaken in dogs but has in general failed in humans (Dees, 1967; Montgomery and Boyce, 1967) because of concomitant stimulation of the sphincteral system. Electrical stimulation using implanted electrodes on the nerve roots of the sacral plexus has been demonstrated experimentally in animals and used clinically in the adult. At present this technique does not appear to be applicable to congenital spinal cord lesions (Grimes and Nashold, 1974; Jonas, Jones and Tanagho, 1975). Electrical stimulation of the pelvic floor by implanted pacemakers was recommended by Caldwell *et al.* (1969). The object is to retain the urine within the bladder as long as the stimulator is active. There have been no long-term reports of successful cures and on basic principles it seems unlikely that this technique would work in the case of neuropathic bladder.

External sphincterotomy

In the neuropathic bladder the internal sphincter is almost invariably open and funnel shaped and presents no obstruction. Nevertheless it is not unusual for the external sphincter to be hyperactive, producing an element of obstruction that can lead to severe upper tract dilatation. This can occur relatively late in the course of the disorder, and often becomes evident in adolescent boys whose X-rays then show gross dilatation of the posterior urethra with filling of the prostatic ducts and sometimes secondary stone formation. Relief of external sphincter obstruction in relation to the neuropathic bladder is therefore important. In the past Y-V plasty of the bladder neck and the external sphincter was recommended (Eckstein, 1977). The development of modern endoscopic instruments has made it possible to perform a transurethral incision of the external sphincter in young children. A single cut may be made through the sphincteral region in the anterior

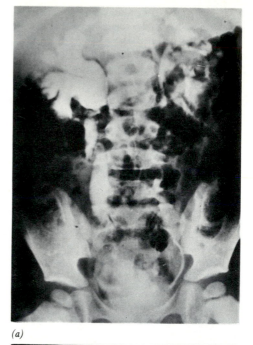

(a)

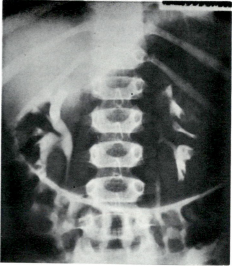

(b)

Figure 27.2. *(a)* Excretory urogram in male patient with myelomeningocele suffering from recurrent urinary tract infection. Note dilated right upper tract. *(b)* Excretory urogram in the same patient 6 months after transurethral resection of the external sphincter showing decreased dilatation of the right upper tract. Infection was eliminated.

midline or this may be supplemented by incisions at 4 o'clock and 8 o'clock which must not be prolonged downwards and thereby risk entering the corpora cavernosa. In postpubertal cases

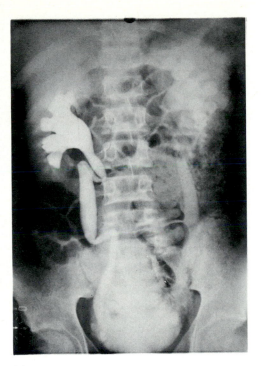

(a)

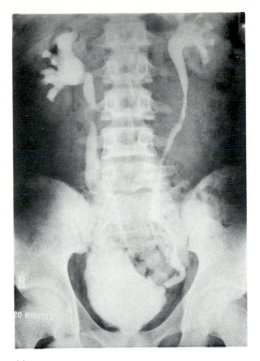

(c)

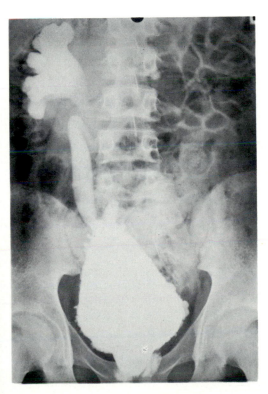

(b)

Figure 27.3. Neuropathic bladder due to sacral myelomeningocele. *(a)* Intravenous urogram in a 13-year-old boy with a recent exacerbation of straining and incontinence. *(b)* Cystogram at the same stage showing hypertrophied bladder, posterior urethral dilatation with filling of the prostatic ducts and right-sided reflux. *(c)* Intravenous urogram 4 months after Otis urethrotomy incision of external sphincter, showing a greatly improved upper tract. The boy had regained urinary control.

the Otis urethrotome may be used at 24 F or 28 F (*Figures 27.2 and 27.3*).

Operative sphincteral reconstruction

Surgical procedures to restore continence in relation to the neuropathic bladder have fascinated urologists for a long time. Sphincteral tightening using either the Young-Dees technique or muscular and fascial slings has been singularly unsuccessful in the authors' experience (*Figure 27.4*). Although incontinence could be cured in approximately 50 per cent of children in whom such procedures were tried, all those who apparently became continent developed severe upper tract dilatation so that

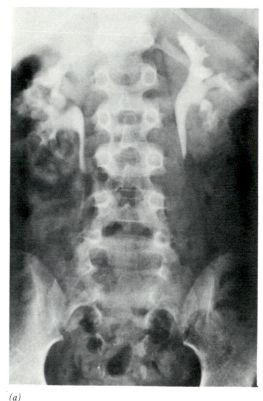
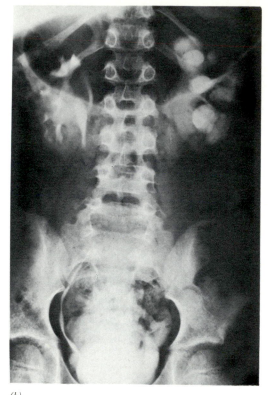

(a)   *(b)*

Figure 27.4. *(a)* Excretory urogram in a girl with neuropathic (spina bifida) incontinence. Note the essentially normal upper urinary tract. *(b)* Same patient. Excretory urogram 18 months after bladder neck tightening procedure which was very successful as far as continence is concerned. Note marked upper tract dilatation (this patient also developed severe urinary tract infection problems). Subsequent urinary ileal conduit diversion resulted in restoration to normality of the upper urinary tract and elimination of infection.

their sphincteral mechanisms had to be destroyed by transurethral resection to prevent progressive upper urinary tract damage. Bladder neck surgery in relation to the neuropathic bladder is therefore not usually recommended (*Figure 27.4*).

Artificial sphincters

An implantable compressible balloon system was devised by Scott, Bradley and Timen (1974) to relieve bladder outflow incontinence. While this operation appears to be reasonably successful in adults with sphincteral injuries, success in paediatric cases with neuropathic incontinence has been in a limited number of patients and not of long duration (Schreiter and Bressel, 1977; Gonzalez and Dewolf, 1979). Even if urinary incontinence can be controlled by such implantable appliances the question of vesicoureteric

reflux on the one hand and of recurrent urinary tract infection on the other still presents a problem in this group of patients with neuropathic bladders.

Appliances

To date there are no satisfactory appliances available for girls with urinary incontinence. One of the major problems in the development of such devices in relation to the female is the fact that the perineum is anaesthetic and any intravaginal appliances occluding the urethra are likely to result in pressure necrosis. However, there have been considerable advances in the development of devices for male children and it is now usually possible to fit a boy aged 5 or over with a suitable penile appliance and collecting bag so as to render him socially continent. Suitable adaptations for collecting urine at night are available. It is significant that a number of adolescent males who were managed very successfully on penile appliances before puberty have come back and requested a urinary diversion so that they no longer have to wear a sheath over the penis. On the whole the authors have acceded to their requests for diversion and we feel that the use of penile appliances may ultimately be limited to prepubertal boys.

Urinary diversion

If the above-mentioned lines of treatment are either inapplicable or unsuccessful, the question of urinary tract diversion has to be considered. Since the nerve supply to the bladder sphincters and the anal sphincters has a common origin it is not possible to perform ureterosigmoid diversion in the child with a neuropathic bladder. Cutaneous diversion in the form of cutaneous ureterostomy, vesicostomy, ileal conduit or colonic conduit must be considered in relation either to the control of incontinence or to uncontrollable urinary tract infection or progressive upper tract dilatation. It must be pointed out that urinary diversion should only be performed in children with neuropathic bladder incontinence if conservative techniques have failed, but it must also be appreciated that cutaneous urinary tract diversion can result in a perfectly acceptable situation as far as long-term survival is concerned. The details of urinary tract diversion are dealt with in Chapter 28. Bauer, Colodny and Hallet (1981) discussed the circumstances in which a child already given an ileal loop may be considered for reversal of diversion.

References

Allen, T.D. (1979) The dysfunctional voider. *Dialogues in Pediatric Urology*, **2**, 3

Bauer S.B., Colodny A.H. and Hallet M. (1981) Urinary undiversion in myelodysplasia: criteria for selection. *Journal of Urology*, **124**, 89

Bors, E. and Comarr, A.E. (1971) Neurological Urology. University Park Press, Baltimore

Caine, M. and Raz, S. (1975) Clinical implications of adrenergic receptors in the urinary tract. *Archives of Surgery*, **110**, 247

Caldwell, K.P.S., Martin, M.R., Flack, F.C. and James, E.D. (1969) An alternative method of dealing with incontinence in children with neurogenic bladders. *Archives of Disease in Childhood*, **44**, 625

Dees, J.E. (1967) Contraction of the urinary bladder produced by electrical stimulation. *In* Neurogenic Bladder (edited by Boyarsky, S.). Williams and Wilkins, Baltimore.p.209

Devens, K., Pompino, H.J. and Kubler, F. (1978) The upper urinary tract in neurogenic bladder without diversion. *Progress in Pediatric Surgery*, **10**, 177

Donker, P.J., Dvoes, J.T.P.M. and Van Ulden, B.M. (1976) *In* Scientific Foundations of Urology, Vol. 2 (edited by Williams, D.I. and Chisholm, G.D.). Heinemann, London. p.32

Duhamel, B. (1956) New operation for congenital megacolon: retro-rectal and transanal lowering of the colon and its possible application to the treatment of various other malformations. *Presse Médicale*, **64**, 2249

Eckstein, H.B. (1968) The Neurogenic Bladder. *In* Paediatric Urology (edited by Williams, D.I.). Butterworths, London. p.371

Eckstein, H.B. (1977) Bladder Neck Y-V Plasty. *In* Surgical Pediatric Urology (edited by Eckstein, H.B., Hohenfellner, R. and Williams, D.I.). Theime, Stuttgart.p.322

Eckstein, H.B. (1979) Intermittent catheterisation of the bladder in patients with neuropathic incontinence of urine. *Zeitschrift für Kinderchirurgie*, **28**, 408

Eckstein, H.B. and Armstrong, S. (1978) Cysto-urethroscopy in infants and children. *Aktuelle Urologie*, **9**, 201

El Badawi, A. and Shenk, E.A. (1974) A new theory of the innervation of bladder musculature. *Journal of Urology*, **111**, 613

Firlit, C.C. (1979) Techniques of urodynamics. *Dialogues in Pediatric Urology*, **2**, 5

Forrest, D.M. (1974) The use of the Foley catheter for long-term urine collection in girls. *Developmental Medicine and Child Neurology*, **16**, Suppl. 32, p.54

Gonzalez, R. and Dewolf, W.C. (1979) The artificial bladder sphincter AS 721 for the treatment of incontinence in patients with neurogenic bladder. *Journal of Urology*, **121**, 71

Grimes, J.H. and Nashold, B.S. (1974) Clinical application of electronic bladder stimulation in paraplegics. *British Journal of Urology*, **46**, 653

Hunt, G.M., Whithycome, J.F.R. and Whitaker, R.H. (1978) The management of urinary incontinence by intermittent catheterisation in children with myelomeningocele. *Zeitschrift für Kinderchirurgie*, **25**, 395

Jeffs, R.D., Jonas, P. and Schillinger, J.F. (1976) Surgical correction of vesico-ureteral reflux in children with neurogenic bladder. *Journal of Urology*, **115**, 449

Jonas, V., Jones, L.W. and Tanagho, E.A. (1975) Spinal cord stimulation versus detrusor stimulation. *Investigative Urology*, **13**, 171

Katona, F. and Eckstein, H.B. (1974) The treatment of the neuropathic bladder by transurethral electrical stimulation: a preliminary report. *Lancet*, i, 780

Lapides, J. (1962) Denervation supersensitivity as a test for neurogenic bladder. *Surgery, Gynaecology and Obstetrics*, **114**, 241

Lapides, J., Dickno, A.C., Silber, S.J. and Lowe, B.S. (1972) Clean intermittent self-catheterisation in the treatment of urinary tract disease. *Journal of Urology*, **107**, 458

Lorber, J. (1971) Results of treatment of myelomeningocele. *Developmental Medicine and Child Neurology*, **13**, 279

Lyon, R.P., Scott, M.P. and Marshall, S. (1975) Intermittent catheterisation rather than urinary diversion in children with myelomeningocele. *Journal of Urology*, **113**, 409

Mayo, M.E., Chapman, W.H. and Shurtleff, D.D. (1979) Bladder function in children with meningomyelocele: comparison of cine-fluoroscopy and urodynamics. *Journal of Urology*, **121**, 458

Montgomery, W.G. and Boyce, W.H. (1967) Problems related to the physiology of micturition in attempting artificial electrical stimulation of the urinary bladder. *In* Neurogenic Bladder (edited by Boyarsky, S.). Williams and Wilkins, Baltimore.p.229

Nathan, P.W. (1976) *In* Scientific Foundations of Urology, Vol. 2 (edited by Williams, D.I. and Chisholm, G.D.). Heinemann, London. p.51

Nicholas, J.L. and Eckstein, H.B. (1975) Endovesical electrotherapy in the treatment of urinary incontinence in spina bifida patients. *Lancet*, ii, 1276

Rehbein, F. (1959) Operation for anal and rectal atresia with recto-urethral fistula. *Chirurgie*, **30**, 417

Schreiter, F. and Bressel, K. (1977) Operative treatment of incontinence secondary to myelodysplasia by an artificial sphincter. *Zeitschrift für Kinderchirurgie*, **22**, 560

Scott, F.B., Bradley, W.E. and Timen, G.W. (1974) Treatment of urinary incontinence by an implantable urinary sphincter. *Journal of Urology*, **112**, 75

Soave, F. (1966) Hirschsprung's disease – technique and result of Soave's operation. *British Journal of Surgery*, **53**, 1023

Stockamp, K. (1977) The neuropathic bladder. *In* Surgical Pediatric Urology (edited by Eckstein, H.B., Hohenfellner, R. and Williams, D.I.). Thieme, Stuttgart. p.315

Sundin, T., Dahlström, A., Norlen, L. and Svedmyr, N. (1977) The sympathetic innervation and adreno-receptor function of the human lower urinary tract in the normal state and after para-sympathetic denervation. *Investigative Urology*, **14**, 322

Swenson, O. (1950). A new treatment for Hirschsprung's disease. *Surgery*, **28**, 371

Williams, D.I. and Nixon, H.H. (1957) Agenesis of the sacrum. *Surgery, Gynaecology and Obstetrics*, **105**, 84

28 Urinary Diversion

J.H. Johnston

Urinary diversion during childhood may be needed either temporarily, when its reversal is planned, or permanently, when because of the need to provide urinary control or to preserve renal function all prospect of retaining the normal urinary pathway has to be abandoned.

Temporary diversion

Temporary diversion of urine can be obtained by the use of catheters or by nonintubated means. The choice of method depends partly on the nature of the urinary tract pathology and partly on the expected duration of urinary drainage.

Intubated diversion

Temporary urinary diversion by tube or catheter is mainly employed following reconstructive operations on the urinary tract and the genitalia. As a preliminary to definitive surgery intubated diversion has a more limited application. Perurethral catheter drainage of the bladder is useful in the infant boy with posterior urethral valves whose bladder is tensely distended and who requires correction of sepsis, dehydration or acidaemia as a preliminary to valve ablation; only infrequently is this drainage needed for longer than 2–3 days. Suprapubic cystostomy is

rarely indicated to provide preoperative drainage. It may be needed under the circumstances stated above in a child with an infravesical obstruction in whom it is not possible to pass a urethral catheter. As a rule a fine polyethylene catheter can be inserted percutaneously through a needle or trocar and commercially produced sterile packs are now available for this purpose.

Tube nephrostomy or pyelostomy may be indicated for therapeutic purposes in acute-on-chronic upper tract obstruction, especially when there is complicating infection and particularly when a solitary functioning kidney is affected. The procedure can also be of value as a prognostic measure, by indicating the volume and quality of urine drained, to aid the decision as to whether or not a kidney of dubious function is worth preserving. The technique required varies with the circumstances. Percutaneous insertion of a fine polyethylene catheter may suffice but such tubes are readily obstructed and have an exasperating tendency to fall out. When drainage is likely to be needed for more than a few days, and in particular when infection exists, it is often safer to insert a 10 F or 12 F flanged catheter through a small flank incision. If tube blockage by pus and the consequent need for irrigation are anticipated, the use of a loop tube nephrostomy is advantageous (*Figure 28.1*). Tube displacement cannot then readily occur and the tube can be replaced if necessary by a railroad technique.

In children tube nephrostomy or pyelostomy is satisfactory as long as its duration does not exceed 2–3 weeks. More prolonged drainage by

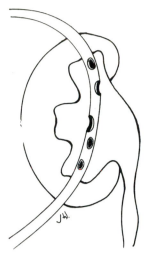

Figure 28.1. Loop tube nephrostomy.

this means is inevitably followed by infection and pyelonephritis because even when a closed system of drainage is employed bacteria can gain entry around the tube. It is necessary therefore to proceed without delay either to the appropriate definitive surgery or to an alternative nonintubated method of diversion.

Nonintubated diversion

Cutaneous loop ureterostomy

Temporary bilateral loop ureterostomies have their main indication in the baby boy when, following endoscopic destruction of posterior urethral valves, the bladder is emptying satisfactorily but there is urinary stasis and infection in the upper urinary tracts which are dilated and decompensated and show ineffective peristalsis. In such circumstances the clinical and biochemical status of the patient fails to improve or even deteriorates and prompt, direct, prolonged kidney drainage is needed (Johnston, 1963). The tortuous ureters characteristic of the infant with urethral valves can be brought easily to the surface. The stomas must be fashioned in the flanks which has the advantages that kidney drainage is direct and that the lower portions of the ureters are left undisturbed in case reconstructive ureteric surgery is needed prior to ureterostomy closure. In pratice further ureteric surgery is rarely necessary. Clinical experience (Johnston and Kulatilake, 1971; Johnston, 1979) and pressure-flow studies (Whitaker, 1973) have shown that in the majority of cases of urethral valves the ureters are not themselves obstructed and that when kidney function is adequate striking improvement in peristaltic activity and in the degree of pelviureteric dilatation, with cessation of vesicoureteric reflux, can occur spontaneously following the relief of the urethral obstruction. On occasions one kidney is found to be nonfunctioning, usually in association with persistent reflux, and nephroureterectomy is then indicated.

Ureterostomy drainage may be needed for weeks or even months. If and when the child's general condition is satisfactory, the adequacy of ureteric and vesical function must be demonstrated by descending ureterography and cystography with fluoroscopy before ureterostomy closure. If necessary the child's bladder can be re-educated by dripping saline through a Foley catheter inserted into the descending limb of the ureterostomy. During closure of loop ureterostomy, which should be performed on one side at a time, redundant ureter is resected. Preferably the ureter above the stoma is excised and the ureter below is anastomosed to the renal pelvis. This avoids the need for a ureteroureteric anastomosis which can be slow to transmit the peristaltic wave.

Infrequently total diversion of urine from the bladder leads to vesical contraction and it can then be difficult, or rarely even impossible, to restore normal urinary tract continuity. For this reason some authors have modified the loop ureterostomy either by fashioning a Y junction (Sober, 1972) or by anastomosing the two limbs of the loop to form a ring (Williams and Cromie, 1975) in order to let some urine reach the bladder (*Figure 28.2*). These methods have the

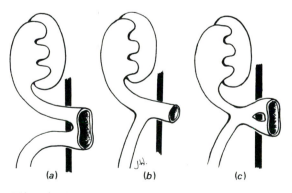

Figure 28.2. Varieties of temporary ureterostomy. *(b)* Loop ureterostomy. *(b)* Ureterostomy-en-Y. *(c)* Ring ureterostomy.

disadvantage that it is impossible to control the volume of urine descending the ureter so that kidney drainage, which is the essential object of the ureterostomy, may prove to be inadequate.

Since its introduction some 16 years ago cutaneous loop ureterostomy has often been overused, sometimes to the point of being abused, in the management of children with upper tract dilatation. It must be emphasized that the procedure is warranted only when there is upper urinary tract stasis that is likely to be prolonged in spite of the elimination of obstructive uropathy, is associated with infection unresponsive to chemotherapy, and is responsible for lack of improvement or even deterioration in the patient's general condition and renal functional status as determined clinically and biochemically. Upper tract dilatation alone is not an indication for the operation.

In the author's experience the need for loop ureterostomy has lessened greatly in recent years and the method is now rarely employed. This is mainly due to improvements in medical management of babies with urethral valvular obstruction. Since urologists have appreciated the high fluid intake that infants with impaired renal tubular function commonly require and since there are now improved methods of controlling infection and of measuring and correcting acid-base and other electrolyte disturbances there has been less indication for diversionary drainage.

Cutaneous vesicostomy

Cutaneous vesicostomy is mainly of value as a temporizing measure in the infant with a neuropathic bladder that is not readily expressible and is retaining urine, causing upper tract dilatation and threatening renal function. Because the procedure is readily reversible it does not jeopardize the possibility of closing the stoma and managing the bladder dysfunction along conservative lines when the child reaches the age at which urinary continence is important. The tendency of the bladder to prolapse through the vesicostomy is reduced by bringing the bladder fundus to the abdominal surface and constructing a stoma no larger than that allowing the passage of a 28 F catheter (Duckett, 1974). Because vesicostomy is employed in children at the napkin stage a collecting appliance is unnecessary.

Permanent diversion

Ureterosigmoidostomy

The first anastomosis between the ureters and the large intestine was performed by Simon in 1852 on a 13-year-old boy with bladder exstrophy and this anomaly and related lesions continue to be the main indications for ureterosigmoidostomy during childhood. Following its introduction in 1911 the Coffey technique was for a long time the standard operation, but it led to a high incidence of ureteric stricture and colorenal reflux causing progressive deterioration of renal function with or without symptoms of obstruction or ascending pyelonephritis.

In 1951 Harvard and Thompson reported a series of ureterosigmoidostomies performed in children with exstrophic bladder in which the 20-year survival rate was only 52 per cent. Subsequently techniques involving a mucosa-to-mucosa ureterointestinal anastomosis along with an antireflux nipple (Mathisen, 1953) or submucosal tunnel (Leadbetter, 1951; Goodwin et al., 1953) have shown improved long-term results. Wear and Barquin (1973) reported a 17 per cent incidence of upper tract deterioration following the Leadbetter (1951) method compared with 40 per cent after the Coffey (1911) technique. Spence, Hoffman and Pate (1975) recorded 29 good long-term results in 37 patients with exstrophy. Altwein, Jonas and Hohenfellner (1977) employed Goodwin's (Goodwin et al., 1953) operation and had an 8.7 per cent rate of renal deterioration among 39 children. Bennett (1973) reported 34 cases of exstrophy diverted by the Leadbetter technique. Five children required conversion to an external diversion because of upper tract changes or rectal incontinence. Urography showed normal appearances in 25 of 28 patients with ureterosigmoidostomies of at least 5 years duration.

The author's experience is of 23 children with ureterosigmoidostomies followed for periods between 2–15 years. Three died: a 1-year-old infant who became severely acidaemic at home and was comatose on readmission and two children who died of recurrent rhabdomyosarcoma following cystectomy. Conversion to an external diversion was needed in three patients: in two because of repeated severe electrolyte upsets and in one because of bilateral upper tract deterioration. Four ureterosigmoid anastomoses in three patients had to be revised due to obstruction. One boy required unilateral ureterolithotomy. Eight patients with uretero-sigmoidostomies and one with a solitary kidney (15 renal-ureteric units) continue to have normal pyelograms and upper tracts on intravenous urography. Six patients, of whom one has a solitary kidney (11 renal-ureteric units), have nonprogressive mild to moderate ureteric dilatation with either no or only slight calyectasis. Two of these children show a unilateral gas pyelogram on radiography indicating the existence of colorenal reflux but they remain symptom-free. One boy has a normal urogram on the left and mild changes on the right, and another has more severe dilatation on the right and mild changes on the left.

Adequate bowel preparation prior to surgery is important in the prevention of local infective complications. In the author's practice the child is put on a low residue diet for 3–4 days. Metronidazole 5 mg/kg body weight and neomycin 250–500 mg are given orally three times daily for 3 days. Bowel washouts with 1 per cent neomycin solution are also employed.

Contraindications

Ureterosigmoidostomy is contraindicated in the patient with anything greater than slight dilatation of the ureters or with overall renal functional impairment. In addition the method obviously cannot be employed in a child with inadequate anal control. This clearly exists with neuropathic disease or in the exstrophy patient who has recurrent complete rectal prolapse, but otherwise it can be difficult to decide whether an anus that can control solid faeces will be able to cope with a volume of urine in the rectum. A history of incontinence during a bout of diarrhoea may be relevant. Sphincteral electromyography has little prognostic advantage over simple clinical inspection and digital examination. Although in the older child the instillation of saline into the rectum is helpful, this is of no value in the uncooperative toddler. In exstrophy cases Hendren (1976) advocated external diversion by colonic conduit as a temporary measure until the child develops improved anal control at the age of 5 or more when the conduit may be anastomosed to the sigmoid colon. However, in the author's experience anal continence of urine must be learned by the patient and some degree of transient incomplete control nearly always follows diversion to the intact colon regardless of the age at which it is performed and the reason

for its performance. As a rule full daytime control is achieved within a few weeks or months but occasional leakage during sleep may continue indefinitely. Faradism to the sphincter, oral ephedrine sulphate 10 mg four times daily or Eskornade in an age-related dose may enhance anal tone and continence. Lomotil (diphenoxylate hydrochloride 2.5 mg and atropine sulphate 0.025 mg per tablet) in a dosage of one tablet three or four times daily may also be helpful.

Complications

ELECTROLYTE AND METABOLIC DISTURBANCES
Hyperchloraemic acidosis and hypokalaemia, which may follow selective absorption of urinary constituents from and loss of potassium into the bowel lumen, are well recognized as possible complications of ureterosigmoidostomy. The disturbances are readily detectable biochemically and can usually be controlled by oral administration of sodium bicarbonate and potassium citrate and by ensuring that the patient empties the bowel of urine at sufficiently frequent intervals. However, regular timed voidings are impossible to organize in the infant and it is in this age group that the most severe electrolyte upsets can occur. For this reason ureterosigmoidostomy is preferably deferred until the child is capable of cooperation in bowel evacuation.

Mild to moderate elevation of the blood urea level is commonly found following ureterosigmoidostomy. This is the result of absorption from the bowel and is not necessarily indicative of renal insufficiency. Rarely osteomalacia develops secondary to metabolic acidosis (Siklos *et al.*, 1979). This condition generally responds to alkali therapy but calciferol supplements may be necessary.

DEFECTIVE BODY GROWTH
Defective body growth has been considered to be a possible ill effect of ureterosigmoidostomy performed during childhood. It has been attributed to chronic acidaemia or to a reduction in intracellular potassium even in the presence of a normal serum potassium level. However, children with bladder exstrophy tend to be smaller than average and their height is generally less than that of normal siblings at the same age and ultimately of the mother or father, regardless of the method of management. Bakker, Van Damme and de Voogt (1977) administered oral

bicarbonate and potassium routinely to their patients following ureterosigmoidostomy and found that in the individual child somatic growth proceeded at the normal rate within the percentile range. Modern opinion concerning skeletal growth during childhood is that nutritional deprivation in the newborn is an important factor in the causation of subsequent small stature. This must raise the question of the advisability of operative intervention for bladder exstrophy during the neonatal period even though, technically, vesical reconstruction is generally more effectively accomplished at this time.

COLONIC TUMOUR

A possible late complication of ureterosigmoidostomy is the development of a colonic neoplasm at the site of ureteric reimplantation. The risk of tumour formation was estimated by Sooriyaarachchi, Johnson and Carbone (1977) to be some 100 times greater than average. Transitional cell carcinoma has been reported (Whitaker, Pugh and Dow, 1971) but more often the tumour is a benign adenomatous polyp or an adenocarcinoma presumed to be derived from the intestinal mucosa. Polyps have been reported in two 16-year-olds and a carcinoma in a 17-year-old respectively 14 and 15 years after colonic diversion (Kozak, Watkins and Jewell, 1966; Markowitz and Koontz, 1966). In the case reported by Shapiro *et al.* (1974) an adenocarcinoma developed at a ureterosigmoidostomy site 14 years after the diversion had been converted to an ileal conduit. The pathogenesis of the neoplastic change is uncertain. Carcinogens excreted in the urine or mechanical trauma acting on a ureteric nipple may be involved. Stewart *et al.* (1981) suggested that the carcinogen N-nitrosamine may be formed when urinary nitrate comes into contact with endogenous amine in the presence of colonic bacteria. The most common presenting symptom is bleeding per anum. Flank pain may result from ureteric obstruction.

It is clear that ureterosigmoidostomy carries an appreciable risk of possible late postoperative complications and that follow-up of the patient is needed indefinitely even in the absence of symptoms. Blood chemistry estimations are required at intervals to detect electrolyte disturbances that may have to be corrected. Whether or not the patient should be kept on a urinary antiseptic is debatable and in the author's prac-

tice lengthy chemotherapy has been employed only if there are symptoms suggestive of ascending infection. Regular urography is needed to determine whether there is upper tract deterioration, which may result from ureteric obstruction or coloureteric reflux, because such complications may require reanastomosis of the ureter to the colon. Uncontrollable electrolyte upsets or the development of bilateral upper tract and renal deterioration may necessitate conversion of the ureterosigmoidostomy to an external diversion. The decision as to whether or not cutaneous diversion is essential for the preservation of renal function can be extremely difficult, especially if the upper tract changes are not severe and the patient is symptom-free. In the author's series moderate ureteric dilatation with no or only mild calyectasis which is shown by repeated studies to be nonprogressive has been considered acceptable and not an indication for reoperation. In a review of Williams' cases Aaronson and Morgan (1979) evaluated 19 patients 3–22 years following ureterosigmoidostomy performed in childhood. All had normal growth and 14 had normal urograms. With 3-hourly voiding daytime soiling was rare but nearly half had lack of full control during sleep.

Other continent diversions utilizing the anal sphincter

Various alternative methods of urinary diversion aimed at producing anal control of urine have been employed in exstrophy patients.

Gregoir and Schulman (1978) revived the Maydl (1894) technique of trigonosigmoidostomy. This procedure obviates the risk of ureteric stricture and the authors found that coloureteric reflux did not occur, surprisingly in view of the known inadequacy of the ureterovesical valvular mechanism in the exstrophic bladder.

Pompino, Singer and Hor (1970) advised closing the exstrophy and the bladder outlet and then creating a fistula between the bladder and the rectum. The Hays-Powell (Hays, Powell and Strauss, 1969) procedure is similar except that a segment of ileum is interposed between the two viscera. Neither method appears to have any advantage over ureterosigmoidostomy and each carries the possibility of anastomotic stricture and of faecal reflux from the bowel to the bladder leading to vesical stone formation and ascending infection of the kidneys.

Boyce and Vest (1952) anastomosed the closed bladder to the isolated rectum with the construction of a proximal terminal colostomy. Since the effect is to provide urinary control at the expense of complete faecal incontinence this method possesses little attraction.

In the Gersuny (1880) operation the ureters are implanted into the isolated rectum and the extremity of the colon is brought anterior to the rectum, or posterior to it in the Heitz-Boyer-Hovelacque (Heitz-Boyer and Hovelacque, 1912) modification, to form a separate faecal orifice within the anal sphincter. The sphincter may prove to be incapable of providing control for the two orifices and in the author's limited experience of the operation it has not been possible to maintain complete separation of the urinary and faecal streams since the intervening septum retracted inwards. However, satisfactory results have been reported by Tacciuoli, Laurenti and Racheli (1977).

Ileal conduit

External urinary diversion by an ileal conduit was introduced by Bricker in 1950 because of the unsatisfactory results being obtained at that time from ureterosigmoidostomy. The essential features of the operation soon became standardized, the main variations being in the technique of ureteroileostomy. Bricker anastomosed the ureters separately to the conduit while others (Wallace 1966; Clark, 1979) found it more convenient to unite the ureters and make a single anastomosis to the extremity of the conduit. Only later did the question of preventing ileoureteric reflux arise.

In children the ileal loop operation is used mainly in the management of the neuropathic bladder due to spina bifida. The optimum position for the stoma must be determined before surgery, attention being paid not only to the avoidance of proximity to abdominal scars and bony prominences but also to postural deformities due to kyphoscoliosis and the position of orthopaedic appliances. It is often advisable to apply the collecting bag containing water to the proposed stomal site for a day or two before operation to ensure satisfactory positioning. In the absence of colonic or rectal faecal loading which requires clearing by enemas no elaborate bowel preparation is needed. However, the patient is preferably kept on a low residue diet for a few days before surgery.

For postoperative follow-up intravenous urography is required routinely 3 months after surgery and subsequently at intervals that vary in length according to the circumstances of the individual patient. At outpatient visits the stoma is catheterized to exclude stomal narrowing and to measure the volume of residual urine (with an adequately functioning conduit draining an undilated upper tract this should not exceed 10 ml).

Results and complications

Many series of ileal conduit diversion in children with long-term follow-up have been reported so that a full evaluation of the efficacy of the procedure is now possible. Early complications such as anastomotic leaks, devascularization of the ureter or the conduit and intestinal obstruction from internal herniation are the results of faulty technique and are avoidable.

STOMAL PROBLEMS
Among the late complications experienced stomal problems figure largely. Phosphatic encrustation of the exposed extremity of the conduit leading to ulceration, metaplasia and scarring is due mainly to alkalinity of the urine either as it is excreted from the conduit or because of decomposition occurring in the appliance. The modern use of disposable polyvinyl collecting bags, especially those with a nonreturn flap valve that prevents the stoma from being bathed with urine even in the supine posture, has reduced the incidence of this complication. Encrustation can be prevented or treated by acidification of the urine with ascorbic acid 1 g four times daily by mouth or with an aspirin tablet or acetic acid in the form of vinegar diluted one in eight with water which is inserted daily into the bag. Peristomal skin ulceration is avoidable by ensuring that the ring flange of the appliance fits closely and accurately around the bowel stoma. For this reason the construction of a projecting nipple elevated about 1.5 cm is preferable to that of a flat stoma since the former facilitates correct application of the flange, particularly by the patient (Jeter, 1976).

Stomal stenosis has been reported in up to 40 per cent of cases (Ray and De Dominico, 1972).

It may occur at the mucosal orifice as a consequence of encrustation and ulceration. Narrowing at skin level can be the result of excising an insufficiently large skin disc at operation or of fibrosis secondary to peristomal excoriation. The conduit may be compressed in its course through the abdominal wall if the aperture formed during surgery is too narrow or if the musculoaponeurotic layers were merely incised in the direction of their fibres instead of being cored out or divided in a cruciate fashion. On occasions a baffle effect that angulates the conduit results from failure to maintain the abdominal layers in their normal alignment while the stomal aperture is being fashioned.

Although a high incidence of stomal stenosis has been reported in the literature, precise definition of this complication is difficult. It is common experience that a very contracted stoma can coexist with an efficiently emptying conduit while on the contrary a wide stoma may be associated with stasis in the loop and inadequate upper tract drainage. Clearly the resistance offered by the stoma must be related to the contractility and propulsive capability of the conduit itself.

CONDUIT MALFUNCTION

Impaired emptying of the conduit may result from the construction of an unnecessarily long loop or from its overgrowth with growth of the child because either can lead to angulation of the bowel segment. The development of annular fibrous strictures in the conduit was reported by Esho *et al.* (1974) and Hardy *et al.* (1977). Their pathogenesis is uncertain; localized areas of devascularization or inflammation secondary to infection or to an autoimmune reaction have been postulated.

In the presence of upper tract dilatation radiological investigation of ileal conduits with fluoroscopic observation commonly demonstrates that peristaltic activity is sluggish, producing churning of the loop content rather than its rapid propulsion through the stoma. Clinical impressions suggest that conduit function tends to deteriorate with time but this was not confirmed by the observations of Minton, Kiser and Ketcham (1964). These authors studied the peristaltic activity of 39 unobstructed ileal conduits employing pressure measurements. Three patterns were found. In the commonest, which occurred in 22 patients, the conduit exhibited periodic forceful contractions ranging in pressure from 10–100 mmHg. Frequent low amplitude contractions were least common, occurring in six patients. In 11 there were irregular weak contractions producing pressures between 1–10 mmHg and associated with delayed loop emptying. The incidence of infection was highest in the last group. Minton, Kiser and Ketcham (1964) found that the peristaltic pattern was inherent in the individual patient, did not change with time and was unrelated to the length of the loop. Their observations suggest that the propulsive efficiency of an ileal conduit and therefore the result to be expected from ureteroileal diversion may be predetermined by the type of peristalsis existing in the intact terminal ileum. However, at present there is no ready means of predicting the form of ileal peristaltic activity before the conduit is constructed.

BIOCHEMICAL DISTURBANCES

Since the contact time between urine and bowel mucosa is shorter with a conduit than with ureterosigmoidostomy symptomatic electrolyte upsets are rare with the former although minor abnormalities can often be detected biochemically. Nevertheless clinical manifestations can occur when there is urine stasis in the conduit and when renal function is impaired so that the kidneys cannot compensate (Castro and Ram, 1970).

Absorption of vitamin B_{12} normally takes place from the terminal ileum and may therefore be defective following the construction of an ileal conduit. No case of resulting megaloblastic anaemia has been reported but Rogers and Steyn (1974) found on investigation that vitamin B_{12} deficiency existed in 28 per cent of their patients after ureteroileostomy.

URINARY TRACT INFECTION AND CALCULUS FORMATION

Urine obtained by catheterization of an ileal conduit commonly gives a positive bacterial culture but this may be due to contamination of the catheter during its passage through the stoma which is generally heavily colonized. More reliable information can be obtained by the double-catheter technique in which an aspirating catheter is passed through an outer protective sleeve (Spence, Stewart and Cass, 1972). Because an adequately functioning conduit empties more frequently than a normal bladder bacterial counts even below 100 000/ml must be taken to indicate the existence of significant bacilluria although the precisely relevant figure is debatable and undecided.

Antibody coating of bacteria obtained from a conduit does not necessarily indicate the existence of pyelonephritis. Woodside *et al.* (1978) considered that the conduit may contribute immunoglobulin to bacteria in its lumen.

Infection with a urea-splitting organism, most often Proteus, may be followed by the development of urinary tract calculi. Stones develop especially when there is upper tract dilatation before the construction of the conduit. Dretler (1973) found that stasis in the conduit enhanced chloride-bicarbonate exchange, leading to chronic bicarbonate loss and consequently to hypercalciuria and increased risk of stone formation.

UPPER URINARY TRACT AND RENAL DETERIORATION

This is the most disquieting aspect of the late results of ureteroileostomy. Deterioration was reported to occur with time in 20, 32, 32, 42, 48, 56 and 77 per cent of initially normal renal-ureteric units in the series of King and Scott (1962), Shapiro, Lebowitz and Colodny (1975), Ray and De Dominico (1972), Susset *et al.* (1966), Scott (1973), Schwarz and Jeffs (1975) and Middleton and Hendren (1976) respectively. Scott (1973) noted that the onset of deterioration could be delayed for up to 7 years following the operation. In some instances obstructive lesions in the stoma or conduit or at the ureteroileal anastomoses may account for upper tract changes and Scott (1973) considered that stomal obstruction may result from faulty application of the bag or from compression by clothing. However, often no obstructive factor can be detected and it has become evident (as already discussed) that the ileal conduit is often a very inefficient propellant of urine and acts more like a urine reservoir than as an extension of the ureters to the abdominal surface. For this reason the question of ascending infection resulting from ileoureteric reflux has become of increasing interest and concern.

ILEOURETERIC REFLUX

Convincing evidence of the deleterious effect of conduitoureteric reflux was produced experimentally by Richie and Skinner (1975). In dogs the right ureter was implanted into an ileal conduit and the left into a colonic conduit, and only with the left ureter was an antireflux technique employed. At 3 months there was a significantly lower rate of pyelonephritic change in the left kidney (7 per cent) than in the right one (83 per cent).

Various techniques of implanting the ureter into the ileum aimed at preventing reflux have been described, for example a submucosal tunnel (Kafetsioulis and Swinney, 1970), a subserosal tunnel (Starr, Rose and Cooper, 1975) and the construction of projecting ureteric nipples (Rege *et al.*, 1974). Bergman and Nilson (1974) and Zinman and Libertino (1975) produced an intussusception in the conduit aimed at preventing reflux from its distal to its proximal portion. Although some success has been reported with these methods, it is generally accepted that an antireflux ureterointestinal anastomosis is more likely to be effective in the thicker-walled colon than in the ileum and for this reason the sigmoid colonic conduit has increased in popularity in recent years.

Sigmoid colonic conduit

One of the earliest exponents of the sigmoid colonic conduit was Mogg who in 1965 recorded a lower incidence of stomal problems than with the ileal loop and noted that whether the conduit was isoperistaltic or antiperistaltic was of no consequence. Mogg used a nipple type of ureterocolostomy that was subsequently shown (Mogg and Syme, 1969) to be effective in preventing reflux in only 50 per cent of cases. Elder, Moisey and Rees (1979) employed the Mogg technique and reviewed 26 patients who had had a colonic conduit constructed during childhood and were followed up for periods between 9–20 years. Stomal stenosis occurred in 61.5 per cent of cases, calculi developed in 16 per cent of renal-ureteric units, 22 per cent of ureters demonstrated stricture and 58 per cent of patients showed colouteric reflux. Fifteen (48 per cent) of 31 renal-ureteric units normal at the time of surgery later deteriorated, as did 13 (87 per cent) of 15 abnormal units. The authors concluded that in their hands the results of the colonic conduit were no better than those obtained with the ileal conduit. They considered that the high incidence of upper tract complications was probably related to the nipple type of ureterointestinal anastomosis and to its failure to prevent reflux.

Other authors have reported happier experiences of the colonic conduit. Morales and Golimbu (1975) described no upper tract deterioration when colouretic reflux was prevented. Altwein, Jonas and Hohenfellner (1977) employed a submucosal tunnel ureteric implantation and noted an 8.3 per cent incidence of late upper tract problems. Hendren (1976) used a similar technique in 26 colonic conduits in children and reported pyelographic deterioration in only one patient in whom one ureter became obstructed and needed reoperation. Low pressure ureteric reflux did not occur in any of his cases but reflux could be induced when there was a high pressure in the conduit.

It is clear that a longer period of review is needed before the late results of the colonic conduit employing an antireflux technique of ureteric implantation can be fully assessed. In the author's experience the indications for this operation are few. An effective reflux-preventing technique requires the implanted portion of ureter to be of virtually normal calibre, either naturally or following operative narrowing of a dilated system. An undilated upper tract is unusual in the child needing an external diversion and the patient with dilated ureters can generally, and preferably, be managed by cutaneous ureterostomy with transureteroureterostomy.

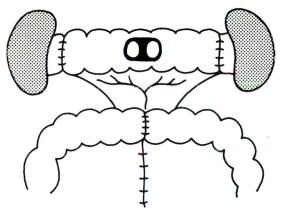

Figure 28.3. Pyelocolonic diversion employing isolated transverse colon with central double-barrelled stoma.

kyphosis whose abdominal wall is virtually nonexistent when he is sitting and whose stoma must therefore be at or near the xiphisternum.

Cutaneous ureterostomy with transureteroureterostomy

With this technique one ureter is brought to the abdominal surface as a terminal ureterostomy in the ipsilateral iliac fossa. The other is passed

Pyelointestinal conduit

When the ureters are severely dilated and show little or no peristalsis on fluoroscopy more direct and more effective kidney drainage can be obtained with a pyelointestinal than with a ureterointestinal conduit. The use of the jejunum for this purpose is contraindicated since it has led to the development of hypochloraemic acidosis, hyponatraemia, hyperkalaemia and azotaemia (Clark, 1974). Bellman and King (1974) employed a pyeloileal diversion but their method has the disadvantage of necessitating a very long conduit. Johnston (1974) described pyelocolonic diversion using the isolated transverse colon. Each extremity of the colon is anastomosed to a renal pelvis and a central double-barrelled stoma is constructed (*Figure 28.3*). The stoma is ordinarily at umbilical level, but a higher siting is possible and can be usefully applied to the patient with severe

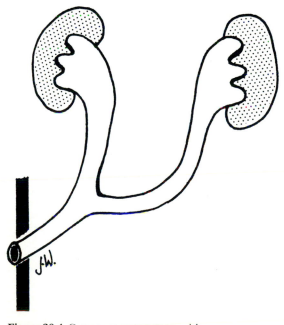

Figure 28.4. Cutaneous ureterostomy with transureteroureterostomy.

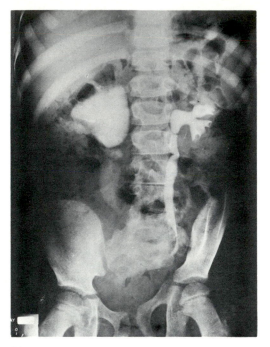

(a)

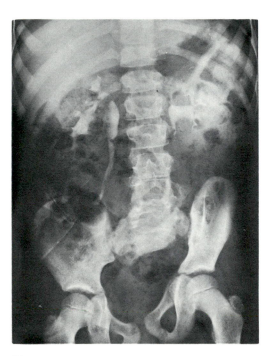

(b)

Figure 28.5. Intravenous urograms in a boy with a neuropathic bladder. *(a)* Before diversion. *(b)* 8 months following right cutaneous ureterostomy with transureteroureterostomy.

posteriorly to the pelvic mesocolon and an end-to-side ureteroureteric anastomosis is performed (*Figure 28.4*; Shapiro, Peckler and Johnston, 1976). To preclude devascularization of the distal portion of the recipient ureter care is needed to avoid division or occlusion of its longitudinally running vessels during the anastomosis. Although the procedure is performed transperitoneally, the entire ureteric system is ultimately retroperitoneal. The operation is a much lesser one than a conduit diversion and it avoids the possible early and late complications associated with the latter. It does require a minimum of one ureter (that forming the stoma) to be at least moderately dilated in order to avoid subsequent stomal narrowing. Since this situation exists in the majority of children needing external urinary diversion the operation has a wide application and in my view is the optimum method available (*Figure 28.5*). Stomal stenosis is avoidable by careful preservation of the ureteric blood supply.

Continent external diversions

Various methods aimed at preventing continual drainage from an external conduit and so avoiding the need for a collecting bag have been devised. Harzmann, Bickler and Ideler (1978) employed a carbon stoma that traversed the abdominal wall and drained an ileal conduit to the exterior; the stoma was spigotted to allow periods of dryness. In the experimental animal Wilhelm *et al.* (1978) implanted a magnetic ring into the subfascial layer around a colonic conduit stoma and incorporated a similar ring into a plastic stoma cap that plugged the stomal lumen. Sullivan, Gilchrist and Merricks (1973) isolated the ileocaecal region, closed the colonic extremity, implanted the ureters into the colon and brought the ileum to the exterior as a stoma. The ileocaecal valve apparently prevented urine leakage, surprisingly in view of its reputation for incompetence during barium enema studies, and the conduit was emptied by intermittent catheterization. Ashken (1974) also employed the isolated ileocaecal area. The ureters were implanted into the ileum with closure of its extremity and an isolated segment of ileum inserted in an antiperistaltic direction connected the colon to the surface. Intermittent catheterization was performed to empty the conduit. The effectiveness of the procedure was frustrated by the tendency of the ileal spout to prolapse.

Regardless of whether or not these reservoir techniques are effective in preventing urine leakage, and there is considerable reason for doubt on that count, the advisability of constructing what is essentially an intermittently obstructed system must be questioned in view of the well known ill effects of impaired conduit drainage on the upper urinary tract and on renal function.

The permanently nonfunctioning bladder

Pyocystis or vesical empyema results from infection and liquefaction of retained desquamated mucosal cells in a nonfunctioning bladder and is a frequent complication of permanent urinary diversion in children. It is especially likely to develop with a trabeculated, incompletely emptying, neuropathic bladder and is much commoner in girls, indicating that ascending infection is an important factor in its causation. A thick yellow foul-smelling discharge occurs from the urethra. Proteus or Pseudomonas are often obtained on culture while on occasions the pus is sterile on routine culture suggesting an anaerobic infection.

The condition may respond to vesical irrigation employing a solution of noxytiolin or, when anaerobic organisms are incriminated, of metronidazole. Often repeated irrigations are needed. In girls free bladder drainage and cure of the complication can be obtained by division of the septum between the vagina and the urethra and bladder (Spence and Allen, 1971). This procedure has largely obviated the need for cystectomy in the female. In the male endoscopic resection of an obstructive bladder outlet or of a spastic external urethral sphincter may provide effective drainage but sometimes cystectomy is required.

The occurrence in a nonfunctioning neuropathic bladder of a transitional cell carcinoma containing areas of squamous metaplasia was recorded by Aaronson (1978) and Silber (1973). The possibility of such a development must be kept in mind when pyocystis does not respond to conservative management. As discussed in Chapter 25, when urinary diversion is needed following closure of an exstrophic bladder cystectomy is indicated because of the possibility of neoplastic change.

References

Aaronson, I.A. (1978) Carcinoma in the bladder left behind. *British Journal of Urology*, **50**, 139

Aaronson, I.A. and Morgan, T.C. (1979) Ureterosigmoidostomy in childhood. *Journal of Pediatric Surgery*, **14**, 74

Altwein, J.E., Jonas, U. and Hohenfellner, R. (1977) Long-term follow-up of children with colonic conduit urinary diversion and uretero-sigmoidostomy. *Journal of Urology*, **118**, 832

Ashken, M.H. (1974) An appliance-free ileo-caecal urinary diversion: preliminary communication. *British Journal of Urology*, **46**, 631

Bakker, N.J., Van Damme, K.J. and de Voogt, H.J. (1977) Follow-up of 13 children with ureterosigmoidostomy. *In* Urinary System Malformation in Children, Vol. 13, No.5 (edited by Bergsma, D. and Duckett, J.W.). Liss, New York. p.193

Bellman, A.B. and King, L.R. (1974) Urinary diversion in children. *In* Reviews in Paediatric Urology (edited by Johnston, J.H. and Goodwin, W.E.). Excerpta Medica, Amsterdam. p.173

Bennett, A.H. (1973) Exstrophy of the bladder treated by uretero-sigmoidostomies: long-term evaluation. *Urology*, **2**, 165

Bergman, B. and Nilson, A.E.V. (1974) Intussusception of the ileal loop: an operative method for preventing urinary backflow in ileal conduits. *Journal of Urology*, **112**, 735

Boyce, W.H. and Vest, S.A. (1952) A new concept concerning treatment of exstrophy of the bladder. *Journal of Urology*, **67**, 503

Bricker, E.M. (1950) Bladder substitution after pelvic evisceration. *Surgical Clinics of North America*, **30**, 1511

Castro, J.E. and Ram, M.D. (1970) Electrolyte imbalance following ileal urinary diversion. *British Journal of Urology*, **42**, 29

Clark, P.B. (1979) End-to-end ureteroileal anastomosis for ileal conduits. *British Journal of Urology*, **51**, 105

Clark, S.S. (1974) Electrolyte disturbance associated with jejunal conduit. *Journal of Urology*, **112**, 42

Coffey, R.C. (1911) Physiologic implantation of a severed ureter or common bile duct into the intestine. *Journal of the American Medical Association*, **56**, 397

Dretler, S.P. (1973) The pathogenesis of urinary tract calculi occurring after ileal conduit diversion. *Journal of Urology*, **109**, 204

Duckett, J.W. (1974) Cutaneous vesicostomy in childhood: the Blocksom technique. *Urological Clinics of North America*, **1**, 485

Elder, D.D., Moisey, C.U. and Rees, R.W.M. (1979) A long-term follow-up of the colonic conduit operation in children. *British Journal of Urology*, **51**, 462

Esho, J., Ireland, G., Balckard, C. and Cass, A. (1974) Late stenosis of bowel segment of iliac conduit (pipe-stem loop). *Urology*, **3**, 30

Gersuny, R. (1880) Cited by Foges (1899) *Weiner Klinische Wochenschrift*, **11**, 999

Goodwin, W.E., Harris, A.P., Kaufmann, J.J. and Beal, J.M. (1953) Open, transcolonic ureterointestinal anastomosis; new approach. *Surgery, Gynecology and Obstetrics*, **97**, 295

Gregoir, W. and Schulman, C.C. (1978) Exstrophy of the bladder: treatment by trigonosigmoidostomy–long-term results. *British Journal of Urology*, **50**, 90

Hardy, B.E., Lebowitz, R.L., Baez, A. and Colodny, A.H. (1977) Strictures of the ileal loop. *Journal of Urology*, **117**, 358

Harvard, R.M. and Thompson, G.J. (1951) Congenital exstrophy of the bladder: late results of treatment by the Coffey-Mayo method of ureterointestinal anastomosis. *Journal of Urology*, **65**, 223

Harzmann, R., Bickler, K.G. and Ideler, V. (1978) The use of pure carbon stomata (biocarbon) in urinary diversion. *British Journal of Urology*, **50**, 485

Hays, D.M., Powell, T.O. and Strauss, J. (1969) Vesicoileosigmoidostomy in the treatment of exstrophy: re-evaluation. *Surgery*, **66**, 1103

Heitz-Boyer, M. and Hovelacque, A. (1912) Creation d'une nouvelle vessie et un nouvel uretere. *Journal of Urology*, **1**, 237

Hendren, W.H. (1976) Exstrophy of the bladder–an alternative method of management. *Journal of Urology*, **115**, 195

Jeter, K.F. (1976) The flush versus the protruding urinary stoma. *Journal of Urology*, **116**, 424

Johnston, J.H. (1963) Temporary cutaneous ureterostomy in the management of advanced congenital urinary obstruction. *Archives of Disease in Childhood*, **38**, 161

Johnston, J.H. (1974) Pyelo-colonic diversion in children. *British Journal of Urology*, **46**, 169

Johnston, J.H. (1979) Vesicoureteric reflux with urethral valves. *British Journal of Urology*, **51**, 100

Johnston, J.H. and Kulatilake, A.E. (1971) The sequelae of posterior urethral valves. *British Journal of Urology*, **43**, 743

Kafetsioulis, A. and Swinney, J. (1970) A study of the function of ileal conduits. *British Journal of Urology*, **42**, 33

King, L.R. and Scott, W.W. (1962) Ileal urinary diversion: success of pyeloileocutaneous anastomosis in correction of hydroureteronephrosis persisting after ureteroileocutaneous anastomosis. *Journal of the American Medical Association*, **181**, 831

Kozak, J.A., Watkins, W.E. and Jewell, W.R. (1966) Neoplastic stomal obstruction: a complication of ureterosigmoidostomy. *Journal of Urology*, **96**, 691

Leadbetter, W.F. (1951) Consideration of problems incident to performance of uretero-enterostomy: report of a technique. *Journal of Urology*, **65**, 818

Markowitz, A.M. and Koontz, P. (1966) The development of colonic polyps at the site of ureteral reimplantation. *Surgery*, **60**, 761

Mathisen, W. (1953) New method for uretero-intestinal anastomosis. *Surgery, Gynecology and Obstetrics*, **96**, 255

Maydl, K. (1894) Uber die radikltherapie der ectopia vesical urinariae. *Wiener Medizinische Wochenschrift*, **25**, 1113

Middleton, A.W. and Hendren, W.H. (1976) Ileal conduits in children at the Massachusetts General Hospital from 1955 to 1970. *Journal of Urology*, **115**, 591

Minton, J.P., Kiser, W.S. and Ketcham, A.S. (1964) A study of the functional dynamics of ileal conduit urinary diversion with relationship to urinary infection. *Surgery, Gynecology and Obstetrics*, **119**, 541

Mogg, R.A. (1965) The treatment of neurogenic urinary incontinence using the colonic conduit. *British Journal of Urology*, **37**, 681

Mogg, R.A. and Syme, R.R.A. (1969) The results of urinary diversion using the colonic conduit. *British Journal of Urology*, **41**, 434

Morales, P. and Golimbu, M. (1975) Colonic urinary diversion: 10 years of experience. *Journal of Urology*, **113**, 302

Pompino, H.J., Singer, H. and Hor, G. (1970) The treatment of exstrophy of the bladder. *Zeitschrift für Kinderchirurgie*, **9**, 85

Ray, P. and De Dominico, I. (1972) Intestinal conduit urinary diversion in children. *British Journal of Urology*, **44**, 345

Rege, P.R., Malik, I.K., Wendel, R.G. and Evans, A.T. (1974) Muscular nipple ureteroileal anastomosis to prevent reflux. *Urology*, **4**, 402

Richie, J.P. and Skinner, D.G. (1975) Urinary diversion: the physiological rationale for non-refluxing colonic conduits. *British Journal of Urology*, **47**, 269

Rogers, A.C.N. and Steyn, J.H. (1974) Vitamin B_{12} absorption in patients with ileal resection. *British Journal of Urology*, **46**, 625

Schwarz, G.R. and Jeffs, R.D. (1975) Ileal conduit urinary diversion in children: computer analysis of follow-up from 2 to 16 years. *Journal of Urology*, **114**, 285

Scott, J.E.S. (1973) Urinary diversion in children. *Archives of Disease in Childhood*, **48**, 199

Shapiro, S.R., Baez, A., Colodny, A.H. and Folkman, J. (1974) Adenocarcinoma of colon at ureterosigmoidostomy site 14 years after conversion to ileal loop. *Urology*, **3**, 229

Shapiro, S.R., Lebowitz, R. and Colodny, A.H. (1975) Fate of 90 children with ileal conduit urinary diversion a decade later: analysis of complications, pyelography, renal function and bacteriology. *Journal of Urology*, **114**, 289

Shapiro, S.R., Peckler, M.S. and Johnston, J.H. (1976) Transureteroureterostomy for urinary diversion in children. *Urology*, **8**, 35

Siklos, P., Davie, M., Jung, R.T. and Chalmers, T.M. (1980) Osteomalacia in ureterosigmoidostomy: healing by correction of the acidosis. *British Journal of Urology*, **52**, 61

Silber, S.J. (1973) Carcinoma in the bladder left behind. *Journal of Urology*, **110**, 675

Simon, J. (1852) Ectopia vesicae (absence of the anterior walls of the bladder and pubic abdominal parietes): operation for diverting the orifices of ureters into the rectum: temporary success, subsequent death, autopsy. *Lancet*, ii, 568

Sober, I. (1972) Pelviureterostomy-en-Y. *Journal of Urology*, **107**, 473

Sooriyaarachchi, G.S., Johnson, R.O. and Carbone, P.P. (1977) Neoplasms of the large bowel following ureterosigmoidostomy. *Archives of Surgery*, **112**, 1174

Spence, B., Stewart, W. and Cass, A.S. (1972) Use of a double lumen catheter to determine bacteriuria in intestinal loop diversions in children. *Journal of Urology*, **108**, 800

Spence, H.M. and Allen, T.D. (1971) Vaginal vesicostomy for empyema of the defunctionalized bladder. *Journal of Urology*, **106**, 862

Spence, H.M., Hoffman, W.M. and Pate, V.A. (1975) Exstrophy of the bladder: long-term results in a series of 37 cases treated by ureterosigmoidostomy. *Journal of Urology*, **114**, 133

Starr, A., Rose, D.H. and Cooper, J.F. (1975) Antireflux uretero-ileal anastomoses in humans. *Journal of Urology*, **113**, 170

Stewart, M., Hill, M.J., Pugh, R.C.B. and Williams, J.P. (1981). The role of N-nitrosamine in carcinogenesis at the ureterocolic anastomosis. *British Journal of Urology*, **53**, 115

Sullivan, H., Gilchrist, R.K. and Merricks, J.W. (1973) Ileocecal substitute bladder: long-term follow-up. *Journal of Urology*, **109**, 43

Susset, J.G., Taguchi, Y., De Dominico, I. and MacKinnon, K.J. (1966) Hydronephrosis and hydroureter in ileal conduit urinary diversion. *Canadian Journal of Surgery*, **9**, 141

Tacciuoli, M., Laurenti, C. and Racheli, T. (1977) Sixteen years experience with the Hertz Boyer-Hovelacque procedure for exstrophy of the bladder. *British Journal of Urology*, **49**, 385

Wallace, D.M. (1966) Ureteric diversion using a conduit: a simplified technique. *British Journal of Urology*, **38**, 522

Wear, J.B. and Barquin, O.P. (1973) Ureterosigmoidostomy: long-term results. *Urology*, **1**, 192

Whitaker, R.H. (1973) The ureter in posterior urethral valves. *British Journal of Urology*, **45**, 395

Whitaker, R.H., Pugh, R.C.B. and Dow, D. (1971) Colonic tumours following uretero-sigmoidostomy. *British Journal of Urology*, **43**, 562

Wilhelm, E., Sigel, A., Hager, T. and Hennig, G. (1978) Technique and results of the colonic conduit, continent by means of a new magnetic stoma seal: an experimental study. *British Journal of Urology*, **50**, 264

Williams, D.I. and Cromie, W.J. (1975) Ring ureterostomy. *British Journal of Urology*, **47**, 789

Woodside, J.R., Reed, W.P., Kiker, J.D. and Borden, T.A. (1978) Antibody-coated bacteria in urine of patients with ileal conduit urinary diversion. *Urology*, **11**, 472

Zinman, L. and Libertino, J.A. (1975) Ileocecal conduit for temporary and permanent urinary diversion. *Journal of Urology*, **113**, 317

29 Urolithiasis : Medical Aspects

T.M. Barratt

Epidemiology

The incidence, the composition and the clinical characteristics of urinary calculi vary greatly from one part of the world to another and from one historical period to the next (Blacklock, 1976). However, it is possible to discern three major epidemiological patterns in childhood (Barratt and Williams, 1974).

In some areas of the world such as Turkey and the Far East (particularly Thailand) childhood urolithiasis is endemic and is very common, especially in boys, accounting for a significant proportion of children admitted to hospital. In these cases the stones are usually found in the bladder and are composed of ammonium acid urate and oxalate. There is evidence implicating dietary factors in their pathogenesis and in particular dependence on a cereal or rice diet (Andersen, 1969). Such stones used to be common in England, notably in rural areas like East Anglia, but their incidence declined in the early part of this century possibly as a consequence of improved standards of nutrition (Lett, 1936).

In the UK and certain other European countries urolithiasis is somewhat less common and occurs with a frequency of 1–2 children per million total population per annum (Ghazali, 1975). Approximately 90 per cent have upper tract calculi composed of organic matrix and magnesium ammonium phosphate, and in the majority of these there is evidence of urinary tract infection with Proteus.

For reasons that are not understood the incidence of such infection calculi varies considerably and is low in, for example, Scandinavia and the USA. In these areas urolithiasis in children is rare and can generally be attributed to metabolic disorders, for instance hypercalciuric states, and especially to distal renal tubular acidosis, hyperoxaluria, cystinuria and disorders of purine metabolism. Additionally in areas where the incidence of calcium stones is high in adults, such as the stone belt of the American South, a few older children may be similarly affected.

Stone composition and formation

Chemical composition

The principal varieties of urinary calculi are shown in *Table 29.1*. Some calculi have many constituents and most struvite (magnesium ammonium phosphate) stones contain apatites (basic calcium phosphates) as well. The presence of calcium atoms renders stones radio-opaque and cystine stones are also radio-opaque due to sulphur content. Nonopaque stones are almost certainly composed of purines.

Chemical analysis of urinary calculi is often inadequately performed in routine hospital laboratories. The wet stone should be dissolved and quantitatively analysed for the main ingredients, namely calcium, phosphorus, magnesium, ammonium, oxalate and urate, and should also be tested for cystine (Westbury and Omenogor, 1970).

Table 29.1   Urinary calculi

Calcium phosphate	hydroxyapatite
	carbonate-apatite
	brushite
	whitlockite
	octocalcium phosphate
Magnesium ammonium phosphate	struvite
Calcium oxalate	whewellite
	wedellite
Purine	ammonium acid urate
	uric acid
	2, 8-dihydroxyadenine
	xanthine
Cystine	

X-ray crystallography has proved an interesting research method and 16 different crystals have been identified (Sutor, 1976) some of which are given in *Table 29.1*.

In addition to crystalline constituents all urinary stones contain a glycoprotein matrix which is particularly prominent in infection calculi (Wickham, 1976). The chemistry of these substances is very complex. Boyce, Stanton-King and Fielden (1962) described matrix substance A which is a glycoprotein of molecular weight 30 000–40 000. Tamm-Horsfall glycoprotein and uromucoid, which are closely related, are also present. This subject requires reinvestigation with modern techniques of glycoprotein chemistry.

Activity products

In spite of a considerable body of research the physicochemical principles underlying the formation of renal calculi remain incompletely understood (Robertson and Nordin, 1976). Precipitation of a salt occurs when the product of the activity of its ionic constituents exceeds a certain critical level, but there are several complexities in such an analysis.

First, it may be difficult to ascertain what proportion of a solute is present in ionized form. For example only 30–60 per cent of urinary calcium is ionized and the remainder is complexed to polyvalent anions such as sulphate, phosphate, oxalate and citrate. Although this proportion may be deduced from a knowledge of the urine composition, 22 complexes have to be considered and the calculations are very elaborate. Secondly it may not be clear which

species of salt is originally precipitated and which ion product is therefore relevant. In the case of calcium phosphate it is probably octocalcium phosphate which converts spontaneously into the less soluble hydroxyapatite. Finally, there are two critical activity products to be considered: the solubility product below which is the undersaturated region where added crystals dissolve, and the formation product above which is the labile region in which spontaneous precipitation occurs. Between the solubility product and the formation product lies the metastable region in which existing crystals grow but precipitation does not occur unless the system is disturbed.

With these considerations in mind it is not surprising that there is a substantial overlap of urinary octocalcium phosphate and calcium oxalate products between stone-forming and healthy individuals. Because of these complex interactions between ions unexpected factors may be important, such as the fact that within the physiological range the activity product of octocalcium phosphate is more influenced by an increase in urinary pH than by an increase in calcium concentration.

Inhibitors of crystallization

The activity products of octocalcium phosphate and calcium oxalate lie in the metastable region in many healthy individuals and so a search has been made for the substances that inhibit precipitation. An inhibitor of the growth of calcium oxalate crystals is found in normal urine and is absent in that of many stone-forming individuals (Robertson and Nordin, 1976) since calcium oxalate microcrystals form spontaneously if the latter is allowed to stand. Low excretion rates of pyrophosphate and citrate and low urinary magnesium/calcium and sodium/calcium ratios have been reported to characterize patients with urinary calculi.

Infection calculi

Presentation

Of children with urinary calculi 75 per cent are less than 5 years at the time of diagnosis with a

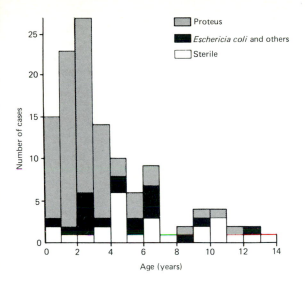

Figure 29.1. Urolithiasis in British children: age and urine culture at presentation. (Reproduced by permission of the editor of *Archives of Disease in Childhood*.)

peak incidence at 2 years. Males make up 80 per cent and 93 per cent have infected urine (*Figure 29.1*; Ghazali, Barratt and Williams, 1973). Presentation is with the usual features of a urinary tract infection, but one that is often resistant to antibiotic therapy. There may also be loin pain and haematuria. Sometimes fragments are passed in the urine. These stones are often very soft and may be described as toothpaste or a discharge. In some children, particularly those with pyonephrosis, the constitutional symptoms of malaise and failure to thrive may be prominent.

The stone is in the upper urinary tract in 85 per cent of cases and usually in the kidney. The left side is involved twice as often as the right and in 15 per cent of patients the calculi are bilateral.

Diagnosis

The cardinal feature of urolithiasis in young children is its association with Proteus infection of the urinary tract. This organism can be isolated from the urine at diagnosis in 75 per cent of patients with stones under 5 years of age. In some patients with sterile urine or *Escherichia coli* infection Proteus may be isolated from the interior of the stone or from the cut surface of the kidney at operation, and in others review of the child's medical history may reveal that the initial infection was with Proteus even though

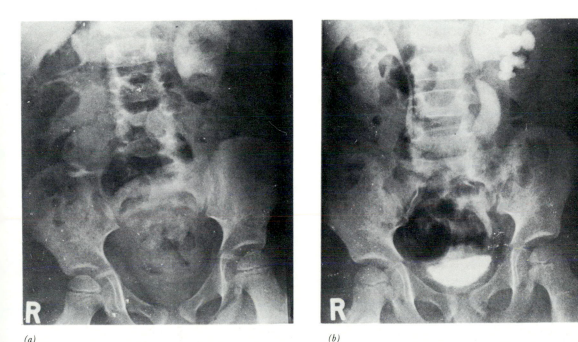

(a)   *(b)*

Figure 29.2. *(a)* A right-sided renal calculus in a girl aged 2 with a Proteus urinary tract infection. *(b)* Intravenous urogram from the same case showing the characteristic dilatation of the lumbar ureter below the stone.

other organisms were subsequently isolated. The diagnosis of stone should be very carefully considered in all children with Proteus infection of the urinary tract (*Figure 29.2*). The stones are usually evident on the plain X-ray taken before intravenous urography, but they may not be very radio-opaque and therefore may not be well visualized especially if there is gaseous abdominal distension. In this case tomography, screening or ultrasound may be very helpful.

Stone composition

There is a large matrix element in these calculi, of which Tamm-Horsfall glycoprotein is a prominent component. The inorganic constituents are struvite (magnesium ammonium phosphate) and apatite (basic calcium phosphate). The significance of the Proteus organism lies in its urease activity. Formation of ammonia from urea elevates the urinary pH which favours the precipitation of calcium phosphate and also leads directly to an increase in ammonium ion concentration thereby raising the magnesium ammonium phosphate ion product.

Associated urological abnormalities

In one third of cases there is an underlying urological malformation other than vesico-ureteric reflux. Of the remainder 35 per cent have reflux preoperatively, but it ceases spontaneously in two thirds of these soon after removal of the calculi so that ureteric reimplantation is only rarely necessary (Ghazali, 1975). Often there is dilatation of the lumbar ureter which may at first suggest obstructive megaureter. This is a consequence of the calculus and recedes rapidly after surgery.

Calcium excretion

In 15 per cent of apparently straightforward infection calculi urinary calcium excretion exceeds 0.15 mmol/kg per 24 h and in another 15 per cent it is between 0.10–0.15 mmol/kg per 24 h. However, the hypercalciuria is of the same order as that observed in other children with urinary tract infection and without stone and it subsides after the calculus is removed, suggesting that the hypercalciuria is an epiphenomenon reflecting immobilization and ill health rather than an underlying metabolic disorder predisposing to stone formation.

Treatment

Stones must be removed surgically. There is no place in children for conservative management of infected calculi because if they are left untreated pyonephrosis may supervene, leading to complete destruction of the kidney. Nephrectomy is necessary on this account in about 10 per cent of cases. Under such circumstances the kidney is found to be full of caseous material, and some cases described as xanthogranulomatous pyelonephritis are really examples of this disease.

The recurrence rate is low, that is less than 10 per cent, and can usually be attributed to failure to remove all the fragments or to persistent Proteus infection (Androulakis *et al.*, 1982). There is no evidence that infection calculi herald a problem of urolithiasis in adult life, although the associated pyelonephritic scarring may be responsible for hypertension and occasionally chronic renal failure.

Pathogenesis

Any hypothesis of the pathogenesis of infection calculi must recognize their close association with Proteus yet explain why children with neurogenic bladder who frequently have Proteus infection are only occasionally afflicted with stone. It must also account for the curious epidemiological characteristics of the disease and the predilection for young male children. At present there is no satisfactory hypothesis dealing with all these features.

Disorders of calcium metabolism

Hypercalcaemia

The hypercalcaemic syndromes of childhood are

complicated more frequently by nephrocalcinosis than by urolithiasis. Causes of hypercalcaemia and nephrocalcinosis or stone in this age group include hyperparathyroidism, vitamin D intoxication, idiopathic hypercalcaemia in its mild and severe forms, hypothyroidism and hypophosphatasia.

Hyperparathyroidism has only rarely been recognized in children (Klein and Haddow, 1975) and usually presents with bone lesions although on occasions it causes renal calculi. It may be part of the endocrine adenomatosis syndrome. Hypothyroidism is easily overlooked as a cause of hypercalcaemia. The diagnosis of vitamin D intoxication may be difficult to establish retrospectively when the plasma calcium level has returned to the normal range. This possibility should be considered in a child with a renal calculus who comes from a country where the administration of vitamin D is haphazard.

Hypercalciuria

Difficulty has been encountered in establishing standards for urinary calcium excretion in healthy children since there may be considerable variation between different nationalities and decades as a consequence of diet or habits of vitamin D prescription. In the older literature there is some uncertainty as well about the technical adequacy of the methods used to measure urinary calcium excretion. Royer (1961) reported the upper limit of calcium excretion to be 0.15 mmol/kg per 24 h (6 mg/kg per 24 h) while in 52 British children aged 1–14 Ghazali and Barratt (1974) found the upper limit was 0.10 mmol/kg per 24 h (4 mg/kg per 24 h). There is considerable diurnal variation in calcium excretion, but a calcium/creatinine concentration ratio greater than 0.1 mmol/mmol (0.25 mg/mg) in the second morning urine specimen strongly suggests hypercalciuria. This simple screening test avoids the problems inherent in 24-hour urine collections in children. It should be recalled that even straightforward surgical operations result in sufficient immobilization to cause hypercalciuria, and so studies of calcium excretion in stone-forming patients should be undertaken either preoperatively or after convalescence.

Urinary calcium excretion is increased in the hypercalcaemic syndromes described above.

Hypercalciuria with normal plasma calcium concentrations may be due to increased gastrointestinal absorption because of vitamin D excess or idiopathic hypercalciuria; to increased bone mobilization of calcium because of immobilization, Cushing's syndrome or neoplastic deposits in bone including leukaemia; or to renal tubular disorders such as Bartter's syndrome, Wilson's disease and renal tubular acidosis.

During immobilization calcium is lost from the skeleton. Children undergoing orthopaedic surgery or with extensive burns are particularly at risk. Even slight activity reduces the negative calcium balance, and a high fluid intake helps to prevent stone formation.

Many children with apparently straightforward infection stones also have hypercalciuria but as already discussed this is probably just an epiphenomenon of a severe infective illness.

Acidification defects

Of the hypercalciuric states described above the paediatric urologist is most troubled by distal renal tubular acidosis since recurrence of calculi is typical in this condition. Distal renal tubular acidosis is characterized by the failure to establish a significant hydrogen ion gradient between the renal tubular fluid and the plasma (Rodriguez-Soriano, 1978). A metabolic acidosis ensues. Because renal failure with divalent anion retention is not present the anion gap is normal and thus the acidosis is associated with hyperchloraemia. There is renal wastage of sodium, potassium and calcium, and defective urine concentration. Citrate excretion is low, especially when assessed in relation to urinary pH. The combination of hypercalciuria, alkaline urine and low citrate excretion favours precipitation of calcium salts. A similar situation is observed with acetazolamide therapy. Osteomalacia or rickets may occur and growth may be poor. In some cases there is a familial pattern suggestive of dominant inheritance, and one variant is associated with nerve deafness.

The combination of nephrocalcinosis and calculi is characteristic of this condition (*Figure 29.3*) although a very similar pattern may be seen in primary hyperoxaluria. Sometimes the stones drop into the ureter and obstruct the flow of urine in which case surgery is necessary. In general the surgical approach should be very

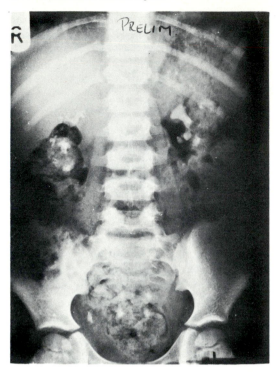

Figure 29.3. Bilateral renal calculi with nephrocalcinosis in a boy aged 4 with distal renal tubular acidosis. He had previously had a left nephrolithotomy and ureterolithotomy. Note the stone at the bottom end of the right ureter.

conservative because of the tendency to recurrence. The diagnosis may be evident from a review of plasma bicarbonate and urinary pH data, and the observation of a urinary pH less than 5.3 (which is often seen in health in the morning urine specimen) excludes the condition. In borderline cases it may be necessary to stress urinary acidification by the administration of ammonium chloride (Wrong and Davis, 1959). If there is urinary tract infection, in particular with a urea-splitting organism such as Proteus, urinary acidification tests cannot be carried out and sometimes it is necessary to defer formal study until the stones have been removed and the infection eradicated.

Treatment consists of the administration of sufficient alkali to neutralize endogenous acid production, that is about 2 mEq/kg per 24 h of sodium or potassium bicarbonate depending on diet. There may be catching up of growth and healing of rickets without any additional vitamin D therapy. Urinary calcium excretion decreases. Unfortunately, stone formation often

continues in spite of seemingly adequate alkali therapy.

Other forms of renal tubular acidosis are not associated with nephrocalcinosis or stone formation.

Disorders of oxalate metabolism

Primary hyperoxaluria

Oxalic acid is an end-product of metabolism. Approximately 15 per cent of urinary oxalate originates from dietary sources and the remainder is derived in more or less equal amounts from the metabolism of glyoxalate and ascorbic acid. Ethylene glycol (antifreeze) and the anaesthetic agent methoxyflurane are also converted to oxalic acid *in vivo*. In health oxalate excretion expressed in terms of anhydrous oxalic acid is 0.2–0.5 mmol/24 h per 1.73 m^2 surface area (20–50 mg/24 h per 1.73 m^2 surface area; Hodgkinson, 1976).

The primary hyperoxalurias are genetically determined conditions characterized by increased urinary oxalate excretion typically above 1 mmol/24 h per 1.73 m^2 surface area, recurrent calcium oxalate nephrolithiasis which usually presents in childhood, nephrocalcinosis and frequently death from end-stage renal failure in early adult life. Small spiky stones form in sterile urine and are often associated with haematuria or renal colic (*Figure 29.4*). While there may be episodes of urinary obstruction the principal cause of renal damage is the precipitation of calcium oxalate within the renal parenchyma. In later stages of the illness there may be oxalate deposition (oxalosis) in other organs as well, notably the cardiac conducting system where it results in arrhythmias.

Type I hyperoxaluria is the commoner variety and is characterized in addition by increased excretion of glyoxalate and glycollate. There is a deficiency of the enzyme 2-oxoglutarate : glyoxalate carboligase which converts glyoxylate and 2-oxoglutarate to 2-hydroxy-3-oxoadipate and thus there is a build-up of glyoxylate and glycollate and increased conversion of glyoxylate to oxalate (Williams and Smith, 1978). In type II hyperoxaluria there is increased excretion of L-glycerate as well. A deficiency of the enzyme D-glycerate dehydrogenase has been described although the pathogenesis of the hyperoxaluria remains uncertain.

There is no satisfactory treatment for either type of hyperoxaluria at present. A few type I patients respond to large doses of pyridoxine but other drugs have not been effective in reducing

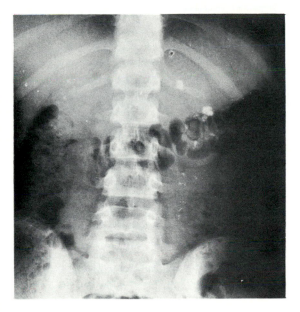

Figure 29.4. Primary hyperoxaluria in a boy aged 8. Oxalate excretion fell from 1.19 to 0.56 mmol/24 h per 1.73 m² surface area in response to pyridoxine 100 mg four times daily.

oxalate excretion. It is obviously appropriate to try to decrease calcium excretion by reduction of dietary calcium in order to lessen the calcium oxalate ion product. It has also been suggested that increased magnesium concentration in the urine tends to inhibit calcium oxalate precipitation. However, it is difficult to influence urinary magnesium excretion by dietary supplementation.

Surgical treatment should be confined to the removal of obviously obstructive calculi and should if anything err on the side of conservatism because recurrence is inevitable. Transplantation has in general been accompanied by the rapid recurrence of oxalate calculi and dialysis by the progression of oxalosis so that these patients have poor prospects on renal replacement programmes.

The majority of adult patients who form calcium oxalate stones, even those with a family history of urolithiasis, do not have primary hyperoxaluria. Many have idiopathic hypercalciuria and this type of calcium oxalate stone is occasionally seen in older children.

Bowel disease

Hyperoxaluria occasionally complicated by renal stones occurs in some patients with bowel disease, particularly that affecting the terminal ileum such as ileal resection or Crohn's disease (Harrison, 1976). Although the mechanism is not certain, it has been observed that bile salts and unsaturated fatty acids promote the absorption of oxalate by the colon. Increased oxalate excretion is seen in some children with coeliac disease but has not to date been reported to be associated with urolithiasis.

Cystinuria

In cystinuria there is defective tubular reabsorption of the dibasic amino acids cystine, ornithine, arginine and lysine from the glomerular filtrate (Thier and Segal, 1978). The transport defect is also present in the gut in some individuals. There is more than one mode of inheritance and three variants are currently recognized. The only clinical abnormality in these children is recurrent formation of urinary calculi. A presumptive diagnosis may be made on the basis of the purple colour that develops when the urine is mixed with cyanide-nitroprusside, and it should be confirmed by further studies of the urinary amino acids with chromatography or high voltage electrophoresis.

Cystine stones can occur in children at all ages. In the very young bladder calculi are not uncommon. Later in childhood renal calculi are predominant and are often large rounded or branched stones in the renal pelvis with multiple calculi in the dilated calyces (*Figure 29.5*). Some cystine stones are passed spontaneously and in cases of renal colic where no explanation is evident the urine should be tested for cystine. All cystine calculi are opaque to X-rays while they are not as dense as many calcium-containing stones and often not as dense as the opaque medium during intravenous urography. If the calculus lies over a transverse process the bone may be visible on X-ray behind the stone.

The attractive simplicity of the view that cystinuria represents a genetic deficiency of the transport system of the dibasic amino acids is threatened by the genetic heterogeneity alluded

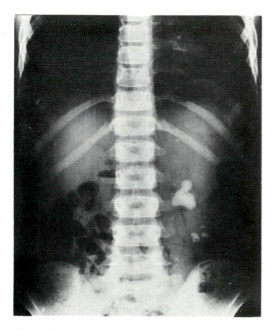

Figure 29.5. Cystine calculi in a boy aged 9.

to above, by the observation that the cystine clearance frequently exceeds the inulin clearance, and by the recognition of phenotypes in which there is an isolated failure of reabsorption of cystine or of the other members of the amino acid group without involvement of cystine (hyperdibasicaminoaciduria).

The solubility of cystine in urine of pH less than 7.5 is about $300 \, mg/\ell$. Above this pH there is a substantial increase in solubility, but it is difficult to maintain the urinary pH consistently in this region with alkali therapy. A quantitative knowledge of cystine excretion enables the minimum safe urine volume to be calculated. In adult patients who excrete about $1 \, g/24 \, h$ this is approximately $4 \, \ell$ daily.

A high fluid intake sustained throughout the day and night prevents the formation of cystine stones and may result in their dissolution. Although the treatment is inconvenient and difficult to follow, it has the merit of being cheap and effective provided that the cooperation of

the patient can be maintained. This is sometimes lost due to the rebellious attitude of adolescence, particularly if it is many years since an episode of renal colic. Alternative treatment with D-penicillamine results in the excretion of mixed cysteine-penicillamine disulphide, which is more soluble than cystine. The drug is expensive and has many side effects, and should be reserved for cases in whom continuous hydration fails. Surgery is occasionally required for the removal of bladder stones and of obstructing renal and ureteric stones, especially if complicated by infection.

Disorders of purine metabolism

Uric acid calculi

Uric acid is a weak acid with a pH of 5.6. Below this pH it exists predominantly in the unionized form which is considerably less soluble than the urate ion. In contrast to calcium phosphate, acid urine favours its precipitation. These stones may develop in situations of uric acid overproduction such as leukaemia or lymphoma, notably after cytotoxic chemotherapy and occasionally as the presenting feature of leukaemia (Nyhan, 1978). Uric acid gravel in both kidneys may lead to acute renal failure without radiological evidence of calculus. Allopurinol and sodium bicarbonate are valuable agents in the prevention of this complication of leukaemia therapy.

On occasions primary gout with uric acid calculi occurs in older children. Another variant is the Lesch-Nyhan syndrome which is a disorder characterized by progressive choreoathetosis, self-mutilation and hyperuricaemia with uric acid calculi. The deficient enzyme is hypoxanthine-guanine phosphoribosyl transferase. Hyperuricosuria with calculus formation may also occur in type I glycogen storage disease although the mechanism is not clear.

In some patients, particularly males of Mediterranean stock, there is a tendency to uric acid stone formation without hyperuricaemia or uricosuria. The syndrome is sometimes familial and is occasionally seen in childhood, but some of these patients may in fact have dihydroxyadenine calculi which are not distinguished from uric acid calculi by routine laboratory techniques.

Dihydroxyadenine calculi

A new inborn error of purine metabolism has recently been recognized. In this, deficiency of the enzyme adenine phosphoribosyl transferase results in the diversion of adenine metabolism to 2, 8-dihydroxyadenine which is relatively insoluble and forms nonopaque stones (*Figure 29.6*; Van Acker *et al.*, 1977; Barratt *et al.*, 1979).

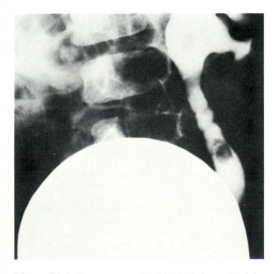

Figure 29.6. Nonopaque calculi in the left renal pelvis and ureter outlined by reflux of contrast medium during cystography. The stones consisted of dihydroxyadenine and the child was shown to have a complete deficiency of adenine-phosphoribosyl-transferase activity. (Reproduced by permission of the editor of *Archives of Disease in Childhood.*)

These stones require specialized chemical analysis to distinguish them from uric acid stones. The diagnosis is important since alkalinization of the urine decreases the solubility of 2, 8-dihydroxyadenine. However, the condition reponds satisfactorily to allopurinol therapy.

Xanthinuria

Xanthinuria is a very rare condition in which there is a deficiency of xanthine oxidase and hence a failure of conversion of xanthine to uric acid. The plasma uric acid concentration is therefore low and because xanthine is relatively insoluble in acidic urine calculi develop which are radiolucent. A xanthine nephropathy may also be precipitated by the use of allopurinol in patients with high uric acid excretion rates.

Investigation of the child with urinary calculi

The extent to which the child with urolithiasis should be screened for metabolic abnormality varies in different clinical circumstances. Thus sterile urine, nephrocalcinosis, recurrence and calculi in older children should lead to close metabolic scrutiny while on the other hand the yield of metabolic diagnoses from screening children with renal calculi and Proteus infection is small.

All children with stone must be screened for cystinuria since the diagnosis may modify the surgical programme because this condition is amenable to medical treatment. Under suspicious circumstances the preoperative 24-hour urinary calcium and oxalate excretions and plasma calcium and uric acid concentrations should be estimated. Quantitative wet stone analysis may prompt further metabolic investigations. A urinary pH of 5.3 or less under any circumstances, either spontaneous or following ammonium chloride loading, excludes the diagnosis of distal renal tubular acidosis. However, if the urine is infected, particularly with Proteus, it may prove difficult to exclude this condition and formal examination of the capacity to acidify the urine should be deferred until the stone has been removed and the urine sterilized. Nonopaque stones are probably purine in nature and require careful investigation by an experienced laboratory.

References

Andersen, D.A. (1969) Historical and geographical differences in the pattern of incidence of urinary stones considered in relation to possible aetiological factors. *In* Renal Stone Research Symposium (edited by Hodgkinson, A. and Nordin, B.A.). Churchill, London. p. 7

Androulakis, P.A., Barratt, T.M., Ransley, P.G. and Williams, D.I. (1982) Urinary calculi in children. *British Journal of Urology*, in press

Barratt, T.M. and Williams, D.I. (1974) Urolithiasis. *In* Encyclopaedia of Urology, Vol.15, Suppl. (edited by Williams, D.I.). Springer-Verlag, Heidelberg. p. 280

Barratt, T.M., Simmonds, H.A., Cameron, J.S., Potter, C.F., Rose, G.A., Arkell, G.D. and Williams, D.I. (1979) Complete deficiency of adenine phosphoribosyltransferase: a third case presenting as renal stones in a young child. *Archives of Disease in Childhood*, **54**, 25

Blacklock, N.J. (1976) Epidemiology of Urolithiasis. *In* Scientific Foundations of Urology, Vol.1 (edited by Williams, D.I. and Chisholm, G.D.). Heinemann, London. p. 235

Boyce, W.H., Stanton-King, J. and Fielden, M.L. (1962) Total non-dialysable solids in human urine: immunological detection of a component peculiar to renal calculous matrix and to urine of calcous patients. *Journal of Clinical Investigation*, **41**, 1180

Ghazali, S. (1975) Childhood urolithiasis in the United Kingdom and Eire. *British Journal of Urology*, **47**, 739

Ghazali, S. and Barratt, T.M. (1974) Urinary excretion of calcium and magnesium in children. *Archives of Disease in Childhood*, **49**, 97

Ghazali, S., Barratt, T.M. and Williams, D.I. (1973) Childhood urolithiasis in Britain. *Archives of Disease in Childhood*, **48**, 291

Harrison, A.R. (1976) Urinary calculi in bowel disorders. *In* Scientific Foundations of Urology, Vol.1 (edited by Williams, D.I. and Chisholm, G.D.). Heinemann, London.p.315

Hodgkinson, A. (1976) Oxalate metabolism and hyperoxaluria. *In* Scientific Foundations of Urology, Vol. 1 (edited by Williams, D.I. and Chisholm, G.D.). Heinemann, London. p.289

Klein, R. and Haddow, J. (1975) Hyperparathyroidism. *In* Endocrine and Genetic Disorders of Childhood and Adolescence, 2nd edn (edited by Gardner, L.I.). Saunders, Philadelphia. p.400

Lett, H. (1936) On urinary calculus with special reference to stone in the bladder. *British Journal of Urology*, **8**, 205

Nyhan, W.L. (1978) Urate nephropathy. *In* Pediatric Kidney Disease, Vol. 2 (edited by Edelmann, C.M.). Little, Brown, Boston. p.894

Robertson, W.G. and Nordin, B.E.C. (1976) Physicochemical factors governing stone formation. *In* Scientific Foundations of Urology, Vol. 1 (edited by Williams, D.I. and Chisholm, G.D.). Heinemann, London. p.254

Rodriguez-Soriano, J. (1978) Renal tubular acidosis. *In* Pediatric Kidney Disease, Vol. 2 (edited by Edelmann, C.M.). Little, Brown, Boston. p.995

Royer P. (1961) Explorations biologique du métabolisme calcique chez l'enfant. *Helvetica Paediatrica Acta*, **16**, 320

Sutor, D.J. (1976) Crystallographic analysis of urinary calculi. *In* Scientific Foundations of Urology, Vol.1 (edited by Williams, D.I. and Chisholm, G.D.). Heinemann, London. p. 244

Thier, S.O. and Segal, S. (1978) Cystinuria. *In* The Metabolic Basis of Inherited Disease, 4th edn (edited by Stanbury, J.B., Wyngaarden, J.B. and Frederickson, D.S.). McGraw-Hill, New York. p.1578

Van Acker, K.J., Simmonds, H.A., Potter, C.F. and Cameron, J.S. (1977) Complete deficiency of adenine phosphoribosyltransferase: report of a family. *New England Journal of Medicine*, **297**, 127

Westbury, E.J. and Omenogor, P. (1970) A quantitative approach to the analysis of renal calculi. *Journal of Medical and Laboratory Technology*, **27**, 462

Wickham, J.E.A. (1976) The matrix of renal calculi. *In* Scientific Foundations of Urology, Vol.1 (edited by Williams, D.I. and Chisholm, G.D.). Heinemann, London. p.323

Williams, H.E. and Smith, L.H. (1978) Primary hyperoxaluria. *In* The Metabolic Basis of Inherited Disease, 4th edn (edited by Stanbury, J.B., Wyngaarden, J.B. and Frederickson, D.S.). McGraw-Hill, New York. p.182

Wrong, O.M. and Davies, H.E.F. (1959) The excretion of acid in renal disease. *Quarterly Journal of Medicine*, **28**, 259

30 Urolithiasis: Surgical Aspects

J.H. Johnston

The surgeon's involvement in the management of the child with urinary calculi concerns not only the removal of stones but also the decision as to whether or not there are pre-existing anatomical lesions that may be responsible at least in part for the formation of the calculi and which, if uncorrected, could lead to stone recurrence after lithotomy.

Whether urinary tract dilatation is the cause or the result of stones is often evident from the intravenous urogram. For example the generally small multiple calculi that occur in a hydronephrosis due to a pelvic outlet obstruction (*Figure 30.1*), in a calyceal diverticulum or in or

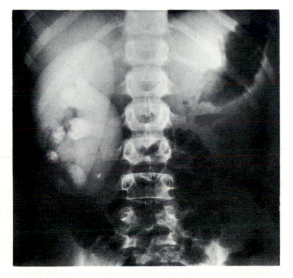

Figure 30.1. Intravenous pyelogram showing multiple small calculi in a solitary hydronephrotic kidney.

above a ureterocele are clearly secondary developments. However, the urogram must be interpreted with caution. As already mentioned (*see* Chapter 29) an infection stag-horn or branched pelvic stone is often associated with moderate dilatation of the ureter which may suggest the existence of a lower ureteric obstruction. Such ureterectasis is, however, entirely the result of muscular hypotonia probably caused by bacterial toxins and it resolves completely when the stone is removed and the infection is eliminated (*see* Chapter 17). When there are stones in a dilated ureter it can be more difficult to distinguish cause from effect, especially if a calculus is impacted near the bladder. The shape of the concretion is helpful. Thus a stone or stones forming an elongated cast of the dilated system infers the presence of a pre-existing obstructed megaureter and the need for appropriate ureteric surgery as well as ureterolithotomy (*see* Chapter 17 and *Figure 17.14*). If the ureter is severely inflamed, as sometimes occurs in such cases, initial surgery is preferably restricted to lithotomy and nephrostomy drainage. Ureteric reimplantation into the bladder can be performed a few weeks later, following antibiotic therapy.

Typically the male infant or toddler with an infection bladder stone has no preceding bladder outlet obstruction and indeed vesical calculus is virtually unknown as a complication of such unequivocal obstructions as posterior urethral valves, even when there is urinary tract infection with Proteus. Nevertheless, vesical stones, which are presumably secondary to urinary stasis, do not occur infrequently as a complication of bladder neck reconstruction for incontinence due to epispadias or of exstrophy closure. On occasions the irritation caused by a bladder stone produces an exaggerated fundal ring on the cystogram which may simulate a congenital hour-glass deformity or a urachal diverticulum.

Vesicoureteric reflux occurs commonly in the child with a bladder stone and rather less often when struvite calculi involve the upper urinary tract. In both circumstances the reflux is frequently due mainly to infection and operative correction need not be considered unless it persists after the stones and the infection have been removed.

Techniques

Renal calculi

Nephrectomy is required mainly in the case of an obstructing pelvic calculus that has led to pyonephrosis and total parenchymal destruction, sometimes with xanthogranulomatous change. The operation can be difficult, notably when there is severe perinephritis, and a subcapsular technique may be unavoidable. Less often nephrectomy is needed for the shrunken kidney, generally with multiple stones, which is shown by excretory urography and scanning with dimercaptosuccinic acid to be nonfunctioning. Johnston and McKendrick (1974) reported that in their series nephrectomy as a primary procedure was necessary in 11 of 146 children with renal stones.

Lower pole partial nephrectomy has been recommended as a virtual routine in the management of the adult with renal calculi. The idea is to remove a dependent sump and promote free drainage to prevent stone recurrence (Papathanassiadis and Swinney, 1966). However, the method has not been extensively used in children. In the author's series the main indication for partial nephrectomy has been impacted calculi in the upper or lower pole associated with severe parenchymal atrophy.

Pyelolithotomy for mobile pelvic stones presents no difficulty. It is often more convenient to open the renal pelvis on its anterior rather than posterior aspect. When the pelvis is first opened the opportunity should be taken to obtain urine for culture. The Gil Vernet (1965) extended sinus technique of intrahilar extrapelvic dissection facilitates the extraction of a branched stone extending into the infundibula but does not help the removal of calyceal stones since the external aspects of the calyces can never be exposed. A stone in a calyx can often be extracted through the open pelvis and a small scoop is generally preferable to the standard calculus forceps since it causes less stretching of the calyceal neck and since the calculus is commonly friable and crumbly.

When there are calculi occupying several calyces as well as the pelvis an extensive longitudinal nephrotomy may be employed. The original bivalve or split kidney operation has been superseded by the anatrophic nephrotomy of Smith and Boyce (1968) which aims at avoiding tissue devascularization by dividing the parenchyma in the plane between the zones of distribution of the anterior and posterior segmental branches of the renal artery. On the renal surface the line of cleavage lies considerably posterior to the lateral convexity of the kidney and is stated to be demonstrable by intravenous injection of methylene blue following occlusion of either the anterior or posterior renal arterial branch; however, not infrequently the colour differences are less than striking. The main renal artery is clamped and, after incision of the capsule, the parenchyma is divided by blunt dissection to minimize damage to intrarenal vessels. The pelvis is entered either through the anterior surfaces of the posterior calyces or directly into its posterolateral margin. After extraction of the calculi and release of the vascular clamp haemostasis is secured by suture-ligation of spurting arteries and of the larger divided veins with fine catgut.

Boyce insisted that water-tight closure of the calyces and the pelvis should be performed with, if necessary, calycorrhaphy to enlarge a stenotic calyceal neck or, when there is extensive calyceal narrowing, calycoplasty by which two calyces are joined together. Other workers (Redman, Bissada and Harper, 1979; Scardino, 1979) have been much less adamant on these points and in the author's experience it is rarely feasible in the kidney of the small child to perform such meticulous intrarenal surgery with confidence. One is always concerned that in attempting precise pyelocalyceal closure or plastic procedures a potentially freely draining calyx may readily be converted into a closed cavity.

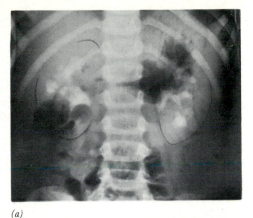

(a)

(b)

Figure 30.2. A 4-year-old boy with extensive bilateral stag-horn calculi. *(a)* Straight film before surgery. *(b)* Intravenous pyelogram 1 year after bilateral anatrophic nephrotomies showing no stone recurrence.

The results of anatrophic nephrotomy without separate closure of the collecting system have been entirely satisfactory in the cases treated by the author (*Figure 30.2*) and also in those of Redman, Bissada and Harper (1979).

In an experimental study in dogs Fitzpatrick *et al.* (1980) compared the effects of various methods of renal lithotomy. They measured the early postoperative clearance rates of creatinine, inulin and para-aminohippuric acid by the kidney and, following sacrifice of the animal, determined the degree of structural damage inflicted by surgery. The extended sinus technique caused no functional or parenchymal tissue loss. Radial nephrotomies, two anterior and one posterior, led to a 20 per cent diminution in function but no significant parenchymal destruction. Anatrophic nephrotomy and bivalve nephrotomy produced respectively 30 per cent and 50

per cent lowerings of clearance rates and considerable loss of kidney tissue. The authors concluded that the optimum method of removing a stag-horn stone is by a combination of the extended sinus approach for the pelvic component and of localized nephrotomies along lines radiating from the hilum to the convexity for intracalyceal calculi not extractable through the renal pelvis.

If it is anticipated that nephrotomy procedures will necessitate lengthy devascularization of the kidney, methods aimed at lowering the renal metabolic rate and so preventing temporary or even permanent impairment of cellular function become important. Renal hypothermia brought about either by heat-exchange coils or by the application of ice sludge externally and the injection of cold saline intrapelvically has been the customary technique. However, it has been shown that the purine nucleoside inosine administered either intravenously or by injection into the renal artery is equally effective at least for a warm ischaemia time lasting up to 1 hour (Wickham *et al.*, 1979).

After the extraction of multiple renal calculi, coagulum pyelolithotomy has been employed to ensure that purulent and matrix material and minute calculus fragments have been entirely removed. Saline solutions of fibrinogen and thrombin are mixed and instilled into the renal pelvis. The resulting clot when withdrawn contains the entrapped residual debris. This method does not have any obvious advantage over the simpler one of vigorous saline irrigation of the pelvis and the calyces.

Whatever method of renal stone removal has been used it is always necessary to employ intraoperative radiography to detect any residual calculi or fragments. Care is needed to ensure that the entire kidney is exposed on the film and it must be remembered that many infection calculi are composed mainly of matrix and may be only slightly radio-opaque, particularly with the customary portable X-ray equipment. The great limitation of standard radiography during surgery is the virtual impossibility of obtaining satisfactory lateral views so that when a calyceal stone remains one cannot readily determine whether it lies in an anterior or a posterior calyx. Cook and Lytton (1977) found intraoperative ultrasound B-scanning, which has the advantage over the previously employed A-scanning of providing a third dimension, to be helpful in the localization of small residual stones. The necessary apparatus is not available in all centres and it appears that considerable experience is needed for accurate interpretation of the ultrasound images.

Nephroscopy using either a paediatric cystoscope or a specifically designed flexible instrument has been advocated for the localization of intracalyceal calculi but even when visibility is perfect, which is by no means invariable, a stone may not be demonstrable when the calyceal neck is undilated. In the absence of facilities for three-dimensional intraoperative radiography (Gil Vernet, 1980) or computed tomography (Wickham, Fry and Wallace, 1980) there is usually no alternative to gentle probing through a pyelotomy. The grating sensation and the sound which occur when a metal implement contacts a stone are unmistakable.

It may not be essential to extract every small calyceal stone in the case of a renal stag-horn calculus. There is a body of opinion that maintains that prolonged potentially traumatic probing may do more damage to renal papillae and hence to the parenchyma than would a residual stone. This philosophy can be a great consolation to the surgeon who has been searching at length and without success. In the author's experience a residual calyceal stone may indeed remain unchanged and cause no demonstrable harm over a period of many years. Nevertheless, in other cases a persistent calculus has led to the continuation of drug-resistant Proteus infection and further stone formation, even to the degree of complete reformation of a stag-horn calculus.

Total stone removal is clearly the ideal, but when a calculus cannot be located a nephrostomy or pyelostomy tube may be left in position after operation with the intention of postoperative stone dissolution by irrigation with a solution of citric acid and various magnesium compounds (Renacidin). This relies on the exchange of the soluble salts for the calcium in the stone. In the past faulty technique led to severe kidney damage in some cases and it is important to ensure that there is free efflux for the irrigant, if necessary by the use of two tubes or a U-tube arrangement, and that urine sterility is maintained either by systemic chemotherapy or by the inclusion of an antibiotic in the solution. The patient's serum magnesium must be monitored to detect possible hypermagnesaemia which would necessitate at least temporary discontinuation of treatment. The normal level of serum magnesium is 1.4–1.8 mEq/ℓ (0.7–0.9 mmol/ℓ).

Occasionally renal stones can be managed without surgery. Recumbency calculi in children who have needed lengthy immobilization for burns or for orthopaedic procedures can be induced to dissolve once ambulation is resumed by treating urinary tract infection and promoting profuse diuresis. In the child with infection stones in a dilated kidney draining into an ileal conduit it has been possible in the author's experience to cause stone dissolution by acidification of the urine and instillation of the appropriate antibiotic solution into the conduit, and thence by ileoureteric reflux to the kidney.

Postlithotomy management

Following the removal of infection calculi the patient is encouraged to promote urinary dilution by a copious fluid intake. The appropriate antibiotic is administered orally for at least 2 months. In deciding the optimum initial form of medication a culture of urine obtained from the renal pelvis at operation is more helpful than one from voided specimens. Proteus organisms elaborate urease which hydrolyses urea to produce ammonia, bicarbonate and alkaline urine. When infection persists after lithotomy acetohydroxamic acid, which is a urease inhibitor, has been employed in an oral dosage in adults of 1 g daily (Griffith *et al.*, 1978). In addition to its main function of preventing stone recurrence this drug also potentiates the antimicrobial effect of chemotherapeutic agents by lessening bacterial virulence.

Ureteric stone

A single oxalate calculus in the lower ureter in an older child, especially a girl in whom a large cystoscope can be inserted, can be extracted with a Dormia basket as in adults. In the much commoner situation of an infection ureteric stone in a smaller child the extractor cannot be passed and ureterolithotomy is needed if there is no prospect of the stone being passed spontaneously. Often in such cases there are in any event coexisting renal calculi requiring surgery, and pyelolithotomy and ureterolithotomy can then be carried out at the same operation and frequently through the same incision. The possibility of there being a preceding lower ureteric obstruction (*see* above) must be kept in mind.

Bladder stone

In children bladder stones are most commonly encountered in very young boys and litholapaxy is not possible because of the small urethral calibre. In adults lithotripsy techniques employing ultrasound or electronic shock waves have been used in recent times to shatter and then fragment the stone. Suitably sized probes are not available for children and there appears to be little need for their development. These methods are time-consuming, not always successful, and not devoid of the risk of causing severe septic complications and bladder injury (Pelander and Kaufman, 1980). They offer no advantage over the eminently simple procedure of suprapubic cystolithotomy.

Urethral stone

Urethral calculus is most commonly encountered as an emergency when a stone impacts just within the urethral meatus in a boy and causes acute urinary retention. Extraction following meatotomy presents little difficulty. A stone situated more proximally can often under anaesthesia be milked manually to a meatal position. A calculus in the prostatic urethra is an occasional occurrence in a boy with a neuropathic bladder and detrusor-sphincter dys-synergia. In this case lithotomy is most easily accomplished by suprapubic cystotomy.

Surgical complications and results

Stone recurrence

As already discussed (*see* Chapter 29) in the absence of an underlying metabolic disorder the postoperative recurrence rate of calculi in children is relatively low when compared with adult series. Williams (1972) reported that in adults

the 5-year, 10-year and 15-year recurrence rates following pyelolithotomy were 8, 37 and 65 per cent respectively; after nephrolithotomy the corresponding figures were 17, 24 and 53 per cent. In the series of children described by Johnston and McKendrick (1974) there was an 8.3 per cent recurrence rate of renal stones over a follow-up period of 1–13 years after pyelolithotomy and/or nephrolithotomy in 95 kidneys. The authors had no doubt that in many instances the recurrences were in fact residual stones that had remained undetected at surgery. The figures support Williams' (Williams and Eckstein, 1968) contention that in the absence of metabolic disease children pass through a phase of stone formation and providing complete calculus clearance is achieved and infection eliminated there is little likelihood of recurrence.

Infundibular stricture

After removal of a branched pelvic stone through a pyelotomy an uncommon complication is the development of an infundibular stricture due to mucosal ulceration by the calculus and causing hydrocalycosis (*Figure 30.3*). When symptoms occur, which is not always the case,

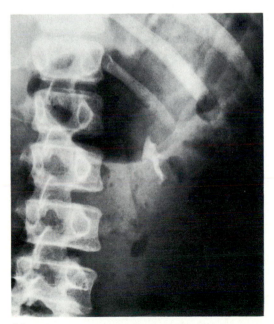

(a)

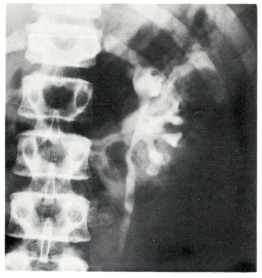

(b)

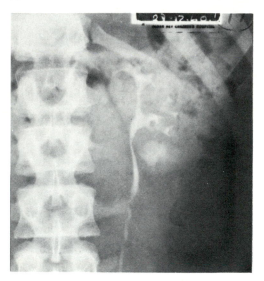

(c)

Figure 30.3. Branched pelvic stone in a 13-year-old boy. *(a)* Straight film. *(b)* Intravenous pyelogram before surgery showing diffuse calyectasis. *(c)* Intravenous pyelogram 2 years after pyelolithotomy by the extended sinus technique showing hydrocalycosis due to stricture of the infundibulum.

treatment generally requires polar partial nephrectomy.

Kidney growth and function

In terms of subsequent kidney growth and function the results of lithotomy for renal calculi in children depend mainly on the severity of the damage inflicted on the parenchyma before treatment. On occasions, even with a branched pelvic stone, the kidney as judged from the intravenous urogram appears to be perfectly normal. In other cases, particularly when a pelvic stone coexists with multiple calyceal calculi, there is already marked parenchymal atrophy and diffuse pyelonephritic scarring at the time of presentation and in such circumstances renal growth and function following stone removal must be expected to be substandard. There is no evidence that nephrolithotomy carries any long-term disadvantages over pyelolithotomy for severe disease. Bartone and Johnston (1977) followed up 19 children, four of whom had bilateral renal involvement, who had had infection stag-horn stones that necessitated extensive nephrotomies. These authors reported that postoperatively growth resumed in all kidneys but in cases with unilateral disease it did so to a lesser degree than in the opposite normal kidney.

References

Bartone, F.F. and Johnston, J.H. (1977) Staghorn calculi in children. *Journal of Urology*, **118**, 76

Cook, J.H. and Lytton, B. (1977) Intraoperative localisation of renal calculi during nephrolithotomy by ultrasound scanning. *Journal of Urology*, **117**, 547

Fitzpatrick, J.M., Sleight, M.W., Braack, A., Marberger, M. and Wickham, J.E.A. (1980) Intrarenal access: effects on renal function and morphology. *British Journal of Urology*, **52**, 409

Gil Vernet, J. (1965) New surgical concepts in removing renal calculi. *Urologia Internationalis*, **20**, 255

Gil Vernet, J. (1980) Cited by Wickham, Fry and Wallace (1980)

Griffith, D.P., Gibson, J.R., Clinton, C.W. and Musher, D.M. (1978) Acetohydroxamic acid: clinical studies of a urease inhibitor in patients with staghorn renal calculi. *Journal of Urology*, **119**, 9

Johnston, J.H. and McKendrick, T. (1974) Urinary calculous disease. *In* Reviews in Paediatric Urology (edited by Johnston, J.H. and Goodwin, W.E.). Excerpta Medica, Amsterdam. p. 349

Papathanassiadis, S. and Swinney, J. (1966) Results of partial nephrectomy compared with pyelolithotomy and nephrolithotomy. *British Journal of Urology*, **38**, 403

Pelander, W.M. and Kaufman, J.M. (1980) Complications of electrohydraulic lithotresis. *Urology*, **16**, 155

Redman, J.F., Bissada, N.K. and Harper, D.C. (1979) Anatrophic nephrolithotomy: experience with a simplication of the Smith and Boyce technique. *Journal of Urology*, **122**, 595

Scardino, P.L. (1979) Editorial. *Journal of Urology*, **122**, 597

Smith, M.J.V. and Boyce, W.H. (1968) Anatrophic nephrotomy and plastic calyrrhaphy. *Journal of Urology*, **99**, 521

Wickham, J.E.A., Fernando, A.R., Hendry, W.F., Whitfield, H.N. and Fitzpatrick, J.M. (1979) Intravenous inosine for ischaemic renal surgery. *British Journal of Urology*, **51**, 437

Wickham, J.E.A., Fry, I.K. and Wallace, D.M.A. (1980) Computerised tomography localisation of intrarenal calculi prior to nephrolithotomy. *British Journal of Urology*, **52**, 422

Williams, D.I. and Eckstein, H.B. (1968) Urinary lithiasis. *In* Paediatric Urology (edited by Williams, D.I.). Butterworth, London. p.323

Williams, R.E. (1972) The results of conservative surgery for stone. *British Journal of Urology*, **44**, 292

31   Urinary Tract Injuries

J.H. Johnston

Closed renal parenchymal injuries

The kidney is more exposed to trauma during childhood than in adult life because it is relatively larger, there is less perinephric fat and it lies in a lower position where it is less well protected by the ribs and the vertebral musculature. Most renal parenchymal injuries arise from direct violence where a fall, a blow to the loin or being run over in a traffic accident compresses the kidney against the ribs or the vertebral column. Often the 11th or 12th rib or the transverse process of a lumbar vertebra is fractured. In traffic accidents other viscera such as the liver, the spleen, the intestine or the lung may be injured by the same force that damaged the kidney and trauma to the head and the limbs often occurs in addition.

Pre-existing renal disease

In a significant number of childhood cases an injured kidney is the site of pre-existing disease. In the series reported by Morse *et al.* (1967), Persky, Forsythe and Forsythe (1964), Smith, Seidel and Bonacorti (1966), Mertz *et al.* (1963) and Esher, Ireland and Cass (1973) the incidence of prior pathology was respectively 10, 23, 22, 17 and 17 per cent. The commonest lesion was hydronephrosis. Several nephroblastomas presented following trauma. A hydronephrotic extrarenal pelvis may be ruptured without parenchymal injury and without the occurrence of macroscopic haematuria.

Classification

Renal parenchymal injuries can be classified into four types (*Figure 31.1*; Nunn, 1962). Renal contusion (*Figure 31.1a*) causes bruising within

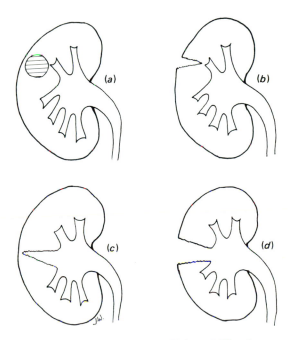

Figure 31.1. Types of closed renal injury. *(a)* Renal contusion. *(b)* Cortical laceration. *(c)* Calyceal laceration. *(d)* Complete parenchymal tear.

369

the parenchyma. Haematuria occurs but the collecting system and the renal capsule remain intact so that there is no bleeding around the kidney and no intrarenal or perirenal extravasation of urine. In cortical laceration (*Figure 31.1b*) bleeding occurs around the kidney or infrequently under the intact capsule. Since the lacerated renal tissue does not excrete urine there is no urine extravasation. When there is calyceal laceration (*Figure 31.1c*) a parenchymal tear communicates with a calyx but does not extend to the capsule. With a complete parenchymal tear (*Figure 31.1d*) the laceration extends from the kidney surface to the collecting system. Blood and urine escape into the perinephric tissues. The severity of the injury ranges from a single tear to virtual shattering of the kidney in which multiple lacerations lead to fragments becoming displaced, devascularized or completely detached.

Diagnosis

The diagnosis of renal injury is based on a history of trauma, the existence of loin pain and tenderness, and the appearance of haematuria. Macroscopic haematuria usually develops soon after the accident, although its onset may be delayed if the urinary excretion rate is depressed as a result of shock or if the ureter is blocked by clot; coexisting injury to the pelvis or the ureter may prevent its occurrence. Elongated clots formed as a cast of the ureter may be passed *per urethram*. Infrequently the accumulation of clot in the bladder causes urine retention. While large amounts of blood or urine in the perinephric tissues lead to a flank mass, often there is such local tenderness and muscular rigidity that accurate palpation is difficult. Diffuse abdominal distension and meteorism may occur as a result of retroperitoneal extravasation causing paralytic ileus. Later on fever is common because of the absorption of blood, and its occurrence does not necessarily indicate the development of infection.

Intravenous urography employing a high dose of contrast medium together with tomography is needed in all cases of renal trauma, even apparently very mild ones, because of the possibility of pre-existing renal pathology. Urography is also advisable in the absence of any clinical evidence of renal injury in patients in whom laparotomy is planned for injuries to intraperitoneal viscera. The investigation should be performed as soon as possible. Delay can be misleading since a simple contusion can then cause nonvisualization of the kidney and simulate a more serious injury. Additionally the onset of gaseous intestinal distension can make radiological interpretation difficult.

On urography attention should be directed not only to the traumatized kidney but also to the presence and the normality or otherwise of the opposite one. Spinal scoliosis concave to the injured side is often present. The injured kidney may show total or partial nonvisualization or there may be pyelocalyceal distortion due to lacerations or the presence of clots. Pooling of contrast medium under the capsule or in the perinephric tissues may be seen with parenchymal tears. A perirenal collection obliterates the psoas line and may displace the ureter. Blood clots may cause filling defects on the cystogram. Rarely, even after the child has been resuscitated and the blood pressure is normal, urography may show bilateral post-shock nephrograms. In these contrast medium accumulates in the renal tubules as a result of a low glomerular filtration rate and increased tubular absorption of salt and water (Pearl and Lilienfeld, 1974).

In recent years selective renal angiography has been increasingly employed in investigating renal injuries. Prior and Williams (1975) advised that the examination is indicated urgently if intravenous urography shows total nonvisualization of the kidney suggestive of a renal pedicle injury or if there is partial nonvisualization indicative of devascularization or detachment of a renal segment. Otherwise, angiography may be required if haematuria persists, if there is persistent poor visualization on urography or if there is uncertainty about the presence of pre-existing disease. Angiography gives precise information concerning the integrity of the renal vascular architecture and can reveal separation or dislocation of parenchymal segments and demonstrate whether or not these have an intact blood supply. However, this investigation does not in most cases allow assessment of the possibility of spontaneous healing of renal lacerations and it does not therefore provide an infallible guide to the need for surgical intervention.

Renal scanning employing ^{99m}Tc-dimercaptosuccinic acid has the advantage over renal angiography that it is less invasive, and it is therefore of particular value in assessing renal trauma in the seriously ill patient with multiple injuries. The flow of the radiopharmaceutical through the renal arteries should be inspected for delayed or absent perfusion which may indicate arterial obstruction. Parenchymal contusions show on the scan as foci of irregular blood flow with reduced uptake of the tracer. Infarcts are seen as areas of absent flow and function. Lacerations are evident as cortical defects and in such cases perirenal extravasation and possibly renal displacement may be demonstrated (O'Reilly, Shields and Testa, 1979).

Treatment

Perirenal haemorrhage from a renal laceration is contained within and tamponaded by Gerota's fascia so that the injury is rarely an immediate threat to life and early operative intervention to control bleeding is seldom needed. The patient should be kept at rest in bed. Frequent observations of pulse rate and blood pressure are required. Repeated abdominal examination is necessary to determine whether any loin mass is developing or increasing in size. The need for blood transfusion is shown by the patient's general condition and haematocrit readings. If perirenal extravasation of blood or urine exists, broad spectrum antibiotic therapy is indicated to prevent infection. The amount and duration of haematuria are themselves of limited value as indicators of the severity and the progress of the injury. However, persisting bright red haematuria is undoubtedly suggestive of continued bleeding while a dark brown discoloration of the urine demonstrates the presence of blood clots in the urinary tract.

When the danger to the patient's life from haemorrhage has passed the salvage of the injured kidney comes to the fore. There is general agreement that renal contusions and lesser lacerations should be managed without surgery. With more severe injuries controversy exists as to whether early operative intervention or an initially conservative approach with the possibility of delayed surgery gives better results.

Series reported by the proponents of the different methods are difficult to compare because the type and the degree of renal trauma and the

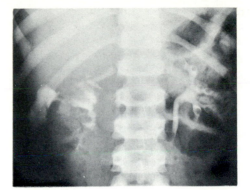

(a)

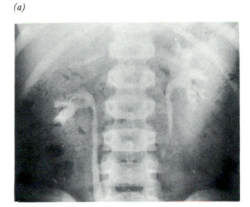

(b)

Figure 31.2. *(a)* Intravenous pyelogram showing a complete parenchymal tear of the right kidney with perirenal extravasation in a 7-year-old boy. There was nonoperative management. *(b)* Intravenous pyelogram 3 months after injury. The kidney shows some calyceal distortion but normal function.

extent and the severity of associated injuries varies greatly. In children it has been the author's experience that the injured kidney has a great capacity for recovery and that even complete parenchymal lacerations generally heal spontaneously with conservative methods alone (*Figure 31.2*). Perusals of the literature give the impression that early intervention, even when begun with the best intentions of repairing the kidney, often ends in the removal of an organ that could have recovered if left undisturbed (Wein *et al.*, 1977). While perirenal urine extravasation is not itself an indication for surgery, exploration is required when leakage is continuing and the urinoma is increasing in size. This may be demonstrated by repeat intravenous urography. The extent of the injury and the precise pathological anatomy are usefully shown preoperatively by angiography and retrograde pyelography, although in most cases the necessity for surgery is apparent from clinical assessment alone.

Surgical technique

On delayed operation the renal parenchyma is not unduly friable and haemorrhage has generally stopped. Nevertheless, generous exposure is indicated with early transperitoneal control of the renal pedicle before Gerota's fascia is opened (Carlton, 1972). Devascularized tissue and blood clot are removed and haemostasis is secured. Renal tears are closed by catgut sutures, if necessary using perinephric fat or omentum to control bleeding. Excision of an ischaemic or detached segment may be needed. When the kidney is extensively lacerated nephrectomy may be unavoidable.

Following traffic accidents the clinical features of renal trauma may be obscured by those of injuries to other abdominal viscera. Blood loss and hypotension may delay the development of haematuria and, if preoperative intravenous urography has not been performed, the kidney injury may be diagnosed only when a retroperitoneal haematoma is seen at laparotomy for intraperitoneal trauma. The decision as to whether or not to explore the kidney must then be based on the apparent severity of the renal injury as judged by the size of the haematoma, the extent of other injuries and the patient's general condition. If the perirenal haematoma is small then it is generally advisable to leave the kidney undisturbed and treat its injury as a separate entity. However, a large or expanding haematoma must be explored following initial control of the renal pedicle. In the critically ill patient with multiple injuries and a severe renal injury nephrectomy may be more prudent than prolonged efforts at surgical repair provided that the opposite kidney is shown to be normal.

Sequelae

When a renal laceration has been treated conservatively or repaired operatively careful clinical and urographic follow-up is needed to detect possible late complications. Hypertension may result from renal ischaemia due to vascular injury or compression of the kidney by perinephric fibrosis following the organization of a haematoma (Page, 1939). Hydronephrosis may develop from scarring obstructing the proximal ureter. As a rule such complications appear within 1 year of injury (Dowse and Kihn, 1963).

An uncommon late sequel to injury is a pararenal pseudohydronephrosis in which a large encysted urinoma forms. The lesion presents clinically as a loin mass, the development of which is often considerably delayed following the trauma. The urinary cyst communicates with the lumen of the pelvicalyceal system. Its persistence is due to an obstruction to pelvic emptying which may have preceded the injury, resulted from it or been caused by compression from the cyst itself. The extravasation is generally restrained by Gerota's fascia and its wall may become calcified. In the case recorded by Sturdy and Magell (1960) the urine burst through the fascia to enter the pelvis and from there extended to the groin and through the sciatic foramen to the sacral region. The diagnosis of pararenal pseudohydronephrosis can be made by intravenous urography; delayed films are often needed. Treatment requires operative relief of the urinary obstruction and closure of the perforation in the urinary tract.

Renal pedicle injuries

Injury to the renal pedicle occurs as a result of its overstretching during a traffic accident when the patient is run over or from a deceleration injury in which he falls from a height. The injury is slightly commoner on the right side and it can occur bilaterally (Toguri *et al.*, 1974). The renal artery or both the artery and the vein may be completely avulsed but bleeding is not necessarily severe, especially in children, and generally stops spontaneously (Watkins, Hirsch and Armour, 1967). With lesser injuries the adventitia and the media of the artery stretch and remain intact while the inelastic intima tears and arterial thrombosis follows. The site of injury is 1–2 cm from the aorta. Haematuria does not occur unless the renal parenchyma is also traumatized. Other abdominal injuries are often present.

On intravenous urography or scanning with dimercaptosuccinic acid there is no excretion by the affected kidney. Aortography demonstrates a short stump of renal artery and so distinguishes the condition from renal agenesis, in which there is also compensatory hypertrophy of the opposite kidney. Owing to the frequent coexistence of other injuries and to inevitable delay in diagnosis the possibility of successful restoration of arterial blood flow by reconstructive vascular surgery or thrombectomy is small. Maggio and Brosman (1978) noted that in 10 kidneys in eight patients which had been reported to be salvaged by operation normal renal function was restored in none. They recommended that the uniformly poor results of surgery should temper heroic efforts and that vascular repair should not be attempted in patients with a normal opposite kidney or with severe injuries elsewhere. If the infarcted kidney is left *in situ*, hypertension is a likely sequel and occurs in more than 50 per cent of cases.

Penetrating parenchymal injuries

Open injuries of the kidney by penetrating external wounds are rare during childhood but may occur as a result of a fall onto a wooden or metal spike. The main danger is primary haemorrhage and operation may be needed for this or for injuries to other viscera. A possible late sequel is an intrarenal arteriovenous fistula.

Needle biopsy of the kidney has been increasingly employed in recent years and carries the risk of causing persistent bleeding into the perinephric tissues or the urinary tract or both. Surgical exploration may be required and on occasions nephrectomy has been necessary. Kalish *et al.* (1974) reported that persisting haematuria following needle biopsy or a penetrating wound may be halted by embolization of the appropriate intrarenal vessel under angiographic control, employing autologous blood clot. The thrombosed vessel recanalizes within 3 months. Alternatively intravenous epsilon-aminocaproic acid may, by inhibiting the urinary fibrinolytic activator urokinase, lead to the cessation of bleeding (Storey, Savdie and Mahoney, 1979).

Perforation or penetration of the renal substance may occur during retrograde catheterization. The possibility is lessened, although not eliminated, if the stylet is withdrawn from the ureteric catheter after the lower ureter has been negotiated. As a rule no ill effects result, even if contrast medium is injected into the parenchyma or the perinephric tissues. Such accidents are readily avoided if retrograde urography is carried out under fluoroscopic control.

Injuries of the ureter

The commonest form of closed ureteric injury is avulsion of the ureter from the renal pelvis. The lesion is caused by overstretching of the ureter as a result of excessive lateral flexion or extension of the spine or of a car wheel crossing the abdomen and displacing the kidney upwards. In the latter case the injury may be bilateral (Boston and Smith, 1975). There is little or no haematuria. A large palpable urinoma forms in the retroperitoneal tissues. Often its appearance is delayed for several days or even some weeks, suggesting that the ureter was not torn immediately but suffered vascular injury which led to its later necrosis and separation. Hypertension because of renal displacement and ischaemia has been recorded (Ribeiro and Quartey, 1976). Intravenous urography shows extravasation of contrast medium.

The ideal treatment is resuture of the ureter to the pelvis by an oblique anastomosis with splinting and temporary nephrostomy. When the gap between the two ends is too wide to allow their approximation it may be possible to join the ureter to the lowest renal calyx (Moloney, 1970). If repair proves impossible, the proximal end of the ureter is ligated and nephrostomy performed. Replacement of the ureter by a segment of intestine can then be considered at a later date.

Penetrating ureteric injuries by stab or gunshot wounds are rare during childhood. Accidental operative trauma is in general easily avoidable since the lack of extraperitoneal fat allows the ureter to be identified without difficulty.

Injuries of the bladder

During childhood the bladder is more of an abdominal viscus than it is in adult life. When full it is therefore more liable to injury of either a closed or an external penetrating type.

Intraperitoneal bladder rupture

This injury occurs when the distended bladder bursts following a blow on the abdomen or a crush injury. The lesion has been reported in a newborn infant in whom abdominal compression occurred during birth (Miller *et al.*, 1960). The tear occurs on the posterior aspect of the fundus. Sterile urine in the peritoneal cavity causes little reaction. The abdomen becomes distended but there is no muscular rigidity and the bowel sounds may be normal. If diagnosis is delayed, self-dialysis may occur so that equilibration between plasma and urine across the peritoneal membrane leads to a fall in the serum sodium and chloride levels and a rise, possibly to a dangerous degree, in the urea and potassium concentrations.

Catheterization is indicated when intraperitoneal bladder rupture is suspected, and some blood-stained urine may be obtained. The diagnosis is best confirmed by cystography with the patient supine which demonstrates intraperitoneal contrast medium in the dependent paracolic gutters and between coils of small intestine. Treatment requires transperitoneal exposure of the bladder. The perforation is closed by suture and the bladder drained by either a suprapubic or a urethral catheter.

Extraperitoneal bladder rupture

Extraperitoneal rupture of the bladder most commonly occurs with injuries causing fracture of the pelvis, especially when the pubic bones or rami are broken. The bladder may be torn by traction on its attachments or may be penetrated by a bony fragment. Urine accumulates around the bladder and, if not drained, may infiltrate the abdominal wall, the scrotum or the thighs. The lower abdomen becomes distended and tender and a boggy pelvic mass is palpable on rectal examination. As a rule micturition is not possible. There is no leakage of blood from the urethral meatus and this distinguishes the injury from a ruptured urethra. The diagnosis is made by cystography following catheterization which shows contrast medium in the perivesical tissues. The bladder is compressed circumferentially by blood and urine into a long narrow ovoid shape (the tear-drop bladder; *Figure 31.3*). A small extraperitoneal bladder perforation

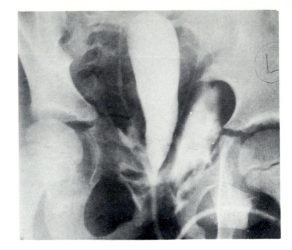

Figure 31.3. Tear-drop bladder. Cystogram in a boy with extraperitoneal bladder rupture.

with little urine extravasation may be managed by urethral catheter drainage alone. Otherwise, exploration is needed with suture of the laceration and drainage of the bladder.

Injuries of the urethra

Intrapelvic urethral rupture

This injury occurs as a complication of fracture-dislocation of the pelvis which most commonly results from a crush injury compressing the pelvis from side to side so that its anteroposterior diameter is increased. As a rule the cause is a traffic accident, and other visceral, bony and soft tissue injuries may be present. Both boys and girls can be affected.

In the male the urethra is most often avulsed at the apex of the prostate, although retrograde urethrography has shown that the injury may involve the urethra both above and below the urogenital diaphragm (Colapinto and McCallum, 1977). The bladder and the prostate retract proximally so that there may be a gap of some inches between the torn urethral ends. Some injuries are incomplete in that a bridge of intact mucosa persists. In young boys in whom the prostate is undeveloped the urethral rupture is often just below the bladder neck and above the verumontanum.

The child is generally severely shocked. A

tender swelling is palpable in the lower abdomen and in the pelvis and dark blood escapes from the urethral meatus. Micturition is not possible. Intravenous urography demonstrates that the bladder lies high in the pelvis and is often compressed by surrounding haematoma. It is now generally agreed, as was first stressed by Mitchell (1968), that catheterization should not be attempted since it is not reliable as a diagnostic measure and carries the risks of introducing infection and causing further damage to the injured urethra. The diagnosis may be confirmed by retrograde urethrography, inserting the nozzle of the syringe containing aqueous contrast medium into the urethral meatus. Periurethral extravasation is seen above or both above and below the urogenital diaphragm (*Figure 31.4a*).

The first therapeutic need is usually resuscitation of the child by blood transfusion. Only when the general state is stable can investigations and specific treatment be undertaken. The management of the injury itself remains a highly contentious matter, with wide disagreement as to whether or not primary correction of the traumatic deformity should be attempted. Mitchell (1968) found that many intrapelvic urethral injuries are incomplete and advocated that the initial treatment should consist only of suprapubic cystostomy. If the rupture is indeed incomplete, healing then occurs without stricture formation, and if a complete rupture is present, the urethral ends approximate spontaneously as the haematoma is absorbed so that the resulting stricture is short and easily treated by reconstructive surgery.

Mitchell's views were reinforced by the reports of Morehouse, Belitsky and Mackinnon (1972) and Morehouse and Mackinnon (1980). Of 27 patients with a ruptured intrapelvic urethra managed by realignment over a catheter 55 per cent were subsequently incontinent and 51 per cent impotent, and all had severe stricture. In 61 cases treated initially by cystostomy alone three incomplete ruptures healed without complications and 58 patients with complete rupture had urethral reconstruction for stricture by the Johanson technique 3 months after injury. Later review revealed no persistent strictures, no incontinence and an impotence rate of less than 10 per cent.

On the other hand Glass *et al.* (1978) found that among 67 males with urethral injury associated with fractured pelvis the best results were

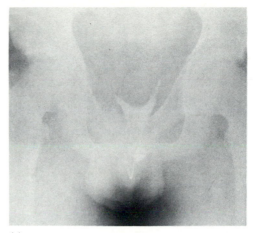

(a)

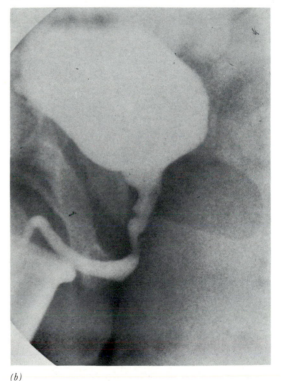

(b)

Figure 31.4. *(a)* Ruptured intrapelvic urethra in a 14-year-old boy. Retrograde urethrogram showing extravasation of contrast below elevated bladder. *(b)* Micturation cystourethrogram of the same patient 5 months after injury demonstrating no stricture and full urinary control.

seen when the two urethral ends were approximated. In four patients stricture was avoided entirely and in 17 others it was short and allowed easy urethroplasty. The most difficult strictures occurred when there was uncontrolled displacement of the torn tissues. These authors considered early surgical repair of the urethral rupture to offer the best chance of minimizing the severity of any subsequent urethral stricture. Primary realignment of the urethra was also employed successfully and advocated by Pierce (1972), Myers and Deweerd (1972), Gibson (1974) and Cranweller *et al.* (1977).

None of the above series made any distinction between prepubertal and postpubertal urethral ruptures. Malek, O'Dea and Kelalis (1977) reported satisfactory results in seven boys treated by urethral approximation over a catheter. The author has had experience of eight boys managed by this method. In only one was the rupture incomplete in that there was a thin strip of dubiously vascularized mucosa between the torn ends.

Technique of repair

The technique is shown in *Figure 31.5*. With the patient in the lithotomy position and with the lower abdomen, the genitals and the perineum exposed, the prevesical space is opened through a midline abdominal incision. Blood and clots are evacuated and the nature of the injury is confirmed. The bladder is opened through its anterior wall. A perineal urethrotomy is performed and a 12 F Foley catheter is passed into the pelvis and thence under direct vision through the proximal urethra into the bladder.

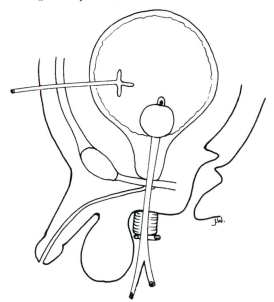

Figure 31.5. Technique of urethral approximation for intrapelvic rupture.

The balloon of the catheter is inflated to about 10 ml and digital traction is applied to the opposite end to bring the two ends of the urethra together. While the pull on the catheter is maintained 2.5 cm adhesive strapping is wrapped around the instrument to produce a large firm mass in contact with the perineal skin. The catheter is transfixed by a safety pin, avoiding the inflating channel, just below the strapping to prevent it slipping. The bladder and the abdomen are closed with suprapubic vesical drainage.

Weight traction on the Foley catheter was formerly employed but is not necessary since approximation of the urethral ends is sufficiently maintained by their compression between the catheter balloon and the perineal strapping. The Foley catheter is removed after 3 weeks. Bougies are passed *per urethram* 1 week later to ensure the absence of stricture before the suprapubic catheter is removed. If all goes well urethral instrumentation is repeated 1 month and 6 months later. The use of a perineal exit rather than a penile urethral course for the Foley catheter permits the use of a larger catheter with a bigger balloon and also eliminates the risk of stricture formation in the vulnerable penile urethra.

In six of the eight boys treated along these lines stricture was completely avoided (*Figure 31.4b*). One developed an annular stricture that was excised through a transpubic approach. The other boy was mismanaged in that a Foley catheter with a 3 ml balloon was employed and excessive weight traction was applied to it after operation. As a result the catheter balloon was drawn through the proximal urethra to lie in the gap between the urethral ends. The resulting stricture was successfully treated by a Badenoch (1950) pull-through operation but the boy subsequently had a severe lack of urinary control which was not improved by a Leadbetter (1964) bladder neck reconstruction. However, continence developed spontaneously at the age of 15. No assessment of potency has been attempted in any of these patients.

Late complications

Impotence is a well recognized complication of intrapelvic urethral rupture. The mechanism of its occurrence is uncertain but it has generally been considered that the traumatic force that leads to the urethral avulsion also causes neural injury and/or vascular damage later followed by thrombosis. Reported results suggest that the method of management may be significant. Employing primary realignment of the torn urethra Morehouse, Belitsky and Mackinnon (1972), Cass and Godec (1978) and Gibson (1970) recorded an incidence of impotence of respectively 51, 38 and 37 per cent. Using early cystostomy with subsequent stricture correction if necessary Morehouse, Belitsky and Mackinnon (1972) reported no impotence in their 11 cases and Johanson (1972) described only four impotent men in a series of 120. Mitchell (1978) considered that the age of the patient is important as regards the likelihood of post-traumatic impotence and he found that the complication is commoner in men over the age of 30 than in younger age groups. Late spontaneous restoration of potency is possible and Gibson (1970) noted that erections could return after an absence of 19 months. The question of financial compensation is obviously relevant to the symptomatology.

As already discussed the incidence of urethral stricture following a ruptured intrapelvic urethra has varied greatly in different reported series, whether the initial treatment was by urethral realignment or by cystostomy alone. In the early weeks after injury intermittent dilatation of a still soft and malleable narrowing can prevent the development of an established stricture. However, in a child or a young adult a life-time of regular bouginage, possibly not always performed by an expert, is a bleak prospect and once a true fibrous stenosis has developed operative treatment is indicated.

The technique required depends mainly on the length of the narrowed segment. Endoscopic urethrotomy is highly effective for an annular stricture (Mitchell, 1978) or for division of the thin shelf that can occur when an S-shaped deformity results from a slight vertical overlap between the proximal and distal ends of the urethra (Glass *et al.*, 1978). Rather longer strictures may be managed by the Badenoch (1950) pull-through technique or by transpubic methods. With the Badenoch operation the bulbar urethra is mobilized and intussuscepted through the prostatic urethra above the stricture. Inadequate freeing of the bulb from the corpora cavernosa can lead to retraction and severe shortening of the penis. Allen (1975) excised the stricture and resutured the urethral ends, having exposed the region by resecting the pubic symphysis. Using a similar exposure and also a perineal approach Waterhouse (1974) mobilized the divided bulbar urethra below the stricture, brought it between the separated corpora cavernosa, and anastomosed it to the prostatic urethra. For more extensive strictures a one-stage island patch urethroplasty (Gardner *et al.*, 1978) or a two-stage scrotal flap urethroplasty (Blandy, Singh and Tresidder, 1968; Turner-Warwick, 1968) is generally needed.

Intrapelvic urethral rupture in the female

The mechanism of the injury is the same as in the male. In girls the urethra is ruptured just above the urogenital diaphragm and the proximal end retracts upwards. In all cases the vagina is torn at the level of the urethral avulsion; in some patients only the anterior wall is involved and in others the laceration is circumferential. If the vaginal injury is not recognized or if first-intention healing is not obtained, urethral and vaginal strictures and a urethrovaginal fistula may follow.

The operative approach is similar to that in the male. The vaginal tear can be demonstrated by inserting a bougie through the introitus, and it is closed with absorbable sutures through the abdominal incision. Reinforcement of the suture line by omentum may be needed and as a rule the omentum can reach the site without formal mobilization. The separated urethral ends are approximated as in the male, using a Foley catheter, and the bladder is drained suprapubically.

Rupture of the bulbar urethra

This lesion is the result of a blow in the perineum or of a straddle injury that compresses the urethra against the pubis. The rupture may be complete or incomplete. There is bleeding from the urethral meatus and a haematoma may develop in the perineum and the scrotum. If the patient micturates, urine extravasation can occur beneath Colles' fascia and extend to the scrotum, the groins and the abdominal wall.

Catheterization should be attempted using a soft rubber catheter. If the catheter passes into the bladder then the urethral injury is clearly incomplete and a small Foley catheter is left in position for 7–10 days. Evacuation of a haematoma may be needed. Urethral bougies are passed 1 month later to ensure the absence of stricture.

If the catheter cannot pass the site of injury, a complete rupture exists. Suprapubic cystotomy is performed and with the patient in the lithotomy position the perineum is explored through a midline incision. The divided urethral ends are exposed, the traumatized extremities are trimmed and the dorsal walls are united using interrupted absorbable sutures. It may be necessary to mobilize the corpus spongiosum from the corpora cavernosa on either side of the injury to allow the urethral ends to come together. Complete closure of the urethral lumen should not be attempted because of the likelihood of its leading to stricture. The ventral wall of the urethra and the overlying part of the wound are left open and packed to heal by secondary intention. When there is loss of tissue so that the torn ends do not come together the skin is sutured to the urethral extremities to form a fistula that can be closed later.

Injuries of the genitalia

Injuries of the penis

During boyhood penile injury may occur when the patient or his colleagues tie a ligature around the organ or pass it through a metal or rubber ring that cannot later be removed because of the development of engorgement and oedema. Unless this is promptly dealt with, distal gangrene may occur or a urethral fistula may form at the site of the constriction. In infants and toddlers similar changes occur when a long hair tightly encircles the circumcised penis several times just behind the coronal sulcus. The hair becomes buried in or through the skin and is usually not visible until surgical exploration is carried out. It is often obvious from the colour that the hair is not from the child but a history can never be obtained as to its origin or how it came to encircle the penis. The likelihood of this condition must be kept in mind in any young child in whom there is swelling and discoloration of the glans penis.

The boy in a hurry to return to play after micturition may catch his foreskin in his fly zipper. A slight attachment can be freed under local anaesthesia. A deeper involvement requires the zipper to be removed from the trousers and a formal circumcision to be performed, removing the foreskin with the attached zipper.

The penile and scrotal skin may be avulsed if the genitals are caught in revolving machinery. If the penis is completely denuded of skin, immediate or delayed skin grafting may be carried out. Alternatively the penile shaft may be buried temporarily under the skin of the lower abdominal wall or the anterior aspect of the scrotum. After some 6 weeks the penis is freed and the dorsal or ventral aspect is covered by abdominal or scrotal skin flaps. Any residual foreskin should be removed since it is liable to persistent oedema. Loss of scrotal skin alone does not usually necessitate immediate grafting because sufficient skin generally remains around the neck of the scrotum to epithelialize and re-cover the scrotal contents.

Iatrogenic injury to the penis is usually the result of circumcision performed by an inexperienced and unskilled operator. The glans may be partly or completely amputated or the penis may slough following the excessive and improper use of diathermy. Occasionally a urethral fistula results from a deeply biting suture inserted to obtain haemostasis in the frenular region or from a ligature tied around the penis to hold a dressing in place.

Injuries of the testis

Rupture of the testis may occur when the organ is compressed against the pubic bone by a kick or a straddle injury. The injury is rare in boys, possibly because testicular retraction is an immediate reflex response to an anticipated blow. Testicular tissue protrudes through the torn tunica albuginea. A haematocele forms and may cause testicular atrophy by compressing the spermatic vessels. Exploration of the scrotum and evacuation of the blood clot are needed together with suture of the laceration in the testicular tunica.

Traumatic dislocation of the testis is generally caused by being run over in a traffic accident. The testis is displaced from the scrotum into the groin, the inguinal canal, the perineum or the thigh. The diagnosis is often delayed and obscured by local haematoma or severe associated injuries. Orchidopexy is indicated when the patient's condition permits.

Injuries of the female genitalia

A straddle injury may lacerate and contuse the vulva and the labia so that evacuation of a haematoma and suturing are often needed. A penetrating genital injury may result from a fall onto a sharp projection. The vaginal wall is commonly perforated and the possibility of injury to the urethra, the bladder, the rectum or the intra-abdominal viscera must always be considered. Radiology of the abdomen and the pelvis may show a retained foreign body or free intraperitoneal gas if the alimentary tract is penetrated. Examination under anaesthesia with cystoscopy, vaginoscopy and proctoscopy is often needed.

Forced sexual intercourse in young girls may lacerate the introitus posteriorly to involve the perineum or even the anus and the rectum.

References

Allen, T.D. (1975) The transpubic approach for strictures of the membranous urethra. *Journal of Urology*, **114**, 63

Badenoch, A.W. (1950) A pull-through operation for impassable traumatic stricture of the urethra. *British Journal of Urology*, **22**, 404

Blandy, J.P., Singh, M. and Tresidder, G.C. (1968) Urethroplasty by scrotal flap for long urethral strictures. *British Journal of Urology*, **40**, 281

Boston, V.E. and Smith, B.T. (1975) Bilateral pelvi-ureteric avulsion following closed trauma. *British Journal of Urology*, **47**, 149

Carlton, C.E. (1972) Early operation in the management of blunt renal trauma. *In* Current Controversies in Urologic Management (edited by Scott, R., Gordon, H.L., Scott, F.B., Carlton, C.E. and Beach, P.D.). Saunders, Philadelphia.p.109

Cass, A.S. and Godec, C.J. (1978) Urethral injury due to external trauma. *Urology*, **11**, 607

Colapinto, V. and McCallum, R.W. (1977) Injury to the male posterior urethra in fractured pelvis: a new classification. *Journal of Urology*, **118**, 575

Cranweller, P.O., Farrow, G.A., Robson, C.J., Russell, J.L. and Colapinto, V. (1977) Traumatic rupture of the supramembranous urethra. *Journal of Urology*, **118**, 770

Dowse, J.L.A. and Kihn, R.B. (1963) Renal injuries: diagnosis, management and sequelae in 67 cases. *British Journal of Surgery*, **50**, 353

Esher, J.O., Ireland, G.W. and Cass, A.S. (1973) Renal trauma and pre-existing lesions of kidney. *Urology*, **1**, 134

Gardner, R.A., Flynn, J.T., Paris, A.M.I. and Blandy, J.P.

(1978) The one-stage island patch urethroplasty. *British Journal of Urology*, **50**, 575

Gibson, G.R. (1974) Urological management and complications of fractured pelvis and ruptured urethra. *Journal of Urology*, **111**, 353

Gibson, R. (1970) Impotence following fractured pelvis and ruptured urethra. *British Journal of Urology*, **42**, 86

Glass, R.E., Flynn, J.T., King, J.B. and Blandy, J.P. (1978) Urethral injury and fractured pelvis. *British Journal of Urology*, **50**, 578

Johanson, B. (1972) Personal communication to Morehouse *et al.* (1972)

Kalish, M., Greenbaum, L., Silber, S. and Goldstein, H. (1974) Traumatic renal haemorrhage treated by arterial embolisation. *Journal of Urology*, **112**, 138

Leadbetter, G.W. (1964) Surgical correction of total urinary incontinence. *Journal of Urology*, **91**, 261

Maggio, A.J. and Brosman, S. (1978) Renal artery trauma. *Urology*, **11**, 125

Malek, R.S., O'Dea, M.J. and Kelalis, P.P. (1977) Management of ruptured posterior urethra in childhood. *Journal of Urology*, **117**, 105

Mertz, J.H.O., Wishard, W.N., Nourse, M.H. and Mertz, H.O. (1963) Injury of the kidney in children. *Journal of the American Medical Association*, **183**, 730

Miller, A.L., Sharp, L., Anderson, E.V. and Emlet, J.R. (1960) Rupture of the bladder in the newborn. *Journal of Urology*, **83**, 630

Mitchell, J.P. (1968) Injuries of the urethra. *British Journal of Urology*, **40**, 649

Mitchell, J.P. (1978) Personal communication

Moloney, G.E. (1970) Avulsion of the renal pelvis treated by ureterocalycostomy. *British Journal of Urology*, **42**, 519

Morehouse, D.D. and Mackinnon, K.J. (1980) Management of prostatomembranous urethral disruption. *Journal of Urology*, **123**, 173

Morehouse, D.D., Belitsky, P. and Mackinnon, K.J. (1972) Rupture of the posterior urethra. *Journal of Urology*, **107**, 253

Morse, T.S., Smith, J.P., Howard, W.H.R. and Rowe, I. (1967) Kidney injuries in children. *Journal of Urology*, **98**, 539

Myers, R.P. and Deweerd, J.H. (1972) Incidence of stricture following primary re-alignment of the disrupted proximal urethra. *Journal of Urology*, **107**, 265

Nunn, I.N. (1962) The management of closed renal injury. *Australian and New Zealand Journal of Surgery*, **31**, 263

O'Reilly, P.H., Shields, R.A. and Testa, H.J. (1979) Urinary tract trauma. *In* Nuclear Medicine in Urology and Nephrology (edited by O'Reilly, P.H., Shields, R.A. and Testa, H.J.). Butterworths, London.p.100

Page, I.H. (1939) The production of persistent arterial hypertension by cellophane perinephritis. *Journal of the American Medical Association*, **113**, 2046

Pearl, M. and Lilienfeld, R.M. (1974) The post-shock nephrogram. *Journal of Urology*, **111**, 391

Persky, L., Forsythe, W.E. and Forsythe, W.E. (1964) Trauma and simulated renal disease. *Journal of Trauma*, **4**, 197

Pierce, J.M. (1972) Management of dismemberment of the prostato-membranous urethra and ensuing stricture disease. *Journal of Urology*, **107**, 259

Prior, J.P. and Williams, J.P. (1975) A study of 137 cases of renal trauma. *British Journal of Urology*, **47**, 45

Ribeiro, B.F. and Quartey, J.K.M. (1976) Traumatic

avulsion of the ureter with obstruction, pseudocyst formation and hypertension. *British Journal of Urology*, **48**, 107

Smith, M.J.V., Seidel, R.F. and Bonacorti, A.F. (1966) Accident-trauma to the kidneys in children. *Journal of Urology*, **96**, 845

Storey, B.G., Savdie, E. and Mahoney, J.F. (1979) Control of bleeding after renal biopsy with epsilon-amino-caproic acid. *British Journal of Urology*, **51**, 68

Sturdy, D.E. and Magell, J. (1960) Traumatic perinephric cyst (pseudohydronephrosis). *British Journal of Surgery*, **48**, 315

Toguri, A.G., Liu, T.T., Bayliss, C., Ameli, F.M. and Deveber, G.A. (1974) Traumatic bilateral renal artery thrombosis. *Journal of Urology*, **12**, 430

Turner-Warwick, R.T. (1968) Repair of urethral strictures in the region of the membranous urethra. *Journal of Urology*, **100**, 303

Waterhouse, K. (1974) Injuries to the urinary tract in children. *In* Reviews in Paediatric Urology (edited by Johnston, J.H. and Goodwin, W.E.). Excerpta Medica, Amsterdam. p.241

Watkins, J.P., Hirsch, J.S. and Armour, T.D. (1967) Traumatic severance of renal artery without death. *Journal of Urology*, **98**, 167

Wein, A.J., Murphy, J.J., Mulholland, S.G., Chait, A.W. and Arger, P.H. (1977) A conservative approach to the management of blunt renal trauma. *Journal of Urology*, **117**, 425

32 Renal Tumours

D. Innes Williams and John Martin

Introduction

Malignant disease in childhood is uncommon, having an approximate incidence of one in 600 children under 15 years of age or one per 10 000 children per year (Manchester Children's Tumour Register, 1968). In developed countries malignant disease is a major cause of death in children aged 1–15 and is only exceeded by deaths from accidents. Acute leukaemia, lymphomas and tumours of the CNS account for more than half the cancers in children. Abdominal tumours, principally neuroblastoma and nephroblastoma, constitute the next most important group.

Many paediatric malignancies are of embryonal nature and a large number have their peak incidence before 5 years of age, for example neuroblastoma, nephroblastoma and acute lymphatic leukaemia. A proportion are associated with congenital malformations or chromosomal abnormalities and, together with an increased familial incidence in some tumours, this suggests that prenatal factors are important in their causation. Knudson (1976) recently proposed a causal hypothesis for childhood cancer in which he suggests that it is dependent upon two discrete mutational events. The first mutation renders the cell precancerous but still capable of normal differentiation and the second transforms the cell into a cancer cell. For some childhood cancers the first mutation is hereditary and only exposure to a second mutagen such as a virus, radiation or a chemical stimulus is required while for others the first event is a somatic mutation.

In both the UK and the USA the incidence of malignant disease in childhood is higher in males, especially in the case of leukaemias, lymphomas and medulloblastoma. The sex incidence in nephroblastoma is equal. Racial differences have been demonstrated for some tumours such as the lower incidence of leukaemia and absence of Ewing's tumour in black children in the USA. There are major geographical variations for many childhood cancers, for instance the high incidence of Burkitt's lymphoma in East Africa. Nephroblastoma by contrast has a relatively uniform worldwide distribution and its incidence has been used as a reference index for epidemiological studies.

Nephroblastoma

Incidence

Nephroblastoma is the commonest single-organ solid tumour outside the nervous system occurring in childhood. Johnston, Mainwaring and Rickham (1969) reported an incidence of one case for every 13 500 births. Morris-Jones (1978) analysed the Manchester Children's Tumour Registry and found a rate of 0.5 cases per 100 000 children per year. These tumours can occur at any age. Most are diagnosed between 6 months and 5 years and very few present in adolescence or adult life. A lesion discovered at birth is more often a mesoblastic nephroma which is a relatively benign disorder and is discussed below, and the older figures relating to Wilms' tumour in the infantile period without taking this diagnosis into account are likely to be inaccurate. The differential incidence in regard to sex and side is insignificant. Bilateral disease has been more frequently recognized in recent years and occurs in 8–12 per cent of cases.

Familial cases have been reported by Fitzgerald and Hardin (1955) and are exceptional. A relationship with other congenital anomalies is frequently commented upon although Berry, Keeling and Hilton (1970) studied embryonic tumours in general and did not find any significant correlation. However, Bond (1975) reported that bilateral nephroblastomas were much more commonly found in children with other anomalies than were unilateral tumours. Aniridia (congenital absence of the iris) is the most important association outside the urinary tract (Woodard and Levine, 1969). This disorder occurs in a familial and a sporadic form, and the latter is more likely to be complicated by nephroblastoma with some 30 per cent of such children developing a tumour usually during the first 2–3 years of life. While hemihypertrophy of the whole body is another related disorder, in lesser degrees this anomaly is hard to define and the incidence of neoplasia has not been worked out. Within the urinary tract tumour may complicate a horseshoe, solitary or duplex kidney. Hypospadias may be associated and a particular syndrome involving pseudohermaphroditism and Wilms' tumour is discussed on page 395. The incidence of congenital anomalies in nephroblastomatosis (*see* p.395) is high but the problems encountered are different from those in true tumours.

Pathology and staging

Nephroblastomas are usually larger than the kidney itself by the time they are recognized and some very large masses are on record. Tumours may arise anywhere in the renal parenchyma and growth is at first expansive, compressing the adjacent renal tissue within a pseudocapsule. Occasionally expansion takes place almost entirely outside the kidney so that at first the tumour appears to be extrarenal in origin (Orlowski, Levin and Dyment, 1980). The tumour mass is lobulated and creamy-white in appearance. Cysts are not uncommon and may contain papilliferous tumour. Cystic degeneration due to necrosis occurs in many patients and considerable haemorrhage is sometimes seen.

The first spread of nephroblastoma takes place locally through the false capsule with infiltration into the renal substance. Further local spread may result in the mass becoming adherent to adjacent structures such as the mesocolon, the spleen and the pancreas. Bloodstream metastasis to the lungs has almost always occurred before this infiltration becomes evident. Lymph-node metastasis occurs relatively often and in late cases there may be a solid tumour mass filling the renal vein and extending into the inferior vena cava and even into the right atrium. Distant bloodstream metastasis occurs to the liver and very rarely to the bones or the superficial tissues. It has recently been suggested (Marsden, Lawler and Kumar, 1978) that bone metastasis is a feature of a particular form of renal tumour different from the classic nephroblastoma. Brain secondaries are very unusual, although they are seen in association with rhabdomyosarcoma of the kidney.

A scheme of staging accepted in recent years is shown in *Figure 32.1*. It should be recognized that there is an element of clinical judgement involved. The decision as to whether the tumour

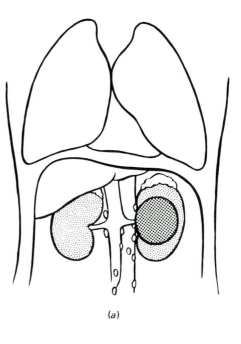

(a)

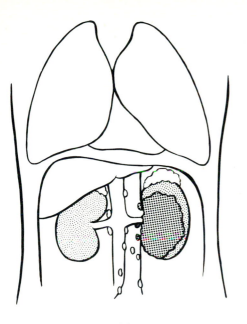

(b)

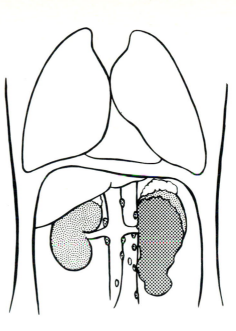

(c)

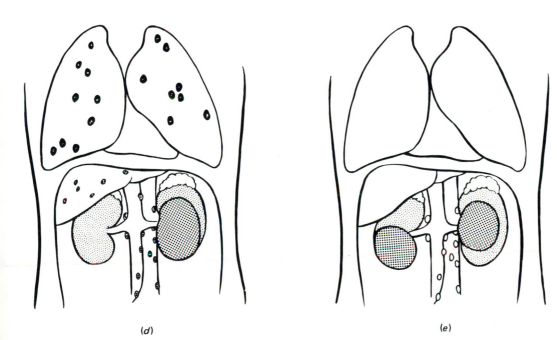

(d)

(e)

Figure 32.1. Staging of nephroblastoma. *(a)* Stage I. Encapsulated tumour: clean nephrectomy, no spread of disease. *(b)* Stage II. Some local infiltration beyond capsule but total surgical removal is possible. *(c)* Stage III. Local extension beyond kidney, peritoneal involvement, multiple lymph-node metastases and tumour spillage. Total surgical removal is unlikely or impossible. *(d)* Stage IV. Metastases in lungs, liver or other distant sites. *(e)* Stage V. Bilateral tumour.

has been totally removed at operation is clearly a difficult one and recently there has been a trend to place all tumours with lymph-node metastasis into stage II.

Bilateral tumours are not infrequently multicentric within one or both of the kidneys, a feature which is rare in unilateral cases. There is a possibility that the second kidney is involved by metastases from the first, but the great majority of cases have no other signs of spread at the time of first presentation. Together with multicentricity, association with other congenital defects and slow evolution as already mentioned this suggests that bilateral nephroblastomas are genuinely multiple primary tumours and may have a different developmental basis. Knudson and Strong (1972) proposed that on analogy with the finding in retinoblastoma a different gene mutation may be involved and that the bilateral disease may conceivably prove to be inheritable.

Histologically a feature of nephroblastomas is embryonic renal tissue in various stages of differentiation. All the tumours contain some undifferentiated renal blastema with masses of loose mesenchyme, collagenous connective tissue, cartilage, and osteoid and adipose tissues. Smooth and striated muscle occurs from time to time. The mixed tumour has always presented a problem to the pathologist grading the degree of malignancy and many attempts to consider multiple factors have failed to give any satisfactory guide to prognosis. With the large amount of material available from controlled trials there has been a revival of interest and some important conclusions have been reached. In particular the results of the first American National Wilms' Tumor Study indicated that the degrees of differentiation and lymph-node involvement are of great prognostic importance. Although there is some disagreement in detail between pathologists, it is in general accepted that several types of unfavourable histology for Wilms' tumours can be identified, including diffuse or focal anaplasia (cellular pleomorphism with hyperchromatic nuclear gigantism and bizarre mitotic figures) and diffuse 'renal sarcoma'. It is not yet apparent whether or not the latter variant is identical to the bone-metastasizing renal tumour described by Marsden, Lawler and Kumar (1978).

Lawler, Marsden and Palmer (1977) analysed the material in the British trial and noted that the degree of tubular differentiation and the presence or absence of glomeruli, cysts and papillary structure were correlated with the clinical stage and with the survival rate. The most significant association was in regard to tubular differentiation so that their group 3+ had a 92 per cent survival rate and their group 0 (no differentiation) had a 58 per cent survival rate. In another study by Beckwith and Palmer (1978) an analysis was made of 427 cases in the American National Wilms' Tumor Study and it was shown that lesions with marked cytological anaplasia and those with predominantly sarcomatous stroma were associated with an unfavourable outcome. Taking these two groups together there was a mortality rate of 57.1 per cent whereas in tumours with neither feature the mortality rate was only 7.1 per cent.

Since children under the age of 2 years are known to have in general a better prognosis, attempts have been made to correlate differentiation with age. Lawler, Marsden and Palmer (1977) were unable to demonstrate that differentiated tumours were more often encountered in younger patients, although there is no doubt that stage I tumours are commoner at this age. Earlier reports on the effects of age are complicated by the inclusion of the neonatal tumour now recognized to be a mesoblastic nephroma, which usually has a very good prognosis. Extremely cystic tumours often cause some difficulty. The disease described as multilocular cyst, cystadenoma or lymphangioma presents clinically as a tumour mass replacing a large proportion of the kidney and enclosed within a single capsule, with the exception that part of it may project as a tongue-like excrescence into the renal pelvis. In its classic form this condition is easily recognized as a benign lesion, but at times the inclusion of some cells suggestive of nephroblastoma in the walls of the cysts gives rise to difficulty in diagnosis (Joshi, Banerjee and Yader, 1977). It appears that the prognosis of the very cystic tumour with a few doubtful cells is almost as good as that of the simple multilocular disease. Bolande (1974) also recognized a type of well differentiated epithelial nephroblastoma in the neonate which he distinguished from mesoblastic nephroma and which has a prognosis as good as that of the cystic form.

Growth rate

The development of nephroblastoma is usually

rapid so that death occurs within 1 year of the first symptoms. A slow evolution is recorded from time to time, particularly in bilateral cases. It is generally believed that the tumour arises in foci of blastema persisting within the fully differentiated renal substance. Once these cells become active, growth is rapid. Thus Rabinowitz and Bagnasio (1970) recorded a case in which no abdominal mass was palpable at birth after a very careful and deliberate search, yet a huge mass was present 3 months later. By contrast Haas and Jackson (1961) described a child in whom nephrectomy was performed at the age of 4 years, lobectomy for metastasis at 9 years and laparotomy for recurrence at 12 years, and death occurred at 14 years. In one of the authors' cases of bilateral disease the child had a unilateral nephrectomy at the age of 2 years with irradiation to the contralateral kidney. She was symptom-free until 19 years when she developed a large mass in the solitary kidney and she died at the age of 25 with multiple metastases.

Collins (1955) suggested that the total growth period of a tumour might be valuable for testing the results of treatment. He postulated that the child's age plus 9 months, representing the gestational period, was the total growth period of the tumour and that if no clinical recurrence had occurred within that time then a permanent cure was likely. Platt and Linden (1964) tested this criterion of cure against a 2-year survival period and found little difference. There were five exceptions to Collins' rule among 83 children and four exceptions to the 2-year survival rule. However, the aggressive use of chemotherapy for recurrences can play havoc with such prognostication.

Clinical features and presentation

In the great majority of cases the child is brought to hospital because the parents or the doctor have observed an expanding abdominal mass or simply an enlarged abdomen. The tumour grows so rapidly that the mass is palpable in well over 90 per cent of those cases diagnosed during life, and probably if the examination were always performed under anaesthesia then 100 per cent would be palpable.

The size of the tumour varies considerably. Smaller tumours have all the usual characteristics of renal masses but larger ones have a less clearly definable origin. They may fill the abdomen to such an extent that they are rendered relatively immobile by their bulk even when not fixed by the infiltration of neighbouring organs.

The tumour is always apt to protrude forwards rather than backwards and when it crosses the midline it usually does so superficially, overlapping rather than infiltrating the region of the great vessels. It is unusual for the tumour to bulge in the loin when the child is sitting up (this feature is seen much more often in neuroblastoma). The mass is hard, heavy and not tender; in most cases it is irregularly lobulated while sometimes there appears to be a single smooth swelling. A taut cystic consistency may be found in rapidly growing tumours which is not easily distinguished from the feel of a tensely obstructed hydronephrosis. The larger tumours are likely to be associated with advanced disease and it has been suggested (Garcia, Douglass and Schlosser, 1963) that where the size exceeds 550 ml the prognosis is poor. Metastases in the liver are found in some cases at the time of the first examination and may form a continuous mass with the primary tumour. Extension of the disease to the para-aortic nodes may be palpable and limits the mobility of the tumour mass.

Abdominal pain is not infrequently associated with an enlarging tumour, although it is seldom severe until there is local infiltration. Vomiting of not very obvious cause sometimes accompanies the pain.

Haematuria is seen in about one third of cases at the time of presentation. It can be due to ulceration of the tumour into the pelvis or can even result from spread down the ureter, but not uncommonly it results from thrombosis and rupture of obstructed veins in the renal sinus and does not necessarily indicate a bad prognosis. In childhood benign causes of haematuria are relatively common and several cases in our series were at first regarded as examples of acute glomerulonephritis because albumin and casts were observed in the urine at the time of the bleed. It is obligatory to perform an intravenous pyelogram in any doubtful case of haematuria.

A mild fever is not uncommon with a nephroblastoma, as in hypernephroma. It occurred in as many as 30 per cent of patients in the series reported by Hastings and Gwinn (1965) and may well accompany haemorrhage into the tumour. Anaemia and loss of weight are features of some cases, and are much more common after metastasis has taken place.

Breathlessness may occur with multiple pulmonary secondaries, but usually the smaller lesions are symptomless.

Hypertension occurs in a proportion of cases, although its incidence has never been satisfactorily worked out since few patients are observed for a sufficiently long period before surgery. The blood pressure almost always falls after nephrectomy (Sukarochana, Tolentino and Kiesewetter, 1972) and in general persistent growth does not lead to any recurrence of hypertension. An exception to this rule was recorded by Cox and Smellie (1955). Veraguth and Chanson (1969) recorded reduction of blood pressure after preoperative irradiation. It is uncertain whether the rise of blood pressure is due to a specific secretion of tumour cells or whether the pressure of the tumour on the blood supply can produce ischaemia of the remaining renal tissue and therefore excessive renin production. Mitchell *et al.* (1970) found a raised plasma renin level in a 22-month-old child with nephroblastoma in whom normal values were recorded after nephrectomy. Sphar, Demers and Sochat (1981) reported another renin-producing Wilms' tumour. The finding of a haemangiopericytoma (Lee, 1970) within the kidney producing hypertension has suggested that similar cells might be present in nephroblastoma.

Spontaneous rupture of nephroblastoma occurs in a few examples. One patient observed in the authors' series had a sudden onset of abdominal pain and signs similar to the perforation of a hollow viscus. The peritoneum was found to contain blood and masses of tumour tissue. A few cases of haemorrhage due to rupture of the tumour into the peritoneal tissues have been recorded.

Varicoceles are a well recognized but rarely observed complication of renal tumours in children. The scrotal veins on the left side are tense rather than truly varicose, yet can form a visible swelling. Ordinarily this presentation is associated with local metastases in the spermatic cord as well as venous obstruction due to the renal tumour mass.

Diagnosis

Usually a combination of clinical palpation and intravenous urography is sufficient to diagnose nephroblastoma and the addition of chest tomography is all that is required for staging. The numerous and complex investigations described below are important in cases where the diagnosis is in doubt or clinical evidence of tumour fixation demands a more thorough assessment of the degree of spread.

Plain X-ray shows a mass lesion in the renal area and good films demonstrate its continuity with the renal outline. Calcification is rare and gives rise to a suspicion of neuroblastoma rather than nephroblastoma. Intravenous urography demonstrates renal enlargement with gross distortion of the calyces, which may be displaced in any direction and even across the midline. These calyces may be hydronephrotic (*Figure 32.2*), although seldom so much as to suggest a

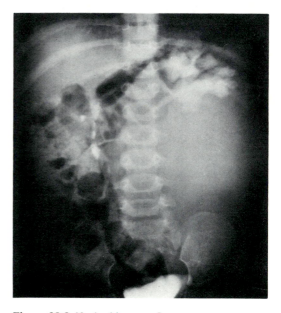

Figure 32.2. Nephroblastoma. Intravenous urogram showing very large tumour mass with hydronephrotic calyces displaced upwards.

congenital obstruction. Often the whole pelvicalyceal system appears enormously enlarged although in reality it is simply stretched out on the surface of a large tumour (*Figure 32.3*). Rarely there is a small expanding lesion (*Figure 32.4*) deforming or obliterating a single calyx, as is often seen in adenocarcinoma in adults. The entire renal mass may be displaced away from the midline by enlargement of the para-aortic nodes. The ipsilateral ureter may show dilatation due to obstructing tumour while displacement of the opposite ureter provides evidence of

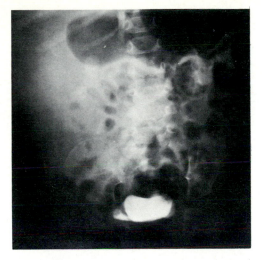

(a)

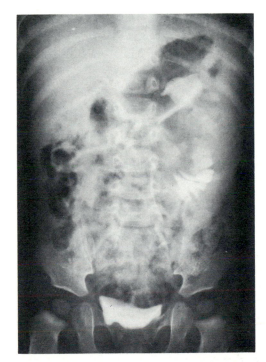

(a)

(b)

(b)

Figure 32.3. Nephroblastoma. Intravenous urograms. Tumour presenting as an abdominal mass in an 11-month-old child. Nephrectomy was performed and followed by radiotherapy and chemotherapy, but there was rapid development of nephrotic syndrome with hypertension and death at 13 months. *(a)* Anteroposterior view. *(b)* Lateral view.

Figure 32.4. Nephroblastoma. Bilateral sequential tumours. Intravenous urograms. *(a)* At 11 weeks showing an expanding lesion in the lower pole of the right kidney and an apparently normal left side. (Nephrectomy is only performed in view of stage I disease in a neonate.) *(b)* At 9 months showing massive tumour in the left kidney.

extensive disease. Infrequently intravenous urograms show no opacification even with a high
dose of opaque medium. This indicates advanced disease and major vascular involvement
which can give rise to diagnostic difficulty and
demands at least an ultrasound scan to differentiate it from a nonopacified hydronephrosis.

A space-occupying lesion within the kidney
and simulating Wilms' tumour can be a cyst, a
hydronephrosis in a duplex system, an abscess
or a tumour of other pathology. Cysts are rare
and are diagnosed without difficulty by ultrasound (*see Figure 2.12*) as are hemihydro-
nephroses. Abscesses and carbuncles are usually
suggested by the history and clinical findings
and generally show as trans-sonic lesions,
although septa may be present. Other tumours,
including cystadenoma or multilocular tumour,
are likely to be diagnosed only after nephrectomy.

Extension of the tumour into the renal vein
and vena cava can be demonstrated by intravenous cavography. Injection of the contrast
medium for intravenous urography can be given
routinely into a leg vein; the immediate films
show the vena cava sufficiently well, even
though often the pressure of the overlying
tumour and some streaming of the blood from
the opposite vein produce a confusing picture. If
vena caval involvement is demonstrated, it is
important to define the upper limit of the
tumour thrombus by superior cavography with
observation of atrial filling.

Arteriography is not so diagnostic in nephroblastoma as in adenocarcinoma (*see Figure 2.5*).
Clark, Moss and de Lorimier (1971) reported
pathological vascularity in more than 90 per
cent of cases; the vessels are tortuous and irregular with some pooling of contrast. Nevertheless
some tumours are avascular while an early
inflammatory disorder such as renal carbuncle
may be vascularized (*see Figure 2.9*). These difficulties together with the by no means negligible
hazards of performing femoral catheterization
for arteriography in infants diminish the usefulness of this investigation.

Renal arteriography is required when bilateral disease (*Figure 32.5*) is demonstrated or suspected, since it is important to define the possible limits of surgery in tumour excision by
partial nephrectomy. Serial investigations by
arteriography and ultrasound may be useful for
judging the response of tumour foci to chemotherapy. Aortography is valuable when there is

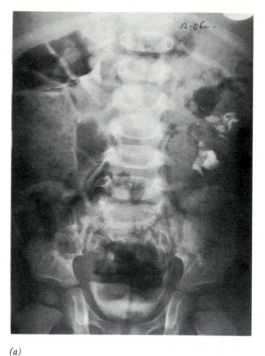

(a)

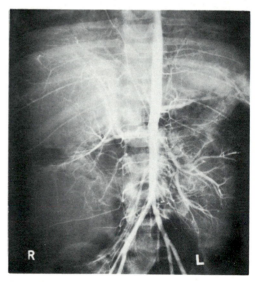

(b)

Figure 32.5. Nephroblastoma. Bilateral
simultaneous tumours in a 15-month-old child with
bilateral flank masses. *(a)* Intravenous urogram. *(b)*
Aortogram.

a large fixed mass of doubtful origin or a functionless kidney on urography. It differentiates
neuroblastoma from other retroperitoneal
tumours such as teratoma.

Percutaneous needle biopsy of the kidney is
resorted to only in cases where the tumour mass

is clearly fixed and inoperable and none of the diagnostic procedures so far described has given any clear indication of the histology of the tumour. The prognosis for adenocarcinoma is very much worse than for nephroblastoma and the precise histological findings can be of value in ordering chemotherapy.

Chest X-rays are vital to staging, although the identification of small secondary deposits often presents difficulties. Fluoroscopy may be valuable while tomography is preferred by many. Ultimately computed tomography may prove the best method of detecting early lung involvement (*see Figure 2.17*). A radiological skeletal survey is required only where neuroblastoma is suspected.

Urine examination reveals nothing except red blood cells, and the presence of pyuria casts doubt on the diagnosis of tumour. Albuminuria and excretion of casts suggest associated renal parenchymal disease of poor prognosis. Radioisotopic scans are seldom necessary except in bilateral cases in which there is doubt about the overall surviving nephron mass.

Routine haematological investigations are undertaken prior to surgery. Anaemia is common and polycythaemia very rare, although it has been recorded, and erythropoietin levels may be relevant in such cases (Kenny, Mirand and Staubitz, 1970). Marrow biopsy is only necessary when there is a possibility of neuroblastoma, and the same can be said for the estimation of urinary catecholamines.

No tumour marker is known for nephroblastoma, but Powars, Allerton and Beierle (1972) identified a circulating mucin and Wallace and Nairn (1972) renal tubular antigens. Further study of these aspects is clearly required.

Liver function tests are needed prior to and during chemotherapy.

Treatment

Many of the major advances in cancer therapy have been introduced in the paediatric field. When improved surgical techniques, better anaesthesia and advances in radiotherapy led to an improving prognosis many patients still relapsed due to the development of distant metastatic disease. Prevention of metastases for many patients awaited the development of systemic therapy with antimitotic drugs in addition to local treatment. Successful chemotherapy for children commenced with Farber's (Farber *et al.*, 1948) use of aminopterin for acute lymphatic leukaemia and was developed by Pinkel *et al.* (1972) in their 'total therapy' approach. Adjuvant chemotherapy for solid tumours in childhood achieved early success in nephroblastoma (Farber, 1966) and rhabdomyosarcoma (Sutow, 1967) and is now used with varying success in most malignant paediatric tumours.

There has been a steady improvement in the survival rates of children with nephroblastoma over the past three decades, reflecting changes in management from surgery alone to surgery plus irradiation to the now general combined approach with surgery, irradiation and chemotherapy. In recent years the development of national and international trials for nephroblastoma such as the American National Wilms' Tumor Study and the MRC and International Society of Paediatric Oncology trials has led to further refinements in therapy. Treatment of large numbers of children with standard protocols has identified groups needing more or less therapy, and detailed pathological studies of patients treated in these trials has helped to identify favourable and unfavourable histological appearances that correlate well with prognosis (Beckwith and Palmer, 1978; Marsden and Lawler, 1978).

The use of several modalities of treatment for childhood cancer has brought about the development of the combined or team approach in the management of these children. This in turn has contributed to higher standards of overall care. With increased survival rates attention has been focused on the quality of life for the patient and his family. This has indicated the need for skilled social support and close cooperation with educational services if emotional and learning difficulties are to be avoided (Peck, 1979).

The need for the development of a skilled team has caused the treatment of children with malignant disease to be concentrated in a number of regional centres where sufficient patients are treated for the team to develop the necessary expertise. Even so most centres on their own are not large enough to evaluate new treatment methods. These are now largely assessed by national bodies such as the American National Wilms' Tumor Study and the UK Children's Cancer Study Group, in which major groups cooperate in clinical studies of new therapeutic approaches. Whenever possible, treatment

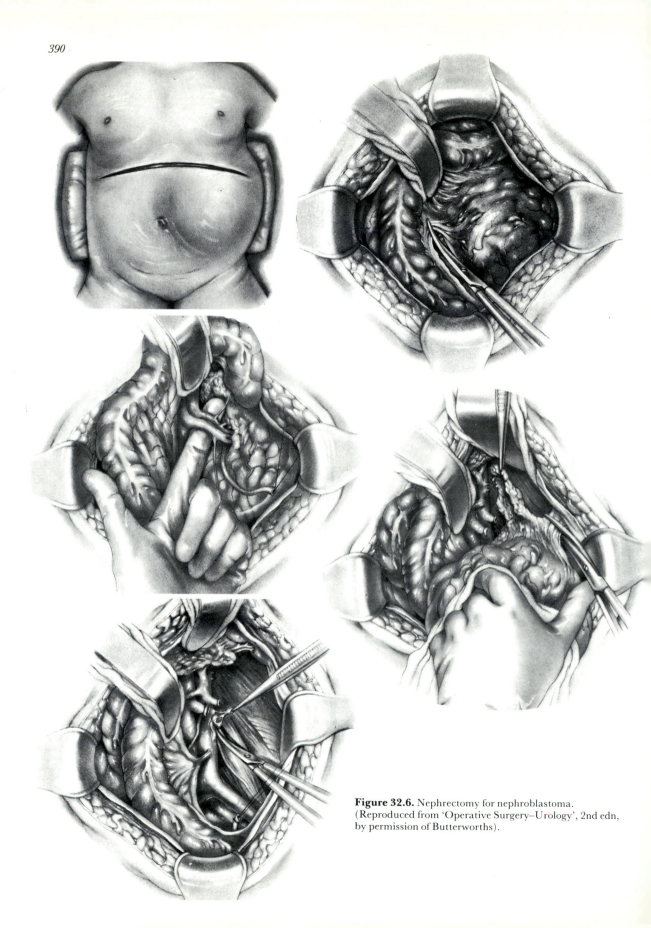

Figure 32.6. Nephrectomy for nephroblastoma.
(Reproduced from 'Operative Surgery–Urology', 2nd edn,
by permission of Butterworths).

should be given following an approved protocol as it has been shown that children treated in such a manner have a significantly increased survival rate (Lennox *et al.*, 1979).

Surgery

Removal of the involved kidney appears to be the one essential form of therapy for all patients with nephroblastoma. It should be undertaken as soon as the diagnosis is established and the full extent of the disease evaluated. In a few patients with very large inoperable tumours or widespread metastases initial surgery may consist of biopsy only and treatment may be commenced with chemotherapy.

For young children a long transverse incision is employed but the thoracoabdominal approach may be preferred for older patients. The principle of ligature of the artery and vein before mobilization is generally accepted and the tumour is removed complete with the surrounding perinephric fat. The steps of the operation are shown in *Figure 32.6*.

An incision is made in the peritoneum lateral to the ascending or descending colon and the bowel is gently mobilized with its mesentery until the area of the renal pedicle comes into view. The ureter is then identified and traced down to the pelvis where it is cut across. The testicular or ovarian vessels are severed at the same time and the ureter is held up so that blunt dissection can proceed behind it to identify and control the pedicle of the kidney. With a finger behind them the vessels are dissected out and a tie is placed first around the artery, even though this is sometimes difficult to expose. The vein is then doubly ligated and cut. If necessary, subsequent ligature and section of the artery can be undertaken once the renal vein and the lymph nodes have been cleared out. The dissection then proceeds upwards keeping the adrenal gland with the kidney and ligating the vessels supplying it. Once all the blood supply is controlled the fascia lateral to the kidney is incised and the kidney together with its perinephric fat is lifted off the renal bed working from below upwards. Care is taken on the left side to dissect free the tail of the pancreas and the splenic vessels. In the ordinary encapsulated case the kidney is then easily removed.

The condition of the para-aortic lymph nodes is inspected and those in the region of the renal pedicle are dissected out and removed. Opinions differ about the need for more radical excision. This is difficult to achieve in many children and in any case small metastases are controlled by chemotherapy.

Difficulty with nephrectomy is encountered in some cases. The size of the tumour alone can make dissection awkward, although it is seldom impossible. Statistically it has been shown that very large tumours have a worse prognosis, but with experience the nephrectomy should not prove too difficult. If the mesocolon is involved by tumour, it may be left attached to the specimen because the marginal colonic vessel is usually sufficient for vascularization of the bowel. The spleen can be removed if it is fixed to the tumour, as can a part of the diaphragmatic muscle. The veins should be inspected for tumour thrombus, and if this is present then a clamp can be placed on the vena cava and the thrombus sucked out. However, at times the tumour thrombus proves to be firmly fixed and invading the venous wall, and it cannot be removed. The tumour itself must always be handled very gently indeed since compression may rupture it. Tumour rupture has a bad effect on prognosis and in experienced hands it occurs only where there is local extension or lymphnode involvement, which are themselves bad prognostic signs.

Radiotherapy

Radiotherapy has long been established as part of the treatment for nephroblastoma. The timing, the size of the field and the dosage have varied considerably. In many European centres preoperative radiotherapy is given but this is not the usual practice in the UK and North America. Although preoperative irradiation has been shown to reduce the incidence of tumour rupture at operation, it does not significantly alter disease-free survival rates (Lemerle, Voute and Tournade, 1976), and there have been a number of misdiagnoses in which a benign condition was irradiated. The more usual practice is to give only postoperative irradiation. This should be commenced as soon as the immediate postoperative period has elapsed, and whenever possible within 10 days of operation.

The field of irradiation should include the tumour bed and a generous margin of at least 2 cm. It should cross the midline medially so that the whole width of the vertebral bodies is included. Whole-abdomen irradiation is no longer considered necessary except in those cases where tumour rupture has led to diffuse peritoneal contamination. When whole-abdomen irradiation is given the opposite kidney should be shielded from the posterior field throughout treatment to prevent radiation nephritis. A satisfactory dosage of radiation is 3000 rads given in 20 fractions over 4 weeks with parallel opposed fields and using megavoltage equipment. The second American National Wilms' Tumor Study used a lower dosage of 2000 rads in 10 or 11 fractions over 2 weeks and this schedule may be sufficient in stage II and III patients who do not have unfavourable histological features. Infants less than 1 year of age are more sensitive to radiotherapy and should be given 50 per cent of the dose for older children. Since the introduction of chemotherapy it is rarely necessary to use preoperative irradiation to make an initially inoperable case operable.

In patients with a right-sided tumour the liver receives a considerable dose of radiation and hepatopathy may occur. This is first evidenced by a rapid fall in the platelet count and may progress to hepatic enlargement possibly simulating rapidly developing liver metastases. Coagulation abnormalities and occasionally liver cell failure may follow. The latter features are more likely to be seen with recall hepatopathy associated with postirradiation chemotherapy.

The results of the first American National Wilms' Tumor Study (D'Angio *et al.*, 1976) indicated that whole-abdomen irradiation did not confer any advantage for relapse-free survival in stage I patients. This group, which has an excellent overall survival rate, should not therefore be given radiotherapy.

Radiotherapy for nephroblastoma causes some bone marrow dysplasia although this is rarely severe. Regular blood counts should be carried out during treatment and the schedule modified if the counts fall below acceptable levels, namely neutrophils less than $1.5 \times 10^9/\ell$ and platelets less than $100 \times 10^9/\ell$. Nausea, anorexia and abdominal discomfort are common symptoms during therapy and should settle rapidly after its completion. Some degree of dysplasia of the soft tissues within the radiation field usually occurs and is rarely serious. Scoliosis may occur following soft tissue damage from both surgery and radiation but it rarely requires active treatment. Irradiation of the

whole width of the vertebral bodies prevents the previously observed more severe degrees of scoliosis. Occasionally patients develop chondromas of the lower ribs producing palpable tumours in some cases. This may cause alarm but no treatment is necessary and the tumours do not progress.

Chemotherapy

The use of antineoplastic drugs should be considered in all cases of nephroblastoma. Four drugs, namely actinomycin D, vincristine, adriamycin and cyclophosphamide, have been shown to have some effect against this tumour. Actinomycin D was first demonstrated by Farber (1966) to improve the survival rate for children with nephroblastoma. Later Wolff *et al.* (1968, 1974) showed the advantage in metastasis-free survival of multiple over single courses of the drug. This was not translated into long-term survival because many of those relapsing after a single course of therapy had their metastases successfully treated. Vincristine was demonstrated to be effective in nephroblastoma by Sullivan *et al.* (1967) and later was used in both the MRC trials and the American National Wilms' Tumor Study. In the former it was shown to be a more effective form of maintenance therapy than actinomycin D (Morris-Jones, 1978) and it was used as the main agent in the second MRC trial. The first American National Wilms' Tumor Study showed that the use of actinomycin D and vincristine together was superior to either drug alone (D'Angio *et al.*, 1976). Adriamycin (Wang *et al.*, 1971) and cyclophosphamide (Sutow, 1967) have been demonstrated to have an effect on nephroblastoma, especially in extensive or metastatic disease. Their role is being assessed and is still far from established.

Actinomycin D is an antibiotic obtained from the genus *Streptomyces*. Its effect is due to interference with RNA synthesis (Goldstein, Slotnik and Journey, 1961). This agent needs to be given by intravenous injection. Traditionally it has been administered in short 5-day courses of 15 µg/kg body weight per day repeated at 6-week to 3-month intervals. It is well tolerated as a single dose of up to 1.5 mg/m² body surface area at 3-week intervals and this method of administration is more acceptable to most patients. In children less than 1 year of age the dose should be halved.

The principal complications of actinomycin D

involve the skin, the gastrointestinal tract and the bone marrow. Skin reactions vary from simple erythema to widespread desquamation. Alopecia is common but temporary. Vomiting is the commonest form of gastrointestinal toxicity and stomatitis and diarrhoea are less frequent. Thrombocytopenia constitutes the main haematological problem.

Vincristine is an alkaloid derived from the common periwinkle *Vinca rosea*. Its principal action is to arrest mitosis at the metaphase in a manner similar to colchicine (Cardinali, Cardinali and Enien, 1963). This does not explain its effect on nondividing nerve cells and its detailed mode of action is complex. Vincristine can only be given by intravenous injection and leakage into surrounding tissues produces a severe chemical burn. The standard dose is 1.5 mg/m^2 body surface area with a maximum single dose of 2 mg. It is usually given not more than once per week for 3–12 weeks.

Toxic effects of vincristine include constipation, which can be avoided by giving regular aperients, alopecia of temporary nature and neurotoxicity. The latter usually starts with depression of the ankle jerk reflexes and may progress to paraesthesiae in the hands and the feet and occasionally to muscular weakness, especially of the dorsiflexors at the ankle. Ptosis and jaw pain are not infrequent but a convulsive disorder associated with inappropriate secretion of antidiuretic hormone is fortunately rare.

Adriamycin is an anthracycline antibiotic derived from *Streptomyces peucetius* and closely related to daunorubicin. It acts by DNA binding and thus inhibiting DNA and RNA synthesis. It is predominantly metabolized in the liver so that impaired liver function delays elimination and can cause exaggerated toxicity. Adriamycin is most effectively given in a dosage of 30–60 mg/m^2 body surface area at 3-week intervals and is usually given in combination with other drugs. Like vincristine it is very vesicant.

Adriamycin causes bone marrow suppression, alopecia, stomatitis and in most cases vomiting for a few hours after its administration. Its most serious form of toxicity is cardiotoxicity which is closely related to the total cumulative dose given. Cardiotoxicity usually takes the form of severe intractable heart failure due to myocardial damage. Serial chest X-rays and ECGs are not helpful in detecting early cardiac damage but serial echocardiograms may be more valuable. Serious cardiotoxicity can be avoided by keeping the total dose of adriamycin below 300 mg/m^2 for children less than 5 years old, 400 mg/m^2 for children aged 5–10 and 500 mg/m^2 for older children.

Cyclophosphamide is an alkylating agent, being a cyclic phosphoramide of nitrogen mustard. It is inert *in vitro* and is activated mainly in the liver to primary metabolites with powerful cytotoxic actions. The drug can be administered orally or intravenously, although experience with childhood tumours has been mainly with the intravenous route and usually in combination with other drugs. The dosage for this route is 300–600 mg/m^2 body surface area given at 3-week or longer intervals.

The principal toxic effects of cyclophosphamide are nausea and vomiting for up to 24 hours after injection, alopecia, bone marrow depression (especially of the granulocyte series) and occasionally haemorrhagic cystitis. The latter presents as haematuria and severe dysuria and can largely be prevented by ensuring the patient maintains a good fluid intake, especially by the intravenous route, for a period after the drug is administered.

The form of chemotherapy indicated in nephroblastoma varies with the stage of the disease. The following suggestions in part follow the treatment used in the current UK Children's Cancer Study Group (1980) Nephroblastoma Study.

STAGE I DISEASE WITH FAVOURABLE HISTOLOGY

These patients have an excellent prognosis with surgery and chemotherapy alone. Both actinomycin D and vincristine as single agents have been shown to be effective. The recommended chemotherapy is intravenous vincristine 1.5 mg/m^2 body surface area weekly for 10 weeks commencing on the day of operation followed by a further five doses at 3-week intervals, giving a total of 6 months treatment. Longer periods of chemotherapy appear unnecessary.

STAGE II DISEASE WITH FAVOURABLE HISTOLOGY

These patients should receive radiotherapy as soon as possible after operation. Vincristine should be given as for stage I patients, that is weekly for 10 weeks and then every 3 weeks up to 6 months. Actinomycin D should be given in addition as a dose of 0.75 mg/m^2 on day 7, followed by 1.5 mg/m^2 at the beginning of week 7 and then every 3 weeks for a further six doses.

It is advisable to give children under 1 year of age half doses of all drugs except the initial dose of vincristine.

As mentioned in the section on radiotherapy recall hepatopathy may occur with right-sided tumours where the liver is included within the radiation field. Attention should be paid to the platelet count and when it falls below $100 \times 10^9/\ell$ the drug doses should be modified.

STAGE III DISEASE WITH FAVOURABLE HISTOLOGY

In these patients a longer course of chemotherapy is indicated. Vincristine and actinomycin D should be given as for stage II patients and both drugs continued at 3-week intervals for 1 year. Whether the addition of a further drug such as adriamycin improves the prognosis is uncertain and needs to be assessed.

STAGE I, II AND III DISEASE WITH UNFAVOURABLE HISTOLOGY

The majority of treatment failures occur in these patients and studies of alternative approaches to therapy are indicated. A reasonable method may include the use of 'second-look' surgery and chemotherapy using all four known effective drugs. Injections of vincristine and cyclophosphamide every 3 weeks alternately with adriamycin or actinomycin D are a schedule well tried with other paediatric tumours and could be utilized for these children. The adriamycin dose should be $40\,\mathrm{mg/m^2}$ and the cyclophosphamide dose $600\,\mathrm{mg/m^2}$ body surface area. Treatment should be continued for 1 year making sure the total cumulative dose of adriamycin does not exceed the levels previously mentioned. Dosages should be modified for children under 1 year old and great care taken with right-sided tumours in the early weeks after radiotherapy.

STAGE IV DISEASE

Although these patients with metastatic disease have a poorer outlook than those at other stages, many, including some with extensive metastases, can be cured. Vincristine should be administered weekly from the day of operation or of biopsy in initially inoperable cases. Radiotherapy should be given postoperatively to the abdomen but not to the lungs because pulmonary metastases may clear with chemotherapy. If lung metastases persist, surgery should be considered when there are only one or two and

whole-lung irradiation given when they are multiple. Chemotherapy should include all four active drugs described above for patients with tumours of unfavourable histological types.

STAGE V DISEASE

The management of patients with bilateral disease must always be individual, using surgery, irradiation and chemotherapy in varying combinations. Radiotherapy should only be administered to one side so as to avoid radiation nephritis. These patients often do better than anticipated and approximately 50 per cent can be cured (Aron, 1974; Bond, 1975).

METASTATIC DISEASE

Nephroblastoma most commonly metastasizes to the lungs and regular chest X-rays should be performed at monthly intervals during the first 2 years after diagnosis. Lung metastases are usually multiple. Where a solitary lesion is seen on a plain chest X-ray, computed or whole-lung tomography should be performed to ensure that the lesion is an isolated one. Surgical excision is the method of choice for one and occasionally two lesions, but multiple tumours should be treated with whole-lung irradiation. Whether surgery is performed or radiotherapy administered, chemotherapy should be given wherever possible and should incorporate drugs not previously used. An attempt should always be made to treat pulmonary metastases since at least 50 per cent of patients can be cured (Martin and Rickham, 1970).

Liver metastases have a much poorer prognosis as do the unusual bone metastases. Alternative chemotherapeutic drugs should be tried in these patients together with local radiotherapy for bone lesions. While the latter can rarely be eradicated, effective pain relief can usually be obtained.

Prognosis

The survival rate in Wilms' tumour has steadily improved over the years. D'Angio, Beckwith and Breslow(1980) give the figures shown in *Table 32.1* for the best arm of the American National Wilms' Tumor Study.

Table 32.1   The survival rate in Wilms' tumour (data from D'Angio, Beckwith and Breslow, 1980)

	4 years recurrence-free (%)	*4-year survival rate (%)*
Nephroblastoma stage I under 2 years	89	94
Nephroblastoma stage I over 2 years	76	98
Nephroblastoma stages II and III	79	84
	2 years recurrence-free (%)	*2-year survival rate (%)*
Nephroblastoma with favourable histology	89	89
Nephroblastoma with unfavourable histology	14	19

Other renal tumours

Nephroblastomatosis

The relationship between true tumours and the pathological condition known as nephroblastomatosis is obscure. In any kidney, and particularly in other parts of one affected by tumour, there may be clusters of primitive undifferentiated cells which Bove, Koffler and McAdams (1969) described as nodular renal blastema. It appears that normally these cells undergo involution. However, proliferation may occur and when the nodules are both large and numerous they can produce a considerable bilateral enlargement of the kidneys which is described as nephroblastomatosis. The disorder is recognized in infants and the urographic appearance is of stretched-out distorted calyces in large kidneys with near-normal function. Arteriographically the characteristic picture is of multiple avascular areas in a lobulated kidney.

Bove, Koffler and McAdams (1969) described an association with trisomy 18. Liban and Kozenitzky (1970) found nephroblastomatosis in a familial syndrome of gigantism, diabetes and a bizarre facies. Cases have been described as bilateral Wilms' tumour by Lee-Tsun and Holman (1961) and Anderson *et al.* (1968). The patient of the latter authors was biopsied and treated by irradiation and was well 5 years later. It may be that no treatment is required and there is little doubt that chemotherapy is preferred at the present time.

Nephroblastoma, nephritis and male pseudohermaphroditism

Several patients with this combination of disorders have been reported (Barakat, Papadoulou and Chandra, 1974) and the incomplete syndrome has also been seen. One of the authors' cases was a boy treated at the age of 2 years for severe hypospadias. Laparotomy was performed for biopsy of the gonads and poorly developed testes were found. Mild albuminuria was noted at the time but not treated. At 4 years he returned with a large nephroblastoma together with nephrotic syndrome and a raised plasma creatinine level. Nephrectomy was performed for an encapsulated tumour but the nephron disorder was progressive with severe hypertension which was ultimately fatal. Unilateral or bilateral nephroblastoma can be accompanied by glomerulonephritis in normal boys and in girls, and in contrast male pseudohermaphroditism may be complicated by the nephron disorder without tumour. The exact nature of the glomerular lesion requires further exploration. The prognosis is poor and there is concern that chemotherapy for the tumour may exacerbate the renal condition.

Congenital mesoblastic nephroma

Congenital or neonatal Wilms' tumours have been reported from time to time and have in general been noted to have a good prognosis. Bolande, Brough and Izant (1967) demonstrated that the majority of these cases are not genuine nephroblastomas but relatively benign tumours which they described as congenital mesoblastic nephromas.

These lesions may be relatively small in an otherwise normal organ or else so large as to replace the kidney entirely. Pathologically the cut surface shows a very tough white or creamy structure with whorls of fibrous tissue (*Figures*

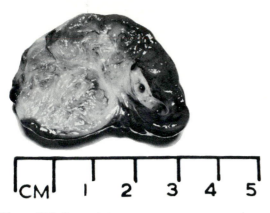

Figure 32.7. Congenital mesoblastic nephroma. Nephrectomy specimen.

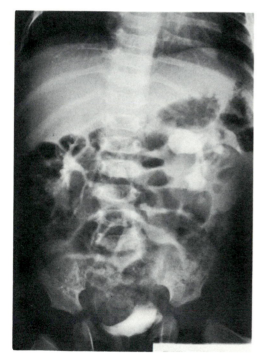

Figure 32.8. Congenital mesoblastic nephroma. Intravenous urogram in a neonate.

32.7 and 32.8). There is no clear-cut capsule separating the tumour from the kidney itself and this feature differentiates mesoblastic nephroma from encapsulated early nephroblastoma. Although a few examples show necrosis or haemorrhage most are entirely solid. Histologically fibrosarcomatous tissue is the most important element. There may be differentiation towards smooth muscle cells and some of these tumours have been labelled leiomyomas.

Peripherally the tumour appears to infiltrate the kidney substance, and tubular structures included at its periphery may be surviving renal elements rather than products of the nephroma itself. Occasionally definite neoplastic tubules and masses of cartilaginous tissue simulate the condition in nephroblastoma. Metastasis is very rare and perhaps does not occur in true examples of the disorder. Two cases of local recurrence in the retroperitoneal area are on record. Involvement of the mesentery can be fatal (Fu and Kay, 1973; Joshi, Kay and Milsten, 1973).

Some tumours appear to be intermediate between congenital mesoblastic nephroma and sarcomatous nephroblastoma, and must be suspected of malignancy when planning treatment (Beckwith, 1974). It is interesting to speculate on the natural history of the typical benign case since many must have passed untreated in early years. Later presentation of leiomyomas and leiomyosarcomas has been reported extremely rarely.

The tumour presents as an exceptionally hard mass in the abdomen of a newborn child. It is sometimes large enough to be obvious at delivery and sometimes found only on routine palpation during postnatal examination. Usually the infants are healthy and without other complaints. Intravenous urography should be postponed until at least 24–48 hours after birth. It shows an enlarged kidney with either a localized expanding lesion or total replacement of the functionless organ. Treatment should be by nephrectomy when the child's general condition is stable. Operation is not urgent. Postoperatively neither chemotherapy nor radiotherapy should be necessary for the typical case. In the past there have been some unfortunate deaths resulting from injudicious use of actinomycin D. Nevertheless, in infants presenting later in the first year or with borderline malignant changes chemotherapy may be considered.

Rhabdomyosarcoma

Among the various tissues found in nephroblastoma striated muscle cells are occasionally seen. Where they predominate some pathologists retain the tumour within the nephroblastoma category while others, for example Malek (1971), regard it as a very specific neoplasm, namely rhabdomyosarcoma. In one such patient aged 4 months treated by one of the authors there proved to be a cerebral metastasis responsible for repeated vomiting. A secondary in the brain is exceptionally rare in Wilms' tumour and separate categorization of rhabdomyosarcoma therefore seems justifiable, although the diagnosis is unlikely to be made until after nephrectomy and treatment does not differ postoperatively. Apart from solid tumours in the kidney, polypoid rhabdomyosarcoma has in the authors' experience extended upwards from a tumour originating in the bladder and associated with vesicoureteric reflux.

Leiomyosarcoma

With the exception of leiomyomatous mesoblastic nephromas very few cases in this category present during childhood. They have been reviewed by Loomis (1972).

Angiomyolipoma

A benign hamartomatous tumour may present as a solitary lesion on very rare occasions at any age. It closely simulates the malignant condition, although certain of its angiographic features may lead to a specific diagnosis (McCullough, Scott and Seybold, 1971). However, in childhood multiple angiomyolipomas occur in the kidneys in cases of tuberose sclerosis. This is a familial disorder characterized by nodular areas of gliosis in the cerebral hemispheres causing epilepsy and mental deficiency ultimately with symptoms of increased intracranial pressure. Other lesions are likely to be found including adenoma sebaceum, that is tumour-like nodules on the face. The renal lesions seldom cause symptoms during childhood but they may reach a considerable size and bleed either into the urine or into the retroperitoneal space. Malignant change is exceptionally rare and since the condition is bilateral treatment is not advised.

Haemangioma

In children as in adults a minute haemangioma is occasionally responsible for recurrent haematuria over a number of years. It is an exceptionally rare cause of such a symptom and the diagnosis should not be accepted without very definite calyceal deformity and arteriographic confirmation. The topic has been reviewed by Peterson and Thompson (1971).

Haemangiopericytoma

A single case of this disorder was reported in a child by Lee (1971). It was a small benign neoplasm producing severe hypertension which was watched over a long period before the minor radiological changes ultimately led to nephrectomy. High plasma renin values were obtained before operation and the blood pressure returned to normal afterwards.

Adenocarcinoma

The typical renal cell carcinoma or hypernephroma can occur at any age, although it is more often seen in older children. A palpable mass and haematuria are the usual presenting symptoms and the distinction from nephroblastoma is unlikely to be made until excision or biopsy. The progress of the disease and the pattern of metastasis is similar to that found in adults. Castellanos, Aron and Evans (1974) reviewed the childhood disease and found little difference from the adult tumour, but possibly a slightly better prognosis where local lymph nodes are involved. Radical nephrectomy is the treatment of choice and chemotherapy has very little place. Radiotherapy should be employed postoperatively.

Lymphosarcoma and leukaemia

Both kidneys may be infiltrated by leukaemic deposits. While the generalized disease is likely to be recognized before the renal manifestations, diagnostic difficulties can arise. The infiltration results in very great renal enlargement without any disastrous deterioration of function and the intravenous pyelogram therefore presents an appearance not unlike that in adult polycystic disease. Treatment is confined to a continuation of chemotherapy.

Transitional cell tumours of the renal pelvis and the ureter

A true transitional cell tumour is an exceptional rarity and apt to be confused with the papillary form of Wilms' tumour. Its presentation is with haematuria and the radiological finding of a filling defect in the renal pelvis, and differs from the adult pattern of the disease. Development may be slow, but the tumours are apt to be malignant (Schlapik, 1943; Koyanagi, Sasaki and Arikado, 1975). Treatment is by nephro-ureterectomy.

Ureteric polyps

Polypoid lesions in the upper end of the ureter, often about 1 cm below the pelviureteric junction, can cause hydronephrosis which closely resembles that of the common congenital obstruction. Although these polyps are not true tumours, at times the filling defect they produce is sufficiently large to be recognizable radiologically (Williams and Neiderhausen, 1963). Treatment consists of excising the section of ureter from which the polyps arise and performing a modified pyeloplasty. Lower down the ureter myomatous polyps can cause obstruction and at times haematuria, and may produce a ureteric intussusception and present at the ureteric orifice. These lesions are commoner in older children and adolescents. They can be excised locally since they have a long narrow stalk.

References

Anderson, E.E., Harper, J.M., Small, M.P. and Atwill, W.H. (1968) Bilateral diffuse Wilms' tumour. *Journal of Urology*, **99**, 707

Aron, B.S. (1974) Wilms' tumor, a clinical study of eighty-one patients. *Cancer*, **33**, 637

Barakat, A.Y., Papadoulou, Z.L., Chandra, R.S. (1974) Pseudohermaphroditism, nephron disorder and Wilms' tumour. *Pediatrics*, **54**, 366

Beckwith, J.B. (1974) Mesenchymal renal neoplasm of infancy revisited. *Journal of Pediatric Surgery*, **9**, 803

Beckwith, J.B. and Palmer, N.F. (1978) Histopathology and prognosis of Wilms' tumour: result from the First National Wilms' Tumour Study. *Cancer*, **41**, 1937

Berry, C.L., Keeling, J., Hilton, C. (1970) Co-incidence of congenital malformation and embryonic tumours in childhood. *Archives of Disease in Childhood*, **45**, 229

Bolande, R.P. (1974) Congenital and infantile neoplasia of the kidney. *Lancet*, ii, 1497

Bolande, R.P., Brough, A.J. and Izant, R.J. (1967) Congenital mesoblastic nephroma of infancy: a report of eight cases and the relationship to Wilms' tumor. *Pediatrics*, **40**, 272

Bond, J.V. (1975) Bilateral Wilms' tumor: age at diagnosis, associated congenital anomalies and possible pattern of inheritance. *Lancet*, ii, 482

Bove, K.E., Koffler, H. and McAdams, A.J. (1969) Nodular renal blastema (definition and possible significance). *Cancer*, **24**, 323

Cardinali, G., Cardinali, G. and Enien, M.A. (1963) Studies of the antimitotic activity of levrocristine (vincristine). *Blood*, **21**, 102

Castellanos, R.D., Aron, B.S. and Evans, A.T. (1974) Renal adenocarcinoma in children: incidence, therapy and prognosis. *Journal of Urology*, **111**, 534

Clark, R.E., Moss, A.A., de Lorimier, A.A. (1971) Arteriography of Wilms' tumor. *American Journal of Roentgenology, Radium Therapy and Nuclear Medicine*, **113**, 476

Collins, V.P. (1955) Wilms' tumor: its behaviour and prognosis. *Journal of the Louisiana Medical Society*, **107**, 474

Cox, P. and Smellie, J.M. (1955) Hypertension and Wilms' tumour. *Great Ormond Street Journal*, **10**, 112

D'Angio, G.J., Evans, A.E., Breslow, N., Beckwith, B., Bishop, H., Fiegl, P., Goodwin, W., Leape, L.L., Sinks, L.F., Sutow, W., Tefft, M. and Wolff, J. (1976) The treatment of Wilms' tumour: results of the National Wilms' Tumor Study. *Cancer*, **38**, 633

D'Angio, G.J., Beckwith, J.B., Breslow, N.E. (1980) Wilms' tumor: an update. *Cancer*, **45**, 1791

Farber, S. (1966) Chemotherapy in the treatment of leukaemia and Wilms' tumour. *Journal of the American Medical Association*, **198**, 826

Farber, S., Diamond, L.K., Mercer, R.D., Sylvester, R.F. and Wolff, J.A. (1948) Temporary remissions in acute leukaemia in children, produced by folic acid antagonist 4-aminopteroylglutamic acid, aminopterin. *New England Journal of Medicine*, **238**, 787

Fitzgerald, W.L. and Hardin, N.C. (1955) Bilateral Wilms' tumour in a Wilms' tumour family: case report. *Journal of Urology*, **73**, 468

Fu, Y.S. and Kay, S. (1973) Congenital mesoblastic nephroma and its recurrence: an ultrastructural observation. *Archives of Pathology*, **96**, 66

Garcia, M., Douglass, C. and Schlosser, J.V. (1963) Classification of progress in Wilms' tumour. *Radiology*, **80**, 574

Goldstein, M.N., Slotnik, I.J. and Journey, L.J. (1961) In vitro studies with HeLa cell lines sensitive and resistant to actinomycin D. *Annals of the New York Academy of Sciences*, **89**, 474

Haas, L. and Jackson, A.D.M. (1961) Wilms' tumour: lobectomy for pulmonary metastasis; a case report. *British Journal of Surgery*, **48**, 516

Hastings, N. and Gwinn, J.L. (1965) Wilms' tumour. *American Journal of Surgery*, **110**, 203

Johnston, J.H., Mainwaring, D. and Rickham, P.P. (1969) Ten years' experience with Actinomycin D in the treatment of nephroblastoma. *Zeitschrift für Kinderchirurgie*, **6**, Suppl. 171

Joshi, V.V., Kay, S., Milsten, R. (1973) Congenital mesoblastic nephroma of infancy: report of a case with unusual clinical behaviour. *American Journal of Clinical Pathology*, **60**, 811

Joshi, V.V., Banerjee, A.K., Yader, K. (1977) Cystic partially differentiated nephroblastoma. *Cancer*, **40**, 789

Kenny, G.M., Mirand, E.A. and Staubitz, W.J. (1970) Erythropoietin levels in Wilms' tumours. *Journal of Urology*, **104**, 758

Knudson, A.G. (1976) Genetics and the aetiology of childhood cancer. *Pediatric Research*, **10**, 513

Knudson, A.G. and Strong, L.C. (1972) Mutation and cancer: a model for Wilms' tumor of the kidney. *Journal of the National Cancer Institute*, **48**, 313

Koyanagi, T., Sasaki, K., Arikado, K. (1975) Transitional cell carcinoma in renal pelvis in an infant. *Journal of Urology*, **113**, 114

Lawler, W., Marsden, H.B. and Palmer, M.K. (1977) Histopathological study of the first Medical Research Council Nephroblastoma Trial. *Cancer*, **40**, 1519

Lee, M.R. (1970) Renin secreting kidney tumours. *Lancet*, ii, 254

Lee, M.R. (1971) Renin secreting kidney tumours: a rare but remediable cause of serious hypertension. *Lancet*, ii, 254

Lee-Tsun, H. and Holman, R.L. (1961) Bilateral nephroblastomatosis in a premature infant. *Journal of Pathology and Bacteriology*, **82**, 249

Lemerle, J., Voute, P.A., Tournade, M.F. (1976) Preoperative versus post-operative radiotherapy; single versus multiple courses of actinomycin D in the treatment of Wilms' tumour. *Cancer*, **38**, 647

Lennox, E.L., Stiller, C.A., Morris Jones, P.H. and Kinnier Wilson, L.M. (1979) Nephroblastoma: treatment during 1970–3 and the effect on survival of inclusion in the first MRC trial. *British Medical Journal*, ii, 567

Liban, E. and Kozenitzky, I.L. (1970) Metanephric hamartomas and nephroblastomatosis in siblings. *Cancer*, **27**, 885

Loomis, R.C. (1972) Primary leiomyosarcoma of the kidney. *Journal of Urology*, **105**, 32

McCullough, D.L., Scott, R. and Seybold, H.M. (1971) Renal angiomyolipoma (hamartoma) : a review of literature and report of 7 cases. *Journal of Urology*, **105**, 32

Malek, T. (1971) Rhabdomyosarcoma alveolare der nieren bei einem 20 monate alten kind. *Zeitschrift für Urologie und Nephrologie*, **64**, 145

Manchester Children's Tumour Register (1968) Problems of children's tumours in Britain. *In* Tumours in Children (edited by Marsden, H.R. and Steward, J.K.). Springer, Berlin. p.1

Marsden, H.B. and Lawler, W. (1978) Bone metastasising renal tumour of childhood. *British Journal of Cancer*, **38**, 437

Marsden, H.B., Lawler, W. and Kumar, P.M. (1978) Bone metastasizing renal tumour of childhood: morphological and clinical features, and differences from Wilms' tumour. *Cancer*, **42**, 1922

Martin, J. and Rickham, P.P. (1970) Pulmonary metastases in Wilms' tumour. *Archives of Disease in Childhood*, **45**, 805

Mitchell, J.D., Baxter, T.J., Blair West, J.R. and McCredie, D.A. (1970) Renin levels in nephroblastoma. *Archives of Disease in Childhood*, **45**, 376

Morris-Jones, P.M. (1978) MRC nephroblastoma trial – results. *Archives of Disease in Childhood*, **53**, 112

Orlowski, J.P., Levin, H.S. and Dyment, P.G. (1980) Intrascrotal Wilms' tumour developing in a heterotopic renal anlage of probable mesonephric origin. *Journal of Pediatric Surgery*, **15**, 679

Peck, B. (1979) Effects of childhood cancer on long-term survivors and their families. *British Medical Journal*, i, 1327

Peterson, N.E. and Thompson, H.T. (1971) Renal hemangioma. *Journal of Urology*, **105**, 27

Pinkel, D., Simone, J., Husto, O. and Aur, R.J.A. (1972) Nine years' experience with "total therapy" of childhood acute lymphocytic leukemia. *Pediatrics*, **50**, 246

Platt, B.B. and Linden, G. (1964) Wilms's tumour: comparison of two criteria for survival. *Cancer*, **17**, 1573

Powars, D.R., Allerton, S.E., Beierle, J. (1972) Wilms' tumor: clinical correlation with circulating mucin in three cases. *Cancer*, **29**, 1597

Rabinowitz, J.G. and Bagnasio, F.M. (1970) Wilms' tumour demonstrating onset and rapid growth. *Journal of Urology*, **103**, 86

Schlapik, D. (1943) Papillary carcinoma of the kidney in childhood. *Urologic and Cutaneous Reviews*, **47**, 283

Sphar, J., Demers, L.M. and Shochat, S.J. (1981) Renin producing Wilms' tumour. *Journal of Pediatric Surgery*, **16**, 32

Sukarochana, K., Tolentino, W., Kiesewetter, W.B. (1972) Wilms' tumor and hypertension. *Journal of Pediatric Surgery*, **7**, 573

Sullivan, M.P., Sutow, W.W., Cangir, A. and Taylor, G. (1967) Vincristine sulphate in the management of Wilms' tumour: replacement of pre-operative irradiation by chemotherapy. *Journal of the American Medical Association*, **202**, 381

Sutow, W.W. (1967) Cyclophosphamide in Wilms' tumor and rhabdomyosarcoma. *Cancer Chemotherapy Reports*, **51**, 407

UK Children's Cancer Study Group (1980) Nephroblastoma Study. Co-ordinators: P.A. Morris Jones and J. Pritchard.

Veraguth, P. and Chanson, J.F. (1969) Arterial hypertension in renal tumours in childhood: the influence of pre-operative radiotherapy. *Helvetica chirurgica Acta*, **36**, 355

Wallace, A.C. and Nairn, R.C. (1972) Renal tubular antigens in kidney tumours. *Cancer*, **29**, 977

Wang, J.J., Cortes, E., Sinks, L.F. and Holland, J.F. (1971) Therapeutic effect and toxicity of Adriamycin in patients with neoplastic disease. *Cancer*, **28**, 837

Williams, D.I. and Niederhausen, W.V. (1963) Les polypes de l'uretère. *Journale d'Urologie et Nephrologie*, **69**, 145

Wolff, J.A., D'Angio, G.J., Hartmann, J., Krwit, W. and Newton, W.A. (1968) Long-term evaluation of single versus multiple courses of actinomycin D therapy of Wilms' tumor. *New England Journal of Medicine*, **290**, 84

Wolff, J.A., Krwit, W., Newton, W.A. and D'Angio, G.J. (1974) Single versus multiple dose actinomycin D therapy of Wilms' tumor. *New England Journal of Medicine*, **279**, 290

Woodard, J.R. and Levine, M.K. (1969) Nephroblastoma (Wilms' tumour) and aniridia. *Journal of Urology*, **101**, 140

33 Neuroblastoma, Teratoma and Other Retroperitoneal Tumours

J.H. Johnston

Neuroblastoma

Apart from tumours of the CNS neuroblastoma is the commonest solid malignancy of childhood, occurring in about one in 30 000 live births. The tumour most often arises from the sympathetic nervous system or its precursors but it may originate from parasympathetic ganglia, dorsal root ganglia of the spinal cord or the neurilemma of peripheral nerves (Beckwith and Martin, 1968). While the most frequent sites of origin are the adrenal medulla and the abdominal sympathetic ganglia the tumour may occur in sympathochromaffin tissue in the neck, thorax or pelvis.

Pathology

In gross appearance a neuroblastoma usually forms a large nodular mass. Areas of haemorrhage and necrosis may be present and cyst formation and calcification are common. Frequently there is extensive local infiltration of adjacent structures and organs. A paravertebral tumour may extend in dumb-bell fashion through an intervertebral foramen. Some two thirds of patients have distant metastases when first seen and the distribution of these varies in different age groups. For example the young infant shows multiple skin secondaries and extensive liver involvement and the older child develops bone metastases, particularly in the skull and the long bones.

Histologically the most rapidly growing tumours are composed of masses of closely packed round cells without any structural arrangement. Early differentiation is shown by rosette-like clusters of cells around central masses of fibrils representing young axons. Some tumours, so-called ganglioneuroblastomas, are further differentiated and contain mature nerve cells and fibres. Since there are all gradations of differentiation even within the same tumour between a primitive neuroblastoma and a mature ganglioneuroma, these lesions must be regarded as the extremes of a spectrum rather than separate entities. Beckwith and Martin (1968) found a better prognosis with the more highly differentiated tumours. The presence of lymphocytic infiltration, indicating an immune reaction to the neoplasm, also implies an improved outlook.

Spontaneous regression

Neuroblastoma is unique in its propensity for spontaneous regression. This phenomenon, which affects both the primary tumour and metastases, is seen mainly in infants and is more likely to occur in girls (Wilson and Draper, 1974). Everson and Cole (1966) recorded 29 examples of neuroblastoma regression in which all the patients were under 2 years of age and 21 were less than 6 months old. In four cases the tumour matured to a benign ganglioneuroma and in the remainder it underwent necrosis and disappeared. Beckwith and Perrin (1963) showed that spontaneous resolution of infantile neuroblastoma is a common occurrence. At routine autopsies in babies they found that *in situ* nodules of neuroblastoma occurred in the adrenals and elsewhere with a frequency some 40 times greater than that of clinically overt tumours.

The mechanisms concerned in spontaneous tumour regression have been extensively studied in recent years. Hellstrom *et al.* (1970) demonstrated that neuroblastoma produces tumour-specific antigens. Colonies of tumour cells are inhibited *in vitro* by the patient's own lymphocytes whether the disease is progressive or not, but not by lymphocytes from other affected patients. The lymphocytes, and in some instances the plasma (Bill and Morgan, 1970), of healthy mothers of children with neuroblastoma also prevent growth of the tumour cells. However, the serum of patients with progressive neuroblastoma possesses a blocking antibody that prevents the lymphocytic effect on the tumour; it is absent in patients cured of the disease. Nerve growth factor (NGF), which is a protein isolated by Levi-Montalcini (1966), may also be involved in the regression process. This factor selectively stimulates the growth of embryonic sympathetic and posterior root ganglia and accelerates cellular differentiation by enhancing the RNA-synthesizing mechanisms. Siebert and Bill (1968) considered that there is a direct relationship between tumour regression and the level of NGF in the patient's serum and Burdman and Goldstein (1964) found high serum levels in children with active neoplasia. These findings were not confirmed by Waghe, Kumar and Steward (1970).

Clinical features

Apart from occasional coexistence with neurofibromatosis, syndactyly or rib abnormalities (Sy and Edmondson, 1968) neuroblastoma unlike nephroblastoma has no special concurrence with any congenital anomalies. The tumour is rarely familial although its occurrence in twins has been recorded (Miller, Fraumeni and Hill, 1968). Chatten and Voorhess (1967) described a family in which four of five siblings were affected and the mother had a markedly increased urinary excretion rate for vanillylmandelic acid (VMA).

Neuroblastoma is a neoplasm of early childhood, the great majority of cases occurring in the first 4 years of life. It is commoner in girls than in boys. Often the tumour is congenital so that secondary deposits may be present at birth and the placenta may contain metastases. Occasionally the mother suffers symptoms of flushing, sweating and tachycardia during pregnancy because of catecholamine secretion by the fetal tumour (Jonte, Wadman and van Putten, 1970).

The presenting features are very variable depending upon the site and the extent of the disease. An adrenal tumour commonly presents as an abdominal mass that extends under the costal margin, is deep and fixed and may stretch across the midline. Haemorrhage into the mass may cause pain and its sudden enlargement; rarely exsanguinating intraperitoneal haemorrhage occurs (Murthy, Irving and Lister, 1978). Paraplegia results if a paravertebral tumour extends through an intervertebral foramen and compresses the spinal cord. A pelvic tumour may displace and obstruct the bladder. Frequently the first symptoms are due to secondary deposits. Thus an infant may present with a hard diffusely enlarged liver or multiple cutaneous nodules. In the older child unilateral proptosis with periorbital haemorrhage due to a retro-ocular deposit is a common manifestation. Bone secondaries may produce limb pains or calvarial swellings. Infrequently the first evidence of neuroblastoma is encephalopathy with ataxia, opsoclonus and myoclonus. Atrophic changes in the cerebellum have been found in such patients at autopsy (Senelick *et al.*, 1973) but the mechanism of the nervous system damage is unknown.

The child with neuroblastoma is often thin, pale, irritable and lethargic. Hypertension due to secretion of catecholamines by the tumour is uncommon. Since the hormones are rapidly converted to inactive metabolites the severe hypertensive episodes and vasomotor effects typical of phaeochromocytoma do not occur.

Diagnosis

Radiography may demonstrate the tumour as a soft-tissue mass, commonly with stippled calcification. With an adrenal tumour the kidney is displaced and often rotated downwards and laterally (*Figure 33.1*). Tumours arising from the

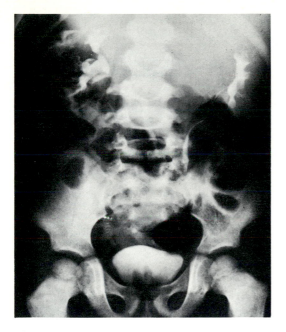

Figure 33.1. Intravenous pyelogram in a case of right adrenal neuroblastoma showing the kidney displaced laterally.

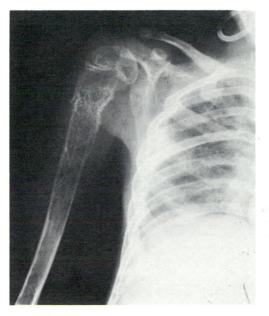

Figure 33.2. Osteolytic secondary deposits from neuroblastoma in humerus.

lumbar sympathetic chain may invade the kidney and distort the pelvicalyceal system. A radiological skeletal survey is indicated to determine if bone secondaries are present: osteolytic changes in the cortex with subperiosteal new bone formation are characteristic (*Figure 33.2*). Radioisotopic bone scans using the gamma camera and ^{99m}Tc-diphosphonate may demonstrate metastases not shown on radiography. The raised uptake of isotope is related to increased osteoclastic or osteoblastic activity. Scanning may reveal hot or cold areas depending upon whether the secondary deposit is purely destructive or is inducing a bone reaction. Extraosseous localization of the isotope may occur in the primary tumour, possibly as a result of excessive calcium concentration in it (Carty, 1979). Marrow biopsy is required because osseous deposits may exist without radiographic or bone-scan evidence.

Haematological examination often shows anaemia. A shift of granulocytes to the left and normoblastaemia are highly suggestive of bone marrow involvement.

Some 75 per cent of neuroblastomas secrete the catecholamines dopamine, noradrenaline and adrenaline and these hormones and their breakdown metabolites VMA and homovanillic acid (HVA) are excreted in excess in the urine. Their measurement is therefore of value in diagnosis and in assessing the effects of treatment. The synthesis and the breakdown of the hormones are shown in *Figure 33.3*. Since the

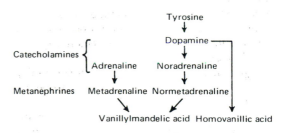

Figure 33.3. The pathway of synthesis and breakdown of the adrenal hormones.

excretion rates show significant diurnal variation a 24-hour specimen of urine provides the most satisfactory estimations. Alternatively using smaller specimens excretion may be related to creatinine output. Very young children have low rates of creatinine elimination so that the upper limit of nontumour VMA levels is higher in children under the age of 18 months than in older children. Normal and highly suspicious levels of excretion are indicated in *Table 33.1*. The normal range of excretion for HVA is 2.5–9 mg/24 hours. False-positive results may be obtained from a child in cardiac failure or

Table 33.1   The excretion rates of catecholamines

Measurement	Normal (μmol/mmol creatinine)	(μg/mg)	Highly suspicious under 18 months (μmol/mmol creatinine)	(μg/mg)	over 18 months (μmol/mmol creatinine)	(μg/mg)
Total catecholamines	0–0.93	0–1.5	2.70	4.5	2.70	4.5
Metanephrines	0–0.57	0–1.0	1.71	3.0	1.71	3.0
Vanillyl mandelic acid	0–5.70	0–10.0	14.25	25.0	6.84	12.0

following surgery or exchange transfusion; the ingestion of vanilla-containing foods such as bananas or ice cream may produce high VMA levels as may degenerative lesions of the CNS (Young and Hosking, 1978). Haemorrhage into the tumour may temporarily lower catecholamine secretion to nondiagnostic levels. A high excretion rate for HVA as compared with VMA generally indicates a high degree of malignancy (Ireland, 1978).

Staging

Staging of neuroblastoma is important as regards treatment and prognosis. The scheme of Evans, D'Angio and Randolph (1971) has been generally accepted and is as follows:
1. Stage I. The tumour is confined to the structure or organ of origin.
2. Stage II. The tumour extends beyond its structure or organ of origin but does not cross the midline of the body. The regional lymph glands may contain metastases.
3. Stage III. The tumour extends in continuity across the midline. The lymph glands may be involved bilaterally.
4. Stage IV. There is widespread disease involving other organs, soft tissues, distant lymph glands and the skeleton.
5. Stage IV-S. Patients who would otherwise be in stage I or II who have distant disease restricted to the liver, skin or bone marrow without radiological evidence of skeletal involvement. Whether or not bone scans may be positive is at present uncertain.

Treatment

In view of the differing manifestations of neuroblastoma in various cases treatment must be individual and related to the stage of the disease. The ideal is complete surgical removal of the tumour, which is possible at stage I and

with less certainty at stage II. Following operation if there is no clinical or radiological evidence of residual neoplasm and if previously raised VMA excretion levels fall to normal then no further treatment is needed. When local extension prohibits total removal as much tumour tissue as possible within the bounds of safety should be excised since adjuvant therapy and the patient's immune reaction are more effective when there is a minimum quantity of neoplastic tissue. With patients in stage IV surgery to the tumour is justified only if the secondary deposits respond well to chemotherapy. When an initially unresectable tumour at stage II or III has shrunk following postoperative irradiation or chemotherapy 'second-look' surgery has been employed to excise residual neoplasm. At such re-explorations the tumour, although smaller, has precisely the same extensions that rendered it irremovable en bloc at the original operation and it is doubtful if much of value is achieved.

Chemotherapy with cytotoxic drugs has been extensively used in the treatment of residual tumour and of metastatic deposits in cases of stage III or IV disease. However, such treatment has not been as effective with neuroblastoma as with nephroblastoma and no specific drug protocol has been evolved. The agents most often used have been vincristine, cyclophosphamide and adriamycin alone or in combination. Razoxane (ICRF 159) induces blood vessel changes in the tumour and may prevent the development of blood-bone metastases. It has been used to potentiate the effect of other drugs.

Irradiation is not required in stage I cases. In stage II cases with subtotal removal of the tumour Koop and Johnson (1971) found it to be of little benefit but in stage III patients the survival rate was improved. Whole-body sequential irradiation was combined with chemotherapy for children with disseminated disease by Green *et al.* (1976) without benefit. Palliative radiotherapy is effective in relieving pain from bone metastases.

Since neuroblastoma has a high rate of spontaneous regression, especially in infancy, and since such regression offers the best prospect of cure various attempts have been made to enhance the patient's immune response to the tumour. Nonspecific stimulation by BCG has been employed with little effect. Specific measures were considered by Bill and Morgan (1970). Because humoral antibodies lethal to the tumour have been demonstrated in some mothers of neuroblastoma patients it was suggested that maternal plasma infusions to the child might be employed therapeutically when the absence of a blocking antibody could be demonstrated by colony inhibition studies. Plasmapheresis to remove the blocking factor has not been effective. Kumar *et al.* (1970) investigated the possible therapeutic role of NGF. It was considered that NGF might cause a neuroblastoma to mature, that anti-NGF might destroy a tumour in the same way as it destroys non-neoplastic sympathetic tissue and that if NGF or anti-NGF became attached to neuroblastoma tissue it might be used as a vehicle for cytotoxic drugs. The administration of NGF to three children with widespread neuroblastoma did not influence the course of the disease. In tumour culture anti-NGF had no effect on cell growth nor did it attach to the tumour tissue.

Stage IV-S cases form a special group. Such patients are usually infants and have a high rate of spontaneous tumour regression. They may be at greater risk from treatment than from the disease, particularly since cytotoxic drug therapy antagonizes the immune response. Martin (1974) advised chemotherapy only if there is bone marrow involvement while Grosfeld *et al.* (1978) found that marrow deposits worsened the outlook. Schwartz *et al.* (1974) reported two patients at stage IV-S who recovered without any specific treatment. Spontaneous maturation to a ganglioneuroma occurred without therapy in the patient of Rangecroft, Lauder and Wagget (1978). In some instances liver enlargement is sufficiently great to cause respiratory distress and vena caval compression and in such cases Schnaufer and Koop (1975) produced a temporary ventral abdominal hernia employing a Silastic patch. The primary tumour is generally small and often cannot be recognized. Because spontaneous regression affects both primary and secondary lesions simultaneously, operation aimed at excising the primary is unnecessary and may be harmful since incomplete removal of the tumour may temporarily depress the immune reaction (Uchino, Hata and Kasai, 1978).

Prognosis

The prognosis for the child with neuroblastoma depends mainly on the site of the tumour, its degree of differentiation and especially the age of the patient and the stage of the disease. The outlook is best when the tumour is highly differentiated, the child presents under the age of 1 year and the stage is I or IV-S.

In their review of 487 cases in the UK Wilson and Draper (1974) found a 23 per cent 3-year survival rate for the whole series. The outlook was best with intrathoracic tumours and worst with adrenal and other abdominal tumours. In children under 1 year old the 3-year survival rate was 48.8 per cent while in those aged 1–2, 2–4, 5–9 and 10–14 the rates were respectively 24.1, 10.1, 16.3 and 13 per cent. Stage I cases had a 59 per cent 3-year survival rate and the rates for stages II, III, IV and IV-S were respectively 46.8, 19.4, 5.0 and 48.7 per cent. Girls had a significantly better 3-year survival rate than boys, namely 30.1 per cent compared with 17.9 per cent. The various factors indicating a good prognosis are to some extent interrelated since most well differentiated tumours are stage I and since stage I and stage IV-S tumours occur predominantly in infants. Tumours in girls tend to have other more favourable features, yet even when comparisons are made within the various categories girls tend to do better than boys. Similarly the younger child has a better prognosis than the older one within a particular stage. The series of Breslow and McCann (1971), taking the disease–free 2-year survival rate in 256 children produced similar prognostic conclusions to that of Wilson and Draper (1974) and better survival figures. The latter do not appear to be dependent upon the different follow-up period because Wilson and Draper reported that nearly all deaths in their series occurred in the first year after diagnosis and that death from the tumour was very unlikely if the patient survived more than 2 years.

High urinary cystathionine levels suggest the existence of metastases (Geiser and Efron, 1968) but cystathionine excretion may be absent in the presence of disseminated disease. Frens, Bray and Wie (1975) noted that high plasma levels of carcinoembryonic antigen were associated with progressive disease and a poor outlook. The existence of radiologically demonstrable bone deposits carries a very ominous prognosis, although recoveries have been reported (Reilly, Nesbit and Krivit, 1968).

Ganglioneuroma

Ganglioneuroma is a benign tumour derived from neural crest ectoderm which may develop in the cervical, thoracic or lumbar sympathetic ganglia or in the adrenal medulla. It is composed of fully differentiated nerve cells and intertwining medullated or nonmedullated fibres. Ganglioneuroma and neuroblastoma represent fully differentiated and undifferentiated extremes of the same species of tumour and intermediate grades or ganglioneuroblastomas can be recognized. According to Willis (1967) every ganglioneuroma begins as a neuroblastoma that later undergoes maturation. Histological proof of progressive tumour differentiation has been obtained by Dyke and Mulkey (1967).

A benign ganglioneuroma produces symptoms mainly by local pressure effects. Increased urinary outputs of catecholamines and their metabolites may occur but the levels are lower than with a neuroblastoma. Some ganglioneuromas or ganglioneuroblastomas are associated with severe persistent diarrhoea, gaseous intestinal distension, hypokalaemia and skin rashes and flushes. It is likely that these effects are due to secretion by the tumour of a vasoactive intestinal peptide, the plasma levels of which are markedly raised (Bloom, 1978). Removal of the tumour promptly cures the symptoms.

Teratoma

A teratoma is a tumour composed of multiple tissues foreign to the part in which it arises. Generally all three germ layers are represented and mature tissue such as brain, bone, skin, hair and teeth may be present. If malignant change

occurs, it may affect several or only one of the components. The tumour is generally partly solid and partly cystic.

Retroperitoneal teratomas arise in the upper abdomen. They are commoner in the female than in the male and usually present during the first year of life as an abdominal swelling producing pressure effects on the alimentary or urinary tract. Radiology shows a soft-tissue mass, often with calcification, which displaces the intestines and the ureters and frequently has an obstructive effect (*Figure 33.4*). Treatment

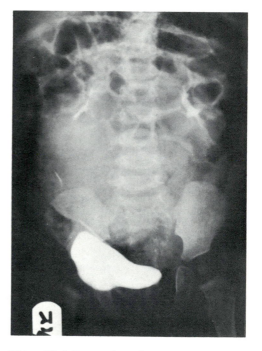

Figure 33.4. Retroperitoneal teratoma displacing the ureters and compressing the bladder. Intravenous pyelogram in a 1-year-old boy.

consists of surgical excision of the tumour. In Arnheim's (1951) collected series 6.8 per cent of retroperitoneal teratomas contained malignant tissue.

A presacral teratoma is a variant of the congenital sacrococcygeal teratoma where the mass is contained within the pelvis, lying anterior to the sacrum, and there is no external swelling. It compresses the rectum and often displaces the bladder and the ureters, leading to upper urinary tract dilatation (*Figure 33.5*). The tumour is three times commoner in girls and there is often a history of twin births in the

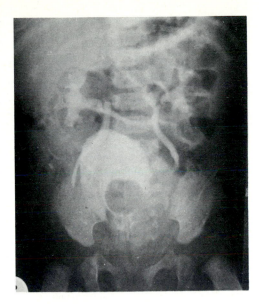

Figure 33.5. Presacral teratoma displacing the bladder upwards and forwards. Intravenous pyelogram in a 9-month-old girl. There is a Foley catheter in the bladder.

Fetus in fetu

In this condition a monozygotic twin is contained as a parasite within the body of its usually otherwise normal sibling. The lesion is distinguished from a teratoma by its possession of a vertebral column and by an appropriate arrangement of limbs and organs in relation to the spine. While the enclosed fetus most commonly lies in the retroperitoneum of the upper abdomen it may be in the pelvis or in the ileal mesentery. The condition presents in early life as an abdominal mass or because of pressure effects on the alimentary tract. Kakizol and Tahara (1972) described a fetus in fetu occupying the scrotum of its brother. As a rule the parasitic fetus is single; however, Lee (1965) reported a case in which three rudimentary fetuses were present. Since the fetus continues to grow with the host its removal is indicated, but the capsule is often densely adherent to its surroundings and in such circumstances it may be prudent to leave it *in situ*.

family. At birth the teratoma is usually entirely benign but malignant change, most commonly in the form of a papillary adenocarcinoma, may develop within a few months. Altman's (1974) review of 405 cases of sacrococcygeal teratoma revealed that the incidence of malignancy was 7 per cent at birth, 37 per cent at 1 year of age and 50 per cent at 2 years. With entirely intrapelvic teratomas where the diagnosis is often made relatively late Arnheim (1951) found an incidence of malignancy of 38 per cent. In Ghazali's (1973) series malignant change occurred in five cases in which the diagnosis was made after 10 months of age, and four of the children died.

In view of this predisposition to malignant degeneration pelvic teratoma requires prompt surgical excision. A transabdominal approach is indicated. The coccyx is intimately attached to the tumour and should be removed in continuity with it, if necessary through a separate perineal incision. Injury to the parasympathetic supply to the bladder, leading to neuropathic dysfunction, may be unavoidable during the difficult dissection of an adherent tumour. If malignant change has occurred, treatment with vincristine and actinomycin D combined with either cyclophosphamide or methotrexate may be curative even in the presence of metastatic deposits in the liver or lungs (Grosfeld, 1976).

Other retroperitoneal tumours

A variety of benign and malignant retroperitoneal tumours of both connective tissue and epithelial origin have been described.

Lymph-node masses due to lymphosarcoma, lymphadenoma or secondary deposits from a testicular tumour may produce a large retroperitoneal swelling that displaces the kidneys or ureters. In each instance the diagnosis is generally clear from other manifestations elsewhere.

Lipomatous tumours may be benign (Harvard, 1953) or malignant (Peeples and Hazra, 1976). Fibrosarcoma and rhabdomyosarcoma occur rarely in the retroperitoneal space. Complete surgical excision is often not possible. In the case of rhabdomyosarcoma encouraging results have been obtained in recent years from cytotoxic drug therapy.

Lymphangioma is a benign tumour usually of large size and presents with diffuse abdominal enlargement. On occasions it may extend into an inguinal hernial sac (Kafka and Novak, 1970). Surgery is needed to relieve pressure effects but the tumour is often widely infiltrating so that total removal cannot be achieved. Retroperitoneal cavernous haemangioma may present as an abdominal swelling similar to that caused by lymphangioma. Bleeding into or around the tumour may occur or thrombocytopenia with generalized haemorrhagic effects may result from platelets becoming trapped within the haemangioma. The latter complication may be controlled and tumour shrinkage obtained by steroid therapy (Kasubuchi, Sawada and Nakamura, 1973). Total surgical excision of the tumour is rarely possible but ligature of feeding vessels may prevent complications and encourage tumour regression. Alternatively, transcatheteric embolization of the principal supplying arteries may be effective.

Haemangiopericytomas arise from pericytes which spiral around blood capillaries. The tumour may be benign or malignant (Kauffman and Stout, 1960).

Malignant paraganglioma is a rare and in general functionally inert tumour derived from the paraganglionic vascular glomera in the retroperitoneal space. Cohen and Persky (1966) described a case in a young boy where the tumour obstructed the ureter and metastasized to the kidney. Olson and Abell (1969) reviewed 21 reported examples.

Retroperitoneal neurofibromas are generally only one manifestation of generalized Von Recklinghausen's disease.

Suprarenal neurilemmoma is a rare lesion that commonly undergoes cystic degeneration. This tumour is frequently large and an abdominal swelling is the usual clinical presentation (Wilson and Middleton, 1975).

Xanthogranuloma of the retroperitoneum was reported in a 2-year-old girl by Bissada and Fried (1973). A yellow mass composed of cholesterol-containing foam cells obstructed the ureter. It is uncertain whether this lesion is neoplastic or inflammatory.

References

Altman, P. (1974) Sacrococcygeal teratomas. *Journal of Pediatric Surgery*, **9**, 389

Arnheim, E.E. (1951) Retroperitoneal teratoma in infancy and childhood. *Pediatrics*, **8**, 309

Beckwith, J.B. and Martin, R.F. (1968) Observations on the histopathology of neuroblastomas. *Journal of Pediatric Surgery*, **3**, 106

Beckwith, J.B. and Perrin, E.V. (1963) In situ neuroblastomas: a contribution to the natural history of neural crest tumours. *American Journal of Pathology*, **43**, 1089

Bill, A.H. and Morgan, A. (1970) Evidence for immune reactions to neuroblastoma and future possibilities for investigation. *Journal of Pediatric Surgery*, **5**, 111

Bissada, N.K. and Fried, F.A. (1973) Retroperitoneal xanthogranuloma: case report and review of the literature. *Journal of Urology*, **110**, 354

Bloom, S.R. (1978) VIP and watery diarrhoea. *In* Gut Hormones (edited by Bloom, S.R.). Churchill Livingstone, Edinburgh, London and New York. p.583

Breslow, N. and McCann, B. (1971) Statistical estimation of prognosis for children with neuroblastoma. *Cancer Research*, **31**, 2098

Burdman, J.A. and Goldstein, M.N. (1964) Long term tissue culture of neuroblastoma: in vitro studies of a nerve growth stimulating factor in sera of children with neuroblastoma. *Journal of the National Cancer Institute*, **33**, 123

Carty, H. (1979) Personal communication

Chatten, J. and Voorhess, M.L. (1967) Familial neuroblastoma: report of a kindred with multiple disorders, including neuroblastoma in four siblings. *New England Journal of Medicine*, **277**, 1230

Cohen, S.M. and Persky, L. (1966) Malignant non-chromaffin paraganglioma with metastasis to the kidney. *Journal of Urology*, **96**, 122

Dyke, P.C. and Mulkey, D.A. (1967) Maturation of ganglioneuroblastoma to ganglioneuroma. *Cancer*, **20**, 1343

Evans, A.E., D'Angio, G.J. and Randolph, J. (1971) A proposed staging for children with neuroblastoma: Children's Cancer Study Group A. *Cancer*, **27**, 374

Everson, T.C. and Cole, W.H. (1966) Spontaneous regression of cancer: a study and abstract of reports in the world medical literature and of personal communications concerning spontaneous regression of malignant disease. Saunders, Philadelphia

Frens, D.B., Bray, P.F. and Wie, J.T. (1975) The carcinoembryonic antigen (CEA) assay: prognostic implications in neural crest tumours. *Pediatric Research*, **9**, 387

Geiser, C.F. and Efron, M.L. (1968) Cystathioninuria in patients with neuroblastoma or ganglioneuroblastoma: its correlation to vanillylmandelic acid excretion and its value in diagnosis and therapy. *Cancer*, **22**, 856

Ghazali, S. (1973) Presacral teratomas in children. *Journal of Pediatric Surgery*, **8**, 915

Green, A.A., Hustic, H.O., Palmer, R. and Pinkel, D. (1976) Total-body sequential segmental irradiation and combination chemotherapy for children with disseminated neuroblastoma. *Cancer*, **38**, 2250

Grosfeld, J. (1976) Benign and malignant teratomas in children; analysis of 85 patients. *Surgery*, **80**, 297

Grosfeld, J.L., Schatzlein, M., Ballantine, T.U.N., Weetman, R.M. and Balhner, R.L. (1978) Metastatic neuroblastoma: factors influencing survival. *Journal of Pediatric Surgery*, **13**, 59

Harvard, B.M. (1953) Retroperitoneal lipoma in children: report of a case and review of the literature. *Journal of Urology*, **70**, 159

Hellstrom, I., Hellstrom, K.E., Bill, A.H., Pierce, G.E. and Young J.P.S. (1970) Studies on cellular immunity to human neuroblastoma cells. *International Journal of Cancer*, **6**, 172

Ireland, J. (1978) Personal communication

Jonte, P.A., Wadman, S.K. and van Putten, W.J. (1970) Congenital neuroblastoma: symptoms in the mother during pregnancy. *Clinical Pediatrics*, **9**, 206

Kafka, V. and Novak, K. (1970) Multicystic retroperitoneal lymphangioma in an infant appearing as an inguinal hernia. *Journal of Pediatric Surgery*, **5**, 573

Kakizol, T. and Tahara, M. (1972) Fetus in fetu located in the scrotal sac of a newborn infant: a case report. *Journal of Urology*, **107**, 506

Kasubuchi, Y., Sawada, T. and Nakamura, T. (1973) Successful treatment of neonatal retroperitoneal haemangioma with corticosteroid. *Journal of Pediatric Surgery*, **8**, 59

Kauffman, S.L. and Stout, A.P. (1960) Haemangiopericytoma in children. *Cancer*, **13**, 695

Koop, C.E. and Johnson, D.G. (1971) Neuroblastoma: an assessment of therapy in reference to staging. *Journal of Pediatric Surgery*, **6**, 595

Kumar, S., Steward, J.K., Waghe, M. Pearson, D., Edwards, D.C., Fenton, E.C. and Griffiths, E.H. (1970) The administration of nerve growth factor to children with widespread neuroblastoma. *Journal of Pediatric Surgery*, **5**, 18

Lee, E.Y.C. (1965) Foetus in foetu. *Archives of Disease in Childhood*, **40**, 689

Levi-Montalcini, R. (1966) Nerve growth factor: its mode of action on sensory and sympathetic nerve cells. *Harvey Lectures*, **60**, 217

Martin, J. (1974) Chemotherapy and urogenital tumours. *In* Reviews in Paediatric Urology (edited by Johnston, J.H. and Goodwin, W.E.). Excerpta Medica, Amsterdam. p.383

Miller, R.W., Fraumeni, J.F. and Hill, J.A. (1968) Neuroblastoma: an epidemiologic approach to its origins. *Journal of Pediatric Surgery*, **3**, 141

Murthy, T.V.M., Irving, I.M. and Lister, J. (1978) Massive adrenal haemorrhage in neonatal neuroblastoma. *Journal of Pediatric Surgery*, **13**, 31

Olson, J.R. and Abell, M.R. (1969) Nonfunctional, nonchromaffin paragangliomas of the retroperitoneum. *Cancer*, **23**, 1358

Peeples, W.J. and Hazra, T. (1976) Retroperitoneal liposarcoma in a child. *Urology*, **7**, 89

Rangecroft, L., Lauder, I. and Wagget, J. (1978) Spontaneous maturation of stage IV S neuroblastoma. *Archives of Disease in Childhood*, **53**, 815

Reilly, D., Nesbit, M.E. and Krivit, W. (1968) Cure of three patients who had skeletal metastases in disseminated neuroblastoma. *Pediatrics*, **41**, 47

Schnaufer, L. and Koop, C.E. (1975) Silastic abdominal patch for temporary hepatomegaly in stage IV S neuroblastoma. *Journal of Pediatric Surgery*, **10**, 73

Schwartz, A.D., Zadeh, M.D., Lee, H. and Swaney, J.J. (1974) Spontaneous regression of disseminated neuroblastoma. *Journal of Pediatrics*, **85**, 760

Senelick, R.C., Bray, P.F., Lahey, E., Van Dyk, H.J.L. and Johnson, D.G. (1973) Neuroblastoma and myoclonic encephalopathy: two cases and a review of the literature. *Journal of Pediatric Surgery*, **8**, 623

Siebert, E.S. and Bill, A.H. (1968) The chick assay test for nerve growth factor in human serum. *Journal of Pediatric Surgery*, **3**, 170

Sy, W.M. and Edmondson, J.H. (1968) The developmental defects associated with neuroblastoma: etiologic implications. *Cancer*, **22**, 234

Uchino, J., Hata, Y. and Kasai, Y. (1978) Stage IV S neuroblastoma. *Journal of Pediatric Surgery*, **13**, 167

Waghe, M., Kumar, S. and Steward, J.K. (1970) Nerve growth factor in human sera. *Journal of Pediatric Surgery*, **5**, 14

Willis, R.A. (1967) Pathology of Tumours, 4th edn. Butterworths, London.p.857

Wilson, C.S. and Middleton, R.G. (1975) Suprarenal neurilemmoma. *Urology*, **5**, 707

Wilson, L.M.K. and Draper, G.J. (1974) Neuroblastoma, its natural history and prognosis: a study of 487 cases. *British Medical Journal*, iii, 301

Young, I. and Hosking, G.P. (1978) Familial neurodegenerative disorders associated with raised urinary vanillylmandelic acid. *Archives of Disease in Childhood*, **53**, 682

34 Tumours of the Lower Genitourinary Tract

D. Innes Williams and John Martin

Although tumours of the lower urinary tract are much less common than renal tumours in children, they are an important group for urological study in view of their considerable mortality rate. Several varieties of neoplasm may be encountered but very few resemble in their presentation the common transitional cell tumour of adults. An appreciation of the peculiarities of childhood malignancy is therefore necessary if a diagnosis is to be reached at a stage when treatment has a reasonable chance of success. The most common tumour is a rhabdomyosarcoma which may arise in a variety of anatomical situations.

Rhabdomyosarcoma

Rhabdomyosarcoma is a malignant connective tissue tumour that includes rhabdomyoblasts, which are the precursors of striated muscle cells, in various stages of differentiation. These tumours occur in a number of locations, for example the orbit, the pharynx, the bile ducts and the genitourinary tract. However, when all these are taken together rhabdomyosarcomas are less numerous than neuroblastomas or nephroblastomas. The third National Cancer Survey (1975) carried out in the USA from 1969–71 found rhabdomyosarcoma had an incidence of 4.5 per million white children under the age of 15 years and accounted for approximately 13 per cent of all solid malignant tumours.

Rhabdomyosarcoma of the lower genitourinary tract occurs most often in the bladder base where it may be polypoid and lobulated (*Figure 34.1*) or solid (*Figure 34.2*). In the male a solid tumour of the bladder base is difficult to distinguish from one arising in the prostate, which is the next most common situation. In girls a vaginal lesion presenting as 'sarcoma botryoides' is well recognized but again tumours may involve the bladder base as well as the urethra and the anterior vaginal wall. Solid rhabdomyosarcomas occur in the broad ligament area in the female and on the periphery of the bladder in the male. These tumours present most often in the age group 2–6 years in contradistinction to the paratesticular rhabdomyosarcomas which are usually seen in late childhood,

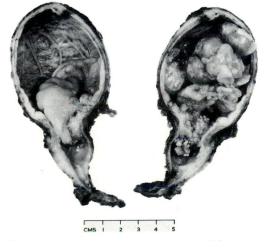

Figure 34.1. Polypoid rhabdomyosarcoma of the bladder, total cystectomy specimen.

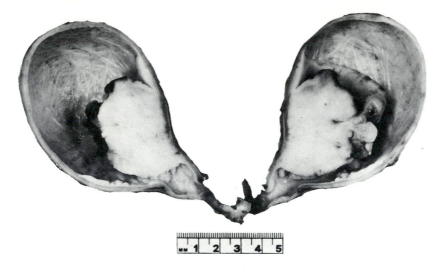

Figure 34.2. Solid rhabdomyosarcoma of the bladder, total cystectomy specimen.

adolescence or early adult life (*see* Chapter 47). Rarely a perineal tumour may have this histology (Hildebrand *et al.*, 1980). The fact that rhabdomyoblasts occur in tumours in these situations where skeletal muscle is ordinarily scanty or absent has caused much speculation, and no satisfactory explanation has yet emerged. Batsakis (1963) suggested that their origin may be found in undifferentiated mesenchyme surrounding the mesonephric duct, and this provides an embryological explanation of their range of occurrence.

Histologically rhabdomyosarcoma can be classified as embryonal, alveolar or pleomorphic (Horn and Enterline, 1958). The embryonal variety is almost always involved in lower urinary tract tumours. It consists of mesenchymal cells with large single hyperchromatic nuclei. Some cells are elongated in a strap or tadpole form with deeply eosinophilic cytoplasm within which longitudinal fibrils and transverse striations can be detected. In the alveolar type smaller compact and rounded cells occur sometimes with transverse striations and with a tendency to align themselves around spaces in a fibrovascular stroma. This form is occasionally observed in the prostate in children (Evans, 1968). The pleomorphic variety is characteristic of the tumour arising in voluntary muscle in adults. An ultrastructural study of childhood rhabdomyosarcoma was reported by Mierau and Favara (1980).

Bladder tumours

Rhabdomyosarcoma of the bladder

Most tumours present during the first 4 years of life and there is a slight predominance of male cases. The polypoid form is more amenable to treatment and fortunately commoner than the solid one. Both forms involve chiefly the bladder base and can extend upwards towards the dome. The growths originate in the submucosal or superficial muscle layers of the bladder. The bulk of the tumour is a mass of pearly-grey lobules. On the periphery it is represented by a thin submucosal plaque with a very clear-cut margin advancing across the bladder. This plaque may extend down the urethra right through the membranous portion of the male duct and for the whole length of the female one. Similar extension occurs upwards into the ureters, although it is not so common. An extension of a vaginal or labial lesion may also involve the bladder by upward growth. Local spread within the pelvis together with lymph-node involvement occurs before distant metastases and many cases are seen while the tumour is still confined to the bladder.

The lobulated form of the tumour within the bladder gives rise to very characteristic symptoms. The child has strangury, an urgent desire to micturate without being able to accomplish the activity, because the lobules descend into the urethra in the same way as a stone. Acute or subacute retention is therefore the presenting symptom and is accompanied by a great deal of pain. Infection is a common complication because of the residual urine, but haematuria is rare unlike the situation in carcinomatous tumours of adults. The obstruction leads to upper tract dilatation and uraemia. Symptoms of renal failure are present in some patients at the time of hospital admission.

Diagnosis

On physical examination the bladder is palpably distended and tense. The swelling does not disappear on catheterization and on rectal examination the bladder is firmer than would be expected in simple retention. Very often the diagnosis can be suspected clinically on these findings supported by a characteristic history.

The intravenous pyelogram shows a variable degree of obstruction. The dilatation of the ureters is clearly of relatively recent onset and they are tense and full, not showing the tortuousity common in the congenital obstructions of childhood. There is almost invariably a widening of the gap between the lower ends of the ureters where the tumour mass has separated them and sometimes the ureters actually turn laterally at their terminations. There are characteristic lobulated filling defects at the base or sometimes throughout the bladder. The appearance of the posterior urethra is important: there is a cone of dilatation maintained by the prolapsed lobules forcing their way down into the urethra. The bladder neck is wide, the urethra narrows somewhere around the verumontanum and filling defects due to lobules can be observed (*Figure 34.3*). These findings are best seen where the intravenous urogram gives an adequate concentration of contrast medium. Injection cystograms are required to show the typical picture when renal failure is advanced.

Radiologically disorders that may cause confusion are ectopic ureteroceles (although the upper urinary tract anomaly should leave no doubt) and the polyps seen in rare inflammatory conditions such as eosinophilic cystitis. Ultrasound reveals the solid element of the tumour and the degree of extravesical spread within the pelvis and the abdomen but it may not differentiate other tumours or hamartomas such as neurofibroma. At cystoscopy the pearly-grey

lobules are easily recognizable unless there is considerable complicating inflammation while the solid tumours of the bladder base are not so easily diagnosed and endoscopic or needle biopsy is essential. Investigations should also include

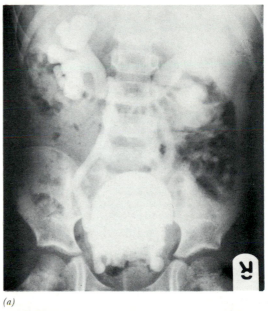

(a)

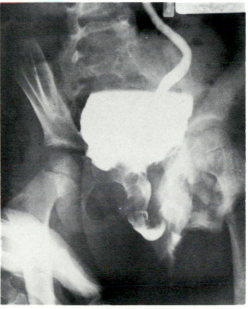

(b)

Figure 34.3. Polypoid rhabdomyosarcoma of the bladder. *(a)* Intravenous urogram showing ureteric obstruction, filling defects in the bladder and widening of the bladder base. *(b)* Micturating cystogram showing lobulated filling defects in the urethra and unilateral reflux.

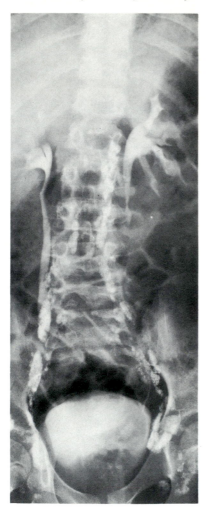

Figure 34.4. Rhabdomyosarcoma of the bladder, combined lymphogram and intravenous urogram showing a filling defect in the bladder but no ureteric obstruction or lymph-node involvement.

a search for distant spread by means of a chest X-ray and a skeletal survey. Lymphography and bone marrow biopsy are required only in doubtful cases (*Figure 34.4*).

Treatment

Pelvic rhabdomyosarcoma faces urologists with the difficult situation of a rare tumour with diverse manifestations and a rapidly changing therapeutic scene. There has been some experience of the possibilities of radical surgery, and combined chemotherapy and radiotherapy have given some spectacular short-term results as

well as a number of severe disappointments where tumours failed to respond. Up to the 1970s it was usually believed that rhabdomyosarcoma was not amenable to radiotherapy, and certainly in those cases where it was tried in doses comparable to those used for nephroblastoma there was very little response from either the primary or metastases. In those early years individual cases were treated by single-drug chemotherapeutic regimens, usually with actinomycin D or vincristine, and it was not easy to see that any improvement followed this line of treatment. More recently it has been demonstrated that rhabdomyosarcoma at any site can respond to multiple-drug chemotherapy combined with radiotherapy in larger doses.

The rapidity with which treatment regimens are developed and altered together with the relative rarity of rhabdomyosarcoma has meant that most reports cover only a small number of cases which have varying manifestations and that little attempt is made to stage the tumours. Thus Razak, Perez and Lee (1977), reporting the great advances made since chemotherapy was introduced, mentioned only 10 examples of all forms of pelvic rhabdomyosarcoma. One out of five patients survived before chemotherapy and five out of five afterwards. Nevertheless, out of the total series four patients had a radical operation, all with a successful result, and therefore the contribution of chemotherapy is more difficult to assess.

The present authors' early cases were reported by Ghazali (1973). The total Great Ormond Street experience between 1945–76 comprised 28 cases of rhabdomyosarcoma of the bladder treated by attempted cystoprostatectomy or cystourethrovaginectomy sometimes associated with hysterectomy. Overall there were 14 survivors from this group. Adjuvant radiotherapy or chemotherapy was administered in only six, largely because the majority of patients presented before the chemotherapy era. Of these six just two survived, in both of whom it is reasonable to believe that the chemotherapy contributed towards the successful outcome since one had a fungating tumour on the abdominal wall. All the survivors had predominantly polypoid tumours and, except for the one case mentioned, did not have histological evidence of spread beyond the scope of operative excision. The dangers of submucous urethral infiltration were recognized early in the series, although before that at least one patient died through failure to excise the urethra down into the bulb. In many cases the anterior vaginal wall alone was removed and in most instances it proved to be free from tumour. Where there was doubt a total hysterectomy and vaginectomy was performed at the same time as cystectomy. Apart from clearance of the obvious lymph nodes in the iliac region no extensive lymph-node dissection was undertaken. In this connection it is interesting to note that Cukier *et al.* (1968) described a method for very radical excision and pelvic clearance with encouraging short-term results. In all five of their cases late recurrence took place after 3 years.

The evolution of rhabdomyosarcoma is sometimes remarkably prolonged either before or after treatment. For example a 3-month-old child was treated by radical cystoprostatectomy for a bladder tumour and had no recurrence until 5 years after operation, when there was a massive regrowth in the pelvis that was rapidly fatal. In another case primary excision by cystoprostatectomy and chemotherapy with vincristine, actinomycin and cyclophosphamide were followed 2 years later by the appearance of a massive left renal tumour. At nephrectomy this proved to be a rhabdomyosarcoma involving the kidney and the upper part of the ureter. The lower ureteric segment adjoining the ileal loop was clear. It must be assumed that seeding of the upper urinary tract had occurred from a polypoid bladder tumour associated with vesicoureteric reflux which had been recognized preoperatively.

In spite of the relative efficacy of surgery for polypoid tumours the recently reported successes of chemotherapy and radiotherapy (Maurer Moon and Donaldson, 1977; Hays, 1980) unquestionably alter the attitude towards a radical operation that leaves the child with a severe disability due to urinary diversion and sterility (although impotence is not necessarily a feature of childhood cystoprostatectomy). Treatment should therefore always involve more than one modality and discussion must include the timing of drug therapy, irradiation and surgery, as well as dosages and techniques. Wherever possible such children should be treated along the lines of an agreed protocol and in a centre with experience of this uncommon tumour.

Radiotherapy

While embryonic rhabdomyosarcoma is less radiosensitive than many other tumours it does respond to larger doses of radiotherapy. This can be used both to assist in reducing the size of initially large tumours that are inoperable or where operation would be mutilating, and to help in achieving local control after incomplete surgical excision.

Irradiation should be administered by megavoltage apparatus or its equivalent. Satisfactory dosages are usually in the range of 4000–6000 rads in 4–6 weeks using daily fractions of 200 rads. Portals should be planned so as to treat the tumour and spare as much as possible of the surrounding tissues. Special care should be taken to shield the heads of the femora and the scrotum. Local side effects are common and are inevitable when irradiation and chemotherapy are given concurrently. They include vigorous local skin reaction, dysuria and proctitis, but usually settle over a few weeks and do not generally cause long-term problems.

Chemotherapy

A number of antimitotic drugs have been demonstrated to have an effect on pelvic rhabdomyosarcoma. Actinomycin D, vincristine and cyclophosphamide are all effective as single agents. Wilbur *et al.* (1975) showed the advantages of combined therapy with these drugs, and many variations have since been used. Adriamycin also has considerable activity against this tumour but has not yet been used widely. Modes of action, methods of administration, dosages and side effects are discussed in Chapter 32.

The authors' experience has been of a form of pulsed combined therapy. Weekly intravenous doses of vincristine $1.5\,mg/m^2$ body surface area and actinomycin D $0.6\,mg/m^2$ body surface area are administered for 6 weeks followed by a similar pulse at 3-week intervals to 2 years. The initial 6 weeks' therapy can be given concurrently with radiotherapy.

Operative techniques

Partial cystectomy, in the very exceptional case to which it is applicable, must be planned individually according to the site of the tumour. A wide excision through healthy tissue is essential and may necessitate incursion upon the bladder neck and reimplantation of the ureter. If the posterior urethra is involved, cystoprostatectomy is preferable.

Total cystectomy can in general follow the technique established for carcinoma of the bladder (Zingg, 1977) although certain features of childhood disease require comment. In the male cystectomy should aim to remove in one piece the urethra as far as the penoscrotal junction and it is therefore preferable to commence the operation from the perineum, freeing and cutting across the urethra distally and pushing it up under the pubic arch. In the female the entire urethra and surrounding labial tissues should be excised together with the anterior wall of the vagina or the entire organ if it is involved. While the uterus itself is not primarily affected hysterectomy may be required where there is vaginal extension. Abdominal dissection within the pelvis is greatly facilitated by splitting the symphysis pubis and retracting the pubic bones laterally. This not only allows more delicate dissection of the tissues anterior to the bladder and the prostate but also gives room for manipulation in the internal iliac region. Lymph-node clearance in the pelvis should accompany cystectomy, although very radical lymph-node dissection at a higher level has not proved justifiable. Urinary diversion by ileal conduit is preferable to other methods since it leaves the pelvis free from any reconstructive surgery that may be affected by later radiotherapy.

Treatment plan

The bladder tumour that is diagnosed early and confirmed by biopsy should first be considered for conservative treatment. Chemotherapy may effect sufficient control to allow local tumour resection with preservation of bladder function, but radiotherapy seldom leaves a field suitable for reconstructive surgery. A reasonable policy is therefore to commence treatment using triple-drug therapy (with or without an indwelling catheter for control of retention) and to observe progress by palpation, ultrasound, radiology and cystoscopy. Complete regression of the tumour is unlikely and needs to be checked by repeated biopsy. Partial regression may enable a partial cystectomy to be performed. A negative response indicates the need for radical surgery and postoperative irradiation. Local recurrence after surgery requires chemotherapy and irradiation and there is very little prospect of effective secondary surgery.

More extensive bladder tumours and tumours of the prostate are best treated by initial combined chemotherapy together with radiotherapy. Surgery is used to deal with any residual disease which is often minimal. This approach avoids mutilating surgery for many patients. However, McDougal and Persky (1980) found that treatment schemes omitting radical operations gave inferior results.

In late cases where distant metastases are already present at the time of diagnosis there should be initial chemotherapy and local treatment should be confined to the relief of symptoms. A good response of metastatic disease to treatment justifies later more aggressive therapy for the primary tumour with surgery and/or radiotherapy.

Transitional cell bladder tumours

Papillary growths of transitional cell origin are exceptionally rare in childhood and are usually relatively benign. Siegel and Pincus (1969) reported a papilloma and reviewed the literature. Castellanos, Wakefield and Evans (1975) discussed malignant tumours. Multiple and recurrent papillary tumours appear to be even rarer than the solitary form. Their presentation is generally with haematuria and the diagnosis is reached from the deformity apparent on the bladder films from intravenous urography and cystoscopy. Endoscopic biopsy and either diathermy excision or open partial cystectomy have been the treatment of choice.

Phaeochromocytoma

Phaeochromocytoma can develop in the bladder wall in children as in adults and can produce paroxysmal hypertension and haematuria (Leestma and Price, 1971).

Hamartoma and benign tumours

Neurofibromatosis can involve the bladder and the urinary tract to a major or minor degree. The generalized disorder is characterized by multiple subcutaneous tumours along the course of the peripheral nerves and by pigmented café-au-lait spots on the skin, neither of which are

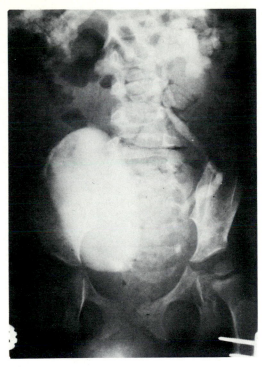

(a)

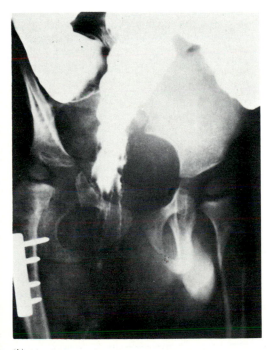

(b)

Figure 34.5. Pelvic neurofibromatosis. *(a)* Intravenous urogram showing displacement of bladder and ureteric obstruction. *(b)* Barium enema showing compressed rectum and bone disorder.

usually evident at birth but appear during the first 2–3 years. Involvement of the skeleton with dwarfism and scoliosis is a common complication while visceral lesions are rare. The bladder may be involved externally by massive plexiform tumours of the lumbar and sacral nerves so that it is displaced upwards (*Figure 34.5*) with a flattened elongated urethra that may become obstructed. In such cases there are also likely to be neurofibromas in the inguinal or labial region and perhaps additionally in the mesentery of the intestine. At other times the disease process affects more specifically the bladder wall and the submucosal layer in particular. Irregular infiltration with neurofibromatous tissue gives the bladder a somewhat trabeculated and sacculated appearance on cystography and endoscopy, although the hamartomatous tissue is much paler in colour than the ordinary bladder trabeculae. Bladder function is often surprisingly well maintained even in the presence of considerable involvement in the neurofibromatous process. In the course of time ureteric obstruction (*Figure 34.6*) is apt to occur as well as retention due to bladder neck rigidity (Carlson and Wilkinson, 1972).

The diagnosis should be suspected from the superficial café-au-lait spots and subcutaneous neurofibromas. Endoscopic biopsy of the bladder gives a positive diagnosis. Treatment should ordinarily be confined to the relief of obstruction where this is present. Progress of the disease is often exceptionally slow and a very conservative approach should be adopted. Simple excision of pelvic masses is seldom required. Occasionally massive involvement of the bladder with complicating sepsis demands cystectomy and urinary diversion.

Myoma

A benign rhabdomyoma of polypoid form in the bladder is easily mistaken for a malignancy. An example was recorded by Russell, Lipin and Gaines (1958) and another occurred in the authors' practice. In all cases there was severe haematuria and an obstructive element. The origin was at the bladder base and there was no resemblance to the simple or fibromatous urethral polyp, which generally arises by a long stalk in the region of the verumontanum. Following biopsy local excision should be sufficient.

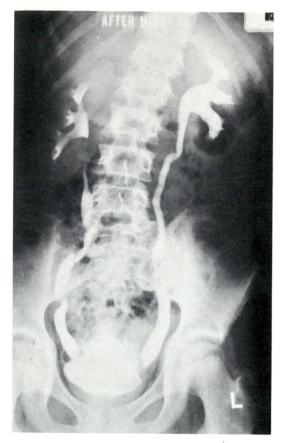

(a)

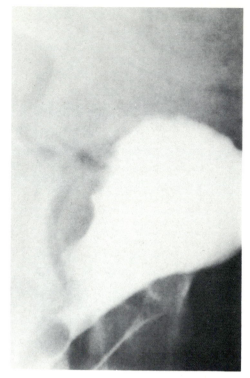

(b)

Figure 34.6. Vesical neurofibromatosis. *(a)* Intravenous urogram showing ureteric obstruction. *(b)* Cystogram showing deformation of posterior bladder wall.

Haemangioma

Like neurofibroma, haemangioma may exist primarily in the connective tissue spaces of the pelvis and only involve the bladder incidentally. Hendry and Vinnicombe (1971) reported 31 patients who presented with haematuria before the age of 20. Such haematuria can be due to a small haemangioma of the bladder, which cystoscopically resembles a transitional cell tumour, or to a large hamartomatous mass involving the entire pelvis. Most haemangiomas show some superficial signs and are usually large enough to produce a deformity on the intravenous urogram. Haemangioma is therefore one of the rarest causes of asymptomatic haematuria. Cystoscopic biopsy is a hazardous procedure since it may precipitate a massive haemorrhage, and open exploration with resection of the involved tissue is advisable.

Partial cystectomy along with excision of the extravesical mass is often possible and is the treatment of choice. Rarely total cystectomy may be required for uncontrollable haemorrhage from a widely diffused haemangioma.

Prostatic tumours
Rhabdomyosarcoma

The exact origin of a solid tumour in the pelvis may be hard to determine but those arising in the prostatic region form clinically a separate group from bladder tumours. The majority of such growths are rhabdomyosarcomas, and while other histological types occur they may all be considered under this heading. A large solid globular mass fills the pelvis, displacing the bladder upwards and stretching the urethra tightly across the surface. The base of the bladder is infiltrated and submucosal extension

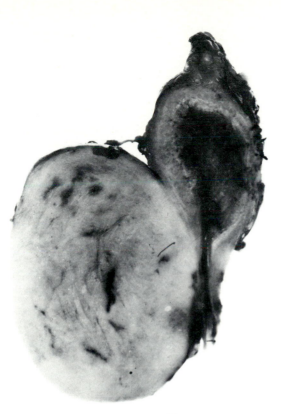

Figure 34.7. Rhabdomyosarcoma of the prostate. Cystoprostatectomy specimen.

needle introduced from the perineum. Other possible swellings in the prostatic area in children include abscess (Williams and Martins, 1960) and utricular cyst (where, however, the swelling tends to ride higher behind the bladder).

The prognosis for prostatic rhabdomyosarcoma is very much worse than for bladder tumours. Tucker (1972) reviewed 53 cases in the literature and found only two survivors. In the authors' series (Ghazali, 1973) there were nine prostatic rhabdomyosarcomas. Primary cystoprostatectomy was possible in only three cases, two of whom were the only survivors from the entire group.

Treatment for prostatic tumours should combine chemotherapy, radiotherapy and surgery on the lines already described for bladder rhabdomyosarcoma. Radical surgery is possible less often because of local extension. A drug regimen associated with radiotherapy may reduce the tumour size, leaving a fixed mass in the pelvis which may or may not contain active neoplasm. In such circumstances prolonged observation and repeated biopsy are preferable to heroic attempts at surgical excision.

occurs along the urethra (*Figure 34.7*). The average age of presentation is greater than in bladder tumours and the growth is usually further advanced with local spread when first seen. Distant metastases are also more likely to be found on initial investigation. As in bladder rhabdomyosarcoma there is a urinary obstruction and retention is a common mode of presentation. The very acute symptoms of bladder cases due to impaction of lobules of tumour in the urethra are absent and the retention appears to be of more gradual origin.

The diagnosis can be readily suspected from the presence of a smooth and firm or tensely cystic mass filling the pelvis and extending upwards into the abdomen. Rectal examination reveals the tumour to be anterior to the bowel, distinguishing it from sacral neuroblastoma or teratoma. Its situation can also be demonstrated by ultrasound. Cystourethrography illustrates the prostatic situation of the tumour and the distortion of the urethra. Endoscopy is usually impossible because of the size of the mass and biopsy of the tumour is best performed by a

Tumours of the penis and the scrotum

Although a papillary adenocarcinoma of the glans penis has been described in an Indian boy aged 2 years (Kini, 1944), these tumours have not been seen by most Western authors. Haemangioma and lymphangioma affecting the penis and scrotum are relatively common.

Cavernous haemangiomas are often small and unnoticed at birth and they either spread or fill out during the first few years so that in the scrotum and the perineum they may reach a considerable size. In this situation they are apt to become ulcerated and infected, but even in the absence of complications most of them sclerose spontaneously in the course of the first 5 years of life and very little treatment is required. Haemangiomas accompanying similar hamartomas of the bladder and the pelvic tissues can present a much more serious problem and can be associated with severe urethral bleeding (*Figure 34.8*). While treatment ordinarily has to be conservative, at times excision of haemangioma-tous masses, ligature of supplying vessels and injection of sclerosing fluids may be required. Matthews (1956) reported an enormous haemangioma involving the whole genital area in which the penis was grossly enlarged. Treatment of such a lesion is difficult and dangerous and Matthews' case suffered fatal air embolism during surgery.

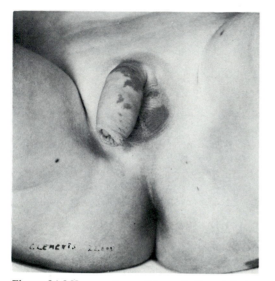

Figure 34.8 Haemangioma of the genitalia and the legs associated with a bleeding haemangioma of the bladder and the urethra.

Small haemangiomas are sometimes seen on the surface of the glans penis and cause no symptoms, although a little bleeding may occur at times. Their appearance can be alarming but treatment should be avoided if possible since there is a reasonable chance of spontaneous regression and active treatment is likely to prove destructive to the epithelium of the glans.

Lymphangioma presents as a soft circumscribed swelling in the skin of the scrotum or penis. It is unsightly but causes little inconvenience. It can be excised without difficulty.

Tumours of the female genital tract

Rhabdomyosarcoma of the vagina

The term sarcoma botryoides has long been employed for the characteristic rhabdomyosarcoma of the vagina when grape-like lobules of

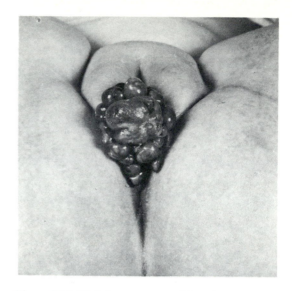

Figure 34.9. Rhabdomyosarcoma of the vulva.

tumour appear at the vulva. As with bladder and prostatic growths vaginal tumours are most likely to occur during the first 3 years of life. Prolapse of the fleshy polypoid masses is usually the initial sign of the disease (*Figure 34.9*). Where they are exposed ulceration occurs leading to haemorrhage and purulent vaginal discharge. There may also be a flat spreading submucosal element to the tumour which involves the urethra and the vulval tissues as well as the vaginal wall. Sometimes polyps are present both in the bladder and in the vagina. Dissemination to the inguinal glands occurs once the vulva is involved but distant metastases are relatively late in appearance. Hilgers, Malkasian and Soule (1970) reviewed the literature and gave a full account of the clinicopathological condition.

The diagnosis is readily made from the appearance of the tumour and from biopsy which is easily performed. While urethral prolapse and prolapsing ectopic ureterocele sometimes give rise to suspicion of sarcoma they are differentiated without difficulty on closer inspection.

As with bladder and prostatic tumours the earlier literature refers chiefly to the success of radical excision of the vagina, the uterus, the bladder and the urethra. More recently (Kumar, Wrenn and Fleming, 1976) reports have emphasized the advantages of less radical surgery combined with chemotherapy and irradiation. Pelvic exenteration is scarcely ever necessary and it may well be possible to excise the length of the vagina with the uterus and the tubes and leave the urinary tract intact. However, in this procedure there is a danger of producing a neuropathic bladder. An even less radical sleeve resection of the vagina may be practicable if there is a preliminary response to chemotherapy. In future treatment will probably follow the lines laid down for bladder rhabdomyosarcoma.

Other tumours

Rare tumours causing vaginal bleeding and polypoid vulval masses in infants have been the subject of some pathological discussion. Examples occurring during the first 2 years of life and arising in the upper vagina or cervix were at one time regarded as adenocarcinomas derived from Gaertner's duct (mesonephromas). More recently it has been recognized (Norris, Bagley and Taylor, 1970; Allyn, Silverberg and Salzberg, 1971) that they can be endodermal sinus tumours of the type found in the ovary or testis with characteristic alpha-fetoprotein production. The majority, including those in the authors' experience, exhibit early metastatic spread and end fatally within 6–9 months. They have been treated by colpectomy with hysterectomy in recent years with the addition of radiotherapy and chemotherapy, and some survivors are now reported (Siegel, Sagerman and Berdon, 1970).

Clear cell carcinomas of the vagina occur in adolescence and Herbst, Kurman and Scully (1972) demonstrated the causative relationship of some of these lesions with excessive maternal oestrogen therapy during pregnancy. Radical surgery and irradiation have been employed.

Carcinoma of the cervix is extremely rare but cases have been reported by Dalley, Dewhurst and Flood (1971).

Paravesical and broad ligament tumours

Solid tumours arising within the fascial planes of the pelvis are sometimes rhabdomyosarcomas, although this diagnosis can scarcely be made without biopsy which is ordinarily undertaken at laparotomy. Such patients present with a pelvic mass displacing the bladder and sometimes obstructing a ureter. The tumour is often adherent to adjacent organs when first diagnosed. In two of the authors' cases there was a very rapid response to chemotherapy and irradiation, leaving a residual mass attached to the bladder wall that could be removed satisfactorily without damage to other organs.

References

Allyn, D.G., Silverberg, S.G. and Salzberg, A.M. (1971) Endodermal sinus tumour of the vagina. *Cancer*, **27**, 1931

Batsakis, J.G. (1963) Urogenital rhabdomyosarcoma: histogenesis and classification. *Journal of Urology*, **90**, 180

Carlson, D.H. and Wilkinson, R.J. (1972) Neurofibromatosis of the bladder in children. *Radiology*, **105**, 401

Castellanos, R.D., Wakefield, P.B. and Evans, A.T. (1975) Carcinoma of the bladder in children. *Journal of Urology*, **113**, 261

Cukier, J., Benhamon, G., Laurent, M. and Boukier, T. (1968) Five cases of sarcoma of the urogenital sinus. *Journal d'urologie et nephrologie*, **74**, 813

Dalley, V.M., Dewhurst, C.J. and Flood, C.M. (1971) Carcinoma of cervix in childhood. *Journal of Obstetrics and Gynaecology of the British Commonwealth*, **78**, 1133

Evans, R.W. (1968) Histological appearance of tumours, 2nd edn. Livingstone, Edinburgh. p.53

Ghazali, S. (1973) Embryonic rhabdomyosarcoma of the urogenital tract. *British Journal of Surgery*, **60**, 124

Hays, D.M. (1980) Pelvic rhabdomyosarcomas in childhood: diagnosis and concepts of management reviewed. *Cancer*, **45**, 1810

Hendry, W.F. and Vinnicombe, J. (1971) Haemangioma of the bladder in children and young adults. *British Journal of Urology*, **43**, 309

Herbst, A.L., Kurman, R.J., Scully, R.E. (1972) Clear cell adenocarcinoma of the genital tract in young females. *New England Journal of Medicine*, **287**, 1259

Hildebrand, H.F., Krivosic, I., Grandier-Vazeille, X., Tetaert, D. and Biserte, G. (1980) Perineal rhabdomyosarcoma in a newborn child: pathological and biochemical studies with emphasis on contractile proteins. *Journal of Clinical Pathology*, **33**, 823

Hilgers, R.D., Malkasian, G.D. and Soule, E.H. (1970) Embryonal rhabdomyosarcoma (botryoid type) of vagina: a clinico-pathological review. *American Journal of Obstetrics and Gynecology*, **107**, 484

Horn, R.C. and Enterline, H.T. (1958) Rhabdomyosarcoma: a clinico-pathological study and classification of 39 cases. *Cancer*, **11**, 181

Kini, M.G. (1944) Cancer of the penis in a child aged two years. *Indian Medical Gazette*, **79**, 66

Kumar, A.P.M., Wrenn, E.L., Fleming, I.D. (1976) Combined therapy to prevent complete exenteration for rhabdomyosarcoma of the vagina or uterus. *Cancer*, **37**, 118

Leestma, J.E. and Price, E.B. (1971) Paraganglioma of the urinary bladder. *Cancer*, **28**, 1063

McDougal, W.S. and Persky, L. (1980) Rhabdomyosarcoma of the bladder and prostate in children. *Journal of Urology*, **124**, 882

Matthews, D.W. (1956) Cavernous haemangioma of the scrotal septum. *Journal of Pediatrics*, **49**, 744

Maurer, M.M., Moon, T., Donaldson, M. (1977) The intergroup rhabdomyosarcoma study; a preliminary report. *Cancer*, **40**, 2015

Mierau, G.W. and Favara, B.E. (1980) Rhabdomyosarcoma in children, ultrastructural study of 31 cases. *Cancer*, **46**, 2035

National Cancer Survey (1975) National Institute Monographs, no. 41. Washington

Norris, H.J., Bagley, G.P. and Taylor, H.B. (1970) Carcinoma of the infant's vagina: a distinctive tumour. *Archives of Pathology*, **90**, 473

Razak, A.A., Perez, C.A. and Lee, F.A. (1977) Combined treatment modalities of rhabdomyosarcoma in children. *Cancer*, **39**, 24

Russell, H.L., Lipin, J.L. and Gaines, J.W. (1958) Tumours of the bladder in infants. *Journal of Urology*, **79**, 823

Siegel, H.A., Sagerman, R., Berdon, W.E. (1970) Mesonephric adenocarcinoma of the vagina. *Journal of Pediatric Surgery*, **5**, 468

Siegel, W.H. and Pincus, M.B. (1969) Epithelial bladder tumours in children. *Journal of Urology*, **101**, 55

Tucker, E.C., (1972) Rhabdomyosarcoma of the prostate. *Journal of Abdominal Surgery*, **14**, 19

Wilbur, J.R., Sutow, W.W., Sullivan, M.P. and Gottlieb, J.A. (1975) Chemotherapy of sarcomas. *Cancer*, **36**, 765

Williams, D.I. and Martins, A. (1960) Peri-prostatic haematoma and prostatic abscess in the neonatal period. *Archives of Disease in Childhood*, **35**, 177

Zingg, E.J. (1977) Radical Cystectomy. *In* Operative Surgery, 2nd edn, Vol. 13 (edited by Rob, C. and Smith, R.). Butterworths, London. p.201

35 Normal and Abnormal Sexual Development

David B. Grant and D. Innes Williams

The wide range of disorders of genital development described in the following chapters are difficult to understand unless they are considered against the background of normal development. This chapter reviews the chromosomal, embryological and endocrine aspects of normal genital development and outlines the variety of clinical conditions that can arise as a result of failure of these mechanisms.

Chromosomal determination of sex

In man the nuclei of all the somatic cells carry 46 chromosomes, namely two sex chromosomes and 22 pairs of autosomes. Gonadal differentiation is governed by the two sex chromosomes, which are a relatively large X chromosome and a much smaller Y chromosome. Individual variation of the size of the Y chromosome is due to differences in the length of the long arm and has no appreciable effect on genital development.

As a result of the two stages of meiotic division each maternal germ cell produces an ovum with a haploid complement of 22 autosomes and one X chromosome and two or three polar bodies (*Figure 35.1*). Similarly each male germ cell produces four spermatozoa each of which carries 22 autosomes and either an X chromosome or a Y chromosome (*Figure 35.1*).

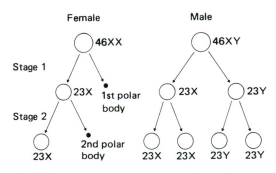

Figure 35.1. Normal meiosis showing schematic disposition of sex chromosomes.

Fertilization of an ovum by an X-bearing cell results in a zygote with a 46 XX diploid karyotype which subsequently leads to ovarian development. Only one X chromosome appears to be necessary for the initial stages of ovarian differentiation (Singh and Carr, 1966). The later stages with formation of primary follicles depend on the presence of both X chromosomes even though one has undergone random inactivation (Lyon, 1961) and is visible only as a small mass of chromatin within the cell nucleus (X-chromatin or Barr body). Clinical studies on patients with different types of Turner's syndrome indicate that genes on both the long and the short arms of the X chromosome are necessary for completely normal ovarian development.

Fertilization of an ovum by a Y-bearing sperm results in a zygote with a 46 XY karyotype which leads to subsequent development of testes and in turn to differentiation and development of male internal and external genitalia. The genes responsible for testicular differentiation are probably carried on the short arm of the Y chromosome but there is debate as to their exact mode of action. It now appears that they may not have a direct role, and there is growing evidence that production of H-Y antigen plays an important part in the process (Wachtel *et al.*, 1975). Sex reversal with the formation of testes in individuals who are H-Y positive and have apparently normal female karyotypes has been well documented in man and in several other species (Wachtel *et al.*, 1976) and may be due to abnormal activity of a testis-regulating gene carried on an autosome. Alternatively some of these cases may be explained by an undetectable translocation of genes from the short arm of a Y chromosome onto either an autosome or one of the X chromosomes.

Chromosome analysis

Chromosome analysis is usually carried out on peripheral lymphocytes incubated in the presence of phytohaemagglutinin to stimulate mitosis. Colchicine, which inhibits mitosis in metaphase, is added to the culture. The cells are ruptured by exposure to a hypotonic solution before they are fixed and stained to show the mitotic figures. Normally about 3 days incubation is required to obtain a reasonable harvest of cells in mitosis, but shorter times are employed if unstimulated bone marrow cells are used. Chromosome analysis can also be carried out on other cell lines such as fibroblasts grown in culture.

During the last 10 years great advances have been made in cytogenetics following the discovery of different staining techniques. Incubation of chromosomes with quinacrine shows multiple bands on fluorescence microscopy (Q banding). The long arm of the Y chromosome fluoresces particularly strongly. Further bands are obtained when the chromosomes are heated at 60° in saline and sodium citrate or treated with trypsin before staining (G banding). In general the Q and G bands correspond with one another. In R banding the results are complementary to Q and G banding. If the chromosomes are incubated with sodium hydroxide and stained with Giemsa solution another set of dark bands are obtained (C banding). Some of these bands may be related to the presence of two types of DNA in each chromosome, that is unique sequence DNA which carries genetic information and repetitious DNA which has no genetic role. During heating or trypsin incubation the repetitious DNA is annealed and thus protected against denaturation during subsequent fixation. As a result it can take up more stain than the denatured unique sequence DNA.

These techniques have allowed much clearer identification of individual chromosomes. They permit recognition of minor abnormalities such as small deletions and inversions which cannot be detected by conventional staining.

Buccal smear examination

Investigation of nuclear chromatin provides an alternative method for evaluating sex chromosome constitution. While the technique gives much less information than chromosome analysis it is relatively rapid and inexpensive because cell culture is not needed. The method originated from the observation that cells in the hypoglossal nucleus of the cat carry a small nuclear mass in females (Barr and Bertram, 1949) and the subsequent discovery that this nuclear chromatin is present in the tissues of other species including man. The nuclei of the cells lining the mouth show this chromatin mass very clearly–in normal girls and women it is seen in about 20 per cent of the cells–and buccal smear examination is widely used to evaluate the sex chromosome pattern.

Buccal smears are of relatively little value for evaluating subjects with complicated sex chromosomal anomalies such as mosaicism or structural changes. As noted above the chromatin represents an inactivated X chromosome and the technique is useful for identifying subjects with only one X chromosome, such as normal males and patients with nonmosaic Turner's syndrome or 45 X/46 XY mosaicism, in whom X-inactivation does not take place and who are chromatin-negative. Subjects with two X chromosomes, for instance normal females and patients with Klinefelter's syndrome, are chromatin-positive. Patients with the unusual condition of more than two X chromosomes, for example 49 XXXXY, have several chromatin masses, the number being one less than the X chromosome complement.

Cells from the buccal mucosa can also be stained with quinacrine to show the presence of a Y chromosome as a highly fluorescent dot within the nucleus. Unfortunately only the long arm of the Y chromosome fluoresces and the short arm which carries the testis-determining genes cannot be identified.

Developmental morphology

The gonads

The gonads are developed upon the urogenital ridges, which are longitudinal structures arising from the mesoderm of the intermediate cell mass and bulging into the coelomic cavity on either side of the root of the mesentery (*Figure 35.2*).

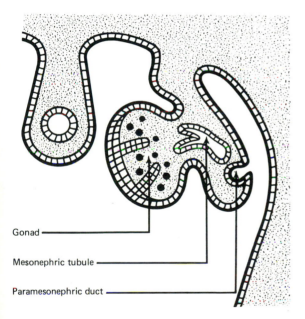

Gonad ——————

Mesonephric tubule ——————

Paramesonephric duct ——————

Figure 35.2. Diagrammatic cross-section of an 11 mm embryo showing the urogenital ridge with the developing gonad, the mesonephric tubule draining into the mesonephric (wolffian) duct and the paramesonephric (müllerian) duct invaginated from the surface.

The first differentiation in the ridges is the appearance of the pronephric and mesonephric tubules and of the wolffian duct which links the tubules and grows caudally to join the cloaca. On the medial aspect of the urogenital ridge

mesoblastic cells differentiate at the cranial extremity to form the adrenal cortical primordium, while in the middle section the cellular condensation that forms the gonadal blastema is evident in embryos of 7–12 mm. The cells that contribute to the formation of the gonad are the mesoblastic primitive coelomic cells, the mesenchymal cells derived from the interstitium of the urogenital ridge, and the primordial germ cells (Jirasek, 1977).

The last-named are of great interest and importance, and identifiable germ cells were recognized by Hertig, Rock and Adams (1956) in an unimplanted human embryo 4½ days old. Between 17–20 days they are found in the endoderm of the allantois and adjacent yolk sac and from this situation they migrate by amoeboid movement to the region of the urogenital ridge. Some are incorporated in the gonadal blastema and others remain extragenital.

The testis

The testis begins to differentiate from the gonadal primordium at 43–49 days (14–20 mm). The process is controlled by the masculinizing gene on the short arm of the Y chromosome. The blastema is divided by thin septa into testicular cords within which the germ cells are incorporated, having lost the pseudopodia associated with their migration. Peripherally these cords become separated from the surface epithelium and centrally they develop into rete cords which interconnect and ultimately join with adjacent mesonephric tubules. The amount of connective tissue increases both on the surface to form the tunica albuginea and around the seminiferous tubules.

At approximately 60 days (32–35 mm) Leydig cells appear and proliferate, reaching their maximum number at about 12 weeks after which they decline. This cellular activity is associated with the production of fetal androgens. The seminiferous tubules enlarge and become coiled. They contain primitive Sertoli cells and spermatogonia derived from the germ cells. Neither of these groups reaches maturity during fetal life, although there is evidence that the Sertoli cells produce antimüllerian hormone which is discussed below. The lumen of the testicular tubules appears during the second half of fetal life and the germ cells which remain on the surface of the testis until this time atrophy. The subsequent descent of the testis into the scrotum is discussed below.

The ovary

The ovary is differentiated somewhat later than the testicle at 45–55 days (18–25 mm). Although irregular epithelial cords are formed within the blastema, they do not separate from the surface and they connect centrally with the mesonephric tubules. In the cortical layer there is an intense proliferation of germ cells which become oogonia. Oocytes appear at 60–65 days and granulosa cells gradually begin to organize around the oocytes to form primordial follicles. At this early stage of the fetal ovary there is no difference between the fetus with a 46 XX complement and one with 45 X. However, the next phase is the formation of a complete layer of follicular cells which requires a double dose of the feminizing determinant on the short arm of the X chromosome so that in 45 X fetuses all the oocytes degenerate.

At birth the ovary exhibits many follicles with a multilayered granulosa, and large vesicular follicles are present at 2–3 weeks of age. These degenerate and disappear during the first 6 months of postnatal life. The child's ovary contains no vesicular but many primary or atretic follicles. Vesiculation reappears at puberty.

The gonadal ducts

The gonadal ducts are derived from the mesonephric and paramesonephric systems. The first to appear in the urogenital ridge is the pronephric duct. As the pronephros soon atrophies its duct is taken over by the mesonephric system and then called the wolffian duct. This grows caudally to reach the cloaca at the 4–5 mm stage. The paramesonephric or müllerian duct arises by invagination of the coelomic epithelium immediately lateral to and closely associated with the wolffian duct. It also grows caudally and then turns medially to cross the wolffian duct ventrally and fuse with its fellow from the opposite side. The fused tip finally reaches the urogenital sinus at 56–60

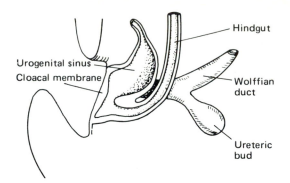

Figure 35.3. The urogenital sinus at 11 mm showing the completion of the urorectal septum, the intact cloacal membrane with the small genital tubercle and the broadening out of the terminal segment of the wolffian duct, which is being taken up into the urogenital sinus.

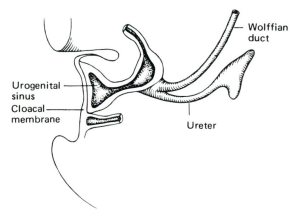

Figure 35.4. The urogenital sinus at 25 mm showing the disappearance of the cloacal membrane, the enlargement of the genital tubercle, the appearance of the fused caudal extremity of the müllerian duct, which now approaches the urogenital sinus, and the loop formation of the wolffian duct becoming separated from the ureteric opening.

days (30–35 mm) and opens between the orifices of the wolffian ducts.

In the male the mesonephric tubules which are alongside the developing gonad become connected to the rete testis to form the vasa efferentia and the wolffian duct is transformed into the epididymis, the vas deferens and the ejaculatory duct with a sacculation forming the seminal vesicle. This process is dependent upon the testicular output of fetal androgen. The male müllerian duct degenerates, at first in the region of the lower pole of the testis in 25–40 mm embryos. The atrophy progressively involves the upper and lower ends, while the extremities may remain cranially to form the appendix testis or hydatid of Morgagni and caudally to contribute to the utriculus masculinus. This degeneration results from the testicular production of anti-müllerian hormone.

In the female the mesonephric tubules which were attached to the developing ovary separate and fragment, occasionally persisting as an epoophoron or paraoophoron. The wolffian duct degenerates, although its caudal extremity may remain as Gartner's duct in the wall of the vagina. The müllerian ducts in the absence of a testicle grow and differentiate to form the fallopian tubes, the uterus and the upper vagina.

The vagina

Up to the 38 mm stage the development of the female urethra differs little from that of the male one. However, the urethral folds on either side of the phallic part of the urogenital sinus do not close and from this stage the sexes diverge. At the 60 mm stage the müllerian tubercle is flattened out and destroyed by two outgrowths of the urogenital sinus, that is the sinovaginal bulbs (Koff, 1933). The epithelium of the bulbs is stratified and the lumina are soon obliterated by the mass of cells. At the same time the tip of the uterovaginal canal (the fused müllerian ducts) is pushed back by the bulbs and becomes stratified and solid. The identity of the sinus and the müllerian derivatives is soon lost in the solid vaginal plate which undergoes rapid proliferation. Wells (1959) believed that the sinovaginal

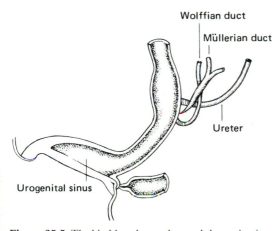

Figure 35.5. The bladder, the urethra and the vagina in a 100 mm female embryo. The urogenital sinus has widened out caudally and the vagina, formed partly from the müllerian duct and partly from the sinovaginal bulbs, has come to open into the vulva.

bulbs are merely the junction of two kinds of epithelium, namely that of the müllerian duct and that of the urogenital sinus.

At the 150 mm stage the cranial end is demarcated by the formation of anterior and posterior fornices while at the lower end the expanding vagina, regaining its cavity, pushes in the posterior wall of the urogenital sinus and extends caudally. Meanwhile the distal urethra becomes shorter and wider until the opening of the vagina is brought near to the surface in the shallow vestibule. The hymen is formed from the anterior paired elements derived from the urogenital sinus in the region of the original evagination of the sinovaginal bulbs and from a posterior median element that represents the compressed posterior wall of the sinus caudal to the opening of the vagina.

It appears that development of the lower end of the vagina occurs in any fetus lacking testicular androgens or with external genital tissues unresponsive to them. Thus in the testicular feminization syndrome the müllerian duct element seems to be suppressed by the testicular output of antimüllerian hormone but the vulva and the lower vagina appear to be normally feminine.

The external genitalia

The form of the external genitalia in the two sexes depends upon both the development of the phallic portion of the urogenital sinus and the growth of the genital tubercle. The latter is derived from the mesoderm that infiltrates between the primitive layers of the cloaca immediately caudal to the umbilical cord. In 10 mm embryos it may be evident in front of the definitive cloacal membrane with folds extending backwards. As this membrane is divided by the urorectal septum into an anterior urogenital portion and a posterior anal portion the anterior urethral folds and posterior anal folds are differentiated. During enlargement of the genital tubercle the pars phallica of the urogenital sinus extends up into it and at the 16–17 mm stage the membrane ruptures, laying the urogenital sinus wide open to the amniotic cavity.

From this stage until the embryo measures 35–40 mm (9 weeks) the appearance of the external genitalia is similar in both sexes. If either endogenous or exogenous androgens are circulating in a fetus with androgen-sensitive genital tissues the phallus continues to grow, the distance between the anus and the urogenital sinus increases, the urethral folds begin to fuse from behind forwards and the labioscrotal folds outside enlarge and fuse in the midline. The male urethra should be completely closed up to the tip of the phallus in fetuses of 90–120 mm (12–14 weeks). Defects before this period can lead to the development of hypospadias. After this period there is a simple growth in length and failure takes the form of micropenis.

Testicular descent

Although no fully satisfactory explanation of the mechanism of descent of the testicle has yet emerged, there have been many detailed descriptions of the process. The reader is referred particularly to Backhouse (1964) and Gier and Marion (1969).

In what is sometimes regarded as the first stage in descent the testis assumes a position inside the inguinal ring largely as a result of differential growth of the posterior abdominal wall structures. Thus in the fourth and fifth weeks of fetal life the cranial part of the mesonephric ridge is degenerating while caudally there is a band of condensed mesenchyme linking the mesonephros to the anterior abdominal wall. With the ascent of the kidney and the unrolling of the body curvature the tethering of this band ensures that the testis assumes a relatively lower position.

During the second stage the mesenchymal band becomes enlarged by infiltration with acid mucopolysaccharide and is called the gubernaculum. Proximally it is attached to the epididymis which has developed from the mesonephric duct and distally it penetrates the inguinal canal around which the abdominal muscles are forming and is anchored to the connective tissue of the scrotum. The peritoneum evaginates beyond the lower pole of the testis to form the processus vaginalis.

The third stage, that is true descent, takes place between 7 months of fetal life and 1 month after birth. The enlarging gubernaculum, the epididymis and the testis covered by the processus vaginalis pass down through the inguinal canal to reach the scrotum. Afterwards the gubernaculum atrophies, the inguinal canal tightens up and the processus vaginalis becomes obliterated.

It is commonly supposed that this process of descent is related to herniation resulting from increased intra-abdominal pressure. To some extent it seems to be under hormonal control since in rats premature descent can be induced by the injection of HCG or dihydrotestosterone (but not testosterone) and conversely inhibited by oestradiol which suppresses pituitary gonadotrophin release (Rajfer and Walsh, 1977). However, in most instances failure of descent appears to be related more closely to mechanical than to hormonal factors.

Endocrine control of genital differentiation

Males

Development of the male external genitalia with differentiation of the accessory ducts and suppression of the müllerian derivatives is completely dependent on the endocrine activity of the fetal testis. Using orchidectomy in fetal rabbits Jost (1953) demonstrated that two separate mechanisms were involved in these processes. Differentiation of the internal ducts and virilization of the external genitalia are brought about by secretion of testosterone by the fetal testis, while a second hormone is necessary for suppression of the müllerian ducts.

Proliferation of Leydig cells in the fetal testis is associated with a marked rise in the plasma testosterone level, which reaches a peak around the end of the first trimester (Siiteri and Wilson, 1974). Differentiation of the external genitalia is probably brought about by dihydrotestosterone, the active metabolite of testosterone, which is produced in the genital tissues by 5-alpha-reductase. The activity of this enzyme in the urogenital sinus increases rapidly during early fetal life, reaching a peak at about 12 weeks when fusion of the genital folds is taking place (Siiteri and Wilson, 1974). Testosterone secretion carries on after the end of the first trimester but its plasma levels fall progressively. This continued secretion of testosterone is probably necessary for further growth and development of the penis after closure of the urogenital sinus. Direct diffusion of testosterone itself down the wolffian ducts is thought to be responsible for their further evolution (Jost, 1953) and an ipsilateral testis is required for the development of the vas deferens.

Both the placenta and the fetal pituitary appear to play important roles in controlling Leydig cell activity (Kaplan and Grumbach, 1976). The initial proliferation of Leydig cells is probably controlled by placental gonadotrophin (HCG) which is present at high concentrations in the fetal circulation at the end of the first trimester and subsequently declines. Pituitary LH and FSH can be detected in the fetal circulation after about 80 days, and these gonadotrophins probably have a major role in regulating testosterone secretion during the latter half of fetal life.

Following the demonstration that the testis is directly responsible for regression of the müllerian ducts and that this effect is not mediated by testosterone (Jost, 1953), Josso defined several aspects of the secretion and the nature of antimüllerian hormone. By incubating müllerian ducts from fetal rats with fragments of testicular tissue she showed that the hormone is secreted by the fetal Sertoli cells and is probably a relatively small polypeptide (Josso, 1972; Blanchard and Josso, 1974). The müllerian structures are only sensitive to the hormone over a limited period of development. It is likely that antimüllerian hormone reaches the target tissue by direct diffusion and that an ipsilateral testis is necessary for involution of the müllerian ducts.

Females

Jost's (1953) demonstration that internal and external genital development follow a normal female pattern after early gonadectomy in fetal rabbits clearly indicates that normal female development is not dependent on the presence of an ovary. It is generally agreed that the ovaries have no significant endocrine role in female genital differentiation.

Postnatal development

Males

In males there is a period of Leydig cell activity soon after birth. Plasma testosterone levels rise to reach a peak at about 8 weeks and then decline over the next 2–4 months (Forest, Cathiard and Bertrand, 1973). The biological significance of this postnatal surge of testosterone secretion, which is mediated by pituitary LH, is still uncertain.

After early infancy Leydig cells are no longer seen and there is no further maturation of the germinal epithelium until the onset of puberty. At this time the testes increase in size, Leydig cells reappear in the interstitial tissues and the seminal tubules develop well defined lumina lined with mature Sertoli cells, spermatogonia, spermatocytes and spermatozoa.

PUBERTY

The first signs of male adolescent development are a slight increase in testicular size with some rugosity of the scrotum followed by the appearance of hair at the base of the penis which starts to enlarge. Standards for normal penile growth were published by Schonfield (1943). Deepening of the voice and occurrence of acne are not seen until puberty is well established, and growth of facial hair is relatively late. A detailed account of these changes and their staging was given by Tanner (1962). Transient gynaecomastia is common, particularly in the early stages of puberty, but is rarely severe enough to require treatment.

There is a wide variation in the age at which male puberty begins. In the UK the average is 11½ years, and while 95 per cent of boys start puberty between 9½–13½ years (Marshall and Tanner, 1970) a small proportion of normal boys show marked delay and may not begin puberty until 15–16 years. The adolescent growth spurt does not usually start in boys until puberty is fairly well advanced.

ENDOCRINE CHANGES

It is now generally accepted that the adrenal glands and the testes both play important roles in the initiation of puberty. During the latter part of the first decade there is a progressive rise in adrenal androgen secretion, particularly of dehydroepiandrosterone and its sulphate (Hopper and Yen, 1975), and there has been speculation that this may be mediated by a specific anterior pituitary hormone. Increased secretion of the pituitary gonadotrophins LH and FSH only becomes evident when the first clinical signs of puberty appear. Serum LH values increase progressively as puberty advances and episodic LH secretion occurs, especially during sleep (Boyar *et al.*, 1974). Plasma testosterone levels rise progressively throughout puberty and there is also a slight rise in plasma oestrogen concentrations (Lee and Migeon, 1975). The exact mechanism that leads to increased FSH and LH secretion is not clear, although it has been suggested that the earlier secretion of adrenal androgens may modulate the feedback mechanisms controlling gonadotrophin secretion.

There seems to be a complex interplay between LH and FSH in bringing about adolescent development. For example there is evidence that the response of Leydig cells to LH is increased by previous exposure to FSH (Sizonenko, Cuendet and Paunier, 1973). Both LH and FSH are needed for normal spermatogenesis and the effect of LH is probably mediated by testosterone which is carried to the germinal epithelium by a specific binding protein, namely androgen-binding protein, in seminal plasma (Ritzen *et al.*, 1973).

Females

At birth numerous secondary and tertiary follicles are found in the ovary but these degenerate in early infancy and only primary follicles are found before puberty. At adolescence follicles at different stages of development and corpora lutea become evident.

PUBERTY
The first signs of puberty in girls are usually the appearance of pubic hair and the onset of breast enlargement. In a small proportion of normal girls pubic hair develops several years before other signs of puberty (premature adrenarche), probably as a result of adrenal androgen secretion. Premature isolated breast development also occurs in some girls (premature thelarche) and is often associated with a follicular cyst of the ovary.

As in males there is wide individual variation in the age at which puberty starts. In the UK 95 per cent of girls start adolescent development between the ages of 8½–13 (Marshall and Tanner, 1969). In contrast to males the phase of rapid adolescent growth occurs in early puberty and the peak height velocity correlates well with the onset of breast development. Menstruation does not usually occur until breast development is fairly well advanced, although in a small

proportion of girls menstrual bleeding is the first sign of puberty. The average age of menarche in the UK is 13½ years and the great majority of girls begin menstruation before the age of 15½ (Marshall and Tanner, 1969). Initial menstrual irregularity is common and is probably due to absence of ovulation with subsequent failure of progesterone secretion by a corpus luteum.

ENDOCRINE CHANGES
As in boys increased secretion of adrenal androgens occurs around the age of 7 years. Increased gonadotrophin secretion cannot usually be detected until the signs of early puberty appear. While development progresses there is a gradual rise in serum LH and FSH levels and the plasma concentrations of oestrone and oestradiol also increase (Winter and Faiman, 1973). When menstruation is established there is a regular cyclical pattern of gonadotrophin secretion with peak serum LH and FSH values at the time of ovulation (Winter, 1973). Plasma oestradiol levels also show cyclical changes with peaks immediately before ovulation. Plasma progesterone concentrations rise after ovulation with the formation of a corpus luteum, and declining oestradiol and progesterone concentrations at the end of each cycle lead to shedding of the endometrium and menstruation.

The exact mechanism controlling the onset of female puberty is not known. It has been suggested that body weight may be an important regulating factor (Frisch and Revelle, 1971). While this is by no means universally accepted, anorexia nervosa and strict dieting are often associated with amenorrhoea.

Clinical disorders of sexual development

Normal genital development depends on a complex interplay of genetic, morphogenic and endocrine factors. The sex chromosomes determine whether the indifferent gonad develops into a testis or an ovary. The anlages for both the male and female genital tracts are laid down during early embryogenesis, and in males these are modified by the endocrine actions of the testes while in females the ovaries have no direct role to play in genital differentiation. Errors at each of these steps can lead to abnormal genital development. Gonadal differentiation may be disturbed, often as a result of a chromosomal anomaly, and development of the primitive genital tracts may be faulty due to a mistake in early embryogenesis. Failure of secretion of testosterone by the fetal testes or impaired tissue sensitivity to the hormone results in incomplete virilization of the external genitalia and the internal ducts. Persistent müllerian structures in males are probably caused by impaired secretion or action of testicular antimüllerian hormone.

Sex chromosomal abnormalities

An abnormality in the number of sex chromosomes is relatively common, particularly for the karyotypes 47 XXY and 47 XYY (Ratcliffe *et al.*, 1970). Such abnormal distribution of the sex chromosomes can occur in either meiosis or mitosis as a result of nondysjunction or anaphase lag. In nondysjunction both sex chromosomes pass to one daughter cell and if this occurs during meiosis all the cells in the resulting zygote have an abnormal sex chromosome complement. Nondysjunction during mitosis results in two or more cell lines with different sex chromosome complements (*Figure 35.6*). The term mosaicism is used to describe this pattern as distinct from chimerism where two cell lines are derived from fusion of two different zygotes. Anaphase lag, which is frequently associated with a structural chromosomal anomaly, leads to loss of a sex chromosome from one of the daughter cells during meiosis or mitosis.

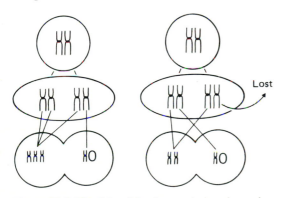

Figure 35.6. Mosaicism following nondysjunction and anaphase lag during mitosis.

Loss of a sex chromosome to give a 45 X karyotype (Turner's syndrome) or acquisition of an extra sex chromosome (for instance 47 XXY or Klinefelter's syndrome and 47 XYY) does not interfere with the early stages of gonadal differentiation and is not associated with genital ambiguity. Similarly, unusual karyotypes such as 47 XXX or 49 XXXXY do not interfere with normal genital development. However, sex chromosomal mosaicism or chimerism usually has marked effects on gonadal differentiation. For example 45 X/46 XY mosaicism leads to the syndrome of mixed gonadal dysgenesis in which a fibrous streak gonad is often associated with a

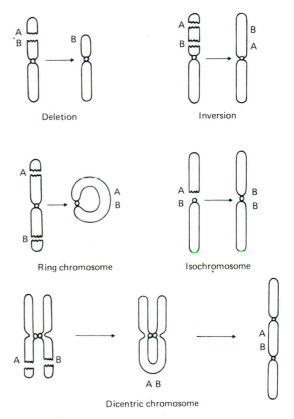

Figure 35.7. Structural abnormalities of the sex chromosome.

contralateral testis, and 46 XX/46 XY chimerism may result in true hermaphroditism. In both these conditions external genital development is almost always abnormal.

A number of structural abnormalities of the sex chromosomes have been described (*Figure 35.7*). In deletions genetic material is lost from either the short arm (p) or the long arm (q).

Breakages at the tips of the long and short arms may lead to refusion with formation of a ring chromosome. Following chromosomal breakage genetic material may be exchanged between chromosomes in a translocation or the order of genes may become altered in an inversion. Isochromosomes have two identical arms derived from either the long arm or the short arm by longitudinal division at the centromere. Dicentric chromosomes have two centromeres and probably arise as a result of fusion of the tips of two homologous chromosomes or daughter chromatids.

These structural abnormalities are often associated with loss of the abnormal chromosome in some cell lines as a result of anaphase lag. They usually lead to the mosaic forms of Turner's syndrome with fibrous streak gonads and normal female external genitalia.

Abnormal gonadal differentiation

Complete failure of gonadal differentiation is not associated with genital ambiguity and produces an entirely female phenotype. This is pure gonadal dysgenesis. Failure of testicular development after an initially normal phase of differentiation with closure of the urogenital sinus and inhibition of the müllerian ducts results in the syndrome of micropenis and rudimentary testes. This is related to failure of testosterone secretion during the last two thirds of gestation and also occurs with fetal gonadotrophin deficiency.

Inappropriate gonadal differentiation, for example the formation of testes in subjects with a female karyotype (XX males) does not usually lead to abnormal genital development. However, hermaphroditism with the formation of both testicular and ovarian tissue is almost always associated with genital ambiguity. The exact cause of hermaphroditism, which is most often associated with a normal 46 XX karyotype, is largely unknown.

Errors in morphogenesis

A number of uncommon but fairly well defined genital abnormalities appear to be the results of errors in morphogenesis of the internal genital ducts or the formation of the urogenital sinus. For example unilateral absence of both the testis and the kidney is well recognized and presumably arises as a result of failure of differentiation of the urogenital ridge. Lack of fusion of the caudal parts of the müllerian ducts leads to absence of the upper vagina and the uterus (Rokitansky anomaly) and less marked errors in morphogenesis cause formation of a duplex or bicornuate uterus or absence of a fallopian tube. These anomalies may also be associated with renal and ureteric malformations. Abnormal differentiation of the cloaca probably accounts for the rare syndrome of female pseudohermaphroditism with rectal agenesis and bladder anomalies. While the causes of these malformations are not known they are probably not due to endocrine factors.

Abnormal androgen metabolism

Failure of normal genital masculinization in the presence of apparently normally developed testes (male pseudohermaphroditism) is thought to be most commonly due to insensitivity of the urogenital tissues to fetal androgens. It can also be caused by a number of enzyme defects that interfere with testosterone biosynthesis. Complete tissue insensitivity, which is considered to be caused usually by absence of intracellular androgen receptors in the genital tissues (Keenan *et al.*, 1974), results in the formation of entirely female external genitalia with a short vagina. The cervix, the uterus and the fallopian tubes are absent, indicating that the secretion of antimüllerian hormone by the testes is normal in this syndrome of complete testicular feminization. In many male pseudohermaphrodites there is some masculinization of the external genitalia and a variable degree of virilization takes place at puberty. Impaired sensitivity of the genital tissues to androgens or delayed maturation of the enzyme 5-alpha-reductase in the fetal tissues have been proposed as possible causes of these syndromes of incomplete testicular feminization.

Masculinization of the female fetus generally occurs as a result of secretion of adrenal androgens in congenital adrenal hyperplasia. However, other causes of female pseudoharmaphroditism have been well documented, for example administration of androgenic hormones during pregnancy (Wilkins *et al.*, 1958) and androgen secretion by a maternal tumour (Verhoeven *et al.*, 1973).

References

Backhouse, K.M. (1964) The gubernaculum testis Hunteri: testicular descent and maldescent. *Annals of the Royal College of Surgeons of England*, **35**, 15

Barr, M.L. and Bertram, E.G. (1949) A morphological distinction between neurones of the male and female, and the behaviour of the nucleolar satellite during accelerated nucleo-protein synthesis. *Nature*, **163**, 676

Blanchard, M.-G., and Josso, N. (1974) Source of anti-Müllerian hormone synthesised by the fetal testis. *Paediatric Research*, **8**, 968

Boyar, R.M., Rosenfeld, R.S., Kapen, S., Finkelstein, J.W., Roffwarg, H.P., Weitzman, E.D. and Hellman, L. (1974) Simultaneous augmented secretion of luteinizing hormone and testosterone during sleep. *Journal of Clinical Investigation*, **54**, 609

Forest, M.G., Cathiard, A.M. and Bertrand, J.A. (1973) Evidence of testicular activity in early infancy. *Journal of Clinical Endocrinology and Metabolism*, **37**, 148

Frisch, R.E. and Revelle, R. (1971) Height and weight at menarche and a hypothesis of menarche. *Archives of Disease in Childhood*, **46**, 695

Gier, H.T. and Marion G.B. (1969) Development of mammalian testes and genital ducts. *Reproductive Biology*, **1**, 1

Hertig, A.T., Rock, J. and Adams, E.G. (1956) A description of 34 human ova within the first 17 days of development. *American Journal of Anatomy*, **98**, 435

Hopper, B.R. and Yen, S.S.C. (1975) Circulating concentrations of dehydroepiandrosterone and dehydroepiandrostone sulphate during pregnancy. *Journal of Clinical Endocrinology and Metabolism*, **40**, 458

Jirasek, J.E. (1977) Morphogenesis and malformation of the genital system. *In* Birth Defects Original Article Series, Vol. 13, No. 2 (edited by Blandau, R.J. and Bergsma, D.). Liss, New York. p.13

Josso, N. (1972) Permeability of membranes to the Müllerian-inhibiting substance synthetized by the human fetal testis in vitro: a clue to its biochemical nature. *Journal of Clinical Endocrinology and Metabolism*, **34**, 265

Jost, A. (1953) Problems of fetal endocrinology: the gonadal and hypophyseal hormones. *Recent Progress in Hormone Research*, **8**, 379

Kaplan, S.L. and Grumbach, M.J. (1976) The ontogenesis of human fetal hormones: luteinizing hormone (LH) and follicle-stimulating hormone (FSH). *Acta Endocrinologica*, **81**, 808

Keenan, B.S., Meyer, W.J., Hadjian, A.J., Jones, H.W. and Migeon, C.J. (1974) Syndrome of androgen insensitivity in man: absence of 5α-dihydrotestosterone binding protein in skin fibroblasts. *Journal of Clinical Endocrinology and Metabolism*, **38**, 1143

Koff, A.K. (1933) Development of the vagina in the human fetus. *Contributions to Embryology of the Carnegie Institute*, **24**, 59

Lee, P.A. and Migeon, C.J. (1975) Puberty in boys: correlation of plasma levels of gonadotrophins, androgens, estrogens and progestins. *Journal of Clinical Endocrinology and Metabolism*, **41**, 556

Lyon, M.F. (1961) Gene action in the X-chromosome of the mouse (Mus musulus L). *Nature*, **190**, 372

Marshall, W.A. and Tanner, J.M. (1969) Variation in pattern of pubertal changes in girls. *Archives of Disease in Childhood*, **44**, 291

Marshall, W.A. and Tanner, J.M. (1970) Variation in pattern of pubertal changes in boys. *Archives of Disease in Childhood*, **45**, 13

Rajfer, J. and Walsh, P.C. (1977) Morphogenesis and malformation of the genital system. *In* Birth Defects Original Article Series, Vol. 13, No. 2 (edited by Blandau, R.J. and Bergsma, D.). Liss, New York. p.107

Ratcliffe, S.G., Stewart, A.L., Melville, M.M., Jacobs, P.A. and Keay, A.J. (1970) Chromosome studies in 3500 newborn males. *Lancet*, i, 121

Ritzen, E.M., Dobbins, M.C., Tindall, D.J., French, F.S. and Nayfen, S.N. (1973) Characteristics of an androgen-binding protein (ABP) in rat testis and epididymis. *Steroids*, **21**, 593

Schonfield, W.A. (1943) Primary and secondary sexual characteristics. *American Journal of Diseases of Children*, **65**, 535

Siiteri, P.K. and Wilson, J.D. (1974) Testosterone formation and metabolism during male sexual differentiation in the human embryo. *Journal of Clinical Endocrinology and Metabolism*, **38**, 113

Singh, R.P. and Carr, D.H. (1966) The anatomy and histology of XO human embryos and fetuses. *Anatomical Record*, **155**, 369

Sizonenko, P.C., Cuendet, A. and Paunier, L. (1973) FSH: Evidence for its mediating role in testosterone secretion in cryptorchidism. *Journal of Clinical Endocrinology and Metabolism*, **37**, 68

Tanner, J.M. (1962) Growth at adolescence, 2nd edn. Blackwell Scientific Publications, Oxford

Verhoeven, A.T.M., Mostbloom, J.L., Van Lousden, H.A.I.M. and Van der Velden, W.H.M. (1973) Virilization in pregnancy co-existing with an ovarian mucinous cystadenoma: a case report and review of virilising ovarian tumours in pregnancy. *Obstetric and Gynecological Survey*, **28**, 597

Wachtel, S.S., Ohno, S., Koo, G.C. and Boyse, E.A. (1975) Possible role for H-Y antigen in the primary determination of sex. *Nature*, **257**, 235

Wachtel, S.S., Koo, G.C., Breg, W.R., Thaler, H.T., Dillard, G.M., Rosenthal, I.M., Dosik, H., Gerald, P.S., Saenger, P., New, M.I., Lieber, E. and Miller, O.J. (1976) Serologic detection of a Y-linked gene in XX males and XX true hermaphrodites. *New England Journal of Medicine*, **295**, 750

Wells, L.J. (1959) Embryology and anatomy of the vagina. *Annals of the New York Academy of Science*, **83**, 80

Wilkins, L., Jones, H., Holman, G.H. and Stempfel, R.S. (1958) Masculinization of the female fetus associated with administration of oral and IM progestins during gestation: non-adrenal female pseudohermaphroditism. *Journal of Clinical Endocrinology and Metabolism*, **18**, 559

Winter, J.S.D. (1973) The development of cyclic pituitary gonadal function in adolescence. *Journal of Clinical Endocrinology and Metabolism*, **37**, 714

Winter, J.S.D. and Faiman, C. (1973) Pituitary gonadal relationships in female children and adolescents. *Paediatric Research*, **7**, 948

36 Abnormalities of the Penis

J.H. Johnston

Phimosis

Phimosis is the condition in which the prepuce cannot be retracted completely behind the glans penis. In the newborn this is a normal state of affairs because of adhesions between the prepuce and the glans. These disappear spontaneously or with a little digital assistance during the second to fourth years of life and the foreskin then becomes retractable. While the child is in napkins the foreskin protects the glans and the urethral meatus from ammoniacal ulceration and for this reason circumcision in the newborn is inadvisable as well as unnecessary. In older boys phimosis develops as a result of scarring and narrowing of the preputial orifice, presumably due to previous ammoniacal excoriation or to splitting of the skin during attempts at forcible retraction. Histological examination of the foreskin shows changes resembling those of balanitis xerotica obliterans but whether these are cause or effect remains uncertain. The stenotic orifice produces ballooning of the foreskin with pain and difficulty in micturition. Circumcision is indicated.

An argument often advanced in favour of routine circumcision in infancy is that carcinoma of the penis is almost (not entirely) unknown in the circumcised while phimosis exists in 40–60 per cent of men with carcinoma (Blandy, 1976). Smegma has been considered to be carcinogenic although there is no experimental proof that this is so. In most cases the phimosis in men with penile cancer appears to be acquired and due to lack of personal hygiene rather than

persistence of the condition since childhood. Carcinoma of the cervix is rare in Jewish women and this has been attributed to the practice of routine male circumcision. Other factors may be concerned, as indicated by the high incidence of cervical neoplasia in Abyssinia where neonatal circumcision is also routine (Leitch, 1970). Aitken-Swan and Baird (1965) showed that there is no difference in the incidence of carcinoma of the cervix in wives of circumcised and uncircumcised men.

Agenesis of the penis

Penile agenesis is the result of absent or incomplete development of the genital tubercle. As a rule the scrotum and the testes are normally formed. The urethra generally opens on the perineum or at or just within the anus and less often on the anterior aspect of the scrotum or above the pubis. In most cases the sex chromosomes are XY but in two examples reported by Sonderdahl, Brosman and Goodwin (1972) there was XX/XXY mosaicism. Other abnormalities involving the upper urinary tract or the rectum and the anus often coexist.

Assignation to the female sex is necessary. Fixation of the median raphe of the scrotum to the underlying fascia produces the appearance of labia. Orchidectomy is needed but its timing is debatable. It may be considered preferable to retain the testes until the child is just prepubertal in order to maintain the normal endocrine relationships of childhood. At the age of puberty oestrogen therapy is instituted (see Micropenis, below). Later vaginoplasty is required, using scrotal skin to line a cavity fashioned anterior to the rectum.

Penile duplication

Two widely separated rudimentary penes each consisting of only one corpus cavernosum with a glans and each epispadiac or without a recognizable urethra are seen with exstrophy of the cloaca. Less severe degrees of penile duplication occur infrequently in association with bladder exstrophy.

Even in the absence of overt exstrophy pubic diastasis is commonly present in cases of double penis and the abnormality is attributed to failure of fusion of the originally paired genital tubercles. Various degrees of the anomaly exist, ranging from partial duplication of the glans to two entirely discrete organs. Complete duplication of the bladder may be present with each hemibladder opening into a separate urethra. Often the two penes are rotated or unequally developed. One or both urethras may be epispadiac or hypospadiac, or one penis may be without a urethra. A bifid scrotum and undescended testes often coexist and especially with the more severe forms of duplication there are often other anomalies such as imperforate anus, colonic duplication, spina bifida and upper urinary tract lesions (Johnson, Carlton and Powell, 1974).

Management of duplex penis depends on the local anatomy, the degree of urinary control that exists and the presence of any abnormalities elsewhere. As a rule the more deformed penis is amputated. In survivors of cloacal exstrophy it may be possible by partially detaching the penile crura from the separated pubes to lengthen each hemipenis sufficiently to allow them to be brought into apposition and skin-grafted to produce an acceptable single organ (*see Figure 25.16*).

Penile cysts and sinuses

In the great majority of boys referred to hospital with the presumptive diagnosis of penile cyst the lesion proves to be a collection of smegma under the prepuce. However, true penile cysts of various types do occur albeit infrequently. With all varieties excision of the cyst presents no difficulties.

Dermoid cysts are the result of implantation of squamous cell rests during closure of the urethral folds and are seen mainly along the line of the penile raphe and less often in the prepuce. Rarely a dermoid is found on the dorsum of the penis. Infection may occur and lead to a sinus discharging sebaceous material.

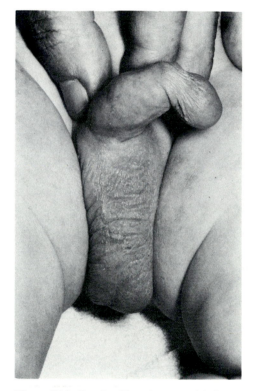

Figure 36.1. Cyst lined by columnar epithelium in the prepuce.

Mucosal subcutaneous cysts lined by columnar epithelium are seen on the ventrum of the penile shaft, the frenular region or the prepuce (*Figure 36.1*). They are believed to be formed from ectopic sequestrated portions of urethral mucosa (Cole and Helwig, 1976).

A parameatal urethral cyst is usually obvious at birth. It is sited on the lateral margin of the urethral meatus, lined by columnar epithelium and filled with clear or cloudy fluid, and is probably the result of obstruction of a parameatal duct.

Buried, concealed or webbed penis, and penile torsion

In obese boys the penis often appears extremely short because it is buried in fat deposits in front of the pubis. Treatment should be directed towards the obesity.

Concealed penis is a congenital anomaly in which the penile skin is not attached normally to the shaft so that on inspection the organ may appear to be entirely absent. When the skin is drawn back it is seen that the penis is of normal size. Phimosis may coexist. The penis itself is normally formed but a similar abnormality of the penile skin can occur with epispadias (*see Figure 25.5*). An improved appearance can be produced by surgical fixation of the skin to the fascia over the pubis and to the base of the penile ventrum (Johnston, 1977).

With webbed penis the scrotal skin extends as a thin fold onto the penile ventrum (*Figure 36.3*).

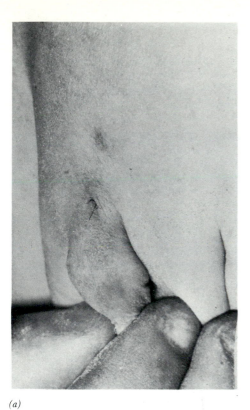

(a)

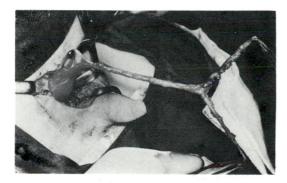

(b)

Figure 36.2. Penile pilonidal sinus in a 3-year-old boy. *(a)* Hair protruding from sinus at base of penis and punctum over pubis. *(b)* Branched tract extending to bladder apex and skin punctum dissected out.

Penile pilonidal sinus is a rare anomaly. In the 3-year-old boy shown in *Figure 36.2* there was a hair-bearing sinus opening at the base of the penile dorsum and a red skin punctum over the pubis. Dissection revealed a long tract that extended from the sinus orifice to the apex of the bladder with a secondary branch going to the skin punctum.

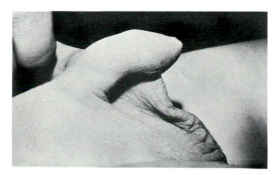

Figure 36.3. Webbed penis.

Although the condition causes no problems during childhood, an extensive penile attachment can cause sexual difficulties in adult life. Treatment consists of simple division and suture of the skin fold. On occasions a broader tongue of scrotum is attached to the penile ventrum in boys with hypospadias. After the scrotum is freed from the penis the raw surface can be covered by a mobilized skin flap derived from the dorsal prepuce (*Figure 36.4*).

Some degree of torsion of the penis around its long axis is commonly seen in association with hypospadias. It is due to anomalous skin attachments and not to any abnormality of the penis itself. Usually a shortened raphe lies on the right lateral aspect of the penis and the organ is rotated so that its ventral surface faces to the

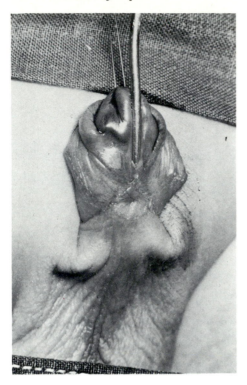

(a)

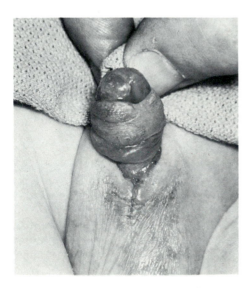

(b)

Figure 36.4. Tongue of scrotum extending to the penile ventrum and causing chordee in a boy with coronal hypospadias. *(a)* Before surgery. *(b)* Following freeing of the scrotum from the penis and utilization of the mobilized dorsal prepuce to cover the raw surface.

patient's left (*Figure 36.5*). Minor degrees of torsion can often be corrected by slight modifications during hypospadias repair. When the rotation reaches 90 degrees the condition needs surgery on its own account. An incision around the base of the penis divides the tissues down to

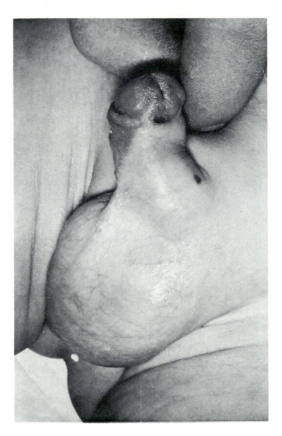

Figure 36.5. Torsion of the penis in a boy with coronal hypospadias. The penis is rotated so that its ventral surface faces left and there is a short raphe on the right of the shaft.

the penile shaft. With the penis rotated into correct alignment the skin is resutured. It is generally possible to release lesser degrees of skin chordee by making the encircling incision include part of the scrotal skin and incorporating this into the skin of the penis.

Micropenis

A short penis is a feature of epispadias with or without associated bladder exstrophy and an undersized organ also occurs with severe degrees of hypospadias, especially when there are underlying endocrinological disorders or chromosomal anomalies. The term micropenis is applicable only to an abnormally short, slender and normally formed penis occurring as a congenital abnormality in a genetic male with a normal wolffian system and without persisting müllerian derivatives.

Aetiology

Penile morphogenesis and subsequent growth during prenatal life are both hormone dependent. During the formative period up to the 14th week the testes are stimulated to secrete androgen by gonadotrophic hormone derived from the placenta. In later fetal life growth of the penis is dependent upon gonadotrophin from the fetal pituitary influencing the testes. Micropenis is the result of a disturbance during the latter period. There are two possible pathogenetic lesions, namely secondary and primary testicular insufficiency.

Secondary testicular failure occurs as a result of disorders of the hypothalamic-pituitary axis. Micropenis and testicular hypoplasia (often with undescended testes) are therefore seen with such lesions as anencephaly, pituitary agenesis, Kallmann's syndrome (Kallmann, Schoenfeld and Barrera, 1944), Noonan's (1968) syndrome, Prader-Willi syndrome (Prader, Labhart and Willi, 1956) and so on. Even in the absence of such gross and usually obvious associated developmental abnormalities Allen (1978) and Walsh *et al.* (1978) have shown that boys with micropenis may have evidence of hypogonadotrophic hypogonadism as indicated by low serum levels of testosterone, LH and FSH. The testes are small and often undescended or impalpable, and biopsies demonstrate Sertoli cells but no germinal elements and only occasional Leydig's cells. A family history of the disorder is frequently obtained.

Primary testicular insufficiency corresponds to the condition of bilateral rudimentary testes, which is a lesion of sporadic occurrence described by Bergada *et al.* (1962). The testes are impalpable clinically. Exploration reveals normal vasa deferentia and epididymides and very small scrotal testes that histologically show only a few scattered tubules containing germinal and

pre-Sertoli cells. In such patients the serum gonadotrophin levels are raised, but not to the degree seen in cases of anorchism, and there is no rise in serum testosterone concentration in response to gonadotrophic stimulation. The reason affected individuals do not suffer from defective penile morphogenesis is unclear. Walsh *et al.* (1978) suggested that less androgen may be required for penile differentiation than for later growth or that steroids of placental origin may provide a substrate for testosterone synthesis during the early phase of development.

Micropenis is also seen in boys with dwarfism due to isolated deficiency of pituitary growth hormone, indicating that this hormone is also necessary for penile growth. Suppression or inhibition of the fetal testis results from the administration of progesterone to the mother during the first trimester of pregnancy and this may be responsible for micropenis in some cases (Smith, 1977). There has been no reported instance in which micropenis was due to a receptor organ failure.

Diagnosis

Since there are considerable variations in the size of the normal phallus at all ages the diagnosis that the organ is abnormally small is to some extent a matter of opinion, and on occasions it can be difficult to persuade parents with unduly high aspirations for their offspring that their boy's rather modest penis is within the range of normality. The various types of pseudo-micropenis, in particular the buried penis in fat boys and the concealed penis resulting from abnormal skin attachments, must be excluded. Feldman and Smith (1975) found that the stretched penile length in full-term newborn boys is 3.5 ± 0.7 cm and Schonfeld (1943) produced a graph showing the normal variations at different ages. Kogan and Williams (1977) diagnosed micropenis when there was extreme discrepancy between general body size and penile size. Even with a very minute phallus the urethra is of adequate calibre so that micturition is unobstructed and instrumentation, if needed, presents no difficulty.

In the absence of obvious hypothalamic-pituitary syndromes with other severe anomalies investigation of the child with micropenis should begin as soon as possible after birth. Chromosome studies are needed to confirm a 46 XY karyotype. Estimation of the serum LH, FSH and testosterone levels and of the response of the latter to HCG stimulation differentiates primary from secondary testicular deficiency. Receptor organ failure can be excluded by determining the response of preputial cells in tissue culture to hormonal stimulation or, more simply, by local application to the penis of 5 per cent testosterone cream three times daily as a therapeutic test significant local growth should be obvious within 2–3 weeks. The patient's mother or any other female applying the cream should wear a rubber glove or finger-stall since absorption of the hormone occurs in both directions.

Treatment

Penile growth may be obtained by the use of systemic testosterone. Harris (1979) employed testosterone oenanthate (Primotestin Depot). Initially 100 mg are given intramuscularly for four doses at intervals of 3 weeks. Further courses are administered throughout childhood. Alternatively 5 per cent testosterone cream can be applied locally. This method produces a rise in serum testosterone and it is clear that the effect of the hormone is systemic, following percutaneous absorption, and not merely local (Jacob, Kaplan and Gittes, 1975). Since the amount of hormone absorbed cannot be predicted intramuscular therapy is preferable because it allows a precise dosage regimen. The increase in penile size produced by treatment persists following its discontinuation, indicating that there has been tissue hyperplasia as well as hypertrophy (*Figure 36.6*; Smith, 1977). Bone growth and osseous maturation are accelerated but later recede to pretreatment levels. Similarly the development of pubic hair is transient.

While increase in penile size during boyhood is important psychologically, it appears likely that early hormonal treatment merely anticipates potential future growth and that in adult life the dimensions of the penis will still be below normal. However, Allen (1978) suggested that if

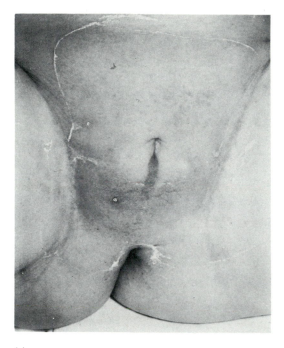

(a)

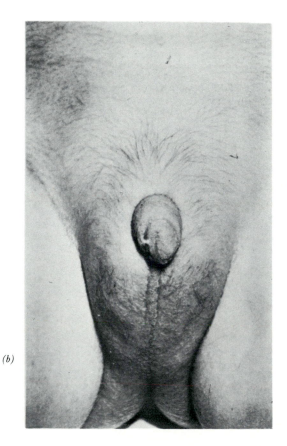

(b)

Figure 36.6. Microphallus. *(a)* Before treatment, aged 2 months. HCG stimulation demonstrated the absence of functioning testes. *(b)* Five months after a course of intramuscular testosterone cenanthate.

therapy is begun very early the boy may be able to recoup some of the growth lost as a result of lack of stimulation *in utero*. Kogan and Williams (1977) found that the prognosis for adequate growth is directly related to the degree of testicular development on clinical assessment. Significant lengthening of the penis can be obtained surgically by partially detaching the penile crura from the puboischial rami and shifting the organ ventrally (Johnston, 1974).

Sex reversal and rearing of the patient as a girl may be contemplated when assessment is completed in early infancy and the penis is severely underdeveloped. A female role may be preferable or unavoidable in the rare case in which there is inadequate response of the penis to hormonal stimulation; otherwise the decision to change the patient's sex, which may seem an easy option in infancy, should not be taken lightly. Unlike many cases of intersex the boy with micropenis does not possess a natural vagina. At the appropriate age the patient needs in addition to oestrogen therapy plastic surgery for construction of an artificial vagina. Even in the best hands this can lead to serious difficulties, disappointments, and physical and emotional stress. Finally the way in which individuals obtain gender identity is by no means completely understood. It has generally been considered that personal psychosexual identification during childhood and at maturity is not an inherent characteristic but is acquired and conforms to the sex of rearing (Money, Hampson and Hampson, 1955). However, Diamond (1965) suggested that, as in lower species, hormonal influences active prenatally may determine a male or female gender orientation and that this is already present when the child is born.

If the patient is brought up as a girl, oestrogen treatment begins at the age that appears appropriate for the individual. Harris (1979) uses daily Enavid containing norethynodrel 5 mg and mestranol 75 μg.

Hypospadias

Embryology and aetiology

At the fourth week of intrauterine life the site of the external genitalia is represented by the cloacal membrane. Lying anterolateral to this are two genital swellings which by the sixth week have fused to produce the midline genital tubercle. The cloacal membrane by then forms the longitudinally disposed urethral groove which is bounded laterally by the urethral folds and sited on the ventral aspect of the tubercle. Opinions differ as to the subsequent stages that lead to the formation of the penile urethra (Gray and Skandalakis, 1972). Johnson (1920) considered that it derived from simple closure from behind forwards of the urethral groove. Glenister (1958) described the sagitally disposed urethral plate, which is an extension into the phallus of endoderm from the cloacal (later urogenital) membrane. In the proximal part of the penis the plate is in contact ventrally with the roof of the urethral groove while more distally it abuts against the ventral ectoderm. Splitting of the urethral plate forms the secondary urethral groove which is continuous with the primary groove. Subsequent fusion of the urethral folds along the shaft of the penis produces the penile urethra. The glandular urethra is formed separately from an ectodermal plate that grows inwards from the tip of the penis. The plate splits on to the ventrum of the glans and later closes so that continuity is produced between the penile and glandular portions of the urethra.

Penile morphogenesis is complete by the 14th week of intrauterine life and requires the stimulus of dihydrotestosterone. This is derived from testosterone produced by the testes under the influence of placental gonadotrophin. Arrested development may be due to a block in the stimulus pathway, the effects on the embryo of inappropriate hormones such as progesterone administered to the mother, or a lack of response of the receptor tissues in the penis. Hypospadias is generally attributed to a failure of fusion of the urethral folds or of closure of the glandular plate. However, the fact that the penile raphe representing the line of union of the folds frequently diverges lateral to the urethral meatus indicates that the precise pathogenesis is probably more complex than a simple failure of tissue fusion.

Hypospadias is one of the commonest congenital anomalies with an incidence between one in 300 and one in 500 live births. Heredity is involved in its causation as shown by its frequent occurrence in brothers and other close male relatives. Twins are often identically affected but on occasions only one has the anomaly, indicating that exogenous as well as endogenous factors are concerned (Ross, Farmer and Lindsay, 1959).

Classification

The various degrees of hypospadias are designated according to the position of the urethral meatus. In each case the prepuce does not encircle the glans and is restricted to the dorsum. Glandular hypospadias where the meatus is on the ventral aspect of an almost normally formed glans is rare. The commonest form of the anomaly is coronal hypospadias in which the orifice lies just proximal to a groove of varying depth on the ventrum of the glans. As a rule there are one or two small blind pits distal to the meatus, and there may be a depression at the penile tip corresponding to the normal meatal position and sometimes leading to a deep sinus lying dorsal to the hypospadiac urethra. Coronal hypospadias and penile hypospadias, where the meatus lies between the base of the penis and the corona glandis, are generally associated with ventral chordee of varied severity. This is due to an insufficiency of skin distal to the meatus, adherence of the skin at this site to the penile tunica albuginea and a relative shortness of the urethra producing a bow-string effect. While the urethral meatus may appear to be stenotic on inspection, instrumentation frequently reveals that its dimensions are adequate.

Penoscrotal and perineal hypospadias are the most severe and least common degrees of the anomaly. There is generally marked chordee due to both inadequacy of skin on the penile ventrum and tight fibrous bands in the tunica albuginea which extend from the meatus to the glans. While the latter are often stated to represent an atrophic abortive corpus spongiosum occasionally a well formed corpus extends distal to the termination of the urethra. With these types of hypospadias the scrotum is bifid. Often the two hemiscrota extend to the dorsum of the base of the penis and they may fuse to surround the penis completely (*see Figure 40.1*). Rarely the scrotum lies entirely anterior to the penis.

Investigation

Any type of hypospadias of whatever severity can be regarded as indicating some degree of intersex. However, in the child with both testicles fully descended the more severe forms of pseudohermaphroditism can be confidently excluded, although enlargement of the prostatic utricle representing a rudimentary vagina is quite common, especially with penoscrotal or perineal hypospadias. If one or both testicles are impalpable, further investigations are needed to examine the possible existence of an intersex state (*see* Chapter 43). Hypospadias with cryptorchidism is a common feature in several multisystem anomaly syndromes. These generally have other obvious clinical manifestations as well as hypogonadism which indicate the diagnosis.

Opinions differ regarding the need for routine intravenous urography in hypospadiac patients with the object of detecting coexisting but silent upper urinary tract abnormalities. Fallon, Devine and Horton (1976) found 10 significant lesions requiring surgical intervention in 160 boys with hypospadias and recommended that all these patients should undergo pyelography. On the other hand Felton (1959) and McArdle and Leibowitz (1975) demonstrated no statistical difference between the incidence of urinary tract anomalies in the general population and in hypospadiac subjects. In the author's practice urography is carried out only in the presence of suggestive symptoms or urinary tract infection.

Treatment

The object of therapy is to construct a straight penis and a meatus as close as possible to the normal site which allows a normal forward-directed urine stream. Culp and McRoberts (1968) stated that it is the basic right of every hypospadiac patient to write his name legibly in the snow. The true result of surgical correction can only be assessed when, after puberty, the patient has outgrown such pastimes and is interested in the copulative and fertilizing capability of his organ as well as his voiding performance. In recent years parents and patients have become increasingly concerned with the cosmetic aspects of hypospadias correction and are anxious for the surgeon to construct a glans of normal appearance containing a glandular urethra with a terminal meatus. However, it is debatable whether such intraglandular urethral constructions are always advisable since it is this segment of the urethra that is most difficult to construct and most prone to complications, in particular stricture formation.

In general surgery should be completed by the age of 5 years. If a two-stage correction is planned, at least 6 months should elapse between operations. Rarely with coronal hypospadias the meatus is severely stenotic so that meatotomy is required in infancy. With any form of hypospadias it is important for the degree of chordee to be determined by examination of the erect penis. In early childhood it is generally possible to induce an erection, or at least sufficient penile turgidity, by compressing the penile crura against the bone and tickling the glans. Alternatively the parents may be asked to view the organ while the child is asleep, when an erection is commonly present. An artificial erection can be produced by applying a tourniquet around the base of the penis and infiltrating one corpus cavernosum or the glans with heparinized saline (Gittes and McLaughlin, 1974). This method is difficult with a very small penis and has the disadvantage that a haematoma or saline blister may be produced so that an interval may be needed between examination and operation. In some cases chordee appears to increase in severity as the child gets older because of discrepancy in growth between the corpora cavernosa and the ventral fibrotic tissue.

According to Culp and McRoberts (1968) some 50 techniques of chordee correction have been reported and over 150 reputedly original methods of urethral construction have been described. It is clear that the ideal procedure which produces maximum correction with the minimum of possible complications has yet to be devised. The following descriptions are of techniques of which the author has had personal experience. With all urethroplasty operations urinary diversion by perineal urethrostomy was carried out by means of a Foley catheter. When nonabsorbable skin sutures were used they were removed 10 days later under general anaesthesia.

Coronal hypospadias without chordee

In this condition the meatus is in an acceptable, although not a normal, position and generally urethroplasty is not needed. The urine stream is often deflected downwards by a skin flap just distal to the meatus which requires division. A broad-nosed artery forceps is applied to the flap for a few moments and the crushed tissue is then cut with fine-pointed scissors. The forward meatotomy must be generous since there is always a tendency for some degree of readherence of the cut edges. Removal of the redundant dorsal foreskin improves the appearance of the penis. If as sometimes occurs the glans is tilted ventrally, correction can be obtained by excising and resuturing a transverse ellipse of tunica albuginea just proximal to the glandular dorsum.

If the parents or the patient are anxious to have a glans of normal appearance with a terminal meatus the Mathieu operation (*see* Williams, 1977) can be employed when there is coronal or distal penile hypospadias without

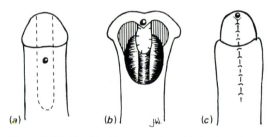

Figure 36.7. The Mathieu operation. *(a)* Outline of the incision on the penile shaft and the glans. *(b)* The skin strip proximal to the meatus is mobilized and sutured to the glandular strip and the glans is separated from the corporal extremities. *(c)* The glans is sutured over the neourethra and the skin incision is closed.

chordee (*Figure 35.7*). It is necessary to preserve carefully the blood supply of the skin flap raised from the penile ventrum, and the mobilization of the glans from the corporal extremities must be sufficiently free to avoid compression of the new glandular urethra when the two halves of the glans are sutured over it. Failure to take these precautions can result in devascularization and stricture of the glandular neourethra and proximal fistula formation.

Coronal and penile hypospadias with chordee

TWO-STAGE OPERATION

The first stage consists of chordee correction (*Figure 36.8*). As a rule there is little or no ventral tunical fibrosis requiring excision. Fixation of each half of the divided prepuce to the ventral aspect of the glans on each side (Crawford,

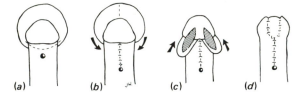

Figure 36.8. First-stage hypospadias correction by the Crawford technique. *(a)* Transverse skin incision between glans and meatus. *(b)* The skin is undermined and dissection dorsal to the urethra allows it to retract proximally. The transverse incision is closed longitudinally and the dorsal prepuce divided vertically. *(c)* Each hemiprepuce is swung to the ventral aspect. An ellipse of epithelium is excised on each side from the hemiprepuce and the glans. *(d)* The raw surfaces are sutured in apposition so that each hemiprepuce is attached to the glans.

1963) facilitates the construction of a terminally sited meatus at the second stage. Some 6 months later the Denis Browne (1949) buried skin strip technique of urethroplasty is performed (*Figure 36.9*). It is sometimes stated that when there is a shortage of skin this method has the advantage that the strip can be made relatively narrow and that the ultimate circumference of the neourethra is greater than the width of the strip. Some animal experimental work supports this contention (Browne, 1953) but clinical experience refutes it and if stenosis is to be avoided then the width of the skin strip must equal the intended urethral circumference. If there is insufficient skin, another technique must be employed. The dorsal relaxation incision should be

routine to ensure complete absence of tension on the suture line.

ONE-STAGE OPERATION
Hodgson (1970) evolved the principle of constructing a neourethra from an isolated skin island vascularized from below. The Asopa (Asopa *et al.*, 1971) modification has the advantages over the original technique that it allows formation of a longer neourethra and produces less bulk on the ventrum of the penis (*Figure 36.10*). The incision partly dividing the base of

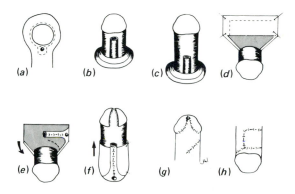

Figure 36.10. The Asopa technique of one-stage hypospadias correction. *(a)* A circumferential skin incision is made proximal to the corona glandis and surrounding the urethral meatus. *(b)* The skin is dissected off the penile shaft. *(c)* Dissection dorsal to the urethra lets it retract proximally and any fibrotic bands are excised. *(d)* The dorsal prepuce is held by skin hooks. Outline of the skin rectangle. *(e)* The skin rectangle is tubularized to form a neourethra. The two layers of surrounding prepuce are separated. Outline of the incision partly dividing the base of the preputial flap. *(f)* The preputial flap is brought around the right side to the ventral aspect of the penis. The neourethra is sutured to the original urethral meatus following spatulation of the latter. A ventral incision is made in the glans. *(g)* The flap is swung forward so that the neourethra lies on the penile ventrum and in the groove in the glans. The new urethral meatus is at the tip of the penis. *(h)* Dorsal view. Often complete skin closure on the dorsum is not possible but epithelialization occurs rapidly.

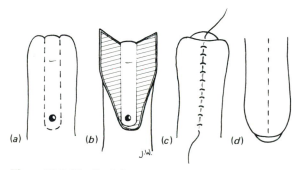

Figure 36.9. The Denis Browne buried skin strip technique of urethroplasty following the first-stage Crawford operation. *(a)* Outline of the skin strip. *(b)* The skin is mobilized on each side from the glans and the penile shaft. *(c)* Skin closure is by continuous subcuticular suture and interrupted skin sutures using 5/0 proline. *(d)* Outline of the dorsal relaxation incision.

the preputial flap must be made with caution. It must be sufficiently long to let the flap come to the penile ventrum without tension, otherwise torsion of the penis results. On the other hand it must be limited so as to avoid jeopardizing the blood supply to the flap. Spatulation of the original urethral orifice is necessary to avoid stricture formation at the site of anastomosis with the neourethra.

Penoscrotal and perineal hypospadias

These cases have severe chordee and a two-stage correction is always necessary. At the first stage (*Figure 36.11*) a modified Byars (1955) operation is employed. All fibrous bands on the penile ventrum must be excised and the urethra freed dorsally so that it can retract proximally. The two layers of the dorsal prepuce are separated to

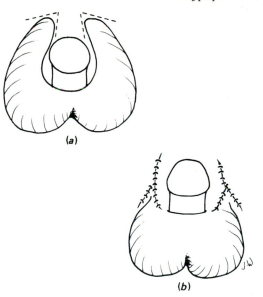

Figure 36.12. Ventral shifting of hemiscrota extending dorsal to the penis. *(a)* An inverted V incision is made on each side. *(b)* The hemiscrota are moved ventrally and the incisions closed as inverted Ys.

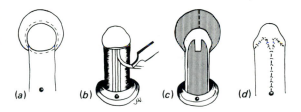

Figure 36.11. First-stage correction of penoscrotal hypospadias with chordee. *(a)* A circumferential incision is made proximal to the corona glandis. *(b)* The skin is reflected off the penis and dissection dorsal to the urethra lets it retract proximally. Fibrous bands in the tunica are excised. *(c)* A triangle of epithelium is excised on each side of the ventrum of the glans. The two layers of the prepuce are separated and the prepuce is divided longitudinally. *(d)* The preputial flaps are sutured on the ventrum.

provide, after longitudinal division, skin flaps sufficiently large to cover the denuded ventral surface.

When the two hemiscrota extend dorsal to the penis it is necessary to displace them ventrally before urethroplasty is performed (*Figure 36.12*). Urethroplasty can be carried out by the buried skin strip technique but the advent of minimally reactive polyglycolic acid sutures has encouraged tubularization of long skin strips. A dorsal relaxation incision does not release tension at the penoscrotal junction and when the suture line crosses this point additional relaxation incisions must be made on each side at the base of the penis (*Figure 36.13*).

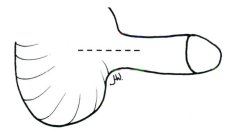

Figure 36.13. Outline of the additional relaxation incision when urethroplasty crosses the penoscrotal junction.

If after completion of chordee correction the urethral meatus is at the base of the penis and there is insufficient penile skin for primary urethroplasty, the Cecil (1952) two-stage urethroplasty can be employed (*Figure 36.14*). When the scrotum is bifid the penis can be attached to one hemiscrotum. After 3 months the penis is freed from the scrotum and the ventrum is covered with scrotal flaps.

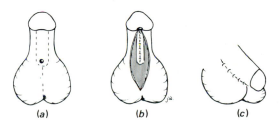

Figure 36.14. Cecil urethroplasty. *(a)* Outline of incision *(b)* The skin strip is tubularized and the skin undermined. *(c)* The raw surfaces on the penis and the scrotum are sutured in apposition.

Complications

The incidence of postoperative complications is minimized by careful surgical technique with complete haemostasis, avoidance of tension on suture lines and meticulous suturing. While surgical experience is clearly important in these respects, even in the hands of an expert there can be no guarantee that complications can be avoided in all cases.

Complications of first-stage chordee corrections are uncommon but devascularization of skin flaps may occur if the technique is faulty. After healing further chordee correction may then be needed.

Fistula

The commonest complication of urethroplasty is fistula formation. The lesion is usually obvious within 2 weeks of surgery and spontaneous healing is a rare occurrence. Although fistula may result from devascularization of flap edges as a result of excessive mobilization or of overuse of relaxation incisions, in the vast majority of cases it is due to tension on the suture line. It is mostly seen with the longer urethroplasties that cross the penoscrotal junction and the commonest site is at the base of the penis since it is at this point that complete elimination of tension is most difficult to achieve.

The incidence of postoperative fistula has varied in different series and with different techniques. Culp and McRoberts (1968) had seven (5.8 per cent) fistulas in 121 cases treated by the Cecil method. Browne (1949) in a personal series of his operation had eight (6.6 per cent) fistulas in 121 cases. Culp and McRoberts (1968) compiled several reported series of the Browne procedure and noted 44 (14 per cent) fistulas in 318 cases. Yarbrough and Johnston (1977) reported seven (7.3 per cent) fistulas in 96 Browne urethroplasties with an incidence of 4.3 per cent in distal penile repairs. It can be suspected that the incidence of fistula is considerably higher in unreported series.

An interval of some 6 months should elapse between urethroplasty and fistula repair. Calibration of the urethra is required to ensure the absence of distal urethral stricture. Urinary diversion by perineal urethrostomy is indicated.

In the case of a small fistula and ample surrounding skin the tract is circumcised and cut off flush with the neourethra. Next 5/0 polyglycolic acid sutures are used to approximate the tissues over the aperture. The skin around the fistula is freely mobilized and it is then usually possible to close the incision, if necessary by raising flaps, so that the skin suture line does not overlie the fistula site. Either polyglycolic acid, nylon or proline 5/0 sutures are satisfactory for skin closure. The edges must be carefully everted to ensure primary healing. A large fistula is best managed by a two-stage Cecil repair (*Figure 36.14*).

Urethral stricture

Diffuse stenosis of the neourethra occurs if the skin strip is too narrow. A localized stricture may develop if an area of devascularization results from inadvisable mobilization of the strip or misuse of diathermy. The former generally requires the neourethra to be laid open and reoperation performed later. When there is a very short stricture localized excision and reanastomosis may be possible.

With the Mathieu method stricture of the intraglandular urethra is a consequence of devascularization of the skin flap. Meatotomy may be sufficient. A longer stenosis must be laid open, in which case a further reconstruction may be needed. Following the use of the Asopa technique stricture can occur at the site of anastomosis between the urethra and the neourethra if spatulation of the former is omitted. The stricture can be excised with reanastomosis by restricted elevation of the original preputial flap on the ventrum of the penis.

Retraction of the meatus

Some degree of retraction and widening of the new urethral meatus causing spraying of the urine stream can occur with many techniques, especially if healing is short of perfection. The complication is most commonly seen with the Cecil procedure. As a rule its existence is obvious at the time of freeing the penis from the scrotum and the opportunity can then be taken to advance the meatus onto the glans.

Urethral sacculation

Saccular dilatation of the neourethra comes about if the skin strip forming it is too wide. Its commonest site is just distal to the original urethral orifice. This complication causes dribbling of urine after micturition. Surgical intervention is rarely needed and the patient is advised to massage the urethra empty at the conclusion of voiding.

Urethral hairs

This complication occurs when hair-bearing skin is used to fashion the neourethra. As a rule no ill effects result but a hair-ball or calculi may form if there is a saccule or diverticulum in which eddying occurs.

Late recurrence of chordee

A long neourethra constructed during childhood may fail to grow and elongate at the same rate as the penis so that after puberty chordee exists during erection. As with a congenitally short urethra correction requires the neourethra to be divided. The two extremities are mobilized to allow them to retract and the penis to be straightened and the resulting fistula is closed some 6 months later.

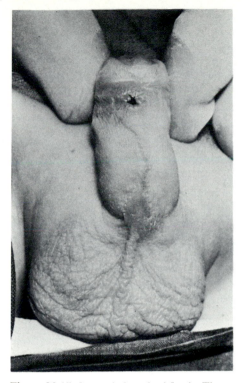

Figure 36.15. Congenital urethral fistula. The fistula is lateral to the penile raphe.

stage procedure. A larger congenital fistula in the penile urethra may be seen in boys with megalourethra (Johnston and Coimbra, 1970).

Congenital urethral fistula

A congenital fistula in the floor of an otherwise intact penile urethra is a rare occurrence. The fistula is sited lateral to the penile raphe and is not readily explicable on the basis of a localized failure of fusion of the urethral folds (*Figure 36.15*). Goldstein (1975) considered that it might be due to a failure of communication between the glandular and penile urethral components. Welch (1979) pointed out that the urethra beyond the fistula is congenitally defective and that simple fistula closure is likely to be followed by recurrence. It is preferable to lay open the distal urethra and to convert the lesion into a hypospadias which is then closed as a second-

Chordee without hypospadias, and congenital short urethra

In these patients the urethral meatus opens at or near its normal position on the glans and there is ventral penile chordee. As a rule the foreskin is restricted to the dorsum of the penis as in hypospadias and the two conditions are clearly embryologically related. From a study of fetuses and premature babies Kaplan and Lamm (1975) showed that chordee is a normal phase during prenatal penile growth and so its persistence represents an arrest of development. Because the formation of the urethral plate and the urethral folds (which are the precursors of the penile urethra) is under the influence of testosterone it has been suggested that when these structures are incapable of responding normally to the hormonal stimulus the urethra and the tissues ventral to it cannot keep pace with the growth of the penis (Goldstein, 1975). Similarly to hypospadias an adequate assessment of the degree of chordee present is possible only when the penis is examined during erection.

In the great majority of cases of chordee without hypospadias the penile urethra is of adequate length and the downwards flexion is caused mainly by insufficiency of skin on the ventrum of the organ. Correction can be obtained by bringing skin to this position utilizing the redundant dorsal prepuce. The technique is similar to the Byars procedure already described for the correction of chordee with hypospadias (*Figure 36.11*). An encircling incision is made just proximal to the glans and the skin is reflected proximally. Often the floor of the distal part of the urethra and the overlying skin are extremely thin and closely adherent to each other so that great care is needed in separating them to avoid opening the urethra. Some mobilization of the dorsal aspect of the urethra from the corpora cavernosa and excision of tunical fibrous bands may be needed to allow full correction. The two layers of the dorsal foreskin are separated and the unfolded preputial flap is divided longitudinally and each half is swung round to cover the denuded penile ventrum.

In a minority of examples of chordee without hypospadias the penile flexion is severe and the urethra is congenitally short. Techniques relying on mobilization of the urethra from the corpora cavernosa do not produce sufficient increase in urethral length and it is necessary to divide the shortened urethra, producing a temporary fistula, to allow the penis to straighten

(*Figure 36.16*). Six months later the fistula is closed by urethroplasty.

Lateral curvature of the penis

In this condition the penis appears normal when flaccid but on erection it bends laterally. There is no fibrosis or Peyronie plaque on the short side and the lesion is attributed to congenital asymmetrical development of the corpora cavernosa. Presentation during childhood is rare. Correction may be obtained by excision with resuture of vertical ellipses of tunica albuginea from the lateral aspect of the corpus spongiosum on the convex side (Gavrell, 1974). The effectiveness of surgery can be assessed during operation by inducing an artificial erection by infiltrating heparinized saline into the penis while a tourniquet is applied around the base.

References

Aitken-Swan, J. and Baird, D. (1965) Circumcision and cancer of the cervix. *British Journal of Cancer*, **19**, 217

Allen, T.D. (1978) Microphallus: clinical and endocrinological characteristics. *Journal of Urology*, **119**, 750

Asopa, H.S., Elhence, I.P., Atri, S.P. and Bansal, N.K. (1971). One stage correction of penile hypospadias using a foreskin tube. *International Surgery*, **55**, 435

Bergada, C., Cleveland, W.W., Jones, W.H. and Wilkins, L. (1962) Variants of embryonic testicular dysgenesis: bilateral anorchia and the syndrome of rudimentary testes. *Acta Endocrinologica*, **40**, 521

Blandy, J.P. (1976) Carcinoma of the penis. *In* Urology (edited by Blandy, J.P.). Blackwell, Oxford. p.1049

Browne, D. (1949) Hypospadias. *Postgraduate Medical Journal*, **25**, 367

Browne, D. (1953) A comparison of the Duplay and Denis Browne techniques for hypospadias operation. *Surgery*, **34**, 787

Byars, L.T. (1955) A technique for consistently satisfactory repair of hypospadias. *Surgery, Gynecology and Obstetrics*, **100**, 184

Cecil, A.B. (1952) Modern treatment of hypospadias. *Journal of Urology*, **67**, 1006

Cole, L.A. and Helwig, E.B. (1976) Mucoid cysts of the penile skin. *Journal of Urology*, **115**, 397

Crawford, B.S. (1963) The management of hypospadias. *British Journal of Clinical Practice*, **17**, 273

Culp, O.S. and McRoberts, J.W. (1968) Hypospadias. *In* Encyclopedia of Urology. Springer, Berlin, Heidelberg, New York. p.307

Diamond, M. (1965) A critical evaluation of the ontogeny of human sexual behaviour. *Quarterly Review of Biology*, **40**, 147

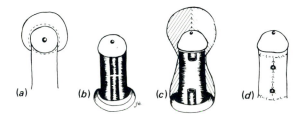

Figure 36.16. First-stage correction of congenital short urethra. *(a)* A circumferential incision is made proximal to the corona glandis. *(b)* The skin is reflected off the penis and the urethra divided. *(c)* The urethra is freed from the corpora cavernosa in each direction. The two layers of the prepuce are separated and the prepuce is divided longitudinally. *(d)* The ventrum of the penis is covered by preputial flaps with formation of urethral fistulas.

Fallon, B., Devine, C.J. and Horton, C.E. (1976) Congenital anomalies associated with hypospadias. *Journal of Urology*, **116**, 585

Feldman, K.W. and Smith, D.W. (1975) Fetal phallic growth and penile standards for newborn males. *Journal of Pediatrics*, **86**, 395

Felton, L.M. (1959) Should intravenous pyelography be a routine procedure for children with cryptorchidism or hypospadias? *Journal of Urology*, **81**, 335

Gavrell, C.J. (1974) Congenital curvature of the penis. *Journal of Urology*, **112**, 489

Gittes, R.F. and McLaughlin, A.P. (1974) Injection technique to induce penile erection. *Urology*, **4**, 473

Glenister, T.W. (1958) A correlation of the normal and abnormal development of the penile urethra and of the infra-abdominal wall. *British Journal of Urology*, **30**, 117

Goldstein, M. (1975) Congenital urethral fistula with chordee. *Journal of Urology*, **113**, 138

Gray, S.W. and Skandalakis, J.E. (1972) The male reproductive tract. *In* Embryology for Surgeons. Saunders, Philadelphia.p.595

Harris, F. (1979) Personal communication

Hodgson, N.B. (1970) A one-stage hypospadias repair. *Journal of Urology*, **104**, 281

Jacob, S.C., Kaplan, G.W. and Gittes, R.F. (1975) Topical testosterone therapy for penile growth. *Urology*, **6**, 708

Johnson, C.F., Carlton, C.F. and Powell, N.B. (1974) Duplication of penis. *Urology*, **4**, 722

Johnson, F.P. (1920) The later development of the urethra in the male. *Journal of Urology*, **4**, 447

Johnston, J.H. (1974) Lengthening of the congenital and acquired short penis. *British Journal of Urology*, **46**, 685

Johnston, J.H. (1977) Other penile abnormalities. *In* Surgical Paediatric Urology (edited by Eckstein, H.B., Hohenfellner, R. and Williams, D.I.). Thieme, Shuttgart.p.406.

Johnston, J.H. and Coimbra, J.A.M. (1970) Megalourethra. *Journal of Pediatric Surgery*, **5**, 304

Kallmann, F.J., Schoenfeld, W.A. and Barrera, S.E. (1944) The genetic aspects of primary eunuchoidism. *American Journal of Mental Deficiency*, **48**, 203

Kaplan, G.W. and Lamm, D.L. (1975) Embryogenesis of chordee. *Journal of Urology*, **114**, 769

Kogan, S.J. and Williams, D.I. (1977) The micropenis syndrome: clinical observations and expectation for growth. *Journal of Urology*, **118**, 311

Leitch, I.O.W. (1970) Circumcision: a continuing enigma. *Australian Paediatric Journal*, **6**, 59

McArdle, R. and Leibowitz, R. (1975) Uncomplicated hypospadias and anomalies of upper tract: need for screening? *Urology*, **5**, 712

Money, J., Hampson, J.G. and Hampson, J.L. (1955) An examination of some basic sexual concepts: the evidence of human hermaphroditism. *Bulletin of the Johns Hopkins Hospital*, **97**, 301

Noonan, J.A. (1968) Hypertelorism with Turner phenotype: a new syndrome with associated congenital heart disease. *American Journal of Diseases of Children*, **116**, 373

Prader, A., Labhart, A. and Willi, H. (1956) Ein syndrom von adipositas, kleinwuchs, kryptorchismus and oligophrenie nach myatonierartigem zustand im neugeborenenalter. *Schweize Medizinsche Wochenschrift*, **86**, 1920

Ross, J.F., Farmer, A.W. and Lindsay, W.K. (1959) Hypospadias: a review of 230 cases. *Plastic and Reconstructive Surgery*, **24**, 357

Schonfeld, W.A. (1943) Primary and secondary sexual characteristics. *American Journal of Diseases of Children*, **65**, 535

Smith, D.W. (1977) Micropenis and its management. *In* Birth Defects Original Article Series, Vol. 13, No.2 (edited by Bergsma, D. and Duckett, J.W.). Liss, New York. p.147

Sonderdahl, D.W., Brosman, S.A. and Goodwin, W.E. (1972) Penile agenesis. *Journal of Urology*, **108**, 496

Walsh, P.C., Wilson, J.D., Allen, T.D., Madden, J.D., Porter, J.C., Neaves, W.B., Griffin, J.E. and Goodwin, W.E. (1978) Clinical and endocrinological evaluation of patients with congenital microphallus. *Journal of Urology*, **120**, 90

Welch, K.J. (1979) Hypospadias. *In* Pediatric Surgery (edited by Ravitch, M.M., Welch, K.J., Benson, C.D., Aberdeen, E. and Randolph, J.G.). Year Book Medical Publishers, Chicago.p.1353

Williams, D.I. (1977) Other methods of hypospadias repair. *In* Operative Surgery: Urology (edited by Williams, D.I.). Butterworths, London.p.359

Yarbrough, W.J. and Johnston, J.H. (1977) Crawford modification of Denis Browne hypospadias procedure. *Journal of Urology*, **117**, 782

37 Abnormalities of the Scrotum and the Testes

J.H. Johnston

Abnormalities of the scrotum

Transposition of the scrotum and the penis, and ectopic scrotum

These conditions result from restricted or abnormal migration of one or both labioscrotal swellings, each of which in the male represents a hemiscrotum.

With complete transposition the penis lies entirely behind the scrotum. A more common disorder is a split scrotum, the two halves of which meet above the penis (*Figure 37.1*). As a rule these abnormalities are associated with

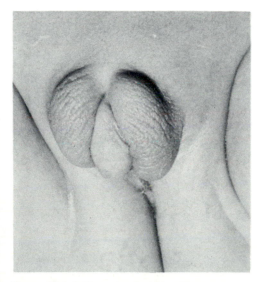

Figure 37.1. Split scrotum in a boy with severe hypospadias.

severe degrees of hypospadias. Correction requires mobilization of each hemiscrotum and its relocation ventral to the penis (*see* Chapter 39).

Ectopic scrotum takes several forms. Wide separation of the hemiscrota is encountered with diphallia in cases of cloacal exstrophy where there is wide diastasis of the pubic bones. Otherwise scrotal ectopia generally involves only one half of the scrotum which is sited in the groin, the iliac fossa or the thigh (*Figure 37.2*). The testis generally accompanies the hemiscrotum to its abnormal position. Treatment involves orchidopexy to the normally placed hemiscrotum and excision of the ectopic one.

An accessory scrotum is a small empty pouch of scrotal tissue attached to the scrotum or the perineum.

Congenital anomalies of the scrotum may occur as isolated lesions but more severe forms are generally associated with malformations of the urinary tract and elsewhere. Bilateral scrotal ectopia is seen in the popliteal pterygium syndrome which is characterized in addition by hypertelorism and cleft lip and palate (Mininberg and Rickman, 1972). Penoscrotal transposition is commonly found with gross degrees of the caudal regression syndrome which comprises absence or severe malformation of the lower spine, imperforate anus and renal agenesis (Miller, 1972).

Scrotal dermoid

An inclusion dermoid cyst lined by squamous epithelium and containing sebaceous material may occur within the scrotal raphe as a result of implantation of cell rests during fusion of the genital swelling. Calculi may form or infection may lead to a discharging sinus (Gupta, Gupta and Khanna, 1974).

Undescended testis

Anatomy

Testicular undescent occurs in two anatomical forms. The first is the incompletely descended testis in which the organ stops somewhere along its normal route of descent (*Figure 37.3*). It may be intra-abdominal, intracanalicular, emergent or sited between the superficial inguinal ring and the scrotal fundus. As a rule the testis lies within a patent processus vaginalis. The second

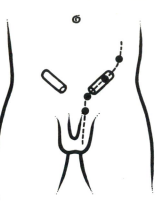

Figure 37.3. Positions of incompletely descended testes.

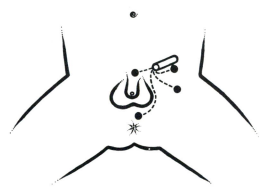

Figure 37.4. Positions of ectopic testes.

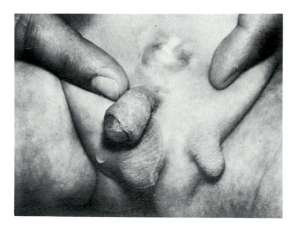

Figure 37.2. Ectopic left hemiscrotum containing a testicle. In addition the umbilicus was low-sited.

type is the ectopic or maldescended testis which is usually not associated with an open processus. It may occupy a pubic, penile, femoral, perineal or most commonly superficial inguinal position where it lies lateral to the superficial inguinal ring deep to Scarpa's fascia (*Figure 37.4*).

With a testis lying in the groin outside the inguinal canal it can quite often be difficult clinically, or even at operation, to make a clear distinction between the two types because the testis has a range of lateral and downwards movement rather than a fixed position. Nevertheless, the distinction is likely to be of prognostic importance. An ectopic testis is generally larger and firmer than an incompletely descended one and its histology shows better tubular development during boyhood (Mack *et al.*, 1961). However, there are no long-term studies available to indicate that childhood orchidopexy gives better results in terms of adult fertility in one or the other type.

A unilateral undescended testis is smaller than the contralateral scrotal organ, although the discrepancy may not be obvious unless both are exposed surgically. Infrequently the scrotal testis opposite an undescended one is hypertrophied and clearly larger than normal even during childhood. The mechanism involved and the teleological reason for such an occurrence before puberty are unknown. When the processus vaginalis is open the testis and the spermatic cord are often suspended within the sac in a mesentery and the local anatomy is frequently distorted. The epididymis and the testis may be widely separated from each other and the vas and its accompanying vessels may descend much lower than the testis and then loop back to join the epididymis. In some cases the ductal anomalies are more severe. Badenoch (1946) described three cases of testicular undescent in which the vasa efferentia were absent on histological study, and similar failures of ductal communication were recorded by Nowak (1972) and Michalek and Krepp (1972). Such abnormalities can easily remain undetected at orchidopexy and it is likely that their incidence is greater than it appears from the numbers reported so that they may contribute significantly to the occurrence of infertility associated with testicular undescent.

Retractile testes

Clinically, undescended testes must be distinguished from retractile ones. Testicular retraction is a normal phenomenon in boys and occurs when the brisk cremasteric contractions of childhood raise the testes to the groins or within the inguinal canal under the stimulus of cold, fear or the sudden grab of an inconsiderate examiner. Retracted testes can usually be manipulated back to the scrotum but they may be mistaken for true undescended testes, particularly in a fat, apprehensive or ticklish patient. Placing the patient in a squatting posture or in a warm bath may be helpful in doubtful cases. The appearance of the scrotum does not aid the distinction because a well formed scrotum or hemiscrotum can coexist with undescended testes and conversely a shallow scrotum can contain normally descended testes. At puberty retractability ceases and the testes take up a permanent scrotal position. From late reviews of patients Puri and Nixon (1977) showed that retractile testes suffer no damage from their frequent sojourns above the scrotum and that in adult life their spermatogenic function is normal. There is little doubt that in the past failure to distinguish between retractile and undescended testes has invalidated many statistics concerning the incidence of testicular undescent during boyhood and this in turn has led to false conclusions being drawn concerning the possibility of late spontaneous descent and the response of undescended testes to hormone treatment.

Pathogenesis

The testis is first recognizable in the 4–5 mm embryo as the genital ridge in the coelomic epithelium medial to the mesonephros. Its prenatal migration within the abdomen is mainly passive due to differential growth of the fetus, but its passage through the inguinal parietes to the scrotum is an active process. The testis is preceded and guided to its ultimate destination by the gubernaculum, which is attached proximally to the lower testicular pole, and is accompanied on its anterior aspect by the processus vaginalis. The proximal portion of the lumen of the processus normally becomes obliterated, leaving the distal part to form the tunica vaginalis. The testes ordinarily reach the scrotum during the eighth month of intrauterine life so that in a normal boy both testes are descended at birth. There are exceptions that are still within the range of normality. For instance a premature baby may be born before full descent exists and even in the full-term infant descent may be somewhat delayed without being pathological (see below).

Hormonal control

The normal migration of the testis from the region of the deep inguinal ring is under complex hormonal regulation and the steps involved were described by Rajfer and Walsh (1977). LH-RH produced by the hypothalamus causes the pituitary to secrete LH and FSH. Following their priming with FSH the fetal testicular Leydig's cells respond to LH and produce testosterone. The latter is converted within the testis by the enzyme 5-alpha-reductase to dihydrotestosterone. This combines with a cytoplasmic protein in the receptor organs in the gubernaculum, the processus vaginalis and the spermatic cord and causes the passage of the testis to the scrotum. Blocks in the hormonal pathway produce various clinical syndromes of which bilateral testicular undescent is a feature.

With anencephaly and pituitary aplasia no pituitary hormones are secreted. In Kallman's syndrome (Kallman, Schoenfeld and Barrera, 1944), which is a hypothalamic anomaly, there is hypogenitalism and anosmia. A deficiency of 5-alpha-reductase is associated with severe degrees of hypospadias. Failure of the target organs to respond to dihydrotestosterone occurs in the testicular feminization syndrome and in Reifenstein's syndrome (Bowen *et al.*, 1965). With all these endocrine disorders there are other easily recognizable and often gross congenital abnormalities as well as undescended testes. It remains uncertain to what degree, if any, hormonal defects are responsible for the common situation in which an otherwise normal boy has one or both testes undescended. Alternative pathogenic possibilities are, first, that the stimulus to the testis is normal but the organ fails to respond because of some intrinsic fault and, secondly, that there is an anatomical obstruction to testicular movement.

Testicular dysgenesis

The concept of a primary, inherent and irreversible but ill defined inadequacy that prevents the testis responding to the normal stimulus to descend originated with Hunter (1762). Other authors (Sohval, 1954; Charny and Wolgin, 1957) also considered that a proportion of undescended testes are of this dysgenetic nature. However, there are no precise histological criteria for the diagnosis of dysgenesis and estimates of its incidence have varied. Mininberg and Bingol (1973) found chromosomal abnormalities in undescended testes in boys with normal blood karyotypes and considered that these were the cause of the failure of descent and also of the predisposition to malignancy. Their findings were not confirmed by other authors (Dewald, Kelalis and Gordon, 1977; Klugo, Van Dyke and Weiss, 1978).

Mack *et al.* (1961) defined the tubular fertility index as the percentage of testicular tubules in which any type of spermatogonia could be identified. Normally this amounts to 80–100 per cent at all ages. Scorer and Farrington (1971) found from histological studies of biopsies that an undescended testis, regardless of the age of the child, has a subnormal tubular fertility index and also a less than normal mean tubular diameter. It is impossible to determine whether these defects, which are most marked in intra-abdominal testes, are primary or secondary to the malposition of the organ without repeating histological examination after the testis has been placed in the scrotum.

Mechanical factors

Inadequate length of the spermatic vessels or the vas deferens, insufficiently wide inguinal rings or a fascial septum across the neck of the scrotum have been postulated to cause cryptorchidism by hindering or obstructing testicular movement. The various lesions cited appear just as likely to be the result as the cause of undescent. In dissections of fetuses Scorer (1962) found that in some instances the gubernaculum was attached to the globus minor of the epididymis or to the vas instead of to the body of the testis and suggested that this may be the basis of the not uncommon situation where the wolffian structures descend farther than the testis. Villumsen and Zachau-Christiansen (1966) pointed out that some undescended testes result from upwards migration of an originally fully descended organ. Among 4300 boys with testes normally descended at birth they found that 69 had 87 testes situated at a higher level at 3 years than at 1 year. Secondary ascent of a testis previously diagnosed as fully descended is an occasional source of embarrassment to the clinician. The mechanism of the phenomenon is obscure and it is presumed to be due to a lag in growth of the spermatic vessels.

Lockwood (1888) considered that an ectopic position resulted from the testis following one of four minor gubernacular attachments to the pubic, perineal, femoral or inguinal regions rather than the main insertion into the scrotum. Schecter (1963) confirmed Lockwood's observations but McGregor (1929) failed to find the gubernacular tails.

Genetic influences and iatrogenesis

Genetic factors are involved in the causation of some cases of cryptorchidism. The occurrence of undescended testes in brothers is quite common and Abrams (1975) described a family in which four of six boys were affected. Hereditary cryptorchidism affecting father and sons may also occur and Wiles (1934) recorded the condition involving three generations.

Iatrogenic cryptorchidism is an occasional complication of inguinal herniotomy performed in infancy or early childhood when the testis becomes adherent to the groin scar.

Associated congenital abnormalities

In addition to the endocrinological disorders already mentioned undescended testes are an invariable occurrence in boys with prune belly syndrome and are a common finding in children with gross lower urinary or alimentary tract abnormalities such as bladder and cloacal exstrophy and imperforate anus. The prevalence of coincidental lesions of the urinary tract in boys with cryptorchidism and no other overt abnormality has been investigated by several authors who performed intravenous urography on their patients. Urological anomalies were found in 10 of 159 (Kelly and Hyland, 1977), six of 45 (Farrington and Kerr, 1969), two of 166 (Waaler and Maurseth, 1976), 14 of 100 (Donohue, Utley and Maling, 1973) and 52 of 400 (Watson, Lennox and Gangai, 1974) patients in different series. Although some of the figures suggest that urinary tract anomalies were present with a greater frequency than would be expected to occur by chance, most of the lesions were of no clinical significance and called for no treatment. In the author's view there is no justification for routine pyelography in boys who present solely because of testicular undescent.

Natural history

Many testes that are undescended at birth reach the scrotum soon afterwards. Villumsen and Zachau-Christiansen (1966) examined 4500 boys at birth and at the ages of 1 and 3 years. They found that in 1.8 per cent of full-term and 17.2 per cent of premature babies one or both testes were undescended at birth and that 75 per cent of these had descended by 1 year at which age the overall incidence of undescent was 0.8 per cent. No testis descended between 1–3 years of age. Scorer's (1964) review produced similar statistics and he concluded that a normal testis results if descent occurs within 6 weeks of birth in a full-term infant or 3 months in a premature baby. With later descent the testis fails to reach the bottom of the scrotum and remains smaller than an opposite scrotal organ.

Formerly it was held that many retained testes descended spontaneously and completely at puberty. This contention has now been discredited. It was based on comparisons made between the estimated incidence of testicular undescent before and after puberty but the figures were invalidated by the failure of observers to distinguish between retractile and true undescended testes during boyhood. More recent statistics have shown that testicular undescent occurs with almost the same frequency in boys as in men. In boys the incidence was found

to be 0.80 per cent by Villumsen and Zachau-Christiansen (1966) and 0.78 per cent by Cour-Palais (1966). In men it has been variously reported as 0.5 per cent (Southam and Cooper, 1927), 0.8 per cent (Baumrucker, 1946) and 0.5–1.0 per cent (Hansen, 1949). Scorer (1964) estimated that cryptorchidism exists in just less than 1 per cent of all males after infancy. Spontaneous complete descent of the testis after infancy is very uncommon and if it does occur, the testis suffers degenerative changes proportionate to its delay in reaching the scrotum. Later spontaneous descent of the testis is not therefore to be expected or desired.

The effects of undescent on the testis

The adult testis is capable of normal spermatogenesis only within a relatively small range of environmental temperature which is regulated by the dartos and cremasteric musculature. There is clinical and experimental evidence (Fridd *et al.*, 1975) that the higher than normal temperature to which an undescended testis is exposed is detrimental not only to production of spermatozoa in the adult but also to tubular development during childhood. Although notable exceptions have been reported (Britton, 1975) in which postpubertal orchidopexy led to spermatogenesis, it is accepted that as a rule irreversible degenerative changes in the retained testis begin soon after puberty and are quickly followed by tubular fibrosis and hyalinization. The Sertoli cells persist longer than the spermatogenic epithelium. Leydig cells remain intact but Kupperman (1963) found that with an intra-abdominal testis interstitial cell degeneration and cessation of testosterone secretion occur at the age of 35–40 years.

There is no uniformity of opinion regarding the age at which degenerative changes begin in an undescended testis. Scorer and Farrington (1971) considered the testis to be histologically abnormal at birth. Others (Robinson and Engle, 1954; Cohn, 1967; Hecker and Hienz, 1967) believed that changes begin at 5 years while Cooper (1929) and Nelson (1951) put it at 3 years and 6–7 years respectively. Hadziselimovic, Herzog and Seguchi (1975) employed electron microscopy of testicular biopsies and reported that tubular degeneration began in the second or third year of life and progressed thereafter. Little information is available concerning the functional potential of an undescended testis with respect to its original position. Generally the more fully descended the testis the more it approaches normal size but Charny and Wolgin (1957) found that the degree of histological degeneration depended on the age rather than the site of the testis. As already discussed a superficial inguinal ectopic testis is usually larger and firmer than an incompletely descended one and Mack *et al.* (1961) observed that histological abnormality was less marked in the former.

The extent to which tubular maldevelopment and dysfunction in an undescended testis are due to an inimical environment acting on a potentially normal organ or to inherent testicular dysgenesis remains unsolved. There is no doubt that an untreated bilaterally cryptorchid patient is almost certainly azoospermic and sterile. In recent years it has become apparent that men with unilateral testicular undescent may similarly be infertile. Hecker and Hienz (1967) found from biopsies that 60 per cent of unilateral descended testes during boyhood showed tubular defects. In the combined series of men with untreated unilateral undescent reported by Mack *et al.* (1961), Scott (1962) and Woodhead, Pohl and Johnson (1973) only 49 (39 per cent) of 125 men were fertile. Woodhead, Pohl and Johnson (1973) and Madersbacher, Kovesdi and Frick (1972) noted that orchidopexy in unilateral cases did not appear to improve fertility. Nevertheless, the combined series of McCollum (1935), Maitland (1953), Hand (1955), Caucci (1966) and Atkinson (1975) showed that 143 (87 per cent) of 164 unilaterally cryptorchid patients who had had orchidopexy during boyhood were fertile. It seems unlikely that the improved fertility rates were due entirely to spermatogenesis in the operated testes and the question arises as to whether an undescended testis depresses the function of an opposite descended one.

Experimental studies concerning this possibility have produced contradictory results. Shirai *et al.* (1966), working with mature dogs found that intra-abdominal placement of one testis caused the other to degenerate and that subsequent orchidopexy restored spermatogenesis. Mengel *et al.* (1977) had similar results with puppies and discovered that degenerative changes in the contralateral testis and to a lesser degree in the operated testis can be prevented by immunosup-

pressive agents, suggesting that an autoimmune mechanism is involved. On the other hand Atkinson (1973) found that in guinea pigs the scrotal testis was unaffected by unilateral induced cryptorchidism.

At present we do not know what proportion of unilateral descended testes have spermatogenic defects, reversible or otherwise. The information available indicates, first, that removal of a unilateral undescended testis should not be lightly undertaken during childhood and, secondly, that a definite assurance concerning future fertility cannot be given in the case of a boy with only one testis in the scrotum.

Complications

Inguinal hernia

In most cases of incomplete testicular descent as distinct from testicular ectopia there is a patent processus vaginalis, but the sac is generally too narrow to allow the entry of abdominal viscera. A clinically obvious hernia is therefore exceptional. When it does occur, it usually appears within the first 2 years of life.

Psychological effects

Some authorities (Lattimer *et al.*, 1974) have considered this aspect to be of vital importance and have advised that it is essential for the cryptorchid boy, or even the boy with retractile testes, to have the testes securely fixed in the scrotum before starting school at the age of 5 years so that he is not exposed to the derision of his colleagues in the kindergarten locker room. In the author's experience boys under the age of 7–8 years, although often very conscious of their phallic dimensions and appearance, are frequently unaware of the existence of their testes and are rarely concerned about testicular position unless parental anxiety is transmitted to them.

Trauma

An undescended testis lying outside the inguinal canal is somewhat more susceptible to external injury than the normal organ which is cushioned by its mobility in the scrotum. However, serious injury during childhood is rare. A perineal testis may be mildly traumatized by sitting on a narrow bicycle saddle.

Torsion

An incompletely descended testis is often suspended by a pedicle inside a patent processus vaginalis and in the past torsion affected undescended testes more often than scrotal ones (Abeshouse, 1936). With the modern tendency for early orchidopexy, torsion of an undescended testis is now uncommon and is seen predominantly in infancy (Johnston, 1965). Torsion of an inguinal testis produces a tender groin swelling that may simulate a strangulated hernia. In children torsion of an abdominal testis is seen infrequently and in adults this complication is preceded by neoplastic change in about 60 per cent of cases (Richie, 1957).

Malignancy

During childhood neoplasia of the testis is rare and its occurrence in an undescended testis is even rarer. Cases were recorded by Gordon-Taylor and Wyndham (1947) and Margolis and Gross (1966) in boys aged respectively 5 months and 2 months. In the adult there is no doubt that an undescended testis is more prone to malignant change than a scrotal organ. Gilbert and Hamilton (1940) found 11 per cent of 7000 testicular tumours were associated with undescent and in other series the corresponding figures ranged from 5.9 per cent of 995 cases (Collins and Pugh, 1964) to 14.3 per cent of 292 cases (Dean, 1935). The risk of testicular cancer in a man with an undescended testis has been estimated to be up to 50 times greater than average. It has generally been considered that an intra-abdominal testis is more prone to malignancy than an undescended testis sited lower down but this was not supported by the studies of Fergusson (1965). The undescended position does not hasten the development of a tumour and in fact the average age of onset of neoplasia is later than in a scrotal testis, in which malignant change occurs most often in the second half of the fourth decade. Although an undescended testis may develop any of the pathological types of testicular tumour, the seminoma is relatively more common and the teratoma relatively less common than in a scrotal testis.

Bringing the testis to the scrotum during boyhood does not eliminate the possibility of malignancy and probably does not lessen the chance. In the series of Gilbert and Hamilton (1940) and Gehring, Rodriguez and Woodhead (1974) 77 of 1000 and 37 of 529 testicular tumours respectively occurred following orchidopexy. A tumour may develop even when the operation is followed by testicular atrophy. Altman and Malament (1967) noted that among their cases of postorchidopexy neoplasia only two patients had undergone the operation before the age of 11 and they suggested that orchidopexy performed before 10 years may prevent malignant change. However, Gehring, Rodriguez and Woodhead (1974) later reported 10 cases of neoplasia developing in men who had had orchidopexy before the age of 10 and they advanced the recommended age of operation to 6 years. Subsequently De Cenzo and Leadbetter (1975) recorded a case of testicular tumour in a 20-year-old man who had undergone orchidopexy at 6 years. It seems likely that placement of the testicle in the scrotum at an early age contributes little if anything to the avoidance of subsequent neoplasia and that the predisposition is inherent in the testis itself.

A similar inborn liability often affects a unilateral descended testis as indicated by the common occurrence of tumour arising in the scrotal testis and not in the undescended one in series of testicular neoplasm associated with unilateral undescent. This was the case in respectively 23 of 840 and nine of 58 such tumours in the studies of Gilbert and Hamilton (1940) and Collins and Pugh (1964) and in 24 per cent in the survey of Gehring, Rodriguez and Woodhead (1974).

The survival rates for men who develop a tumour in an undescended and especially an abdominal testis are considerably lower than those when a scrotal testis is affected. While orchidopexy does not prevent malignancy it is nevertheless of benefit in that it allows earlier diagnosis if and when a tumour develops. A particular hazard of testicular malignancy after orchidopexy is the occurrence of metastases in the inguinal lymph nodes due to surgical alteration of the normal lymphatic drainage.

The increased liability of the undescended testis to neoplasia and the failure of orchidopexy to prevent it appear at first sight to indicate a need for wholesale removal of such organs. Nevertheless tumour of the testis is relatively rare. In the Merseyside Hospital Region the incidence of testicular tumours in 1973 was 1.7

per 100 000 males per annum while that of carcinoma of the rectum, the bladder, the prostate, the colon, the stomach and the bronchus was respectively 18.3, 22.5, 23.4, 25.3, 35.0 and 123.0 per 100 000 males. It is clear that the risk for the cryptorchid man, even if much greater than average, is still relatively small. Tibbs (1961) estimated that there is one chance in 66 of a man developing a tumour in an undescended testis during an adult life span of 50 years. The undescended testis cannot therefore be regarded as a precancerous lesion and orchidectomy with the sole object of preventing malignancy is unjustified during childhood.

Recently Krabbe *et al.* (1979) drew attention to the existence of testicular carcinoma *in situ* in adults who had undergone orchidopexy during childhood. Leadbetter (1979) reported similar histological changes in a biopsy from a macroscopically normal undescended testis in a 12-year-old boy and suggested that testicular biopsy should be performed routinely during orchidopexy. However, whether or not the tubular cells in a prepubertal testis are abnormal is a rather subjective matter so that a confident prognosis concerning their potential for malignancy can be extremely difficult.

Treatment

Investigation and management of boys with unilateral or bilateral impalpable testes are discussed below (see Monorchism and Anorchism).

The object of treatment of cryptorchidism is to obtain a scrotal position for the testis sufficiently early to allow it to reach its maximum potential. Hormone therapy or operation may be employed.

Hormone treatment

Intramuscular gonadotrophin injection for testicular undescent was introduced in the 1930s and for some years was considered to be highly effective. Thompson and Heckel reviewed the literature in 1938 and found that hormone therapy was stated to be successful in inducing testicular descent in 65 per cent of bilateral and 47 per cent of unilateral cases. Later it became clear that the selection of patients had been indiscriminate and that many of the successes

claimed were in boys with retractile testes (Rea, 1951). Having carefully excluded these Ehrlich *et al.* (1969) reported that gonadotrophin treatment produced descent in 38 per cent of bilateral and 16 per cent of unilateral cases. Illig *et al.* (1977) administered either LH-RH or placebo intranasally in a double-blind trial and stated that the hormone led to complete descent in 38 per cent of testes, to an improved position in 28 per cent and to no change in 19 per cent. Success was independent of age but lower undescended testes gave better results than higher ones. It is interesting to note, and indicative of the degree of subjectivity involved in defining the position of a boy's testis, that the authors recorded an improved position in 25 per cent of testes in boys given placebo. Pirazzoli *et al.* (1973) also employed LH-RH as a nasal spray and recorded that it led to descent in seven of 22 boys with unilateral undescent. They found that the hormone produced no rise in the serum gonadotrophin level whether or not it was effective, and it is difficult to understand why descent occurred in the successful cases.

The aim of hormone therapy is to induce a limited degree of premature puberty. Sexual precocity and early epiphyseal closure have been known to occur as side effects, as have degenerative changes in the retained testis (Charny and Wolgin, 1957; Whitaker, 1970). Gonadotrophins are clearly indicated in the treatment of hypogonadotrophic hypogonadism and may be useful when given as a brief preoperative course to facilitate a difficult orchidopexy (Jeffs, 1978). As a definitive method of treatment in a boy without overt endocrinopathy they are effective in only a minority of cases, carry the possibility of producing undesirable consequences and with modern surgical and anaesthetic techniques have no advantages whatever over orchidopexy.

Orchidopexy

The timing of orchidopexy may be determined by the development of a complication such as a hernia or torsion but usually it is a matter of choice. Although some authorities (Scorer and Farrington, 1971) have claimed that degenerative changes in the testis begin at or before birth, orchidopexy in infancy can be a tricky procedure with a possibility of damaging the delicate testicular vessels. In the author's view the operation is preferably deferred until the age of 4–5 years when the tissues are stronger and the operation is easier and safer for the testis. In bilateral cases it is advisable to leave an interval of some months between operations, unless the first orchidopexy is very easily performed, since the result obtained on the first side may influence the method to be employed on the second.

TECHNIQUE

The essential feature of the operation is freeing the spermatic cord from its surroundings so that it can be lengthened sufficiently to let the testis come into the scrotum without tension. The inguinal canal is opened through a groin incision, the cremaster is incised and the testis and the cord are mobilized. During the division of gubernacular remnants below the testis care is needed to avoid injury to an elongated epididymis or vas deferens. A patent processus vaginalis is opened and divided transversely just above the testis; its proximal part is separated from the cord, ligated at the level of the deep ring and excised.

Most of the cord lengthening obtainable is achieved by dividing the suspensory ligament of Browne (1949), which is a firm fascial band that extends upwards and laterally from the cord at the level of the deep inguinal ring. Often the ligament can be divided at more than one level as the cord lengthens. If further elongation is needed, the fascia transversalis forming the posterior wall of the inguinal canal can be incised to let the cord move medially and so eliminate its angulation at the deep ring. Division of the inferior epigastric vessels is not necessary. In the majority of cases these measures are sufficient to let the testis reach the scrotum. When they are not the incision can be extended upwards and laterally and the spermatic vessels can then be freed almost to their origin and the vas mobilized to the bladder base. However, the extensive intra-abdominal dissection frequently gives very little extra length.

Fowler and Stephens (1959) reaffirmed the experience of former observers that the vasal vessels alone are often sufficient to vascularize the testis so that the spermatic vessels can be safely divided when they are too short to let the testis reach the scrotum. Fowler and Stephens' (1959) method is applicable to those cases in which the vas and its vessels form a loop below the testis. Division of the short spermatic vessels and possibly also one or two of the vascular arcades that cross the loop from one limb to the other allows the vas to be straightened and the testis to descend fully. Great care is needed to avoid injury to the vasal vessels during the dissection of a hernial sac, and before the spermatic vessels are finally divided the adequacy of the testicular blood supply must be assured by applying a vascular clamp for some minutes. If doubt exists, one of the subtunical testicular vessels may be incised and the bleeding observed.

Similar division of the spermatic vessels can be employed successfully with high intra-abdominal testes such as in the prune belly syndrome; in this case the vessels are very short and the vas is correspondingly long (Johnston, 1977). Woodard and Parrott (1978) found that when operation is performed in infancy orchidopexy may be possible in cases of prune belly syndrome without dividing the spermatic vessels. Silber and Kelly (1976) performed autotransplantation of intra-abdominal testes by joining the testicular vessels to the internal iliac or inferior epigastric ones using a microvascular technique.

The literature is replete with descriptions of methods of fixing the testis in the scrotum. Nevertheless, this aspect of the operation is of very little importance provided that adequate cord lengthening is achieved. The author's technique is to bring the testis out through a small scrotal incision and then replace it. The scrotal incision is closed with fine catgut sutures which also pick up the testicular tunica albuginea. Postoperative application of elastic bands or temporary fixation to the thigh is contraindicated. When the testis reaches the scrotum easily such traction is unnecessary and when it does not these methods stretch the spermatic cord and may endanger the vascularity of the testis. In any event the ingenious small boy generally frustrates the object of the exercise because he quickly learns that by flexing and adducting his thigh he can relax the traction and relieve the discomfort it causes.

If the testis does not reach the scrotum after complete freeing of the cord it may be fixed by suture in its lowest position and re-explored after an interval of some 6 months. Remobilization is then often successful in achieving sufficient cord length. The second stage of the operation is much easier when, at the first stage, the cord and the testis are wrapped in a thin sheet of Silastic to prevent their adherence to surrounding tissues. If the testis still cannot be made to descend at the second operation, orchidectomy is indicated when the opposite testis appears clinically normal. Otherwise the testis should be retained so that its hormonal function is preserved.

Results

Unless both testes atrophy following operation the results of orchidopexy are satisfactory from the endocrinological viewpoint. At puberty full masculinization occurs and subsequently the plasma testosterone levels are those of a normal adult male, although the serum gonadotrophin levels, especially that of FSH, are generally raised (Corriere and Lipschultz, 1977).

The principal object of orchidopexy is to achieve useful spermatogenesis in the testis and the results of the operation must be judged by this criterion. A gross surgical blunder is obvious clinically when the testis undergoes post-operative atrophy. The incidence of this complication has ranged from 50 per cent (Aird, 1949) to 2 per cent (Snyder and Chaffin, 1955). Gross and Jewett (1956) reported that over 90 per cent of their orchidopexies gave good results in terms of postoperative testicular position, size and consistency, but Charny and Wolgin (1957) found that clinical excellence can coincide with spermatogenic insufficiency. The latter authors studied testicular biopsies before and after orchidopexy and considered the results of the procedure so dismal that it was rarely, if ever, worth performing. However, they were investigating patients who had undergone a modification of the now obsolete Torek thigh-fixation operation. Following the use of a modern technique Kiesewetter, Shull and Fetterman (1969) found an improved histological appearance in 25 of 29 testes.

Atkinson, Epstein and Rippon (1975) considered that raised levels of LH and FSH in adults after orchidopexy indicated a poor prognosis as regards fertility. However, apart from postoperative testicular biopsies the results of orchidopexy can be assessed only in bilateral cases by the patients' paternity, spermatozoa counts or both. Since 1960 the results of eight series of men who had undergone bilateral orchidopexy during boyhood have been reported (Bergstrand and Qvist, 1960; Maier and Spann, 1962; Scott, 1962; Knauth and Potempa, 1963; Hohenfellner

and Eisenhut, 1964; Bramble *et al.*, 1974; Atkinson, 1975; Werder *et al.*, 1976). While a total of 48 (34.3 per cent) of 140 patients were stated to be fertile there were considerable individual variations. Hohenfellner and Eisenhut (1964) had no fertile patient among 15 and at the other extreme 14 (56 per cent) of Bergstrand and Qvist's (1960) 25 patients were fertile. Although the discrepancies between the results are difficult to explain, it is apparent that many authors could trace only a minority of their patients.

Both retrospective and prospective studies are extremely difficult to carry out since the functional result of orchidopexy may not be known until 20 or 25 years have elapsed. As a consequence prognostication remains difficult. In addition there is at present very little information concerning the possible effects of successful orchidopexy, leading to fertility, on the succeeding generation. The latter aspect may become increasingly important in future.

Monorchism

Unilateral congenital absence of the testis is commoner than bilateral absence, the former occurring in one in 5000 males and the latter in one in 20000 (Goldberg, Skaist and Morrow, 1974). Monorchism may be due to testicular agenesis but the local anatomy often indicates that a testis was present at one period of intrauterine life and subsequently vanished, perhaps as a result of a vascular accident such as torsion. Union between the testis and the epididymis occurs towards the end of the sixth month of fetal life and depending upon the timing of the destructive lesion the testis and its ducts may be affected separately or jointly.

When one testis is impalpable it is important to distinguish between testicular absence and high testicular undescent because malignant change affecting an abdominal testis may reach an advanced stage before it becomes clinically apparent. The position and the size of the opposite testis and the state of the upper urinary tract do not help the distinction since anomalies can occur in either case. Goldberg, Skaist and Morrow (1974) found that 10 of 39 boys with monorchism had other genital lesions such as hypospadias or contralateral cryptorchidism and that urography showed ipsilateral upper urinary tract abnormalities in five of 14 cases. Renal agenesis is associated with congenital absence of the mesonephric duct and therefore of the ureter and the vas deferens, but the testis in such cases can develop normally.

It may be possible to demonstrate the presence of an intra-abdominal testis or the position that a now-infarcted testis previously occupied by transfemoral aortography and selective testicular arteriography (Ben-Menachem, Deberardinis and Salinas, 1974). Weiss, Glickman and Lytton (1977) found gonadal venography more valuable, although difficulty may be experienced in catheterizing the right spermatic vein from the vena cava. The spermatic vein is recognizable by the pampiniform plexus at its termination. From animal experiments Bruschini *et al.* (1977) suggested that it may be possible to locate a hidden testis by scintigraphy following the administration of ^{131}I-LH. Often the question of testicular absence or intra-abdominal testicular retention can be resolved only by surgical exploration.

At operation to detect an impalpable testis through an inguinal approach the spermatic vessels and the vas deferens may be found to enter the inguinal canal or the scrotum, where they end blindly or in a small adherent fibrous nodule representing the relic of an infarcted testis. An abdominal testis is most commonly situated intraperitoneally just within the deep inguinal ring. Frequently a loop of vas deferens or an elongated epididymis may extend lower into a patent processus vaginalis and may at first sight be mistaken for the testis. When inguinal exploration is negative the incision must be extended by incising the musculature lateral to the deep inguinal ring and opening the peritoneum more widely. If the testis is not found intraperitoneally or retroperitoneally, the presence or otherwise of the vas deferens and the spermatic vessels must be determined. Theoretically the vessels are a more constant guide to the testis than the vas, but when the organ is missing as a result of previous atrophy they are often extremely small and it can be difficult to decide whether a particular leash is indeed representative of the testicular blood supply. Since the testis and its ducts may be wide apart the finding of a blind-ending vas is not proof of an absent testis. Similarly the absence of the vas is not necessarily indicative of testicular agenesis (Tibbs, 1961).

An extended inguinal incision with good relaxation and retraction allows a wide examination of the ipsilateral side of the pelvis and the lower abdomen. When the testis remains undetected and the spermatic vessels cannot be identified with certainty there is little justification for carrying out a more comprehensive search through a separate laparotomy or flank incision. If a testis exists, it may occupy almost any intraperitoneal or retroperitoneal position and even an extensive exploration remains inconclusive if the organ is not located.

Anorchism

Bilateral congenital absence of the testes is rare. When it occurs in a phenotypic male with a 46 XY karyotype, as is usually the case, it is presumed to be the result of testicular infarction and atrophy occurring later than the 14th week of fetal life at which time penile morphogenesis is complete. This hypothesis is supported by the common operative finding of blind-ending vasa deferentia and spermatic vessels. It is possible that some cases of anorchia are examples of true testicular agenesis and that extratesticular Leydig's cells along the route of testicular descent may have produced sufficient testosterone to promote normal penile development and growth during fetal life and even perhaps some degree of masculinization at puberty (Kirschner, Jacobs and Fraley, 1970). However, the anorchic patient cannot increase his testosterone output to normal levels and eunuchoid features appear.

During childhood anorchism can be distinguished from high cryptorchidism by the existence in the former of raised serum gonadotrophin levels and by the demonstration of no rise in serum testosterone following the administration of HCG. Kogan (1979) advised that under the age of 1 year, between 1–2 years and over 2 years the dosage of HCG should be 500, 1000 and 1500 units respectively given intramuscularly every other day for three doses. The serum testosterone level is measured prior to HCG stimulation and on the day following the last injection.

Anorchism requires the administration of testosterone at the appropriate age. Harris (1979) employed testosterone oenanthate (Primotestin

Depot) 250 mg intramuscularly every 2–3 weeks. The degree of masculinization obtained depends upon the timing of the testicular ablation. In the anorchic boy with normal prepubertal penile dimensions castration clearly occurred no later than during late intrauterine life and normal adult growth of the penis, potency and deepening of the voice are to be expected from androgen replacement therapy. However, the growth of hair on the face, axillae and trunk is often slow to appear and may be permanently defective. The patient's sense of masculinity is enhanced by the insertion of testicular prostheses. The Lattimer design Silastic prosthesis filled with silicone gel, which is available in various sizes, provides a testis with a natural look and feel.

Polyorchism

Duplication of the testis is the result of transverse division of the genital ridge during embryogenesis. Each of the duplicated testes is therefore smaller than normal and as a rule one is smaller than the other. The spermatic vessels bifurcate to reach each moiety and usually each testis has its own epididymis which joins a single vas deferens. A very small supernumerary testis may have no ductal connections. One or both testes may be undescended and torsion may occur. Testicular duplication is commoner on the left side.

The duplicated testes may be palpable clinically but more often the condition is only discovered at surgery for hernia repair or for orchidopexy. A testis without ducts is usually dysplastic and orchidectomy is then indicated. Otherwise both testes should be retained. Although the patient of Jichlinski and Ward-McQuaid (1963) was infertile, many of the duplicated testes reviewed by Mehan, Chehval and Ullah (1976) showed active spermatogenesis.

Transverse testicular ectopia and synorchism

In the rare abnormality of transverse ectopic testis both testes lie in the same hemiscrotum.

The ectopic organ is more often the right one. Each testis has its own spermatic vessels and vas deferens, and those related to the ectopic testis originate on the appropriate side of the abdomen and pass anterior to the bladder to descend through the opposite inguinal canal.

With synorchism the testes are joined to form one mass. The fused testis may be in one or other side of the scrotum or intra-abdominal. Association with renal fusion in the form of a cake or horseshoe kidney may occur.

Testicular ductal anomalies

The testicular ductal system is derived from the mesonephric duct which also gives origin to the ureteric bud at about the fourth week of intrauterine life. Union between the epididymis and the testis occurs at the end of the sixth fetal month. Failure of development of the mesonephric duct leads to congenital absence of the vas deferens, the seminal vesicle and the epididymis and also to ureteric and renal agenesis. Lesions involving the mesonephric duct after the fourth week affect the testicular ducts alone. Since the embryogenesis of the testis is unrelated to that of its ducts the testis may be normally formed and fully descended. Developmental testicular ductal anomalies take several forms and there may be either complete absence of the vas and the seminal vesicle or else segmental or total vasal atresia. The lesions are commonly bilateral and Hanley (1955) found nine men with bilateral absence of the vasa in a series of 148 patients with azoospermia.

Testicular ductal anomalies associated with cryptorchidism are discussed above. In boys with cystic fibrosis the vas is frequently absent or represented by a solid fibrous cord. It is likely that these lesions are due to secondary atrophy consequent upon the viscid mucus secretions of the disease rather than to a primary developmental abnormality.

Union between the ureter and the vas deferens is a rare occurrence. It may result from failure of that part of the mesonephric duct below the ureteric bud to become incorporated into the wall of the urogenital sinus or alternatively from an unusually high origin of the ureteric bud on the mesonephric duct. The

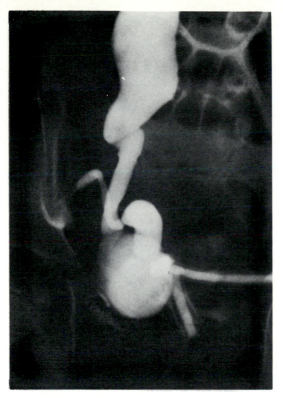

Figure 37.5. Union of the ureter and the vas deferens. Cystogram in a 6-year-old boy who presented with right epididymitis in an undescended testis. There is reflux to the right ureter and vas. The related kidney was dysplastic and afunctional.

ureteric orifice, which in these cases is in fact the opening of the mesonephric duct, often has a high and lateral position in the bladder. Vesicoureteric and ureterovasal reflux are therefore commonly present and urinary tract infection and epididymitis may be the presenting symptoms (*Figure 37.5*). In other cases the ureteric ductal orifice is at the normal bladder site on the trigone or in the posterior urethra. The seminal vesicle is absent. Frequently the related kidney is dysplastic and afunctional yet in some reported cases it is normal (Schwarz and Stephens, 1978). Other urinary tract anomalies and also anorectal lesions are commonly present and the ipsilateral testis may be incompletely descended. Bilateral union between the vasa and the ureters was reported by Redman and Sulieman (1976) and has been seen in cases of cloacal exstrophy (Johnston and Kogan, 1974). In one of the patients of Gibbons, Cromie and Duckett (1978) the vas deferens opened into the bladder separately from the ureter.

Scrotal rests

An accessory spleen attached to the upper pole of the testis is a rare cause of a left-sided scrotal swelling. The condition is due to an adhesion forming between the two closely adjacent organs during embryogenesis. The scrotal splenunculus may be discrete or there may be a transperitoneal cord of tissue, partly splenic and partly fibrous, connecting it to the spleen. Clinically a testicular tumour may be simulated. Attachment of the splenic rest to the spleen may prevent normal descent of the testis.

A small yellow nodule of adrenocortical tissue is quite often found attached to the spermatic cord or lying free in the tunica vaginalis at herniotomy or orchidopexy. Such a rest is rarely of sufficient size to be palpable clinically.

References

Abeshouse, B.S. (1936) Torsion of spermatic cord: report of three cases and review of the literature. *Urological and Cutaneous Review*, **40**, 699

Abrams, H.J. (1975) Familial cryptorchidism. *Urology*, **5**, 849

Aird, I. (1949) A Companion in Surgical Studies. Livingstone, Edinburgh

Altman, B.L. and Malament, M. (1967) Carcinoma of the testis following orchidopexy. *Journal of Urology*, **97**, 498

Atkinson, P.M. (1973) The effect of unilateral experimental cryptorchidism and subsequent orchidopexy upon maturation of the contralateral scrotal testicle of the guinea-pig. *British Journal of Surgery*, **60**, 258

Atkinson, P.M. (1975) A follow up of surgically treated cryptorchid patients. *Journal of Pediatric Surgery*, **10**, 115

Atkinson, P.M., Epstein, M.T. and Rippon, A.E. (1975) Plasma gonadotrophins and androgens in surgically treated cryptorchid patients. *Journal of Pediatric Surgery*, **10**, 27

Badenoch, A.W. (1946) Failure of urogenital union. *Surgery, Gynecology and Obstetrics*, **82**, 471

Baumrucker, G.O. (1946) Incidence of testicular pathology. *Bulletin of the US Army Medical Department*, **5**, 312

Ben-Menachem, Y., Deberardinis, M.C. and Salinas, R. (1974) Localisation of intra-abdominal testes by selective testicular arteriography: a case report. *Journal of Urology*, **112**, 493

Bergstrand, C.G. and Qvist, O. (1960) Die Prognose Chronischer Erkrankungen. Springer, Berlin

Bowen, P., Lee, C.S.N., Migeon, C.J., Kaplan, N.M., Whalley, P.J., McKusick, V.A. and Reifenstein, E.C. (1965) Hereditary male pseudohermaphroditism with hypogonadism, hypospadias and gynecomastia (Reifenstein's syndrome). *Annals of Internal Medicine*, **62**, 252

Bramble, F.J., Houghton, A.L., Eccles, S., O'Shea, A. and Jacobs, H.S. (1974) Reproductive and endocrine function after surgical treatment of bilateral cryptorchidism. *Lancet*, ii, 311

Britton, B.J. (1975) Spermatogenesis following orchidopexy in adult life. *British Journal of Urology*, **47**, 464

Browne, D. (1949) Treatment of undescended testicle. *Proceedings of the Royal Society of Medicine*, **42**, 643

Bruschini, H., Hattner, R., Okerlund, M. and Tanagho, E.A. (1977) Feasability of localising ectopic testes by I^{131} labelled luteinising hormone scintigraphy. *Urology*, **9**, 657

Caucci, M. (1966) Clinical and statistical appraisal of seven hundred orchidopexies. *International Surgery*, **45**, 218

Charny, C.W. and Wolgin, W. (1957) Cryptorchism. Cassel, London

Cohn, B.D. (1967) Histology of the cryptorchid testis. *Surgery*, **62**, 536

Collins, D.H. and Pugh, R.C.B. (1964) The pathology of testicular tumours. *British Journal of Urology*, **36**, Suppl.1

Cooper, E.R.A. (1929) The histology of the retained testis in the human subject at different ages and its comparison with the scrotal testis. *Journal of Anatomy*, **64**, 5

Corriere, J.N. and Lipshultz, L.I. (1977) Endocrinologic and radiographic evaluation of cryptorchid testes. *In* Birth Defects Original Article Series, Vol. 13, No. 5 (edited by Bergsma D. and Duckett, J.W.). Liss, New York.p.275

Cour-Palais, I.J. (1966) Spontaneous descent of the testicle. *Lancet*, i, 1403

Dean, A.L. (1935) Teratoid tumours of the testis. *Journal of the American Medical Association*, **105**, 1965

DeCenzo, J.M. and Leadbetter, G.W. (1975) Early orchidopexy and testis tumours. *Urology*, **5**, 365

Dewald, G.W., Kelalis, P.P. and Gordon, H. (1977) Chromosomal studies in cryptorchidism. *Journal of Urology*, **117**, 110

Donohue, R.E., Utley, W.L.F. and Maling, T.M. (1973) Excretary urography in asymptomatic boys with cryptorchidism. *Journal of Urology*, **109**, 912

Ehrlich, R.M., Dougherty, L.J., Tomashefsky, P. and Lattimer, J.K. (1969) Effect of gonadotropin in cryptorchism. *Journal of Urology*, **102**, 793

Farrington, G.H. and Kerr, I.H. (1969) Abnormalities of the upper urinary tract in cryptorchism. *British Journal of Urology*, **47**, 77

Fergusson, J.D. (1965) Proceedings of the 13th Congress of International Society of Urology. Livingstone, Edinburgh

Fowler, R. and Stephens, F.D. (1959) The role of testicular vascular anatomy in the salvage of high undescended testes. *Australian and New Zealand Journal of Surgery*, **29**, 92

Fridd, C.W., Murphy, J., Linke, C.A. and Bonfiglio, T.A. (1975) Response of rat testis to localised induced hyperthermia. *Urology*, **5**, 76

Gehring, G.G., Rodriguez, F.R. and Woodhead, D.M. (1974) Malignant degeneration of cryptorchid testes following orchidopexy. *Journal of Urology*, **112**, 354

Gibbons, MD., Cromie, W.J. and Duckett, J.W. (1978) Ectopic vas deferens. *Journal of Urology*, **120**, 597

Gilbert, J.B. and Hamilton, J.B. (1940) Studies in malignant testis tumours: incidence and nature of tumours in ectopic testes. *Surgery, Gynecology and Obstetrics*, **71**, 731

Goldberg, L.M., Skaist, L.B. and Morrow, J.W. (1974) Congenital absence of testes: anorchism and monorchism. *Journal of Urology*, **111**, 840

Gordon-Taylor, G. and Wyndham, N.R. (1947) On malignant tumours of the testis. *British Journal of Surgery*, **35**, 6

Gross, R.E. and Jewett, T.C. (1956) Surgical experiences from 1222 operations for undescended testis. *Journal of the American Medical Association*, **160**, 634

Gupta, S.K., Gupta, S. and Khanna, S. (1974) Dermoid cyst of scrotal raphe containing calculi. *British Journal of Urology*, **46**, 348

Hadziselimovic, F., Herzog, B. and Seguchi, H. (1975) Surgical correction of cryptorchidism at 2 years: electron microscopic and morphometric investigations. *Journal of Pediatric Surgery*, **10**, 19

Hand, J.R. (1955) Undescended testes: report of 153 cases with evaluation of clinical findings, treatment and results of follow-up to 33 years. *Transactions of the American Association of Genito-Urinary Surgeons*, **47**, 9

Hanley, H.G. (1955) The surgery of male infertility. *Annals of the Royal College of Surgeons of England*, **17**, 159

Hansen, T.S. (1949) Fertility in operatively treated and untreated cryptorchidism. *Proceedings of the Royal Society of Medicine*, **42**, 645

Harris, F. (1979) Personal communicaton

Hecker, W.C. and Hienz, H. (1967) Cryptorchidism and fertility. *Journal of Pediatric Surgery*, **2**, 513

Hohenfellner, R. and Eisenhut, L. (1964) Evaluation of fertility in cryptorchidism. *International Journal of Fertility*, **9**, 575

Hunter, J. (1762) Observations on the state of the testis in the fetus and on the hernia congenita. *In* W. Hunter Medical Commentaries, Part 1. Millar, London.p.75

Illig, R., Kollman, F., Barkenstein, M., Kuber, W., Exner, G.U., Kellerer, K., Lunglemeyr, L. and Prader, A. (1977) Treatment of cryptorchidism by intranasal synthetic luteinising hormone releasing hormone. *Lancet*, ii, 518

Jeffs, R.D. (1978) Personal communication

Jichlinski, D. and Ward-McQuaid, N. (1953) Duplication of the testis and infertility. *Journal of Urology*, **90**, 583

Johnston, J.H. (1965) The undescended testis. *Archives of Disease in Childhood*, **40**, 113

Johnston, J.H. (1977) Prune belly syndrome. *In* Surgical Paediatric Urology (edited by Eckstein, H.D., Hohenfellner, R. and Williams, D.I.). Thieme, Stuttgart.p.239

Johnston, J.H. and Kogan, S.J. (1974) The exstrophic anomalies and their surgical reconstruction. *In* Current Problems in Surgery. Year Book Medical Publishers, Chicago

Kallman, F.J., Schoenfeld, W.A. and Barrera, S.E. (1944) The genetic aspects of primary eunuchoidism. *American Journal of Mental Deficiency*, **48**, 203

Kelly, D.G. and Hyland, J. (1977) The evaluation of intravenous pyelography in undescended testis. *In* Birth Defects Original Article Series, Vol. 13, No.5 (edited by Bergsma, D. and Duckett, J.W.). Liss, New York. p.287

Kiesewetter, W.B., Shull, W.R. and Fetterman, G.H. (1969) Histologic changes in the testes following anatomically successful orchidopexy. *Journal of Pediatric Surgery*, **4**, 59

Kirschner, M.A., Jacobs, J.B. and Fraley, E.E. (1970) Bilateral anorchia with persistent testosterone production. *New England Journal of Medicine*, **238**, 240

Klugo, R., Van Dyke, D.L. and Weiss, L. (1978) Cytogenic studies of cryptorchid testes. *Urology*, **11**, 255

Knauth, H. and Potempa, J. (1963) Cryptorchidism and fertility. *Urologia Internationalis*, **15**, 77

Kogan, S.J. (1979) A false negative HCG test? *Society for Pediatric Urology Newsletter*, January 10

Krabbe, S., Berthelsen, J.G., Volted, P., Eldrup, J., Shakkeback, N.E., Eyben, F.V., Mauritzen, K. and Nielsen, A.H. (1979) High incidence of neoplasia in maldescended testes. *Lancet*, i, 999

Kupperman, H.S. (1963) Human Endocrinology. Davis, Philadelphia

Lattimer, J.K., Smith, A.M., Dougherty, L.T. and Beck, L. (1974) The optimum time to operate for cryptorchidism. *Pediatrics*, **53**, 96

Leadbetter, G.W. (1979) Incipient germ cell tumor and

cryptorchid testis. *Society for Pediatric Urology Newsletter*, 2 May

Lockwood, C.G. (1888) Development and transition of the testis, normal and abnormal. *Journal of Anatomy and Physiology*, **22**, 505

McCollum, D.W. (1935) Clinical study of the spermatogenesis of undescended testicles. *Archives of Surgery*, **31**, 290

McGregor, A.L. (1929) The third inguinal ring. *Surgery, Gynecology and Obstetrics*, **49**, 273

Mack, W.S., Scott, L.S., Ferguson-Smith, M.A. and Lennox, B. (1961) Ectopic testis and true undescended testis: a histological comparison. *Journal of Pathology and Bacteriology*, **82**, 439

Madersbacher, H., Kovesdi, S. and Frick, J. (1972) Fertility in unilateral cryptorchidism. *Der Urologe*, **11**, 210

Maier, W. and Spann, W. (1962) Die Bedentung der rechtzeitigen behandlung des hodenhochstands für die fertilitat. *Deutsche Medizinsche Wochenschrift*, **87**, 697

Maitland, A.I.L. (1953) Maldescent of the testicle. *Glasgow Medical Journal*, **34**, 170

Margolis, I.B. and Gross, C.G. (1966) Tumor of undescended testicle in an infant. *Journal of the American Medical Association*, **199**, 944

Mehan, D.J., Chehval, M.J. and Ullah, S. (1976) Polyorchidism. *Journal of Urology*, **116**, 530

Mengel, W., Moritz, P., Huttmann, B. and Hecker, W.C. (1977) Investigations into the changes in the descended testis in unilateral cryptorchism. *Zeitschrift für Kinderchirugie*, **22**, 369

Michalek, H.A.L. and Krepp, J. (1972) Failure of urogenital union with secondary amputation of the epididymal tail: a case report with complete review of the literature. *Journal of Urology*, **107**, 436

Miller, S.F. (1972) Transposition of the external genitalia associated with the syndrome of caudal regression. *Journal of Urology*, **108**, 818

Mininberg, D.T. and Bingol, N. (1973) Chromosomal abnormalities in undescended testes. *Urology*, **1**, 98

Mininberg, D.T. and Rickman, A. (1972) Bilateral scrotal testicular ectopia. *Journal of Urology*, **108**, 652

Nelson, W.O. (1951) Mammalian spermatogenesis: effect of experimental cryptorchidism in the rat and non-descent of the testis in man. *Recent Progress in Hormonal Research*, **6**, 29

Nowak, K. (1972) Failure of fusion of epididymis and testicle with complete separation of the vas deferens. *Journal of Pediatric Surgery*, **7**, 715

Pirazzoli, P., Zappilla, F., Bernardi, F., Villa, M.P., Aleksandrowicz, D., Scandola, A., Stancari, P., Cicognani, A. and Cacciari, E. (1973) Luteinising hormone releasing hormone nasal spray as therapy for undescended testicle. *Archives of Disease in Childhood*, **52**, 235

Puri, P. and Nixon, H.H. (1977) Bilateral retractile testes: subsequent effects on fertility. *Journal of Pediatric Surgery*, **12**, 563

Rajfer, J. and Walsh, P.C. (1977) Testicular descent. Birth Defects Original Article Series, Vol. 13, No. 2 (edited by Blandau, R.J. and Bergsma, D.). Liss, New York. p.107

Rea, C.E. (1951) Fertility in cryptorchids. *Minnesota Medicine*, **34**, 216

Redman, J.F. and Sulieman, J.S. (1976) Bilateral vasalureteral communication. *Journal of Urology*, **116**, 808

Richie, J.L. (1957) Torsion of an intra-abdominal testicle. *American Journal of Surgery*, **94**, 672

Robinson, J.N. and Engle, E.T. (1954) Some observations on the cryptorchid testis. *Journal of Urology*, **71**, 726

Schecter, J. (1963) An investigation of the anatomical mechanisms of testicular descent. MA thesis. Johns Hopkins University, Baltimore

Schwarz, R. and Stephens, F.D. (1978) The persisting mesonephric duct: high junction of vas deferens and ureter. *Journal of Urology*, **120**, 592

Scorer, C.G. (1962) The anatomy of testicular descent – normal and incomplete. *British Journal of Surgery*, **49**, 357

Scorer, C.G. (1964) The descent of the testis. *Archives of Disease in Childhood*, **39**, 605

Scorer, C.G. and Farrington, G.H. (1971) Histological studies of the undescended testis. *In* Congenital Deformities of the Testis and Epididymis. Butterworths, London.p.58

Scott, L.S. (1962) Fertility in cryptorchidism. *Proceedings of the Royal Society of Medicine*, **45**, 1047

Shirai, M., Matsushita, S., Kagayama, M., Ichijo, S. and Takeuchi, M. (1966) *Tohoku Journal of Experimental Medicine*, **90**, 363

Silber, S.J. and Kelly, J. (1976) Successful autotransplantation of intra-abdominal testis to the scrotum by microvascular technique. *Journal of Urology*, **115**, 452

Snyder, W.H. and Chaffin, L. (1955) Surgical management of undescended testes: report of 363 cases. *Journal of the American Medical Association*, **157**, 129

Sohval, A.R. (1954) Testicular dysgenesis as an etiologic factor in cryptorchidism. *Journal of Urology*, **72**, 693

Southam, A.H. and Cooper, E.R.A. (1927) Pathology and treatment of the retained testis in childhood. *Lancet*, i, 805

Thompson, W.O. and Heckel, N.J. (1938) Precocious sexual development from an anterior pituitary-like principle. *Journal of the American Medical Association*, **110**, 1813

Tibbs, D.J. (1961) Unilateral absence of the testis: eight cases of true monorchism. *British Journal of Surgery*, **48**, 601

Villumsen, A.L. and Zachau-Christiansen, B. (1966) Spontaneous alterations in position of the testes. *Archives of Disease in Childhood*, **41**, 198

Waaler, P.E. and Maurseth, K. (1976) Cryptorchidism: is routine intravenous pyelography indicated? *Archives of Disease in Childhood*, **51**, 324

Watson, R.H., Lennox, K.W. and Gangai, M.P. (1974) Simple cryptorchidism: the value of the excretory urogram as a screening method. *Journal of Urology*, **111**, 789

Weiss, R.M., Glickman, M.G. and Lytton, B. (1977) Venographic localisation of the non-palpable undescended testis in children. *Journal of Urology*, **117**, 513

Werder, E.A., Illig, R., Torresani, T., Zachmann, M., Baumann, P., Ott, F. and Prader, A. (1976) Gonadal function in young adults after surgical treatment of cryptorchidism. *British Medical Journal*, iv, 1357

Whitaker, R.H. (1970) Management of the undescended testis. *British Journal of Hospital Medicine*, **4**, 25

Wiles, P. (1934) Family tree, showing hereditary undescended right testis and associated deformities. *Proceedings of the Royal Society of Medicine*, **28**, 157

Woodard, J.R. and Parrott, T.S. (1978) Orchidopexy in the prune-belly syndrome. *British Journal of Urology*, **50**, 348

Woodhead, D.M., Pohl, D.R. and Johnson, D.E. (1973) Fertility of patients with solitary testes. *Journal of Urology*, **109**, 66

38   Acquired Lesions of the Penis, the Scrotum and the Testes

J.H. Johnston

Paraphimosis, balanitis, meatal ulceration and stenosis

Paraphimosis occurs when a tightish foreskin is retracted behind the glans and cannot be returned. Pain and oedema make the situation worse. If manipulative reduction is not possible, the tight skin ring corresponding to the preputial orifice must be divided under anaesthesia to allow the foreskin to be drawn forwards. Circumcision is usually needed later when the swelling has settled.

Bacterial balanoposthitis results from infection of smegma and epithelial debris under the foreskin. The acute episode generally settles quickly with antimicrobial therapy. Occasionally a dorsal slit in the prepuce is needed for drainage. Unless the foreskin is readily retractable following the freeing of adhesions, circumcision is required to prevent recurrence.

Balanitis xerotica obliterans is an uncommon progressive sclerosing lesion of unknown causation which involves the epithelium of the foreskin and of the glans penis in adults. Pruritus and burning discomfort occur and involvement of the urethral meatus leads to severe stenosis and dysuria. Mikat, Ackerman and Mikat (1973) described what they considered to be the youngest reported example of balanitis xerotica obliterans in an 11-year-old boy in whom the disease was restricted to the prepuce. However, the pathological preputial changes they recorded are those found almost invariably in prepubertal boys with severe phimosis. It remains uncertain whether the changes represent a specific lesion causing the phimosis or are the result of long-standing exposure of the tissues to urine.

Meatal ulceration is seen in infants following circumcision when ammonia formed in the napkin as a result of faecal organisms causing the breakdown of urea produces excoriation of the urethral orifice. Pain and bleeding occur on micturition. Healing is encouraged and pain relieved by the application of a local anaesthetic cream such as lignocaine. If possible, napkins should be discontinued in the meantime. Later recurrence of ammoniacal irritation is prevented by the use of barrier creams and by frequent napkin changes.

Infrequently meatal stenosis is present with hypospadias. In the author's experience it is unknown in children born with a normally sited meatus and a fully formed foreskin except in the circumcised, particularly those circumcised in infancy. The stenosis results from the healing of a meatal ulcer. Straining on voiding, a narrow stream and slowness in bladder emptying are the presenting symptoms. Meatotomy is needed. Since the foreskin has been removed methods that advance penile skin into the incised meatus are rarely practicable. The preferred technique is to crush the ventral aspect of the glandular urethra with a broad artery forceps and then divide the devascularized tissue. The meatal enlargement should be generous because some degree of renarrowing is likely. Readherence of the edges of the meatotomy can be prevented by the frequent application of petroleum jelly. Measures such as passing a dilator through the meatus or forcibly drawing apart the margins at frequent intervals are often prescribed to the parents but less often practised because the patient is generally uncooperative.

Lymphoedema

Nonfilarial lymphoedema restricted to the penis is rare during boyhood. A low grade streptococcal infection has been incriminated (Vaught, Litvak and McRoberts, 1975) but the causation

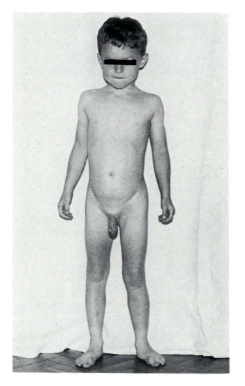

Figure 38.1. Penile lymphoedema in a 6-year-old boy. The condition resolved spontaneously.

is frequently obscure and on occasions self-inflicted trauma cannot be excluded. In the 6-year-boy shown in *Figure 38.1* the condition resolved spontaneously over a period of some months. Persistent lymphoedema may require excision of the thickened tissue together with skin grafting.

Priapism

Priapism is a painful persistent penile erection without sexual excitation and is due to engorgement of the corpora cavernosa. The corpus spongiosum and the glans remain soft and unaffected. Impotence may be a late consequence. In boys the condition is seen most commonly as a complication of haematological diseases.

In sickle cell anaemia the vascular engorgement and the stagnation that occur in the erectile tissues with a normal penile erection during sleep or masturbation lead to increased oxygen extraction from the blood and to crystallization of haemoglobin S. The sickled red blood cells cause sludging and further impede venous return from the penis so that a vicious circle is created. Treatment consists of rapid transfusion of packed red blood cells in sufficient quantity to double the haemoglobin level. The normal cells carry oxygen to the cavernous tissues and so reduce sickling and sludging. As the sickled cells are released into the general circulation the penis becomes flaccid. Operative intervention by venous shunting is rarely needed. As a complication of leukaemia priapism occurs most often in the chronic granulocytic type associated with a high white blood cell count in the peripheral blood. Treatment is that of the underlying cause. The erectile tissue engorgement resolves as the white blood cell count falls on appropriate chemotherapy. Nonspherocytic haemolytic anaemia caused by deficiency of glucosephosphate isomerase may lead to priapism during a haemolytic episode (Goulding, 1976).

Priapism has been reported to result from lipid infiltration of the cavernous tissue in Fabry's disease, which is a glycosphingolipid liposis caused by a genetically determined enzyme deficiency (Wilson, Klionsky and Rhamy, 1973). There is an angiomatous type of skin rash and renal insufficiency due to lipid infiltration of the kidneys. Plasma transfusion is indicated to supply the necessary enzyme.

Priapism secondary to thrombosis of the cavernous tissue has occurred in boys following a straddle injury to the perineum (Oppenheimer, 1976) and as a complication of mumps with or without orchitis (Katz, Politano and Scandiffio, 1976). Needle aspiration of the corpora cavernosa and irrigation with heparinized saline may be effective if performed early. Otherwise a shunting procedure is needed. The corpora cavernosa are most conveniently drained into the flaccid glans penis. For this purpose a renal biopsy or similar cutting needle is inserted into a corpus through the glans and one or more segments of the intervening septum are resected. Since the vascular spaces in the two corpora intercommunicate only one need be drained. This technique has largely superseded the former open operations in which a corpus cavernosum was anastomosed to the corpus spongiosum or the proximal end of the divided internal saphenous vein.

In infants rubbing the penis during bathing or cleansing often induces an erection which may persist for some time afterwards. The continuing penile rigidity is not painful, the organ is not tender and unlike true priapism the condition is not pathological and carries no untoward sequelae.

Fat necrosis in the scrotum

Fat necrosis in the scrotum may occur in boys after swimming in very cold water. A hard nontender mass of organizing necrotic fat and inflammatory exudate forms below each testis. The condition resolves spontaneously and no active measures are called for (Donohue and Utley, 1975).

Idiopathic scrotal oedema

This acute oedematous swelling is of rapid onset and involves one or infrequently both sides of the scrotum in prepubertal boys. The affected hemiscrotum becomes swollen, firm and bright pink in colour. Commonly the swelling extends to the groin or the perineum and on occasions the penis becomes oedematous (*Figure 38.2*). There is little or no pain but local tenderness is present. If surgical exploration is performed because of diagnostic uncertainty, the oedema is seen to be confined to the subcutaneous tissues. The testis and the epididymis are macroscopically normal and testicular biopsy shows no histological abnormality.

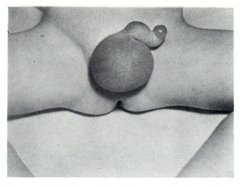

Figure 38.2. Acute right-side scrotal oedema. The swelling extended to the groin and the penis.

The aetiology is obscure. Although the appearance is that of a low grade cellulitis there is usually no fever, the total white blood cell count is normal and the oedema fluid is sterile on culture. An allergic phenomenon similar to angioneurotic oedema has been postulated (Evans and Snyder, 1977) and this hypothesis is supported by the occasional (but not invariable) existence of eosinophilia. The localized nature of the lesion and its characteristic distribution indicate that a hypersensitivity reaction cannot be the entire explanation.

While idiopathic scrotal oedema may resemble intrascrotal torsion or epididymitis the absence of pain, the extension of the swelling beyond the scrotum and the sounds heard with the Doppler stethoscope (see Torsion of the spermatic cord, below) generally allow the distinction to be made. The acute condition subsides almost as rapidly as it appears and is usually entirely gone within 2 days. Occasionally some skin discoloration persists longer. No treatment is needed. Recurrent attacks have been recorded (Johnston, 1968).

Acute scrotal gangrene

Fournier's scrotal gangrene is a rare lesion that can occur at any age. In children it may follow systemic diseases with cutaneous manifestations such as measles or chickenpox (Werner and Falk, 1964). Various organisms may be causative and streptococci, staphylococci, *Proteus vulgaris* and *Clostridium welchii* and other anaerobes have been incriminated in different cases. An obliterative endarteritis leads to necrosis of the overlying skin. The disease is usually of sudden onset with severe general effects of chills, fever and toxaemia. The scrotum becomes swollen, glossy and red and subcutaneous emphysema precedes cutaneous gangrene. The process may spread to involve the skin of the penis or the abdominal wall. Treatment consists of prompt administration of both a broad spectrum antibiotic and metronidazole, to cover anaerobic organisms pending the results of bacterial culture. Multiple scrotal incisions are indicated to relieve tension. Even if almost the entire scrotal skin is lost, regeneration often occurs from the base so that skin grafting is rarely required unless the abdominal wall is affected.

Varicocele

Secondary varicocele may occur on either side and is the result of compression or intraluminal occlusion of the spermatic vein by a retroperitoneal tumour. The veins in the pampiniform plexus are distended even in the lying position.

While primary varicocele is almost always left-sided, rarely it is bilateral. Mild to moderate degrees of the condition are quite common in boys before and at puberty and Oster (1971) found 5.7 per cent of 10 year olds and 19.3 per cent of 14 year olds were affected. In the majority of such cases the varicocele resolves spontaneously. Hanley and Harrison (1962) showed that the veins principally affected are the cremasteric system lying in and external to the cremasteric fascia. The system communicates with the pampiniform plexus of the spermatic vein and drains into the inferior epigastric vein, and to a lesser degree into the superficial external pudendal vein.

In adults varicocele is a recognized cause of infertility because it lessens the temperature differential between the abdomen and the scrotum. In boys the condition is usually symptomless apart from the presence of the swelling. On occasions the left testis is obviously smaller and softer than the right one.

Most cases of boyhood varicocele require no treatment. Since the condition generally disappears spontaneously and since depression of spermatogenesis in persistent cases may not be

of sufficient severity to impair fertility prophylactic surgery against later infertility is unwarranted. However, operation is indicated if the ipsilateral testis is hypotrophic. The proximal end of the cremasteric plexus should be divided between ligatures through a high scrotal incision. If some of the veins of the pampiniform plexus are enlarged, they should be ligated individually (Hanley and Harrison, 1962).

Torsion of the spermatic cord

Torsion of the spermatic cord has two peak incidences, one in the perinatal period and the other around puberty. With a fully descended testis three anatomical types can occur.

In supravaginal torsion the cord twists above the tunica vaginalis so that strangulation involves the serous sac and its contents. This type is seen mainly in early infancy at which time the tunica has only a loose attachment to the scrotal wall, but it has also been described in older boys (Johnston, 1968).

Intravaginal torsion is the commonest variety of torsion. The intravaginal anatomy is abnormal. The tunica vaginalis covers the epididymis entirely and extends high on the spermatic cord so that the testis and the epididymis hang on a narrow vascular pedicle and may lie in a horizontal position when the patient stands (Angell, 1963). Twisting of the pedicle leads to strangulation of the testis and the epididymis.

Torsion of the mesorchium between the testis and the epididymis is rare and can occur only when the testis and the epididymis are widely separated. Vascular changes affect the testis alone.

Torsion during boyhood

The immediate pathogenesis of intravaginal torsion is uncertain. A strong contraction of the spirally arranged cremaster fibres may be the exciting cause. Although a history of recent injury or unusual physical exertion may be obtained, it is doubtful whether these factors are significant because symptoms often begin when the boy is at rest or asleep. The right and left testes are affected with equal frequency and the twist in the pedicle may be in either direction. Spontaneous correction is possible. If the torsion persists, vascular occlusion leads to haemor-rhagic testicular infarction. Bilateral simul-taneous torsion is a rare occurrence.

Clinical features

The onset of symptoms is often gradual rather than dramatically abrupt and pain may be experienced first in the central abdomen, the iliac fossa or the groin so that intra-abdominal pathology is simulated. There is often a history of similar milder attacks that resolved spon-taneously. On examination the testis is swollen, firm and exquisitely tender. In the early stages a skin dimple may be present in the hemiscrotal fundus (Ger, 1969) but this is obscured as the scrotal wall becomes reddened and oedematous. If the torsion is not released then the testis may undergo atrophy or, alternatively, sloughing and secondary infection may lead to discharge of necrotic material through a scrotal sinus.

Diagnosis

Testicular torsion must be distinguished as a matter of urgency from other acute scrotal swell-ings. Acute epididymitis is uncommon during childhood and when it is of sufficient severity to resemble torsion it is generally associated with symptomatic urinary tract infection and with organic pathology in the lower urinary tract. Mumps orchitis is rare in the prepubertal boy and is nearly always preceded by parotitis. Idiopathic scrotal oedema causes local tender-ness with little or no pain and the swelling and discoloration extend beyond the scrotum. In cases of torsion of the testicular appendix it may be possible to determine by palpation and trans-illumination that the tender swelling lies above and is distinct from the testis itself. The vasculi-tis of the Henoch-Schoenlein syndrome may involve the scrotum and the testis and closely resemble torsion. As a rule the cutaneous, arthritic and nephrological manifestations of the disease precede the scrotal lesion. Nevertheless diagnostic precision is rendered difficult by the fact that vasculitis may cause the development of torsion (Loh and Jalan, 1974).

Because the abnormal local anatomy that predisposes to intravaginal torsion is commonly bilateral Angell (1963) advised that a patient with suspected torsion should be examined when standing since a horizontal lie in the

opposite testis supports the diagnosis. However, it is not easy to determine the precise lie of a testis in a child when the opposite organ is swollen and extremely tender.

Radionuclide imaging employing the Anger camera and intravenous ^{99m}Tc as pertechnetate can be used to evaluate the vascularity of the scrotal contents and so differentiate hyperaemic, avascular and normally vascularized lesions. Facilities for the examination must often be planned several hours in advance so that it is of limited value in an emergency. The Doppler stethoscope detects ultrasound waves reflected back from flowing blood. The speed of move-ment of the blood cells determines the pitch and the intensity of the sound and the instrument therefore indicates whether a hyperaemic or an avascular scrotal condition exists. On occasions the Doppler stethoscope demonstrates a blood flow even when the testis is totally infarcted, possibly because of reactive hyperaemia in the surrounding tissues, and the investigation is not completely reliable for differential diagnosis (Nasrallah, Manzwe and King, 1977). If doubt exists regarding the nature of the pathology in a boy with an acute scrotal swelling surgical ex-ploration is always warranted.

Treatment

Manipulative reduction of spermatic cord tor-sion may be possible when the diagnosis is made early. The testis is gently rotated clockwise and counter-clockwise and then in the direction in which movement is freer until pain is relieved. In most cases the testis is too tender to allow this method of management and operation is re-quired urgently. The testis is exposed through a scrotal incision and the cord untwisted. Usually the tunica albuginea must be incised to allow the parenchyma to be examined. If the testis is friable or remains black then orchidectomy is needed but if the colour improves, and especial-ly if active bleeding occurs, the organ can be retained. The tunica albuginea must be sutured to the dartos muscle at three or four sites to prevent recurrence of torsion. When doubt ex-ists as to the viability of the testis its preserva-tion is warranted because Leydig cells, which have a greater resistance to ischaemia than the seminiferous tubules, may survive and function. Schneider, Kendall and Karafin (1975) consi-dered testicular fluorescence to be helpful in indicating the potential for recovery. Sodium fluorescein is injected intravenously and the testis is viable if it shows a light green fluorescence when exposed to ultraviolet light.

Whether the affected testis is retained or removed it is essential to perform prophylactic orchidopexy on the opposite side since the anatomical abnormalities predisposing to torsion are bilateral in at least 50 per cent of cases (Johnson, 1960). The contralateral testis is exposed through the scrotum and the tunica albuginea is fixed to the dartos by three or four sutures.

The possibility of salvaging the testis depends mainly on the rapidity with which the torsion is released. When the condition has been present for more than some 12 hours orchidectomy is generally unavoidable. However, the effect of cord torsion depends upon its degree as well as its duration so that a late diagnosis does not entirely preclude the possibility of testicular recovery. Although a testis may appear at operation to be worth preserving, it is commonly found to be atrophic, even to the degree of being impalpable, a few months later. Krarup (1978) recorded that this was the case with 19 of 28 saved testes in his series. He also noted that spermatozoa counts were low in men who had had unilateral torsion, suggesting the existence of a bilateral testicular abnormality.

Perinatal torsion

Torsion presenting in the newborn infant is typically of the supravaginal type. There is a bluish discoloration within the scrotum and the testis is enlarged and hard but usually not tender. The child's general condition is unaffected. In most cases it is likely that the torsion occurred prenatally even though the swelling may not have been noticed until some time after birth. Bilateral intrauterine testicular torsion has been recorded (Atallah, Ippolito and Rubin, 1976). Because the diagnosis is generally made late, opportunities for saving the testis are rare and in most cases it is doubtful whether surgical exploration is worth performing. While there is less likelihood of subsequent contralateral torsion than there is with intravaginal torsion nevertheless it seems prudent to make sure by performing orchidopexy on the other side.

Torsion of the testicular and epididymal appendices

Torsion of the intrascrotal relics of the mesonephric and paramesonephric ducts most commonly affects the appendix of the testis (one of the hydatids of Morgagni) which is a small pedunculated nodule attached to the upper pole of the testis or to the groove between it and the globus major of the epididymis. The precipitating cause of the torsion is obscure although some cases have followed physical exertion. Bilateral torsion has been described in which the appendices may twist simultaneously or sequentially (Litvak, Melnick and Leberman, 1964). Torsion of the hydatid is most common around puberty. Pain is referred to the scrotum, the abdomen or the groin and followed by swelling and redness of the hemiscrotum. The enlarged appendix may be palpable as a tender pea-sized swelling above the testis and may be demonstrable by transillumination. If a confident diagnosis can be made, no active measures are needed; the symptoms subside in a day or two and the infarcted appendix atrophies. In many cases a clear distinction from testicular torsion is not possible and exploration is needed. Treatment then consists of excision of the appendix.

Torsion of the paradidymis, the vas aberrans or the inconstantly present appendix of the epididymis is rare but examples of each type have been reported (Scoglund, McRoberts and Rayde, 1970).

Idiopathic infarction of the testis

This condition is seen mainly in the newborn infant, when its clinical features are identical with those resulting from testicular torsion. Occasionally it is bilateral. When the scrotum is explored infarctive changes are found to affect the tunica vaginalis and the testis while the spermatic cord is normal and no torsion is present. It is possible that the lesion is the result of spontaneous correction of a pre-existing torsion that had already caused irreversible ischaemic changes. Jung, McGaughey and Matlak (1980) suggested that neonatal polycythaemia and hyperviscosity may be causative.

Localized testicular infarction involving only part of the testis is a rare occurrence in older boys (Johnston, 1960; Shapiro *et al.*, 1977). Its aetiology is unknown and intratesticular haemorrhage resulting from trauma or from vascular rupture due to straining may be responsible. In the acute state the condition closely resembles testicular torsion and later a neoplasm may be simulated.

Vasculitis

In boys with Henoch-Schonlein purpura the vasculitis may involve the scrotal contents and cause acute swelling and discoloration simulating an inflammatory lesion or torsion. The diagnosis is generally clear when the typical skin rash and the arthritic and nephrological manifestations of the syndrome are already present. Occasionally the scrotal lesion appears first (Eadie and Higgins, 1964) and rarely the vasculitis may cause the development of torsion (Loh and Jalan, 1974).

Testicular strangulation with incarcerated hernia

Incarcerated inguinal hernia in young infants commonly causes strangulation of the testis by compressing the spermatic vessels against the fibrous sheath around the cord. Clinically it may be possible to palpate the enlarged tender testis below the hernia. The prevention of infarction requires prompt reduction of the hernia by manipulation, taxis and if necessary operation.

Epididymitis

Acute bacterial epididymitis is uncommon in boys. In the young child it is seen as a complication of urinary tract infection, as a rule only when there are local anatomical abnormalities that allow infection to spread along the lumen of the vas deferens. Epididymitis is often the presenting symptom in cases of ectopic ureter opening into the vas or the seminal vesicle or of union between the vas and the ureter. It may also follow indwelling urethral catheterization, especially after endoscopic fulguration of urethral valves, and is a not uncommon complication of imperforate anus with rectourethral fistula. In both these conditions urethrovasal reflux, presumably resulting from distortion of the orifices of the ejaculatory ducts, may be demonstrable on micturating urethrography.

Nonspecific epididymitis in the absence of urinary tract infection and similar to that seen in army recruits may occur in older prepubertal boys. Urethrovasal reflux is seldom seen radiologically but the condition is nevertheless believed to be due to retrograde flow of sterile urine along the vas. From urodynamic studies in such patients Koff (1976) found that 50 per cent had uninhibited detrusor contractions associated with failure of relaxation of the external urethral sphincter. In such circumstances urine may be forced from the urethra into the ejaculatory duct. Other patients had a large capacity bladder and Koff (1976) considered that when the bladder was full passive opening of the vesical neck and reflux to the vas may occur as a result of the intra-abdominal pressure being raised during physical exertion.

Sterile epididymitis is often subacute and the enlarged epididymis may be palpable as an elongated swelling distinct from the testis. The acute scrotal swelling produced by infective epididymitis can closely simulate testicular torsion but the presence of pyuria and bacilluria, fever, leukocytosis and other symptoms referable to the urinary tract should clarify the diagnosis. As discussed above, although the Doppler stethoscope provides diagnostic aid the information obtained must be considered in conjunction with the other clinical features and the laboratory results. If doubt remains as to whether the scrotal lesion is due to infection or to testicular torsion, operative exploration is fully justified.

Treatment of bacterial epididymitis is by the antibiotic appropriate to the urinary tract infection. A scrotal abscess may require incision. Recurrence of sterile epididymitis may be prevented by the patient ensuring that he empties his bladder completely before undertaking physical activity. In subjects with uninhibited detrusor contractions the administration of relaxant drugs such as propantheline bromide (Probanthine) may be effective.

Mumps orchitis

Mumps orchitis is rare during boyhood. While the complication generally develops a few days after the onset of parotitis, it occasionally precedes it. As a rule the condition is unilateral. The main late effect is testicular atrophy of variable severity. There is no treatment of proven value. Steroids and stilboestrol have been employed but their value is uncertain. Incision of the tunica albuginea to relieve tension within the testis was formerly recommended. However, the procedure is of doubtful benefit and if several of the subtunical end-arteries are divided, it may even promote the development of atrophy.

Abdominoscrotal disease

During early childhood the processus vaginalis commonly has a narrow patent lumen so that intraperitoneal exudates may find their way to the scrotum without previous clinical evidence of a hernia or hydrocele. Peritonitis, urinary ascites or intraperitoneal bleeding from an injured viscus may therefore lead to an acute scrotal swelling because of the presence of pus, urine or blood in the tunica vaginalis. In infants and young children the scrotal lesion may be the most conspicuous clinical feature. In the child with a ventriculoperitoneal shunt to control hydrocephalus CSF may similarly collect in the scrotum.

Meconium hydrocele is the result of a prenatal bowel perforation that allows meconium to escape into the peritoneum and the processus vaginalis. If the perforation remains open, bacterial peritonitis develops postnatally. The bowel may heal spontaneously and the only clinical sign is then the presence at birth of a swollen and discoloured scrotum. Radiography shows speckled calcification of the intraperitoneal and intrascrotal meconium. Treatment

involves removal of the meconium through scrotal incisions.

Spermatic venous thrombosis

Coolsaet and Weinberg (1980) reported the occurrence of thrombosis of the spermatic vein of unknown causation in three boys. The condition was diagnosed by venography or at surgical exploration and caused testicular pain and swelling and discoloration of the cord and the scrotum. It simulated testicular torsion, idiopathic scrotal oedema and inflammatory lesions.

References

Angell, J.C. (1963) Torsion of the testicle: a plea for diagnosis. *Lancet*, i, 19

Atallah, M.W., Ippolito, J.J. and Rubin, B.W. (1976) Intrauterine bilateral torsion of the spermatic cord. *Journal of Urology*, **116**, 128

Coolsaet, B. and Weinberg, R. (1980) Thrombosis of the spermatic vein in children. *Journal of Urology*, **124**, 290

Donohue, R. and Utley, W.L.F. (1975) Idiopathic fat necrosis in the scrotum. *British Journal of Urology*, **47**, 331

Eadie, D.G.A. and Higgins, P.M. (1964) Apparent torsion of the testicle in a case of Henoch-Schoenlein purpura. *British Journal of Surgery*, **51**, 634

Evans, J.P. and Snyder, H.M. (1977) Idiopathic scrotal oedema. *Urology*, **9**, 549

Ger, R. (1969) The scrotal dimple in testicular torsion. *Surgery*, **66**, 907

Goulding, F.J. (1976) Priapism caused by glucose phosphate isomerase deficiency. *Journal of Urology*, **116**, 819

Hanley, H.G. and Harrison, R.G. (1962) The nature and surgical treatment of varicocele. *British Journal of Surgery*, **50**, 64

Johnson, N. (1960) Torsion of the testis: a plea for bilateral exploration. *Medical Journal of Australia*, **1**, 653

Johnston, J.H. (1960) Localised infarction of the testis. *British Journal of Urology*, **32**, 97

Johnston, J.H. (1968) The testicles and the scrotum. In Paediatric Urology (edited by Williams, D.I.). Butterworths, London.p.450

Jung, A.L., McGaughey, H.R. and Matlak, M.E. (1980) Neonatal testicular infarction and polycythaemia. *Journal of Urology*, **123**, 781

Katz, E.R., Politano, V. and Scandiffio, M. (1976) Priapism: an unusual complication of parotitis without orchitis. *Journal of Urology*, **115**, 613

Koff, S.A. (1976) Altered bladder function and non-specific epididymitis. *Journal of Urology*, **116**, 589

Krarup, T. (1978) The testes after torsion. *British Journal of Urology*, **50**, 43

Litvak, A.S., Melnick, I. and Leberman, P.R. (1964) Torsion of the hydatid of Morgagni. *Journal of Urology*, **91**, 574

Loh, H.S. and Jalan, O.M. (1974) Testicular torsion in Henoch-Schoenlein syndrome. *British Medical Journal*, ii, 96

Mikat, D.M., Ackerman, H.R. and Mikat, K.W. (1973) Balanitis xerotica obliterans: report of a case in an 11 year old and review of the literature. *Pediatrics*, **52**, 25

Nasrallah, P.F., Manzwe, D. and King, L.R. (1977) Falsely negative Doppler examinations in testicular torsion. *Journal of Urology*, **118**, 194

Oppenheimer, R. (1976) Priapism in an 8 year old boy treated by spongiocavernosum shunt. *Journal of Urology*, **116**, 818

Oster, J. (1971) Varicocele in children and adolescents: an investigation of the incidence among Danish school children. *Scandinavian Journal of Urology and Nephrology*, **5**, 27

Schneider, H.C., Kendall, A.R. and Karafin, L. (1975) Fluorescence of the testicle: an indication of viability of spermatic cord after torsion. *Urology*, **5**, 133

Scoglund, R.W., McRoberts, J.W. and Rayde, H. (1970) Torsion of testicular appendages: presentation of 43 new cases and a collective review. *Journal of Urology*, **104**, 598

Shapiro, S.R., Rabinovitz, J., Konrad, P. and Tesluk, H. (1977) Focal infarction of the testicle in a child simulating testicular tumour. *Journal of Urology*, **118**, 485

Vaught, S.K., Litvak, A.S. and McRoberts, J.W. (1975) The surgical management of scrotal and penile lymphoedema. *Journal of Urology*, **113**, 204

Werner, H.J. and Falk, M. (1964) Acute gangrene of the scrotum in an 8 year old. *Journal of Pediatrics*, **65**, 133

Wilson, S.K., Klionsky, B.L. and Rhamy, R.K. (1973) A new etiology of priapism: Fabry's disease. *Journal of Urology*, **109**, 646

39 Male Intersex Disorders and Male Hypogonadism

Frank Harris and J.H. Johnston

The conditions described in this chapter are associated with clinically obvious undermasculinization or intersex in the XY genotypic male. Female (XX) intersex is discussed in Chapter 48. Those disorders of intersex characterized by chromosomal mosaic patterns, such as XY/XO and XY/XX, are considered in the chapter on true hermaphrodites (Chapter 45).

Clinical expression of undermasculinization may vary from a mild degree of hypogenitalism in an obviously male phenotype to the severest expression where the genotype XY is the only indication of male sex. The latter group includes the complete forms of the testicular feminization syndrome which do not present with ambiguous genitalia or problems of intersex. However, mention is made of this disorder as it represents in certain instances one end of a spectrum of pathogenetic mechanisms of sexual differentiation.

The syndromes of male intersex and undermasculinization are bedevilled by frequent changes in the eponymous nomenclature as the underlying causes become known. In this chapter eponyms are restricted to the dysmorphogenic syndromes that include intersex or undermasculinization as a feature.

Normal sexual differentiation is dealt with in Chapter 35. *Table 39.1* presents a working approach to the classification of causes of undermasculinization and male intersex.

Table 39.1 Classification of XY undermasculinization

Pathogenesis	*Cause*	
Defects in steroid biosynthesis	Deficiency of 20,22-desmolase	
	Deficiency of 20α-hydroxylase	salt-losing syndromes
	Deficiency of 22α-hydroxylase	
	Deficiency of 3β-steroid dehydrogenase	
	Deficiency of 17α-hydroxylase	non-salt-losing syndromes
	Deficiency of 17,20-desmolase	
	Deficiency of 17-oxosteroid reductase	
Failure of target tissue response	Deficiency of 5α-reductase	
	Abnormalities in 5-dihydrotestosterone cytosol receptors	
	Defect in intranuclear 5-dihydrotestosterone action	
	High binding affinity of β globulin for testosterone	
Failure of fetal pituitary		
Multiple congenital malformation syndromes		
Drugs during early pregnancy		
Miscellaneous		

Defects in steroid biosynthesis

Male intersex accompanies only those defects in steroid biosynthesis that involve pathways leading to androgen formation (*Figure 39.1*). Because some of the pathways and/or enzymes are common to both glucocorticoid and mineralocorticoid synthesis, infants with male intersex may exhibit clinical features of life-threatening acute adrenocortical insufficiency. Consequently the clinical priority is to exclude an associated salt-losing syndrome (*Table 39.1*). In these babies the

Deficiency of 20, 22-desmolase, 20-alpha-hydroxylase and 22-alpha-hydroxylase

The above deficiency states are discussed together since all three enzymes are necessary for the synthesis of pregnenolone from cholesterol (*Figure 39.1*) and can give rise to the so-called congenital adrenal lipid hyperplasia of Prader and Gurtner (1955) and Prader and Siebenmann (1957). These authors described male infants with ambiguous external genitalia, severe salt wasting and adrenal cells filled with

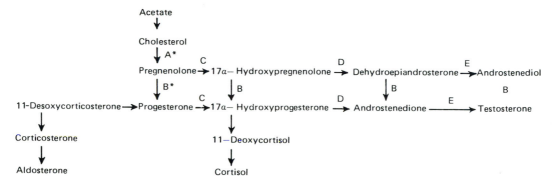

Figure 39.1. Diagram of steroid biosynthesis illustrating the sites of known enzyme defects that lead to failure of testosterone biosynthesis. The defects are common to both the adrenal cortex and the testes. Testicular androgens are derived via a Δ^5 pathway and adrenal androgens are synthesized via a Δ^4 pathway (Δ^5 = unsaturated carbon bond). A = 20α-hydroxylase, 22α-hydroxylase and 20,22-desmolase; B = 3β steroid dehydrogenase; C = 17α-hydroxylase; D = 17,20-desmolase; E = 17-ketosteroid reductase (17β-hydroxysteroid dehydrogenase). Asterisks indicate association with salt-losing syndromes (adrenal insufficiency).

enzyme deficiency causes inadequate secretion by the adrenal cortex of aldosterone and cortisol in addition to decreased formation of testosterone and its metabolites.

The clinical features of acute adrenal insufficiency may be insidious in onset. The newborn infant may present with intermittent vomiting and mild diarrhoea and then rapidly develop severe hyponatraemic dehydration with shock, acidosis and hypoglycaemia. Plasma electrolyte investigations characteristically show hyponatraemia, hypochloraemia, gross hyperkalaemia, an elevated blood urea level and a low pH with a reduced standard bicarbonate concentration. Immediate treatment consisting of rehydration with intravenous saline and replacement therapy with parenteral glucocorticoids and mineralocorticoids should be given. In symptomatic infants, however mild the symptoms, treatment should not be delayed in order to obtain urine for diagnostic purposes.

cholesterol. Although the syndrome is generally thought to be due to the 20,22-desmolase (lyase) deficiency, Degenhart (1971) and Kirkland *et al.* (1973) reported male infants with ambiguous genitalia and probable 20-alpha-hydroxylase deficiency. These patients are unable to synthesize glucocorticoids, mineralocorticoids and androgens, and die in infancy because of the adrenocortical insufficiency. In males the clinical picture is usually of such severe undermasculinization that the infants appear to be phenotypic females.

Deficiency of 3-beta-steroid dehydrogenase

This enzyme is necessary for the biosynthesis of progesterone (*Figure 39.1*) and deficiency thus leads to failure of glucocorticoid, mineralocorticoid and testosterone production with a clinical

Table 39.2 Pattern of urinary steroid excretion in enzyme defects of biosynthesis in the testis and the adrenal gland

Enzyme deficiency	Pregnetriol	Pregnanetriol	17-Keto-steroids	17 Hydroxy-corticosteroids	Dehydro-epiandrosterone	Andro-stenedione	Testosterone	Aldosterone
20, 22-Desmolase 20α-Hydroxylase 22α-Hydroxylase	All adrenocortical and testicular steroids grossly decreased							
3 β-Steroid dehydrogenase	Normal	Normal	Normal/ increased	Decreased	Increased	Decreased	Decreased	Decreased
17α-Hydroxylase		Slightly increased	Slightly decreased	Slightly decreased	Decreased	Decreased	Decreased	Decreased*
17,20-Desmolase		Normal		Normal	Decreased	Decreased	Decreased	
17-Oxosteroid reductase		Increased			Increased	Increased	Decreased	

*Increased corticosterone.

picture of male intersex and adrenal failure (Bongiovanni, 1961, 1962). Some androgen may be synthesized via the pathway of pregnenolone-1 7-hydroxypregnenolone-dehydroepiandrosterone to androstenediol (*Figure 39.1*) and so there may be less undermasculinization in some cases. Clinically affected male infants may have a small penis with a proximal urethral opening and failure of labioscrotal fusion, and thus may be no different from infants with undermasculinization from other causes. These babies tend to die early from the concomitant severe adrenocortical insufficiency and salt losses, although several have survived into childhood (Parks *et al.*, 1971; Jänne *et al.*, 1974). Urinary steroid analysis reveals elevated levels of pregnenolone, pregnenetriol and dehydroepiandrosterone, and low levels of progesterone, pregnanediol and 17-oxosteroids (*Table 39.2*).

Deficiency of 17-alpha-hydroxylase

In males 17-alpha-hydroxylase deficiency presents with a spectrum of undermasculinization resulting from a variable degree of failure of steroid biosynthesis to proceed from pregnenolone and progesterone to 17-hydroxypregnenolone and 17-hydroxyprogesterone respectively (*Figure 39.1*). Consequently there are reduced levels of testosterone and cortisol and increased levels of 11-desoxycorticosterone and corticosterone, which do not require 17-alpha-hydroxylase for their biosynthesis (*Table 39.1*). These infants do not have salt-losing states. New (1970) reported the first affected male, in whom a partial deficiency of the enzyme was demonstrated. The patient presented with ambiguous external genitalia and failed to virilize at puberty, developing gynaecomastia. Clinically these

males can be indistinguishable from patients with partial testicular feminization due to failure of peripheral testosterone action.

Deficiency of 17, 20-desmolase

This enzyme converts both 17-alpha-hydroxypregnenolone and 17-alpha-hydroxyprogesterone to dehydroepiandrosterone and androstenedione respectively. The first family with a disorder due to its deficiency was described by Zachman *et al.* (1972). Two XY cousins had ambiguous genitalia and bilateral incompletely descended testes and a maternal XY 'aunt' was similarly affected. Breast development was not reported, but gynaecomastia would not be anticipated if the enzyme deficiency were complete because oestrogen would not be synthesized (*Figure 39.2*; Goebelsmann *et al.*, 1974).

Deficiency of 17-ketosteroid reductase (17-beta-hydroxysteroid dehydrogenase)

In the first report of this disorder two XY siblings were described with ambiguous genitalia and inguinal testes (Saez *et al.*, 1971, 1972). At puberty the patients, who had been raised as girls, became virilized with clitoral enlargement and male pubic hair distribution and developed breast enlargement. These two subjects were unable to convert androstenedione to testosterone (*Figures 39.1 and 39.2*). Goebelsmann *et al.* (1973), Knorr, Pidlingmaier and Engelhardt (1973) and Givens *et al.* (1974) described further XY patients with ambiguous genitalia in whom

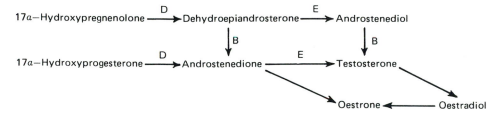

Figure 39.2. Simplified scheme of oestrogen (C17) biosynthesis from androgens (C19). B = 3β-steroid dehydrogenase; D = 17,20-desmolase; E = 17-oxosteroid reductase (17β-hydroxysteroid dehydrogenase).

a deficiency of 17-ketosteroid reductase resulted in low plasma testosterone levels with raised plasma androstenedione and oestrone concentrations (*Table 39.2*). Breast enlargement is not a constant feature in these case reports. When given HCG 2000 iu on alternate days for three doses such infants should respond with a disproportionate increase in plasma androstenedione and oestrone levels compared to plasma testosterone and oestradiol concentrations.

Failure of target tissue response–androgen resistance

It is now clear that there is a series of target tissue defects which may impair response to testosterone and may be complete or incomplete (*Table 39.3*). These clinical syndromes have a confusing and changing series of eponyms, for example Reifenstein's syndrome, Lub's syndrome and Wilson's type I and type 2 syndromes.

Table 39.3　Failure of target tissue response

Clinical syndrome	Endocrine-metabolic defect
Complete testicular feminization	5α-Reductase deficiency
	Abnormal
Incomplete testicular feminization (XY intersex or undermasculinization)	5-dihydrotestosterone cytosol receptors
	Defect in nuclear 5-dihydrotestosterone action
	High binding affinity of β-globulin for testosterone

Unlike other steroid hormones testosterone acts as a prohormone and must be reduced by the enzyme 5-alpha-reductase to 5-alpha-dihydrotestosterone in order to exert its biological action. This reaction takes place in the cytoplasm of the target tissue cells where 5-alpha-dihydrotestosterone is taken up by a receptor protein to form a complex which is transferred to an intranuclear acceptor protein. This nuclear acceptor complex of protein and 5-alpha-dihydrotestosterone is bound to DNA and then further synthesis of nuclear protein is stimulated (Griffin and Wilson, 1980).

The degree of androgen resistance resulting from target tissue defects is variable and a spectrum of clinical disorders is encountered that ranges from the complete testicular feminization syndrome through male intersex with ambiguous genitalia to recognizably male infants with undermasculinization.

Complete testicular feminization syndrome

These patients do not present with ambiguity of phenotypic sex and are only discussed briefly in this chapter as a preliminary to the further discussion of so-called incomplete testicular feminization syndromes. The diagnosis of complete testicular feminization may be suspected in the young phenotypic female infant if bilateral masses are found in the labia or a gonad (testis) is present in an inguinal hernia. Approximately half of these patients have inguinal hernias but few females with inguinal hernias have complete testicular feminization (Jagiello and Atwell, 1962). In a rare instance the diagnosis was made from an antenatal amniocentesis finding of an XY karyotype followed by observation of a female phenotype at birth (Williams, 1979). The sex of the fetus had not been revealed to the parents at the time of amniocentesis.

If the diagnosis of complete testicular feminization cannot be made at birth then the usual sequence of events is for the patient to present as a teenager with primary amenorrhoea. At that time the phenotypic appearance and demeanour are obviously female with normal to relatively large breasts. Scanty pubic and axillary hair may be present. While the external genitalia are those of a normal female the vagina may be vestigial and present as a dimple or a short blind pouch. There is no uterus or cervix. The testes may be intra-abdominal or anywhere along the anatomical pathway of normal descent, and they produce male age-appropriate levels of testosterone.

A considerable body of literature has accumulated concerning the aetiology of complete testicular feminization. Simpson (1976) reviewed the then current theories including the possibilities of a high protein-binding affinity of beta-globulin for testosterone, a deficiency of 5-alpha-reductase and an abnormality of intracellular binding of 5-alpha-dihydrotestosterone or of nuclear transcription. The disorder is inherited as either a sex-linked (X-linked) recessive or a male limited autosomal dominant trait. Many familial examples have been reported and it appears that the phenotype is constant in any kindred; that is complete and incomplete testicular feminization have not occurred in the same family.

The risk of gonadoblastoma occurring in a dysgenetic gonad resides primarily in the presence of tissue containing Y chromosomes. Hence the possibility of neoplastic change in a dysgenetic intra-abdominal gonad is greater in XY individuals than in XO ones such as in Turner's syndrome. The number of reported cases of gonadoblastoma (and hence its incidence) is lower than one might expect from its pre-eminence in clinical discussion. Scully (1970) reviewed 74 cases and a similar number have been reported as individuals or in small series. The vast majority of phenotypic females with gonadoblastoma have gonadal tissue containing Y chromosomes. A very small number of patients have a leukocytic XX karyotype or are chromatin positive (de Bacalao and Dominiquez, 1969; Talerman, 1971). However, this does not preclude the presence of Y chromosomal fragments in the affected gonadal tissue (Khodr *et al.*, 1979). Familial incidence of gonadoblastoma in XY gonadal tissue has been recorded on a number of occasions. Genetically determined forms of XY intersex with a partial or complete female phenotype are therefore at risk (Cohen and Shaw, 1965; Talerman, 1971; Ionescu and Maximilian 1977).

Subjects with complete testicular feminization are reared as females and medical management is confined to counselling, gonadectomy and vaginoplasty when necessary. While there is general agreement that the gonads should be extirpated the timing of gonadectomy is controversial. When there is no doubt that the patient has complete testicular feminization and the testes are not obvious then they may be left *in situ* until after the onset of breast development. It is commonly alleged that breast development with the testes *in situ* is better than that obtained with postgonadectomy oestrogen therapy. The authors believe that the gonads should be removed early if there is any doubt about partial virilization occurring at puberty, the masses are obvious and likely to be traumatized, or the continued presence of the gonads is injuring parental acceptance of the patient's female gender role.

Incomplete testicular feminization syndrome

This syndrome is a nosological bag of worms. Clinically these patients present with a spectrum of signs ranging from recognizably underdeveloped male to completely ambiguous external genitalia (*Figure 39.3*). They have bilateral

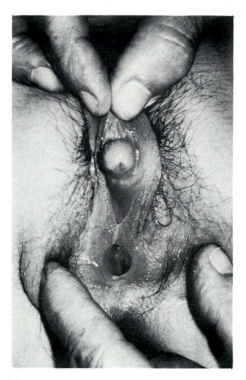

Figure 39.3. Clinical photograph to demonstrate and record salient clinical features in a patient with XY karyotype diagnosed as having probable deficiency of 17-ketosteroid-reductase.

testes and at puberty develop both male (phallic enlargement and hair) and female (breasts) secondary sexual characteristics. There are no female internal genitalia and normal male testosterone levels are present.

Familial occurrence of this undermasculinization syndrome has been reported under a number of eponyms (Reifenstein, 1947; Gilbert-Dreyfus, Sebaoun and Belaisch, 1957; Lubs, Vilar and Bergenstal, 1959; Wilson *et al.*, 1974). It is likely that the earlier case reports include patients who today would be shown by current techniques to have an enzyme deficiency in androgen synthesis. A suggested pathogenesis of incomplete testicular feminization is based on the concept of partial target tissue resistance due to incomplete 5-alpha-reductase deficiency, a partial intracytoplasmic dihydrotestosterone binding defect, or a partial intranuclear transcription defect. The authors conclude that at present the term incomplete testicular feminization syndrome serves no useful purpose. These patients should be grouped under the generic name of male (XY) intersex or undermasculinization syndrome, except for those in whom a specific cause is found.

Management of incomplete testicular feminization can be exceedingly difficult. Even if phallic size is reasonable at the time of presentation the androgen unresponsiveness in the child reared as a boy leads to severe hypogenitalism and impotence. The alternative is assignment to the female sex with a commitment to reconstructive vaginoplasty following phallic resection and gonadectomy.

Pseudovaginal perineoscrotal hypospadias

This type of male intersex was given its descriptive title by Nowaskoski and Lenz (1961) and should be clinically recognizable and therefore distinguishable from the other disorders mentioned. At birth these infants are often assigned to the female sex and reared as girls until puberty when they develop significant virilization. There is no breast development. The external genitalia characteristically consist of a clitoris-like phallus, a perineal urethral orifice and a further pseudovaginal perineal orifice that ends blindly. The testes have the same appearance histologically as undescended gonads.

Patients with these features have been described as having androgen-sensitive pseudohermaphroditism (Jirasèk, 1971), incomplete male pseudohermaphroditism type II (Walsh *et al.*, 1974) and familial perineal hypospadias (Grumbach and Van Wyk, 1974). An autosomal mode of inheritance has been shown. Imperato-McGinley *et al.* (1974) and Walsh *et al.* (1974) demonstrated a deficiency of 5-alpha-reductase in their patients with pseudovaginal perineoscrotal hypospadias. As anticipated plasma testosterone levels are normal.

The diagnosis of pseudovaginal perineoscrotal hypospadias due to 5-alpha-reductase deficiency can be confirmed soon after birth by direct assay of enzyme activity in perineoscrotal or preputial tissue or in fibroblast culture. This permits the correct assisgnment of sex of rearing, which should be male.

Fetal pituitary (gonadotrophin) deficiency

Observations in animals by Jost (1972) suggest that intrauterine gonadotrophin deficiency should cause undermasculinization or male intersex. There is little evidence of this occurring in the human fetus and leading to male intersex at birth. Clement *et al.* (1976) demonstrated that fetal Leydig's cells can be stimulated by chorionic gonadotrophin and this may account for the development of external genitalia in anencephalic male infants. However, Siler-Khodr, Morgenstern and Greenwood (1974) and Park, Aimakhu and Jones (1975) reported examples of male intersex attributable to intrauterine gonadotrophin deficiency. Hypogenitalism of a clearly male phenotype has been recognized with either isolated congenital gonadotrophin deficiency or gonadotrophin deficiency in combination with a congenital lack of growth hormone.

Multiple congenital malformation syndromes

Undermasculinization of the external genitalia may occur in association with a large number of congenital malformation or dysmorphology syndromes (Smith, 1970). The associated genital abnormality varies in severity from a mild degree of hypospadias to such severe underdevelopment of the external genitalia that on external examination the true sex may be in doubt (*Table 39.4*). In most of these dysmorphogenetic states the nongenital malformations are the primary indication for obtaining a karyotype which additionally serves to confirm the genetic sex of the patient. A number of the disorders are lethal in early childhood and/or accompanied by severe mental retardation, for

Table 39.4 Syndromes of congenital malformations associated with undermasculinization

---

*Pseudohermaphroditism with Wilms' tumour and renal anomalies
*Smith-Lemli-Opitz syndrome
*Opitz syndrome
*Camptomelic dwarfism
*Meckel syndrome
*Brachioskeletal-genital syndrome
*Mental retardation and cardiomyopathy syndrome
  Noonan's syndrome
  Ullrich-Feichtiger syndrome
  Trisomy 13
  4p− syndrome
  Dp+ syndrome
  18q− syndrome
  Prader-Willi syndrome
  Seckel birdheaded dwarf
  Aarskog syndrome
  Cornelia de Lange syndrome

---

*Undermasculinization may be severe enough for the external genitalia to be considered ambiguous or intersexual.

example trisomy 13, camptomelic dwarfism, Cornelia de Lange syndrome and Smith-Lemli-Opitz syndrome. Under these circumstances a low clinical priority may be placed on invasive and intensive investigation and management. Nevertheless each patient should be assessed and treated on his merits and this usually requires a combined approach by the paediatrician and the surgeon.

The association of male intersexuality and renal pathology is of particular interest. Wilms' tumour has been reported in male pseudohermaphrodites (Le Maree *et al.*, 1971; Stump and Garrett, 1954; Di George and Harley, 1966) while a further small group of male intersex patients had Wilms' tumour in association with glomerulonephritis (Drash *et al.*, 1970; Spear *et al.*, 1971; Barakat *et al.*, 1974). Two males with intersex described by Barakat *et al.* (1974) developed typical nephrotic syndrome without Wilms' tumour. In some reported cases the blood karyotype was XY, but a chromosomal XX/XY mosaic has been recorded (Denys *et al.*, 1967) and so it is recommended that in addition skin and gonad should be submitted for chromosome analysis. The above association led Barakat *et al.* (1974) to speculate that the renal elements of the syndrome originate at that early stage of embryogenesis when the genital anomaly arises. At present there is no indication as to

the basic defect that is common to male intersex, renal neoplasm and glomerulonephritis.

Drugs in early pregnancy

A small number of male infants whose mothers had been prescribed progesterone during early pregnancy have been reported to have penile or perineoscrotal hypospadias. A wide variety of progesterones have been implicated including medroxyprogesterone, 17-alpha-hydroxy-progesterone, caproate and norethisterone (Aarskog, 1970; Summitt, 1972). A causal relationship has not yet been established by this small number of reported cases. It is possible that other drugs may also lead to varying degrees of undermasculinization and have the capability of destroying the fetal gonad if given during very early pregnancy. Heller and Jones (1964) described ovarian dysgenesis resulting from busulphan administered during pregnancy.

Miscellaneous disorders

There are individual infants and children in whom the aetiology of XY intersex or under-masculinization remains obscure even after most intensive investigation. Lockhart *et al.* (1979) drew attention to the mechanical factors in embryological failure that may lead to findings of pseudovaginal perineoscrotal hypospadias.

Introduction to clinical examination

Differentiation *in utero* of the external genitalia into the normal male phenotype requires the presence and the action at the correct time of a number of hormones and factors and also the appropriate response from the target tissue. Defects or deficiencies in this process have the common outcome of undermasculinization which may vary in degree from hypospadias alone to a perineum that is so undifferentiated as to cast doubt on the patient's genotypic sex.

The optimum time for the detection of genital anomalies is at birth when the infant is examined routinely. At this time the clinical assessment must include a committed examination of the external genitalia and not just a cursory inspection. In all infants the inguinal and perineal regions are inspected and felt for hernias and palpable masses. In male infants the presence of descended testes is established. The scrotum is evaluated for complete fusion and texture, the phallus is palpated to confirm the presence of corporal tissue and the prepuce is inspected. The presence of any unusual pigmentation should be recognized. The position and patency of the anus are checked and the median raphe is examined.

A number of infants with ambiguous external genitalia or significant undermasculinization present after the newborn period and occasionally as late as early adolescence. The clinical assessment of such patients must take into account the additional features of development that are age dependent.

Clinical history

A family history is taken, paying attention to relatives with known genital abnormality, unmarried or childless relations and unusual patterns of pubertal development. Regarding the propositus the mother is asked about details of the conception (for instance infertility and use of fertility agents), her pregnancy (for example bleeding and administration of hormonal agents), and intercurrent infections and self-administered drugs. In the case of older children enquiries are made as to the sex of rearing and the gender role.

Clinical examination

A general assessment is made of the state of hydration, physical growth (length/height and weight) and nutrition. Any pigmentation or extragenital malformations are noted. Systematic examination must include blood pressure measurement.

Local examination

Genital examination should take account of the morphology and the size of the phallus; the site of the urethral orifice; fusion of the labioscrotal folds to form a scrotum and the presence of rugae; and any gonadal masses in the scrotum, the labioscrotal folds or the inguinal region. The presence of an orifice in the perineal midline is detected by examination from the base of the phallus along the median raphe to the anus. Rectal examination and assessment of the pelvic contents, for example for the presence of a uterus, are performed and the voiding of urine is observed.

In older patients, namely adolescents, the degree and the type of secondary sexual characteristics are assessed according to the Tanner (1962) classification regarding the quantity and distribution of pubic hair and the size and nature of breast development. Adequate assessment of the child's gender identity and gender role must be carried out by a member of the team with appropriate training and experience.

The clinical features of undermasculinization are rarely specific enough to indicate the precise aetiology, although they may present clues to the pathogenetic mechanism as follows:
1. A 'gonad' palpable in the inguinal region or the labioscrotal folds is most likely to contain testicular XY tissue
2. Abnormal pigmentation suggests a form of the adrenogenital syndrome occurring in a masculinized XX female
3. Breast development (gynaecomastia in XY intersex patients) at puberty suggests either defects in testosterone action and an unopposed oestrogen effect or a block in androgen biosynthesis that nevertheless permits oestrogen production, for example 17-ketosteroid-reductase deficiency (*Figure 39.2*).

The disorders discussed in this chapter are by definition in patients with an XY karyotype of the blood, the skin and the gonads.

The investigations listed in *Table 39.5* present a series of studies that allow the clinician to establish a diagnosis and therefore proceed to make decisions on therapy. In the immediate newborn infant the presence of falling plasma sodium and bicarbonate levels and rising plasma potassium and urea levels in an infant with male intersex immediately suggests one of the three proximal enzyme defects in steroid biosynthesis that lead to salt-losing states. (Estimation of plasma cortisol concentration by

Table 39.5   Investigations in male intersexual patients

Blood and skin karyotype
Urea and electrolytes
Urinary excretion of 17-oxogenic steroids and 17-oxosteroids
   with androgen fractionation for dehydroepiandrosterone,
   pregnanetriol and androstenedione
Plasma testosterone, plasma oestradiol and urinary steroid
   responses to intramuscular HCG
FSH/LH-RH stimulation for plasma LH and FSH, plasma
   testosterone and plasma β-oestradiol
*Nitrogen retention in response to testosterone

Examination under anaesthesia

Urethroscopy } with contrast X-rays
'Vaginoscopy' }
Gonadal biopsy, if necessary by laparotomy, for histology
   and karyotype and *in vitro* steroid synthesis studies
Prepuce and/or labioscrotal biopsy for assay of 5α-reductase
   activity
Clinical photography

*If incomplete or partial testicular feminization is suspected.

fluorimetric methods can yield misleading results because certain precursors fluoresce highly yet are only present in small amounts.) Plasma assays for the specific precursors in these defects are unavailable generally outside the steroid reference research laboratories. A prompt start should be made to obtain accurate 24-hour collections of urine. In male intersex patients without salt-losing disorders androgen fractionation is required in addition to total steroid estimation (*Table 39.2*).

The authors have found FSH/LH-RH stimulation of plasma LH and FSH relatively uninformative as an indication of testicular failure in very young patients. A short course of HCG 1500 iu daily for 3 days followed by analysis for plasma testosterone and beta-oestradiol, and urinary steroid C19 and C18 fractions can provide more useful data on the presence of the testis and its ability to produce testosterone and can shed more light on the level of an enzyme defect. Zachman (1972) described the use of a single dose of HCG 5000 iu/m^2 and analysis of the urine output for the following 6 days.

Examination under anaesthesia by a clinician experienced in these disorders is a valuable diagnostic tool. This opportunity is used to obtain detailed information about the genital and urethral anatomy, and also to procure tissue for histological examination of the gonad if it is palpable and accessible in the inguinal region or labioscrotal fold. Material for chromosome studies and under appropriate circumstances for *in vitro* synthesis studies can be obtained in addition. A small skin biopsy from labioscrotal, scrotal or preputial tissue can be incubated with testosterone C14 to test for dihydrotestosterone production. In some patients a laparotomy is necessary for gonadal biopsy. Good quality clinical photographs provide the best notation of the findings (*Figure 39.3*).

Treatment

Specific drug treatment of testosterone deficiency states

If the pathogenesis of the undermasculinization is the result of inadequate testosterone production then testosterone should be administered provided that a phallus is present. There are no firm guidelines available for an optimum and proven treatment regimen with respect to dosage and duration of treatment. The authors favour an initial 6-week course of testosterone esters by intramuscular injection with follow-up assessment of their effect on phallic size, the pubic hair and the scrotum, and the labioscrotal skin. The external genital changes following treatment should be graded according to the staging described by Tanner (1962). Notes are also made of unwanted effects such as acceleration of bone age as shown by wrist radiographs and acneiform changes. The appearance of pubic hair is a fair and early test of testosterone responsiveness. An alternative mode of treatment is HCG injection twice weekly in cases shown to be responsive to the hormone. There are no controlled studies of the relative efficacy of these regimens. The unproven hypothesis of an early sensitive period for androgen responsiveness of these tissues recommends early commencement of treatment and its continuation throughout childhood with short courses of testosterone.

General counselling

It is not unknown for the clinician to overlook the parents' need for repeated in-depth counselling about their infant's problem. The clinical interest engendered by these relatively uncommon and complex disorders tends to overshadow the necessity for the time-consuming process of passing on information and advice. The many taboos surrounding discussion by adults of their own sexual problems are to some extent present as well with parents concerning their infant's genital anomaly. It is therefore up to the clinician to introduce the sexual aspects of male intersex for discussion and to anticipate many of the unvoiced concerns that the parents may feel. In the authors' experience parents rarely ask whether their child is more likely to become a homosexual or be promiscuous or be in any way psychosexually abnormal, although these uncertainties cause them serious unvoiced concern. A common area of confusion is the difference between fertility and virility.

It is the authors' practice to maintain regular follow-up of these children and their parents in the paediatric endocrine clinic. Over a period of time parents are more readily able to confide their fears and ask for advice. Parents are urged to maintain confidentiality about their child's intersex without causing them to feel that there is any shame or disgust attached to the disorder but basing the recommendation on the child's need for privacy now and later in life. Information of these disorders is not passed on to community-based child health or school health services unless there is a special indication. The view is taken that these children can be perfectly well educated at school without teachers or social workers being informed of their diagnosis.

In the genetically determined disorders, and most of the conditions in this chapter are hereditary, there is a need for genetic counselling. The majority of the enzyme disorders are autosomal recessive traits while a few are X-linked dominant. Under these circumstances the risks range from one in four to one in two with any pregnancy. The genetic aspects of the disorders require careful explanation because some parents assume that the abnormality in the child's genitalia is the result of their own sexual and/or psychosexual practices. Contrary to the general view that the public is well informed about sex it is the authors' experience that it is singularly ill informed about the biology of sexual differentiation.

Male intersex or undermasculinization characterized by testosterone unresponsiveness and absent phallus

It is recommended that these unfortunate males be reared as females and registered or reregistered as female infants as soon as possible after birth. If needed, phallic recession should be carried out early. In testosterone-unresponsive disorders the gonads may either be removed in infancy or left *in situ* until after adolescence. Many of these children have either a vestigial vagina or only a dimple that requires major reconstructive surgery at a later date. It is the authors' view that reconstructive surgery in an otherwise phenotypic female provides a more acceptable quality of life than a male gender role and identity with gross male hypogenitalism. However, each patient needs to be judged on the individual clinical, psychosocial and psychosexual features. The above views represent the general policy practised in our clinic. Additionally the age of presentation modifies the approach and options that are available. The older the child at the time of presentation the more restricted are the chances for sex reversal (Money and Ehrhardt, 1972).

Change of sex on a birth certificate in England

In those rare instances where a change from the initial registered sex is necessary parents may be assisted by the following advice on initiating the procedure. Because they may feel inhibited from approaching the counter at the local Births Registration Office they are recommended to arrange by letter an appointment to see in private the local Superintendent Registrar of Births. The parents require from the clinician in charge a brief letter certifying the clinical need for reassignment of sex. The local Superintendent Registrar takes the process to the Registrar General who may authorize a new birth certificate and amend the original entry on the NHS computer.

Hypogonadism

For the purposes of this section the discussion of hypogonadism is confined to the problem of phenotypic males presenting as teenagers with symptoms and signs of hypogonadism (*Table 39.6*). Commonly these teenage boys are referred because of a delay in the onset of puberty.

Table 39.6 Clinical features of hypogonadism causing delayed puberty

Absence of erections, nocturnal emissions and libido
Lack of facial, axillary and pubic hair
Persistence of juvenile voice
Sitting:standing height less than 1:2
Prepubertal external genitalia (small penis and scrotum)
Small or absent testes

The initial sign of male pubertal onset is testicular enlargement to a testicular volume of 4 ml+ measured using the Prader orchidometer. The mean age for this is approximately 12 years with a range of 10–14 years for the third and 97th centiles in British boys. This testicular enlargement is accompanied by an increase in size of the scrotum with reddening of the scrotal skin. Tanner (1962) developed a widely accepted staging method for pubic hair and

Table 39.7 Staging of puberty

	External genitalia	Pubic hair
Stage I	Preadolescent	Preadolescent
Stage II	Enlargement of testis, scrotal skin reddens with some rugosity	Sparse growth of long slightly pigmented hair, straight or curled at base of penis
Stage III	Enlargement of penis, initially mainly in length, further growth of testis and scrotum	Considerably darker, coarser and more curled hair spreads sparsely over junction of pubes
Stage IV	Increase in size of penis with growth in breadth and development of glans, testis and scrotum larger, scrotal skin darkened	Hair adult in type, area covered less than in adult and not on medial surface of thighs
Stage V	Genitalia adult in size and shape	Hair adult in quantity and type and on medial surface of thighs
Stage VI		Hair spreads up linea alba

Table 39.8 Causes of delayed puberty

Idiopathic or constitutional delay in puberty	
Hypergonadotrophic hypogonadism	Congenital anorchia
	Acquired anorchia
	Klinefelter's syndrome
Hypogonadotrophic hypogonadism	Craniopharyngioma, pituitary adenoma
	Postcerebral irradiation (cerebral tumours)
	Postmeningitis (tuberculous)
	Post-traumatic
	Kallmann's syndrome (anosmia, cryptorchidism, deafness)
	Prader-Willi syndrome (hypotonia, later obesity, mental subnormality)
	Laurence-Moon-Biedl syndrome (retinitis pigmentosa, polydactyly, obesity, mental subnormality)
	Isolated gonadotrophin deficiency

external genital development during puberty (*Table 39.7*). This clinical scheme facilitates serial assessments by the same or different observers.

The causes of delayed puberty are listed in *Table 39.8*. So-called constitutional delay in puberty is the most common reason in males for late onset of secondary sexual characteristics. These boys usually present with both short stature and sexual immaturity (*Figure 39.4*). The pattern of physical growth in this disorder includes a height at or below the third centile with a previously normal growth velocity for age. Skeletal maturation is appropriate for height age and not chronological age. A family history of delayed puberty is not uncommon and the expectation is for these patients eventually to attain normal stature. However, some boys are genetically small in addition to the delayed onset of the pubertal growth spurt. In this case the eventual onset of a growth spurt does not take them above the third centile. Patients with constitutional delay in puberty may yield a hypogonadotrophic response to FSH/LH-RH and therefore on this test may be indistinguishable from those with permanent hypogonadotrophic hypogonadism. The diagnosis of the former is essentially a clinical one and investigations other than accurate measurement of growth and skeletal maturation should be deferred pending further longitudinal assessment over a period of many months.

Management of teenagers with constitutional

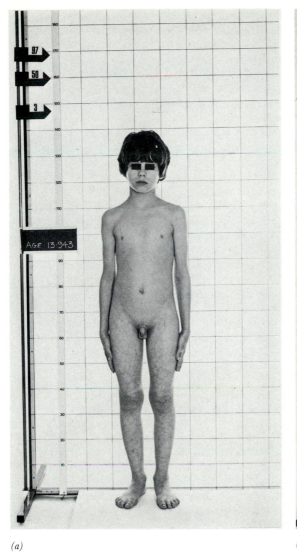

(a)

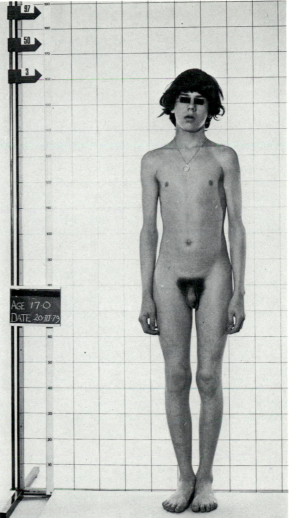

(b)

Figure 39.4. *(a)*Constitutional delay in puberty presenting at 13.9 years with hypogenitalism and short stature. *(b)* Follow-up at 17.0 years after supportive treatment by counselling alone and no hormone therapy.

delay in growth and puberty is based on counselling and support. Hormone therapy is indicated exclusively in boys sustaining severe psychological pressures because of their physical and sexual immaturity. A short course of HCG 1500 iu twice or three times a week by injection to induce the appearance of some pubic hair and genital enlargement may provide sufficient respite until puberty begins spontaneously.

The further causes of hypogonadism listed in *Table 39.8* may be divided conveniently into hypogonadotrophic and hypergonadotrophic hypogonadism. In the absence of clinical features such as anorchia or evidence of intracra-

nial disease the definitive investigations include the FSH/LH-RH and HCG stimulation tests to ascertain the status of the pituitary-gonadal axis. In hypergonadotrophic hypogonadism both basal plasma FSH and LH levels are elevated and there is an exaggerated plasma response to FSH/LH-RH (*Figure 39.5*). In hypogonadotrophic hypogonadism the basal plasma FSH and LH levels are low and may or may not increase depending whether the primary defect is in the hypothalamus or the pituitary. With the former the administration of FSH/LH-RH may cause a rise in plasma FSH and LH concentrations whereas in the latter the pituitary is unable

Plasma FSH (ng/ml)　　　Plasma LH (ng/ml)

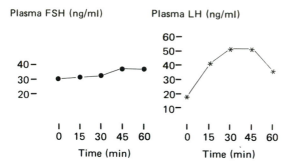

Figure 39.5. Mean plasma FSH and LH levels from four males referred with hypogonadism following failed orchidopexy for bilateral cryptorchidism (100 μg FSH/LH-RH was given intravenously). Note the high basal levels and the exaggerated and sustained response characteristic of hypergonadotrophic hypogonadism.

to respond and plasma FSH and LH levels remain low.

HCG may be used to assess the integrity of the testis in boys with delayed onset of puberty. After three daily injections of HCG 1500–2500 iu the plasma testosterone level should exceed twice the pretest value. Additional investigations may include testing of other pituitary functions, skull radiography, computed tomography and chromosome analysis.

Management

The following recommendations should be considered against the background of a specific

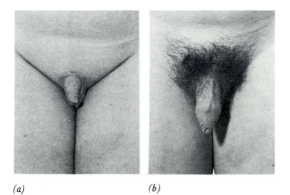

(a)　　　　　　　　　*(b)*

Figure 39.6. *(a)* A patient with hypergonadotrophic hypogonadism referred following failed bilateral orchidopexy in early childhood. Treatment was intramuscular injection of testosterone esters. *(b)* Follow-up photograph after 1 year's treatment.

diagnosis. The general approach to the management of these boys includes a serious commitment to explain the disorder and its implications for potency and fertility to the patient (depending on his age and ability to understand) and his parents. At or around the average age of onset of puberty in the patient's peer group androgen provides the most easily managed form of replacement therapy to induce pubertal changes. A mixture of testosterone esters (propionate, phenylpropionate, isocaproate and decanoate) can be given as an oily solution by intramuscular injection every 3–4 weeks (*Figure 39.6*). After pubertal changes have been achieved it may be desirable in patients with hypogonadotrophic hypogonadism to intermittently replace the testosterone by HCG. This may avoid testosterone-induced depression of testicular function and allow fertility to be achieved by using HCG at a later age. Patients with anorchia require insertion of testicular prostheses. This procedure should be done at a stage when the scrotum has developed sufficiently to contain a prosthesis with a volume of more than 12 ml on each side.

Surgical aspects

Male intersex

Many relevant aspects of the surgical management of the undermasculinized or intersex male are discussed in other chapters.

Male role

When a male role is to be followed in a child with a severely hypospadiac phallus treatment is along the lines described for perineal hypospadias (*see* Chapter 36). Orchidopexy or the insertion of testicular prostheses may be needed (*see* Chapter 37).

Very often such cases have a persistent relic of the müllerian uterovaginal canal. This may take the form either of a closed cyst or more commonly of a tubular vagina-like enlargement of the prostatic utricle which communicates with the posterior urethra and acts like a urethral diverticulum (*Figure 39.7*). The size of the anomaly is unrelated to the degree of penile malformation (Morgan, Williams and Pryor, 1982). Similar relics of the müllerian duct may occur in males

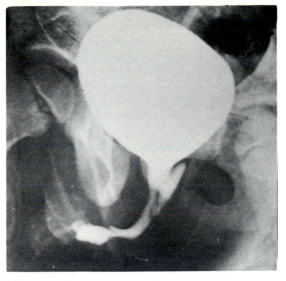

(a)

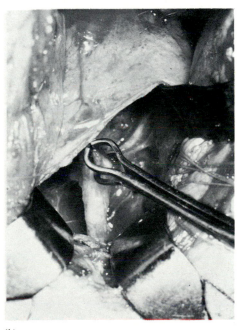

(b)

Figure 39.7. Diverticular prostatic utricle in a hypospadiac boy causing recurrent epididymitis. *(a)* Micturating cystourethrogram. *(b)* Diverticulum (held in forceps) exposed by transvesical approach splitting the trigone.

pouch during voiding may produce dribbling after micturition as the diverticulum re-empties into the urethra. Recurrent infection with urethral bleeding can be a problem and epididymitis may occur as a consequence of urethrovasal or diverticulovasal reflux. On occasions an intradiverticular calculus forms. Often a swelling is palpable on rectal examination. A diverticulum is generally demonstrable by its filling with contrast during micturating cystourethrography. Otherwise endoscopic catheterization of the orifice followed by retrograde injection is needed.

Surgical removal of a müllerian ductal cyst or diverticulum is needed only if troublesome complications occur. Operative exposure of the lesion transabdominally can be extremely awkward and dissection from the perineum or through a parasacral pararectal approach is hardly less difficult and carries the risk of damage to the nervi erigentes or the urethral sphincters. Exposure is most readily achieved transvesically. After the bladder is opened anteriorly in customary fashion the trigone is incised vertically to open the retrovesical and retrourethral spaces (*Figure 39.7*). In some instances the vasa deferentia open into the müllerian relic or are intimately adherent to its wall so that division of the vasa may be unavoidable.

Female role

In a male intersex patient with a poorly developed phallus a female upbringing is necessary. Surgery to the genitalia requires either removal or recession of the phallus, depending upon its size, and vaginoplasty to open the vaginal introitus onto the perineum. The technique is similar to that described in Chapter 44 for girls with the adrenogenital syndrome.

Intra-abdominal or intracanalicular gonads containing cells bearing a Y chromosome must be excised because of their malignant potential. Such organs occur in complete and incomplete forms of the testicular feminization syndrome and the timing of gonadectomy has already been discussed. Technically little difficulty is experienced. When the gonads can be manipulated into inguinal hernias they are readily removed with excision of the hernial sacs through separate groin incisions. When they are entirely intra-abdominal a transperitoneal approach is indicated.

with normal external genitals and the condition is presumed to represent a minor degree of the persistent müllerian duct syndrome (see below) and to be of similar aetiology.

The ductal anomalies are frequently asymptomatic but reflux of urine into a diverticular

Management of the absent or rudimentary vagina in the XY child to whom a female role has been allocated is deferred until the patient is past the age of puberty and is fully motivated to cooperate in the appropriate therapy. The hypoplastic vagina in the testicular feminization syndrome may be gradually increased in depth and calibre by the use of Pyrex tubes of graduated size (Frank, 1938). Starting with the smallest one the tubes are firmly pressed into the vagina by the patient until the largest can be accommodated. When the vagina is nonexistent, as may occur in the more masculinized forms of target organ failure, surgical intervention is needed. The techniques available are discussed under Congenital absence of the vagina (*See* Chapter 40).

The persistent müllerian duct syndrome

This condition was originally described by Nilson (1939) as hernia uteri inguinalis and affects phenotypic males with a 46 XY karyotype. The penis is normally formed but one, or more commonly both, testes are undescended, often with an associated clinically apparent inguinal hernia. There is thus no clinical evidence of intersexuality and the abnormalities are generally discovered only at operation for hernia repair and/or orchidopexy. The testes are macroscopically normal and vasa deferentia are present although the epididymides may be absent or malformed. On each side there is a fallopian tube joining a small uterus and an upper vagina which is shown by subsequent endoscopic or radiological investigations to open into the posterior urethra. As already discussed there are lesser degrees of the anomaly in which only the vagina is represented. Histologically the testes show no abnormality during early childhood while in older children or adults tubular immaturity and hypoplasia have been found (Sloan and Walsh, 1976).

The condition results from either absent or deficient secretion of antimüllerian hormone by the fetal testes or an unusually high resistance of the müllerian duct to the hormone. Since the penis is normally formed the prenatal secretion of testosterone must have been normal or at least adequate. Familial incidence of the syndrome has been recorded (Sloan and Walsh,

1976). The pattern of inheritance is considered to be through either an X-linked recessive or an autosomal dominant trait.

Treatment is essentially that of the undescended testes. Gonadotrophin therapy is generally ineffective and orchidopexy, which may have to be in two stages, is required. However, Pappis *et al.* (1979) found it impossible to get the testes to the scrotum without dividing the vasa deferentia. Removal of the uterus and the vagina is not required unless they become distended by secretions or else fill with urine during micturition and cause persistent urinary tract infection, possibly with stone formation, or urine dribbling after voiding. Such complications are uncommon.

Normal virilization is to be expected at puberty and fertility has been reported in some instances (Young, 1951). In others spermiograms have shown azoospermia, a diminished total count, and reduced mobility or an increased number of atypical forms. The incidence of neoplasia in the testes is no greater than that in cryptorchidism in general and no case of malignancy of the uterus has been reported.

References

Aarskog, D. (1970) Clinical and cytogenetic studies in hypospadias. *Acta Paediatrica Scandinavica*, Suppl. p.203

Barakat, A.Y., Papadopoulou, Z.L., Chandra, R.S., Hollerman, C.E. and Calcagno, P.L. (1974) Pseudohermaphroditism, nephron disorder and Wilms' tumour: a unifying concept. *Pediatrics*, **54**, 366

Bongiovanni, A.M. (1961) Unusual steroid pattern in congenital adrenal hyperplasia: deficiency of 3β hydroxy-dehydrogenase. *Journal of Clinical Endocrinology and Metabolism*, **21**, 860

Bongiovanni, A.M. (1962) The adrenogenital syndrome with deficiency of 3β hydroxy-steroid dehydrogenase. *Journal of Clinical Investigation*, **41**, 2086

Clement, J.A., Reyes, F.I., Winter, J.S.D. and Fairman, C. (1976) Studies on human sexual development, III: fetal pituitary and serum and amniotic fluid concentrations of LH, HCG and FSH. *Journal of Clinical Endocrinology and Metabolism*, **42**, 9

Cohen, M.M. and Shaw, M.W. (1965) Two XY siblings with gonadal dysgenesis and a female phenotype. *New England Journal of Medicine*, **21**, 1083

de Bacalao, E.B. and Dominiquez, I. (1969) Unilateral gonadoblastoma in a pregnant woman. *American Journal of Obstetrics and Gynecology*, **105**, 1279

Degenhart, H.J. (1971) A study of the cholesterol splitting enzyme system in normal adrenals and in lipoid adrenal hyperplasia. *Acta Paediatrica Scandinavica*, **60**, 611

Denys, P., Malvaux, P., Van Den Berghe, H., Tanghe, W. and Proesmans, W. (1967) Association d'un syndrom anatomo-pathologique; de pseudo-hermaphrodisme masculin, d'une tumeur de Wilms, d'une nephropathie parenchymateuse et d'un mosaicisme XX/XY. *Archives Française de Pédiatrie*, **24**, 729

DiGeorge, A.M. and Harley, R.D. (1966) The association of aniridia, Wilm's tumour and genital abnormalities. *Archives of Ophthalmology*, **75**, 796

Drash, A. Sherman, F., Hartmann, W.H. and Blizzard, R.M. (1970) A syndrome of pseudohermaphroditism, Wilms' tumour, hypertension and degenerative renal disease. *Journal of Pediatrics*, **76**, 585

Frank, R. (1938) Formation of an artificial vagina without operation. *American Journal of Obstetrics and Gynecology*, **35**, 1053

Gilbert-Dreyfus, S., Sebaoun, A.C. and Belaisch, J. (1957) Etude d'androgynordisme avec hypospadias grave, gynaecomastic et hyperostrogénie. *Annals d'Endocrinologie*, **18**, 93

Givens, J.R., Wiser, W.L., Summitt, R.L., Kerler, I.J., Anderson, R.N. Pittaway, D.E. and Fish, S.A. (1974) Pseudohermaphroditism and deficient testicular 17 ketosteroid reductase. *New England Journal of Medicine*, **291**, 938

Goebelsmann, U., Horton, R., Mestman, J.H., Arce, J.J., Nagata, Y., Nakamura, R.M., Thorneycroft, I.H. and Mishell, D.R. (1973) Male pseudohermaphroditism due to testicular 17β hydroxy-steroid dehydrogenase deficiency. *Journal of Clinical Endocrinology and Metabolism*, **36**, 867

Goebelsmann, U., Davajan, U., Israel, R., Mestman, J.H., Mishell, D.R. and Zachman, M. (1974) Male pseudohermaphroditism consistent with 17, 20 desmolase deficiency. *Gynecological Investigation*, **5**, 60

Griffin, J.E. and Wilson, J.D. (1980) The syndromes of androgen assistance. *New England Journal of Medicine*, **302**, 198

Grumbach, M.M. and Van Wyk, J.J. (1974) Disorders of sex differentiation. *In* Textbook of Endocrinology, 5th edn (edited by Williams, P.H.). Saunders, Philadelphia. p.423

Heller, R.H. and Jones, H.W. (1964) Production of ovarian dysgenesis in the rat and human by busulphan. *American Journal of Obstetrics and Gynecology*, **89**, 414

Imperato-McGinley, J., Guerrero, L., Gautier, T. and Petersen, R.E. (1974) Steroid 5α-reductase deficiency in man: an inherited form of male pseudohermaphroditism. *Science*, **186**, 1213

Ionescu, B. and Maximilian, C. (1977) Three sisters with gonadoblastoma. *Journal of Medical Genetics*, **14**, 194

Jagiello, G. and Atwell, J.D. (1962) Prevalence of Testicular Feminization. *Lancet*, i, 329

Jänne, O., Perheentupa, J., Vünikka, L and Vinko, R. (1974) Testicular endocrine function in a pubertal boy with 3β hydroxysteroid dehydrogenase deficiency. *Journal of Clinical Endocrinology and Metabolism*, **39**, 206

Jirasèk, J.E. (1971) Development of the Genital System and Male Pseudohermaphroditism. Johns Hopkins University Press, Baltimore, Maryland

Jost, A. (1972) A new look at the mechanisms controlling sex differentiation in mammals. *Johns Hopkins Medical Journal*, **103**, 38

Khodr, G.S., Cadena, G.D., Ong, T.C. and Siler-Khodr, T.M. (1979) Y-Autosome translocation, gonadal dysgenesis and gonadoblastoma. *American Journal of Diseases of Children*, **133**, 277

Kirkland, R.T., Kirkland, J.L., Johnson, C.M., Horning, M.G., Librik, L. and Clayton, G.W. (1973) Congenital lipoid adrenal hyperplasia in an eight year old phenotypic female. *Journal of Clinical Endocrinology and Metabolism*, **36**, 488

Knorr, F., Pidlingmaier, F. and Engelhardt, D. (1973) Reifenstein's syndrome, a 17β-hydroxysteroid-oxireductase deficiency? *Acta Endocrinologica*, Suppl. 173. p.37

LeMaree, B., Lautridon, A., Urvoy, M., Renault, A., Fonlupt, J., Davy, J., Ardouin, M. and Coutel, Y. (1971) Un cas d'association de nephroblastome avec aniridie et malformations genitales. *Archives Française de Pédiatrie*, **28**, 457

Lockhart, J.L., Kineger, R.P., Stevens, P.S. and Glenn, J.F. (1979) Mechanical genital maldevelopment presenting as pseudovaginal perineoscrotal hypospadias. *Journal of Urology*, **121**, 655

Lubs, H.A. Vilar, O. and Bergenstal, D.M. (1959) Familial male pseudohermaphroditism with labial testes and partial feminization: endocrine studies and genetic aspects. *Journal of Clinical Endocrinology and Metabolism*, **19**, 1110

Money, J. and Ehrhardt, A. (1972) Man and Woman, Boy and Girl: The Differentiation and Dimorphism of Gender Identity from Conception to Maturity. Johns Hopkins University Press, Baltimore, Maryland

Morgan, R.J., Williams, D.I. and Pryor, J.P. (1982) Müllerian duct remnants in the male. *British Journal of Urology*, in press

New, M.I. (1970) Male pseudohermaphroditism due to 17α-hydroxylase deficiency. *Journal of Clinical Investigation*, **49**, 1930

Nilson, O. (1939) Hernia uteri inguinalis bein manne. *Acta Chirurgica Scandinavica*, **83**, 231

Nowaskoski, H. and Lenz, W. (1961) Genetic aspects in male hypogonadism. *Recent Progress in Hormone Research*, **17**, 53

Pappis, C., Constantinides, C., Chiotis, D. and Dacou-Voutetakis, C. (1979) Persistent Müllerian duct structures in cryptorchid male infants: surgical dilemmas. *Journal of Pediatric Surgery*, **14**, 128

Park, I.J., Aimakhu, V.E. and Jones, H.W. (1975) An etiologic and pathogenetic classification of male hermaphroditism. *American Journal of Obstetrics and Gynecology*, **123**, 505

Parks, G.A., Bermudez, J.A., Anast, C.S., Bongiovanni, A.M., and New, M.I. (1971) Pubertal boy with the 3β hydroxysteroid dehydrogenase defect. *Journal of Clinical Endocrinology and Metabolism*, **33**, 269

Prader, A. and Gurtner, H.P. (1955) Das syndrom des pseudohermaphroditismus masculinus bei kongenitaler nebennierenrinden-hyperplasia ohne androgenüberproduktion (adrenaler pseudohermaphroditismus masculinus). *Helvetica Paediatrica Acta*, **10**, 397

Prader, A. and Siebenmann, R.E. (1957) Nebennereninsuffizieng bei kongenitaler lipoidhyperplasie den nebennieren. *Helvetica Paediatrica Acta*, **12**, 569

Reifenstein, E.C. (1947) Hereditary familial hypogonadism. *Clinical Research*, **3**, 86

Saez, J.M., de Peretti, E., Morera, A.M., David, M. and Bertrand, J. (1971) Familial male pseudohermaphroditism with gynaecomastia due to a testicular 17 ketosteroid reductase defect: studies in vivo. *Journal of Clinical Endocrinology and Metabolism*, **32**, 604

Saez, J.M. Morera, A.M., de Peretti, E. and Bertrand, J. (1972) Further in vivo studies in male pseudohermaphroditism with gynaecomastia due to a testicular 17 ketosteroid reductase defect (compared to a case of testicular feminization). *Journal of Clinical Endocrinology and Metabolism*, **34**, 598

Scully, R.E. (1970) Gonadoblastoma: a review of 74 cases. *Cancer*, **6**, 1340

Siler-Khodr, T.M. Morgenstern, L.L. and Greenwood, F.C. (1974) Hormone synthesis and release from human fetal adenohypophysis in vitro. *Journal of Clinical Endocrinology and Metabolism*, **39**, 891

Simpson, J.L. (1976) Disorders of Sexual Differentiation. Academic Press, London

Sloan, W.R. and Walsh, P.C. (1976) Familial persistent Müllerian duct syndrome. *Journal of Urology*, **115**, 459

Smith, D.W. (1970) Recognizable patterns of human malformation. *In* Major Problems in Clinical Pediatrics, Vol. 8. Saunders, Philadelphia

Spear, G.S., Hyde, T.P., Gruppo, R.A. and Slusser, R. (1971) Pseudohermaphroditism, glomerulonephritis with the nephrotic syndrome and Wilms' tumour in infancy. *Journal of Pediatrics*, **79**, 677

Stump, T.A. and Garrett, R.A. (1954) Bilateral Wilms' tumour in a male pseudohermaphrodite. *Journal of Urology*, **72**, 1146

Summitt, R.L. (1972) Differential diagnosis of genital ambiguity in the newborn. *Clinical Obstetrics and Gynecology*, **15**, 112

Talerman, A. (1971) Gonadoblastoma and dysgerminoma in two siblings with dysgenetic gonads. *Obstetrics and Gynecology*, **38**, 416

Tanner, J.M. (1962) Growth at Adolescence, 2nd edn. Blackwell, Oxford

Walsh, P.C., Madden, J.D., Harrod, M.J., Goldstein, J.L., MacDonald, P.C., and Wilson, J.D. (1974) Familial incomplete male pseudohermaphroditism, type 2. *New England Journal of Medicine*, **291**, 944

Williams, A.J. (1979) Prediction of fetal sex: a cautionary tale. *British Medical Journal*, iii, 767

Wilson, J.D., Harrod, M.J., Goldstein, J.L., Hemsell, D.L. and MacDonald, P.C. (1974) Familial incomplete male pseudohermaphroditism, type I. *New England Journal of Medicine*, **290**, 1097

Young, D. (1951) Hernia uteri inguinalis in the male. *Journal of Obstetrics and Gynaecology of the British Commonwealth*, **58**, 830

Zachman, M. (1972) The evaluation of testicular endocrine function before and in puberty: effect of a single dose of human chorionic gonadotrophin on urinary steroid secretion under normal and pathological conditions. *Acta Endocrinologica*, Suppl. 70, p.164

Zachman, M., Vollmin, J.A., Hamilton, W. and Prader, A. (1972) Steroid 17, 20- desmolase deficiency: a new cause of male pseudohermaphroditism. *Journal of Clinical Endocrinology and Metabolism*, **1**, 369

40   Female Genital Tract Anomalies

J.H. Johnston

Embryology

The paramesonephric (müllerian) ducts appear one on each side as invaginations of the coelomic epithelium during the sixth week of intrauterine life. They grow caudally, crossing and then progressing medial to the mesonephric ducts until between the 25–30 mm stages their lower ends come into contact with each other and with the posterior wall of the urogenital sinus. Here they produce a localized intraluminal bulge, namely the müllerian tubercle, between the mesonephric ductal orifices. The septum between the coapted portions of the müllerian ducts later breaks down to produce the single lumen of the uterovaginal canal. The proximal portion of each duct forms the ipsilateral fallopian tube.

Subsequently the uterovaginal canal retracts cranially and the mesoderm between it and the urogenital sinus elongates and thickens to form the solid vaginal cord. At 10 weeks sinovaginal bulbs proliferate from the endoderm of the urogenital sinus to produce the vaginal plate which infiltrates and replaces the vaginal cord. The plate canalizes at the fifth month of fetal life so that the uterovaginal canal communicates with the lumen of the urogenital sinus.

At the same time as these developments are taking place the urogenital sinus becomes shallower and by the time they are complete the urethral meatus and the original site of the müllerian tubercle, now the orifice of the vagina, are on the vulva. The vulva itself represents the remains of the urogenital sinus while the hymen is a partition between the sinus and the caudal end of the canalized vaginal plate.

The extent to which the müllerian ducts contribute to the formation of the vagina has long been a matter of dispute. Hunter (1930) was of the opinion that they formed the entire organ. Koff (1933) believed that the lowest one fifth of the vagina derived from the sinovaginal bulbs and the upper four fifths from the ducts. Fluhman (1960) considered that urogenital sinus endoderm formed the mucosa but not the musculature of the whole of the vagina and the cervical canal, basing his view on histochemical as well as anatomical studies.

Congenital absence of the vagina

Complete absence of the vagina is the result of aplasia of the uterovaginal canal and the vaginal plate. On occasions vaginal epithelium can be recognized histologically in the rectovesical septum and the condition is then more accurately described as extreme vaginal hypoplasia. The external genitalia are of normal appearance except that the vaginal opening is absent or represented only by a shallow depression.

As a rule the ovaries are normal while the uterus and the fallopian tubes, which are also of müllerian ductal origin, are rudimentary. Urinary tract anomalies such as unilateral renal agenesis, ureteric duplication, ureterocele and pelvic ectopic kidney are common and occur in up to 51 per cent of cases in recorded series (Bryan, Nigro and Counseller, 1949). Consequently urological investigation is always indicated. Anorectal lesions such as imperforate and ectopic anus frequently coexist, as do skeletal abnormalities involving the ribs and the cervical and thoracic vertebrae. The latter were found in four of 23 patients with congenital vaginal absence reported by Chawla, Bery and Indra (1966).

Vaginal agenesis is generally discovered shortly after birth on routine neonatal examination of the genitalia. A buccal smear and possibly sex chromosomal evaluation may be needed if there is clinical suspicion of the testicular feminization syndrome, which sometimes presents a similar appearance. In the absence of hydrocolpos the distinction between vaginal agenesis and imperforate hymen or inferior vaginal atresia can generally be made by bimanual pelvic examination with a finger in the rectum. With the latter conditions the vagina is palpable as a thickened cord of tissue. It may be possible to insert a needle into the vaginal cavity through the vulva and demonstrate it radiologically following the injection of contrast medium.

Since the uterus is usually severely hypoplastic in cases of congenital vaginal absence intrauterine menstruation is very unlikely. However, Huffman (1968) advised that when the child is 7–8 years old, following the induction of a pneumoperitoneum, radiology should be carried out to confirm the rudimentary nature of the internal genitals and the normality of the ovaries. Alternatively peritoneoscopy or exploratory laparotomy may be employed for this purpose.

In the usual case in which there is no functioning uterus construction of an artificial vagina should be deferred until the patient is postpubertal, anxious to undertake sexual intercourse, and therefore fully motivated to cooperate in the appropriate therapy. The nonsurgical formation of a vaginal canal by the patient intermittently pressing Pyrex tubes of gradually increasing size firmly into the vulva over a period of months was evolved by Frank (1938) and has been reported to be successful (Huffman, 1968). The method is most likely to be effective when there is already a shallow vaginal depression. Considerable patience, persistence and determination are undoubtedly needed. In the McIndoe (1950) procedure a cavity is created by dissection between the urethra and the bladder in front and the rectum behind and lined with split skin grafts. The patient must subsequently keep a mould of appropriate size in position but even so shortening and stenosis of the vagina are common complications. The construction of an artificial vagina from an isolated segment of sigmoid colon was described by Pratt and Smith (1966). Satisfactory results have been reported in spite of some aesthetic drawbacks resulting from the continuous discharge of mucus from the vulva. Williams (1964) reported the simpler technique of vulvovaginoplasty in which a skin-lined cavity is constructed from local flaps external to the vulva. There is no tendency to contracture and although the artificial vagina has little resemblance to the normal organ it is stated to allow satisfactory intercourse for both partners.

Vaginal atresia

With this rare anomaly the lowest part of the vagina is congenitally absent. The condition is presumed to result from failure of canalization of the vaginal plate while the uterovaginal canal develops normally. The vulval appearance is identical with that in vaginal agenesis, but since the upper vagina is patent and the uterus functional the distinction (see above) is important. While hydrocolpos has not been recorded with vaginal atresia haematocolpos and haematometra develop with the onset of ovarian activity. Surgical intervention is needed, employing a combined abdominoperineal approach. Mobilization and downward displacement of the vagina are carried out from above. From below the atretic vaginal segment is cored out and lined with skin flaps raised from the perineum to allow the vaginal lumen to communicate with the exterior.

Genital tract duplication

Total failure of union of the paramesonephric ducts leads to both complete duplication of the vagina and uterus didelphys. The anomaly is

Imperforate hymen, vaginal septum and cervical atresia

In most instances congenital genital tract obstructions of this nature present clinically either in the newborn infant or at puberty.

Hydrocolpos

Hydrocolpos is encountered in the newborn baby when vaginal obstruction coincides with excessive secretion by the fetal cervical and vaginal glands under the stimulus of maternal oestrogen. The obstructive agent may be an imperforate hymen or a septum situated at a higher level.

Septa most commonly occur at the junction of the middle and upper thirds of the vagina but the precise level can be difficult to determine when the upper portion of the vagina is distended by accumulated fluid. Antell (1952) believed that all vaginal occlusions are of septal type, resulting from a failure of communication between the lumina of the uterovaginal canal derived from the paramesonephric ducts and the vaginal plate originating from the urogenital sinus. He considered that an imperforate hymen is in fact a low sited septum and that the true

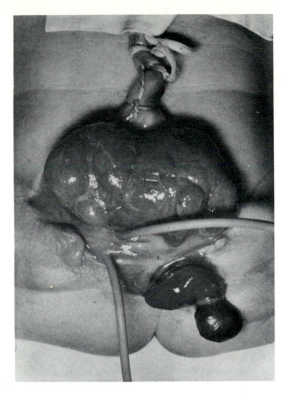

Figure 40.1. Double vagina in a newborn girl with bladder exstrophy. The catheterized vaginas lie in the sagittal plane and both are on the right of the midline. There is also rectal mucosal prolapse with localized strangulation.

rare and most commonly encountered in association with exstrophic lesions, especially exstrophy of the cloaca (*Figure 40.1*). Double vaginas might be expected to lie symmetrically on either side of the midline but often they are both on one side, are askew or occupy anterior and posterior positions so that the existence of the second vagina may readily be overlooked during childhood. Vulval duplication in association with vaginal and uterine duplication is extremely rare; as a rule gross abnormalities coexist which involve the pelvic viscera and other systems and prevent the child's survival. Incomplete union of the müllerian ducts causes septate vaginal duplicity and bicornuate uterus and frequently one hemivagina is larger than the other. Surgical intervention for genital duplication is seldom needed during childhood unless there are coexisting obstructive anomalies. However, a localized vaginal septum may be usefully divided if it is discovered during endoscopic examination under anaesthesia.

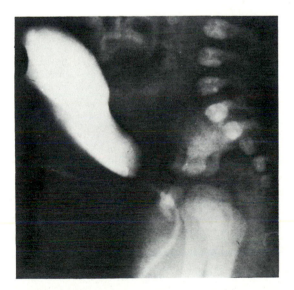

Figure 40.2. Lateral cystogram in a neonate with hydrocolpos. The bladder is displaced upwards and forwards from the pelvis.

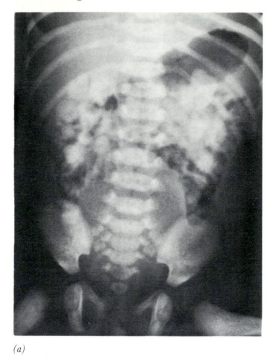
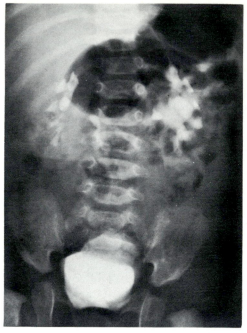

(a)   *(b)*

Figure 40.3. Intravenous urograms in a girl with hydrocolpos. *(a)* Dilated upper tracts before treatment. *(b)* Undilated tracts 1 year after incision of the imperforate hymen.

hymen can be recognized as a separate structure, especially after the obstructing membrane has been incised. Septal vaginal obstruction may have a familial incidence, the anomaly being inherited as a simple autosomal recessive disorder. An association with polydactyly has been reported (Dungy, Aptekar and Cann, 1971).

With hydrocolpos the vagina, to a lesser degree the uterus (hydrometra) and sometimes in addition the fallopian tubes (hydrosalpinx) are distended with a serous, milky or mucinous fluid. Histologically the liquid contains desquamated epithelial cells, leukocytes and erythrocytes. The dilated genital tract displaces the bladder from the pelvis (*Figure 40.2*) so that vesical retention with dribbling micturition and upper urinary tract dilatation may develop (*Figure 40.3*). Pressure on the rectum can lead to incomplete low intestinal obstruction and on occasions the legs become swollen and cyanotic from compression of their venous drainage.

The baby is found at birth to have a tense lower abdominal mass due to the distended vagina. With an imperforate hymen or a low septum a bulging membrane is seen at the vulva

and becomes more prominent when the abdominal mass is compressed (*Figure 40.4*). When the obstruction is caused by a high vaginal septum the introitus appears normal and vaginoscopy is needed for diagnosis. Rarely leakage of fluid through the fallopian tubes into the peritoneal cavity causes plastic peritonitis (Ceballos and Hicks, 1970).

When the vaginal occlusion is at the introitus the genital tract is easily emptied by a cruciate incision of the obstructing membrane. Pervaginal division of a high thick vaginal septum is hazardous because injury to adjacent viscera may occur due to anatomical distortion. In such cases laparotomy is indicated. The anterior wall of the distended vagina is opened and after the fluid has been removed by suction the septum can be divided from below under intraluminal guidance from above.

Ramenofsky and Raffensberger (1971) pointed out that a high obstructive vaginal septum is often associated with persistence of the urogenital sinus, when the urethra opens high on the anterior vaginal wall below the septum (*Figure 40.5*). Simple division of the septum may then subsequently result in pooling

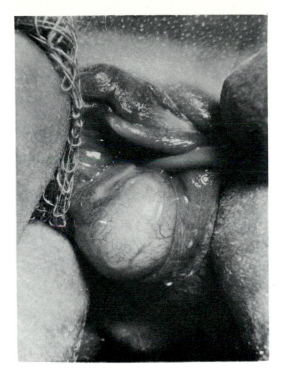

Figure 40.4. Bulging imperforate hymen in a newborn baby with hydrocolpos.

of urine in the dilated vagina and persistent urinary tract infection. These authors recommended an abdominoperineal operation at which the vagina is brought to the vulva and opened posterior to the original introitus. The urogenital sinus then becomes an extension of the true urethra to the exterior. In such cases coexisting urethral anomalies may be present in the form of stenosis causing obstruction or of severe dilatation leading to incontinence. Their management is discussed in Chapter 23. Following evacuation of a hydrocolpos normal bladder emptying is rapidly restored when there are no associated urethral anomalies and upper tract dilatation generally resolves promptly.

Hydrocolpos may occur as an isolated anomaly but often there are other congenital lesions affecting the genitourinary tract, the anus and the rectum, or the lumbosacral spine. The possibility of such coexisting pathology must always be considered and the appropriate investigations performed. In cases of persistence of the cloaca or the urogenital sinus hydrocolpos may occur in the absence of any obvious vaginal obstruction as a result of urine accumulation.

Haematocolpos

Haematocolpos is generally a consequence of an imperforate hymen in a child in whom prenatal vaginal and cervical secretions were not produced in sufficient volume to cause hydrocolpos. At puberty menstrual fluid accumulates in the vagina and often also in the uterus and the fallopian tubes. The patient shows breast and pubic hair development and gives a history of primary amenorrhoea with either intermittent monthly pain or a continuous ache with monthly exacerbations. Difficulty with micturition may result from bladder displacement. Examination reveals a lower abdominal and pelvic mass and a bulging membrane occluding the introitus. Sometimes intra-abdominal menstruation produces signs of peritoneal irritation so that appendicitis may be simulated.

Treatment consists of division of the membrane and release of the accumulated blood. A broad spectrum antibiotic is advisable until the discharge ceases in order to prevent infection which might cause salpingitis and subsequent tubal obstruction. In the absence of such a complication normal fertility can be anticipated.

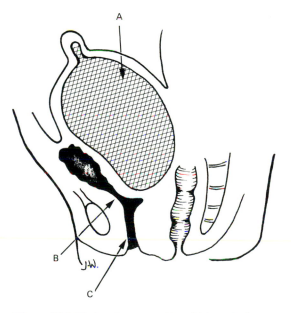

Figure 40.5. Hydrocolpos caused by a high vaginal septum associated with a persistent urogenital sinus. A = hydrocolpos; B = urethra; C = urogenital sinus.

Cervical atresia

Atresia of the cervix uteri is the rarest form of congenital female genital tract obstruction. The cervix is extremely small and the external os is represented by a shallow dimple. The anomaly usually presents at the menarche with the development of haematometra. Treatment consists of the construction of a cervical canal by the passage of a trochar. The uterus is drained by catheter until the discharge ceases. Regular dilatation is likely to be necessary to prevent stenosis. If and when the patient becomes pregnant cervical insufficiency may be a problem.

Vaginal cyst

A cyst projecting into the vagina and through it at the vulva may arise from Gärtner's duct of the epoophoron, which is a relic of the mesonephric duct that descends on each side from the broad ligament through the cervical musculature and down the lateral wall of the vagina to terminate at the level of the hymen. As a rule the cyst is present at birth and it is then often sufficiently large to necessitate its removal. An abdominal approach is required. The condition must be distinguished from other cystic vaginal and vulval protrusions such as those caused by an ectopic ureterocele, an imperforate hymen, a paraurethral cyst or a urethral diverticulum. Careful evaluation of the local anatomy, if necessary under anaesthesia, and urological investigation are therefore always indicated.

Hymenal polyp

Because of the prenatal effect of maternal hormones, at birth the hymen is often thick and oedematous and on occasions its posterior aspect forms a round or elongated polyp; Berglen and Selander (1962) found 60 examples in 1000 newborn girls. Since spontaneous involution occurs no treatment is needed when the diagnosis is assured. In some cases a sarcoma botryoides, which has been reported to occur in the newborn (Ober, Smith and Roullard, 1958), is simulated. Excision of the polyp and histological study are then necessary.

Combined and associated anomalies

Developmental anomalies of the female genital tract are often multiple and duplications, obstructions and urogenital sinus abnormalities may coexist in a variety of ways. Sometimes diagnostic difficulties arise when genital tract obstruction involves only one half of a duplex system. Pain and an abdominal mass may then develop at puberty while menstruation occurs normally from the unobstructed hemiuterus.

Other abnormalities consequent upon maldevelopment of the hind end of the embryo are often present. Uterovaginal lesions are frequently found in association with ectopic or stenotic anus, rectal agenesis, persistence of the cloaca, bladder or cloacal exstrophy, and lumbosacral spinal defects with neurological involvement. As a rule the extragenital anomalies form the presenting clinical feature. Even in the absence of other pelvic visceral and vertebral lesions the upper urinary tract is often abnormal and urological investigation is indicated as a routine.

References

Antell, L. (1952) Hydrocolpos in infancy and childhood. *Pediatrics*, **10**, 306

Berglen, N.E. and Selander, P. (1962) Hymenal polyps in newborn infants. *Acta Paediatrica Scandinavica*, Suppl. 135, p.28

Bryan, A.L., Nigro, J.A. and Counseller, V.S. (1949) One hundred cases of congenital absence of the vagina. *Surgery, Gynecology and Obstetrics*, **88**, 79

Ceballos, R. and Hicks, G.M. (1970) Plastic peritonitis due to neonatal hydrometrocolpos; radiologic and pathogenic observations. *Journal of Pediatric Surgery*, **5**, 63

Chawla, S., Bery, K. and Indra, K.J. (1966) Abnormalities of urinary tract and skeleton associated with congenital absence of vagina. *British Medical Journal*, i, 1398

Dungy, I.C., Aptekar, R.G. and Cann, H.M. (1971) Hereditary hydrometrocolpos and polydactyly in infancy. *Pediatrics*, **47**, 138

Fluhman, C. (1960) The developmental anatomy of the cervix uteri. *Obstetrics and Gynaecology*, **15**, 62

Frank, R. (1938) Formation of artificial vagina without operation. *American Journal of Obstetrics and Gynecology*, **35**, 1053

Huffman, J.W. (1968) Congenital anomalies of the female genitalia. *In* The Gynecology of Childhood and Adolescence. Saunders, Philadelphia.p.169

Hunter, R. (1930) Observations on development of human female genital tract. *Carnegie Institute Contributions to Embryology*, **22**, 91

Koff, A. (1933) Development of the vagina in the human fetus. *Carnegie Institute Contributions to Embryology*, **24**, 61

McIndoe, A. (1950) The treatment of congenital absence and obliterative conditions of the vagina. *British Journal of Plastic Surgery*, **2**, 254

Ober, W.B., Smith, J.A. and Roullard, F.C. (1958) Congenital sarcoma botryoides of vagina; report of two cases. *Cancer*, **11**, 620

Pratt, J.H. and Smith, G.R. (1966) Vaginal reconstruction with a sigmoid loop. *American Journal of Obstetrics and Gynecology*, **96**, 31

Ramenofsky, M.L. and Raffensberger, J.G. (1971) An abdomino-perineal vaginal pull through for definitive treatment of hydrometrocolpos. *Journal of Pediatric Surgery*, **6**, 381

Williams, E.A. (1964) Congenital absence of the vagina: a simple operation for its relief. *Journal of Obstetrics and Gynaecology of the British Commonwealth*, **71**, 511

41 Acquired Female Genital Disorders

J.H. Johnston

Adherent labia minora

Labial adherence is a consequence of intertrigo or mild trauma eroding the delicate epithelium of the vulva of the young child. Although the condition is occasionally seen in infancy, it is not congenital and Finlay (1965) found no example among 5000 newborn girls. The labia may be fused over almost their entire extent, leaving

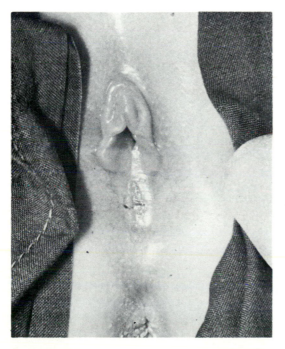

Figure 41.1. Adherent labia minora in a 4-year-old girl.

only a small gap close to the clitoris (*Figure 41.1*), but more often the union is restricted to the region of the posterior commissure. While an extensive labial adherence may cause dysuria, frequently the child is asymptomatic and is referred because she is thought to have vaginal agenesis. The adhesions can be freed by twice-daily application of 0.01 per cent dienoestrol cream for a period of some 2 weeks which produces thickening and keratinization of the epithelium and prevents recurrence. To avoid pseudo-isosexual precocity, therapy should be discontinued as soon as it is seen to have been effective.

Prolapse of the genitalia

Genital procidentia is rare during childhood. In a normal newborn infant it may follow a difficult or impacted breech presentation. Otherwise it occurs in association with myelodysplasia causing paralysis of the supporting levator musculature or with bladder or cloacal exstrophy where there is a wide gap in the pelvic diaphragm (*Figure 41.2*). In neonatal cases the prolapsed cervix and vagina rapidly become swollen and engorged so that a neoplasm may be simulated. Incomplete bilateral ureteric obstruction is common and leads to upper tract dilatation (*Figure 41.3*). Treatment consists of manual reduction of the prolapse following which the legs are bound together for a few weeks. In the otherwise normal infant there is no tendency to recurrence. Operative intervention with repair of the pelvic floor may be needed for recurrent prolapse in children with exstrophy or spina bifida.

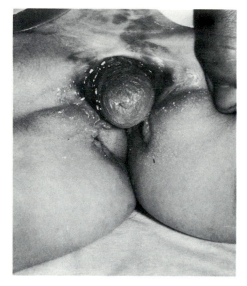

Figure 41.2. Vaginal prolapse in a girl who had had bladder exstrophy.

Clitoral balanitis

As in the male, balanitis may result from infection of retained secretions under an adherent prepuce. Treatment is by freeing the adhesions, usually under general anaesthesia, and removing the accumulated smegma. On occasions a dorsal slit in the prepuce is needed. Readherence of the foreskin can be prevented by local application of 0.01 per cent dienoestrol cream but prolonged hormone treatment must be avoided because of its possible systemic effects.

Leukorrhoea

Leukorrhoea is a normal occurrence in the newborn girl because of the influence of maternal hormones on the fetal cervical and vaginal glands. There is a white mucoid discharge and sometimes uterine bleeding occurs as a withdrawal phenomenon. The condition resolves after the first few days of life. A similar white

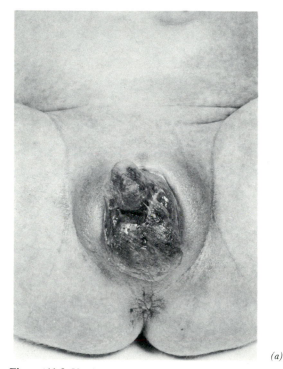

(a)

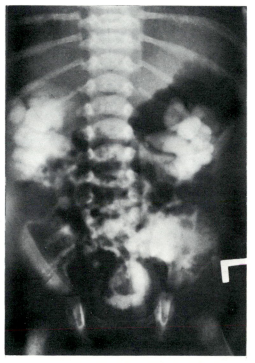

(b)

Figure 41.3. Uterine prolapse in a neonate. There was complete recovery after reduction. *(a)* Clinical picture. *(b)* Intravenous urogram.

discharge is common in girls approaching the menarche. Leukorrhoea is readily distinguished from an infective process by the clinical features and by the fact that the discharge is seen histologically to contain desquamated epithelial cells with no pus cells. Reassurance is all that is needed.

Vaginal foreign body

The presence of a foreign body in the vagina should be suspected when there is a persistent malodorous green discharge especially if it is blood stained. A large body may be visible on inspection of the vulva or palpable on rectal examination but as a rule vaginoscopy under anaesthesia is required for diagnosis. An illuminated paediatric proctoscope allows satisfactory viewing. The foreign bodies most commonly found in young girls are pellets of wool or paper derived from clothing or toilet paper which presumably enter the vagina inadvertently. In older girls a variety of objects, sometimes of an obviously phallic shape, are encountered and there is little doubt that their insertion was deliberate, although an admission is seldom obtained.

Figure 41.4. Vaginal calculus in a 5-year-old girl who had Proteus urinary tract infection but no causative local anatomical abnormality. *(a)* Straight film of pelvis. *(b)* Oblique view of cystogram showing stone behind the bladder.

Vaginal calculus

Vaginal calculi composed of triple phosphate are encountered mainly in severely retarded bed-ridden incontinent children as a result of ammoniacal decomposition of urine accumulated in the vagina. Less often a stone forms as a result of introital stenosis or when an ectopic ureter opens on the vulva or into the vagina. Rarely as in the child illustrated in *Figure 41.4* a vaginal calculus develops in association with Proteus urinary tract infection and there is no demonstrable causative anatomical abnormality.

Nonspecific vulvovaginitis

Because of stimulation by maternal hormones the lining of the vulva and the vagina at birth resembles that of the adult and the secretions are acid. Soon afterwards the epithelium becomes thin and the reaction changes to alkaline so that resistance to infection is lowered. Bacteria

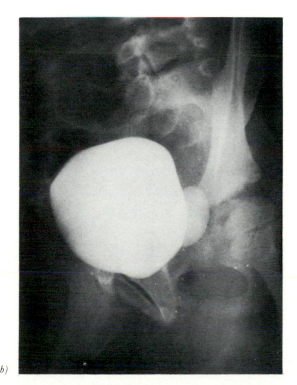

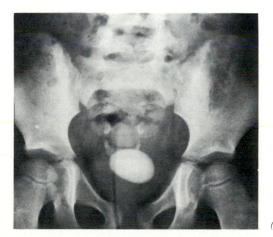

(a)   *(b)*

gain entry easily between the poorly developed labia of small girls and vulvovaginitis may result and is often caused by organisms that elsewhere are of low pathogenicity.

A variety of bacteria may be incriminated. Haemolytic or nonhaemolytic streptococci, pyogenic or nonpyogenic staphylococci, diphtheroids, Proteus or *Escherichia coli* may be cultured. Sometimes a mixed infection exists. Various causative factors may be involved. Faecal organisms may enter the vulva as a result of contamination from dirty underclothes or from inadequate cleansing of the anus after defaecation and vulvovaginitis sometimes follows an attack of diarrhoea. Threadworm infestation is often carried to the vulva by scratching. Excoriation of the epithelium by the use of bubble-baths or antiseptic soap or solutions can allow secondary infection to develop. In some instances attacks of vulvovaginitis coincide with upper respiratory tract infections and are considered to be due to staphylococci or streptococci carried to the vulva by the fingers. In spite of the fact that the vagina is often filled with urine during micturition in small girls urinary tract infection is rarely causative of vulvovaginitis. Conversely, although ascent of organisms from the vulva is commonly considered to be responsible for the development of urinary tract infection in girls, such infection is a very infrequent complication of vulvovaginitis.

The clinical features of nonspecific vulvovaginitis vary in severity. There may be acute symptoms of vulval soreness and profuse discharge, especially when the causative bacteria are haemolytic streptococci or pyogenic staphylococci. Alternatively there may be merely a persistent or intermittent yellow discharge. In acute infections the vulva is swollen and reddened. Vaginal discharge can be induced by massage with a finger in the rectum. Instrumental examination of the vagina is not well tolerated by small girls and such investigations require general anaesthesia. Swabs must be taken of the vulval exudate for bacterial culture and sensitivity tests and of the perianal skin for the detection of threadworm ova. Histological examination of the discharge is required if there is clinical suspicion of trichomoniasis or moniliasis.

Acute episodes of vulvovaginitis resolve rapidly following the use of the appropriate antibiotic and gentle but thorough cleansing of the vulva. However, recurrence of the discharge with or without other symptoms is common and when this occurs or when from the outset the symptoms have been subacute the possibility of a vaginal foreign body must be considered, particularly if the discharge is foul smelling or blood stained.

In the absence of a foreign body various measures may be required to avoid recurrence of vulvovaginitis. Attention is directed to local cleanliness and prevention of faecal contamination of the vulva and the child is instructed to wipe the anus in a posterior direction after defaecation. While frequent bathing is indicated antiseptics and detergents must be avoided. Twice-daily changes of underclothing are advisable and cotton rather than nylon knickers should be worn since the latter, being nonabsorbent, encourage vulval maceration. Antibiotic creams applied to the vulva may be effective or solutions may be instilled into the vagina using an eyedropper. Intravaginal manoeuvres such as douching or the insertion of pessaries are best avoided in young girls. Threadworm infestation is treated by oral piperazine phosphate and standardized senna (Pripsen). One 10 g cachet in the child over 6 years or two thirds of a cachet in the younger child is generally curative. Because the worms may still be in the larval stage when the drug is first taken a follow-up dose 2 weeks later is advisable.

When vulvovaginitis does not respond to the above measures oestrogen therapy may be employed. The hormone causes thickening of the mucosa and acidification of the vaginal secretions so that resistance to infection is increased. Local therapy is generally effective. Intravaginal pessaries may be used but Gray and Kotcher (1961) found it sufficient to apply 0.01 per cent dienoestrol cream to the vulva and the vestibule alone. Therapy should be discontinued when the discharge ceases in order to avoid general hormonal effects but further treatment may be needed if infection recurs.

Specific vulvovaginitis

Gonococcal vulvovaginitis

Gonorrhoea of nonvenereal origin formerly occurred in residential schools and institutions where the disease was introduced by an infected adult and spread by clothing and towels.

Although such outbreaks are now rare, the increased incidence of gonorrhoea in the adult population has led to a rise in the number of isolated cases of childhood gonococcal vulvovaginitis. A profuse yellow discharge occurs and there is vulvar redness and swelling. The infection may spread to the rectum or be transferred to the eyes, causing conjunctivitis. Bartholinitis and salpingitis which are common complications in adults are rare in children.

The diagnosis is confirmed by the isolation of *Neisseria gonorrhoea* from the discharge. Bacterial culture is necessary for confirmation since other Gram-negative intracellular diplococci such as *N. sicca* can also cause vulvovaginitis. The antibiotic sensitivity of the organism must be determined and most cases respond to penicillin. As a rule cultures become sterile after a few days treatment but repeated negative swabs over a period of 2 months are needed before the child can be considered free of infection. During this time autoinfection of the conjunctivas must be prevented by the instillation of penicillin drops, and the possibility of transferral of the infection to others through contaminated fomites must be kept in mind and the appropriate measures taken. The source of the gonococcus, who is usually an adult, must be sought and treated. Girls allergic to penicillin can be treated by tetracycline.

Mycotic vulvovaginitis

Vulval infection by *Candida albicans* is liable to occur in children being treated by a broad spectrum antibiotic which allows proliferation of the monilia in the intestine. A white curdy discharge develops and the vulval mucosa and the surrounding skin are red, shiny and oedematous. White plaques of mycelia may be present, especially within the vagina. The diagnosis is confirmed by histological examination of a wet smear.

Treatment involves discontinuation of the antibiotic if possible. Nystatin is administered orally and applied locally. One tablet of 500 000 units is given by mouth three times daily for 7 days and nystatin ointment 100 000 units/g is applied to the affected parts. If vaginitis exists, nystatin suspension 100 000 units/ml is instilled with a dropper.

Trichomoniasis

Trichomonal infection is rare in childhood but is occasionally encountered in girls just before puberty. There is a thin, yellow and often frothy discharge. The diagnosis is confirmed by histological demonstration of the trichomonad in a film of the exudate. In most cases oral metronidazole (Flagyl) is curative when one 250 mg tablet is taken three times daily for 1 week. Persistent or recurrent infection is less common in the child than in the adult, in whom reinfection is generally of venereal origin. If trichomoniasis recurs, intravaginal metronidazole is indicated.

Herpetic vulvitis

Herpes simplex virus may infect the vulva and produce characteristic small grey vesicles that later ulcerate. There is no specific treatment. Local cleanliness is needed to avoid secondary bacterial infection and analgesic ointment may be required to relieve the burning discomfort. As with labial herpes some patients are prone to recurrent attacks.

Condylomata acuminata

Condylomata acuminata are warty growths on the genital skin and mucosa believed to be caused by viral infection. Single or multiple papillomas occur, particularly on the inner aspects of the labia, and on occasions a large cauliflower-like mass forms. Individual condylomas can be destroyed by diathermy cauterization or by application of a carbon-dioxide-snow pencil under general anaesthesia. For larger masses 20 per cent podophyllin in tincture of benzoin may be applied. Care is required to keep the irritant material from coming into contact with the surrounding normal skin or being transferred to the conjunctivas. The solution must be allowed to dry following its application and is washed off 2 hours later.

Infectious granuloma

This takes the form of a sessile or pedunculated vascular swelling similar to that seen on the lips.

It involves mainly the labia majora. Treatment is by surgical excision or diathermy coagulation.

Gangrenous vulvitis

Phagedenic infections of this type are analogous to Fournier's gangrene of the scrotum and are now rare. They may be encountered in ill nourished neglected children and debilitating illness predisposes to them. Anaerobic organisms, spirochaetes or streptococci may be cultured from the discharge. Treatment involves attention to the child's general condition and administration of the appropriate antibiotic. Incision and drainage or desloughing are commonly needed.

Vaginal lymphorrhoea

In this rare condition, which results from anomalous development of the intra-abdominal lymphatic system, there is a continuous or intermittent discharge of chylous fluid from the uterus and the vagina. Large incompetent lymph trunks in the retroperitoneum allow retrograde flow from the cisterna chyli which drains lacteals from the alimentary tract. Commonly the patient has associated cutaneous angiomas, and the lymphorrhoea may be accompanied or followed by lymphoedema of the external genitalia or the legs and possibly by chylous vesicles in the skin. As a rule the loss of fat is not of sufficient severity to lead to nutritional problems. Diagnosis of the causative pathology is by retrograde lymphangiography. Treatment comprises ligation of the dilated incompetent lymph vessels on the posterior abdominal wall and in the pelvis.

References

Finlay, N.V.L. (1965) Adhesions of the labia minora in childhood. *Proceedings of the Royal Society of Medicine*, **58**, 929

Gray, L.A. and Kotcher, E. (1961) Vaginitis in childhood. *American Journal of Obstetrics and Gynecology*, **82**, 530

42   Turner's Syndrome

Frank Harris

Introduction

Turner's syndrome in infancy, childhood and adolescence has a variable genotype and phenotype but its cardinal clinical features are shortness of stature and lack of pubertal change due to gonadal dysgenesis. The findings are usually accompanied by XO monosomy while in about a quarter of cases there is XO/XX mosaicism or a structurally abnormal X chromosome (for example XiX or XXq-). The various genotypes leading to the syndrome probably occur with a frequency higher than one in 2000 live female births. Some 5 per cent of abortuses have a 45 XO chromosomal constitution, thus seemingly making Turner's syndrome commonly lethal for the embryo. Surviving embryos with this abnormality have a far more favourable prognosis than the high incidence of abortion suggests.

Gonads

Gonadal dysgenesis is the pathological hallmark of Turner's syndrome. The dysgenetic transformation results from loss or abnormality of one of the X chromosomes. Normal and continuing ovarian development requires both X chromosomes to be present and structurally complete. In some cases X monosomy (genotype XO) can represent the loss of a Y chromosome before differentiation of the gonad. The single X chromosome has been shown to be maternal in the majority of patients. In the newborn the gonad in Turner's syndrome is characterized by the initial absence of ova and follicles. The tissue in the broad ligament is mainly vascularized stroma. Neoplasms can arise from these streak gonads and are of the dysgerminoma type. However, their precise incidence while unknown appears to be very low.

Clinical features

The clinical features of Turner's syndrome are conspicuous for the variability encountered in patients who share a similar karyotype (*Table 42.1*). The spectrum of clinical signs ranges from all the classic stigmas (Turner, 1938) to short stature as the sole presenting abnormality in the

Table 42.1   Abnormalities commonly encountered in Turner's syndrome

Short stature	++++
Gonadal (ovarian) dysgenesis	++++
Coarctation	+
Broad chest and widely spaced nipples	+++
Lymphoedema	+++
Cubitus valgus	+++
Unusual facies	+++
Low posterior hairline, webbed neck, triple hair peak	+++
Renal anomalies	++
Hand and nail abnormalities	++++

++++ = >90%; +++ = >75%; ++ = >50%; + = >20%

509

prepubertal subject. Although the cardinal clinical features, firstly of gonadal dysgenesis causing sexual infantilism and secondly of short stature are associated, the former does not cause the latter.

Affected babies are moderately small, of birthweight 2000–3000 g. During the neonatal period the clinical diagnosis is usually made from the findings of oedema of the dorsa of the hands and the feet, loose cervical skin folds and deepset convex fingernails and toenails. Some authors consider the facies of the infant with Turner's syndrome to be diagnostic because of the presence of an antimongoloid slant of the eyes and of epicanthic folds with a deep infra-orbital fold running laterally from them. The ears are prominent. There may be micrognathia, which is usually mild, and a high arched palate. A major associated congenital anomaly is coarctation of the aorta which occurs in about 15–20 per cent of patients. Idiopathic hypertension may also be seen. The kidney is a common site of further malformations such as horseshoe kidney, renal agenesis and hydronephrosis which are found in about half the subjects. Consequently an intravenous pyelogram should be obtained in all diagnosed cases. The external genitalia are invariably normal and the uterus and the fallopian tubes are present.

After the neonatal period and before puberty patients with Turner's syndrome usually present to paediatricians because of short stature or failure to thrive as evidenced by poor linear growth. Particularly in this age group the stigmas of the disorder may be exceedingly variable (*Figure 42.1*). All girls with significantly short stature should therefore undergo chromosome analysis. In most instances a peripheral blood leukocyte culture is adequate for establishing the diagnosis. However, in a small proportion of cases the abnormal cell line is demonstrable only in skin or gonadal tissue from patients with

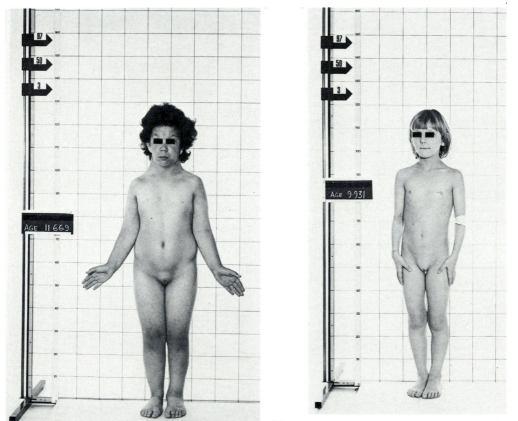

(a)

(b)

Figure 42.1. (a)Classic appearance of Turner's syndrome in a girl aged 11.6 years with karyotype 46 XO. (b) A girl aged 9.9 years with karyotype 46 XO who presented with short stature. Note the absence of gross stigmas of Turner's syndrome.

XX/XO and other mosaic genotypes. Buccal smear examination for chromatin body (Barr body) counts is not adequate for diagnosis of Turner's syndrome since mosaicism and structurally abnormal X chromosomes are not readily seen on this procedure. Careful clinical examination usually reveals some stigmas, albeit minor, if the syndrome is present.

In classic cases the young girl is short but not underweight for age. There is webbing of the neck and a low nuchal hairline with a triple hair peak. The facies may have the features found in newborns. The chest is wide and shield-shaped and the nipples are placed anterolaterally rather than anteriorly on the chest. The limbs may demonstrate persistence of the lymphoedema causing a puffy appearance of the hands and the feet. The fourth metacarpal may be short resulting in the fifth and fourth fingers being of similar length. This can be demonstrated by placing a spatula over the heads of the metacarpals with the fist clenched. If the fourth metacarpal is short, the edge of the spatula touches both the third and fifth metacarpal heads. Normal looking girls with short stature may exhibit gonadal dysgenesis with monosomy X or mosaicism. Careful examination often reveals minor stigmas such as deepset convex nails (*Figure 42.2*), a triple occipital hair peak and multiple naevi.

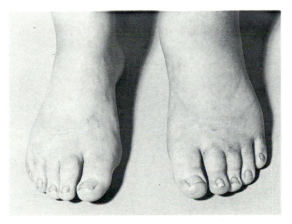

Figure 42.2. Typical concave and deepset toenails in Turner's syndrome. Note the puffiness of the dorsum of the feet. The patient has an XO karyotype and is 11.6 years.

The degree of short stature is of variable severity but is commonly three standard deviations below the mean for age. Short parents tend to have the shorter girls with Turner's syndrome. Rarely gonadal dysgenesis occurs with normal stature and no associated somatic

abnormalities. A very uncommon presentation of the syndrome is found in girls of short stature with breast development, menstruation and abnormalities of an X chromosome, for example a 46 XXq- genotype (*Figure 42.3*).

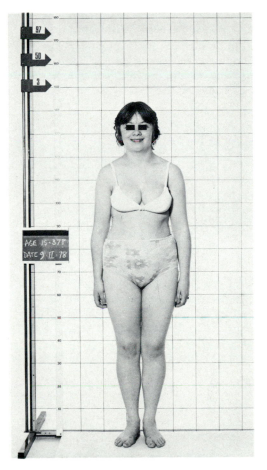

Figure 42.3. Turner's syndrome with breast development and menstruation. This patient presented with short stature and deepset nails. The karyotype was 46 XXq-.

Another group of affected girls only present in their teens because of failure to achieve any evidence of the secondary sex characteristics that are oestrogen dependent. Some poor growth of pubic hair may be present and is due to adrenocortical activity. The external genitalia are structurally those of a normal female but relatively infantile. There is no breast tissue and the nipples and the areolas are underdeveloped and unpigmented. Further clinical examination reveals other stigmas of Turner's syndrome which may be present to a lesser or greater extent. The thyroid gland should be examined for enlargement because there is an association with autoimmune thyroiditis. At the age of normal onset of puberty these patients have the endocrine biochemical pattern of hypergonadotrophic hypogonadism (*Figure 42.4*).

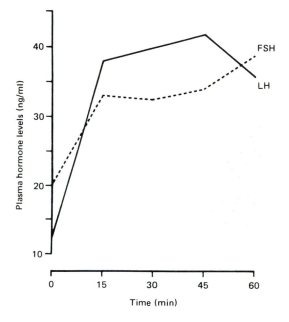

Figure 42.4. Plasma LH and FSH levels following intravenous FSH/LH-RH 100 μg in a 15-year-old girl with Turner's syndrome. Note the high basal levels and the exuberant response which is sustained for 60 minutes post injection.

Radiological features found in Turner's syndrome include changes in the hand and the wrist, the skull, the thorax, the axial skeleton and the long bones (*Table 42.2*).

Table 42.2   Radiological changes in Turner's syndrome

Hand and wrist	Short fourth metacarpal
	Madelung's deformity
	Mild delay in skeletal maturation
Spine	Scoliosis
	Vertebral fusion
Long bones	Coarse trabeculation
	Medial exostosis of tibia
Skull	J-shaped sella turcica
Thorax	Broad chest
	(Rib notching and cardiomegaly in
	coarctation)
Intravenous pyelograms	Various malformations

Management

In infancy and childhood general management consists of giving adequate counselling to the parents about the shortness of stature. The parents and the child need to be prepared for the stresses and strains of impaired growth, particularly from the early teenage years onwards. For instance the small size of the child for her age may cause her teachers to permit underachievement from a misguided sense of concern. Additionally the parents, and at an appropriate time the patient, must be given what is in their judgment an adequate explanation of the patient's gonadal status and its implications for pubertal development and fertility. In exceptional circumstances some patients, namely those with a mosaic genotype or a structurally abnormal X chromosome (for example XXq-), spontaneously develop pubertal changes and rarely even become pregnant. Specific therapy is directed towards any treatable malformations, for instance coarctation of the aorta, and judicious attempts to improve the more gross causes of unusual appearance resulting from webbed neck and protruding ears.

At or around the pubertal age of the girl's peer group or of an older sister substitution therapy is commenced with a combined oestrogen-progestogen preparation (norethynodrel 5 mg and ethinyloestradiol 0.075 mg) for 21 days and then recommenced after breakthrough menstrual bleeding. The author does not recommend initial continuous oestrogen priming therapy nor the sole use of oestrogens as replacement therapy. Anabolic steroids have been employed with the aim of inducing a growth spurt prior to oestrogen-progestogen replacement. Oral oxandrolone 0.10–0.25 mg/kg per day has been administered for 6–12 months (Moore *et al.*, 1977; Urban *et al.*, 1979). The total number of patients reported on this treatment is still relatively small and it is not entirely certain that the induced accelerated growth leads to an improved final height. The author's experience of such androgen therapy has been disappointing. Although the side effects are minimal and tolerable the benefits are at best small and the potential, if not actual, risks great.

Studies of neuropsychological function in Turner's syndrome have demonstrated impaired performance in word fluency, visuomotor coordination, visual memory and motor learning (Waber, 1979). The evidence for the presence of a deficiency in space-form perception is equivocal (Money and Alexander, 1966). In the author's experience the above characteristics have not proved to be a major problem of clinical management. In general children with Turner's syndrome appear remarkably passive and stoical in the clinical setting.

References

Money, J. and Alexander, D. (1966) Turner's syndrome: further demonstration of the presence of specific congenital deficiencies. *Journal of Medical Genetics*, **3**, 47

Moore, D.C., Tattoni, D.S. Ruvalcaba, M.D., Limbeck, G.A. and Kelley, V.C. (1977) Studies of anabolic steroids: effect of prolonged administration of oxandrolone on growth in children and adolescents with gonadal dysgenesis. *Journal of Pediatrics*, **90**, 462

Turner, H.H. (1938) A syndrome of infantilism, congenital webbed neck and cubitus valgus. *Endocrinology*, **23**, 566

Urban, M.D., Lee, P.A., Dorst, J.P., Plotnick, L.P. and Migeon, C.J. (1979) Oxandrolone therapy in patients with Turner's syndrome. *Journal of Pediatrics*, **94**, 823

Waber, D.P. (1979) Neuropsychological aspects of Turner's syndrome. *Developmental Medicine and Child Neurology*, **21**, 58

43 Sexual Precocity

Frank Harris

The medical literature is replete with terms such as complete and incomplete sexual precocity, true sexual precocity, true precocious puberty, precocious pseudopuberty and pubertas praecox. Using these names the subject has been reviewed by a number of authors (Jolly, 1955; Cloutier and Hayles, 1970; Reiter and Kulin, 1972). However, while all children with precocious puberty have sexual precocity not all children with sexual precocity have precocious puberty (*Table 43.1*). Therefore the correct use of

Table 43.1 Sexual precocity

Precocious puberty
Nonpubertal isosexual precocity including thelarche and
  pubarche
Heterosexual precocity

---

terms is important and the preferred nomenclature is outlined in *Figure 43.1*. Further discussion in this chapter adheres strictly to the terminology in *Table 43.1* and *Figure 43.1*.

The approach to management of a child with secondary sexual characteristics is dependent on

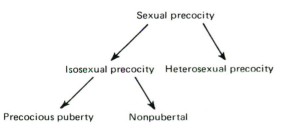

Figure 43.1. Flow scheme to demonstrate the preferred nomenclature in sexual precocity.

the history and the clinical signs. The premature development of secondary sexual changes may be either isosexual or heterosexual. When the changes are appropriate to the phenotypic sex they are isosexual and when inappropriate they are heterosexual (*Table 43.2*). If the changes described by the parents are confirmed to be appropriate for the sex of the patient then the differential diagnosis of isosexual precocity is pursued (*Tables 43.3 and 43.4*). The presence of isosexual maturation is considered precocious before the age of 8 years in girls and 10 years in boys. Heterosexual changes are abnormal at any age, although the finding of a mild degree of temporary breast enlargement in pubertal males is so frequent it should be approached as a normal variation of pubertal male development.

Tanner (1962) devised a widely accepted staging scheme for pubertal development (*Table*

Table 43.2 Isosexual and heterosexual changes

	Males	*Females*
Isosexual changes	Enlargement of penis	Breast development
	Enlargement and pigmentation of scrotum	Female distribution of pubic and body hair
	Male distribution of pubic and body hair	
	Deepening of voice	
Heterosexual changes	Gynaecomastia	Clitoral enlargement
		Male distribution of pubic and body hair
		Deepening of voice

515

Table 43.3   Causes of precocious puberty*

Constitutional (idiopathic)	
Neurogenic	Tumours (hamartomas and neoplasms particularly in hypothalamic and pineal areas)
	Phakomas (tuberous sclerosis and neurofibromatosis)
	Hydrocephalus
	Postmeningitis
	Postcerebral trauma
	Postcerebral irradiation
Treated congenital adrenal hyperplasia	
Hypothyroidism	
Russell-Silver syndrome**	

*All characterized by elevated FSH and LH levels and mature response to FSH/LH-RH.
**No known FSH/LH-RH studies.

Table 43.4   Nonpubertal isosexual precocity

Males	Congenital adrenal hyperplasia
	Testicular tumours (androgen producing)
	Adrenocortical carcinoma or adenoma
	Anabolic steroids
	McCune-Albright syndrome
	Hepatoma/teratoma*
Females	Ovarian tumours (granuloma cell or theca cell)
	Adrenal carcinoma or adenoma (oestrogen producing)
	Exogenous oestrogens
	Premature thelarche
	Premature pubarche
	McCune-Albright syndrome
	Teratoma*

*Gonadotrophin-like polypeptide-secreting tumours.

43.5). The Prader orchidometer has made possible a more uniform assessment of testicular volume (*Figure 43.2*).

Isosexual precocity

Precocious puberty

Precocious puberty describes the syndrome of isosexual precocity occurring as a result of premature hypothalamic-pituitary-gonadal maturation which may be due to a number of causes. The cardinal feature is the maturation of the hypothalamic-pituitary-gonadal axis and

Table 43.5   Staging of pubertal development (data from Tanner, 1962)

a. Stages of breast development

Stage 1	Preadolescent; elevation of papilla only
Stage 2	Breast bud palpable; elevation of breast and papilla as a small mound
Stage 3	Further enlargement and elevation of the breast and areola; no separate contour
Stage 4	Projection of areola and papilla to form a mound beyond the breast contour
Stage 5	Mature breast; papilla projects but areola recedes into the breast contour

b. Stages of pubic hair development

Stage 1	Preadolescent; vellus over pubes not further developed than that over abdominal wall
Stage 2	Sparse growth of long slightly pigmented downy hair, straight or slightly curled, chiefly at base of the penis or along labia
Stage 3	Considerably darker, coarser and more curled hair spreads sparsely over junction of pubes
Stage 4	Hair adult in type; area covered still considerably smaller than in adult; no spread to medial thighs
Stage 5	Hair adult in quantity and type with distribution of the horizontal (or classically feminine) pattern; spread to medial surface of thighs but not up linea alba or elsewhere above the base of the inverse triangle

c. Stages of boys' genital development

Stage 1	Preadolescent; testes, scrotum and penis about same size and proportion as in early childhood
Stage 2	Enlargement of scrotum and testes; skin of scrotum reddens and changes in texture; little or no enlargement of penis at this stage
Stage 3	Enlargement of penis, which occurs at first mainly in length; further growth of testes and scrotum
Stage 4	Increased size of penis with growth in breadth and development of glans; testes and scrotum larger; scrotal skin darkened
Stage 5	Genitalia adult in size and shape

this serves to distinguish precocious puberty from other forms of nonpubertal isosexual precocity.

Precocious puberty is an uncommon disorder and its incidence is unknown because paediatric endocrine clinics tend to attract patients from an undetermined population base. The Endocrine Clinic at Alder Hey Children's Hospital registered 15 new patients with precocious puberty over a 5-year period (1975–80) from an indeterminate catchment area. The majority of patients are girls by a ratio of 13:2. At the Mayo Clinic 96 children with the diagnosis of sexual precocity were seen over a 30-year period (Sigurjonsdottir and Hayles, 1968).

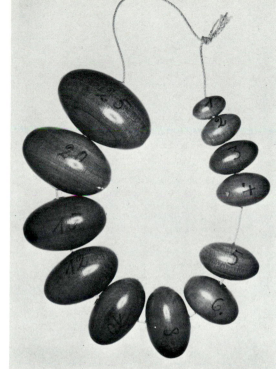

Figure 43.2. The Prader orchidometer.

Diagnostic criteria

The initial age for considering the diagnosis of precocious puberty is somewhat arbitrary. According to Tanner (1962) less than 3 per cent of the normal population of girls develop the first pubertal changes before the age of 9 years and less than 3 per cent of normal boys before 9.5–10 years. In practice children with isosexual precocity referred for management are usually younger than 8 years of age. Parents and family doctors appear to exercise some degree of selection based on their own perception of what constitutes normal development and how they imagine the young patient will cope. The diagnostic criteria for precocious puberty are summarized in *Table 43.6*. By definition the sexual precocity must be isosexual. Therefore male patients should exhibit testicular enlargement, pubic hair and maturation of the external genitalia. The voice may deepen and the musculature may become prominent. Female patients should show breast enlargement and appropriate distribution of pubic hair and may

Table 43.6 Diagnostic criteria of precocious puberty

Isosexual precocity
Onset in males at less than 10 years and in females at less than 8 years
Testicular volume greater than 4 ml
Accelerated height velocity and skeletal maturation
Pubertal response to gonadotrophin-releasing factor

have vaginal bleeding. Children of both sexes may demonstrate acne. While in most cases the progression of the pubertal development is in the normal order it is not only early in onset but also accelerated through the various stages (see *Table 43.5c* for staging of male genital development, *43.5b* for pubic hair development in both sexes and *43.5a* for breast development).

In boys the presence of isosexual precocity and bilateral testicular enlargement enables a firm clinical diagnosis of precocious puberty to be made because the gonads can be readily palpated as enlarged, that is greater than 4 ml. However, a few boys have been described with nonpubertal isosexual precocity and bilateral testicular tumours or bilateral aberrant adrenal tissue in the adrenogenital syndrome simulating precocious puberty because of the testicular enlargement (Rezek and Hardin, 1955; Schoen, Di Raimondo and Dominguez, 1961).

In girls the maturation of the gonads in the sense of having responded to hypothalamic-pituitary stimulation cannot be assessed on physical examination. Consequently the diagnosis of precocious puberty is less firm in girls when made on clinical findings alone because isosexual precocity including vaginal bleeding may result from local ovarian pathology such as tumour.

The first clinical evidence of precocious puberty may appear as early as within the first year of life and at any time thereafter. In girls the initial signs are development of the breasts and appearance of pubic hair with acceleration of growth. The development of sexual maturity may then proceed to vaginal bleeding which becomes cyclical. In boys the development of enlarged testes is accompanied by enlargement of the scrotum and the penis with typical pubic hair growth.

Constitutional precocious puberty

In idiopathic (cryptogenic) or constitutional precocious puberty there are no clinical signs other than those of a normal but premature onset of puberty. This particular form of the condition occurs far more commonly in girls than in boys by perhaps more than 10 to one.

Children with precocious puberty in the absence of any other endocrine disorder usually demonstrate obviously accelerated somatic and skeletal growth (*Figure 43.3*). Hence their size at presentation may be around or even above the 97th centile for height and weight. The skeletal

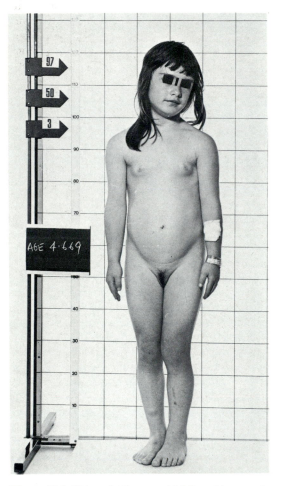

Figure 43.3. Girl aged 4½ years with idiopathic precocious puberty. Her height is above the 97th centile and there is breast and pubic hair development.

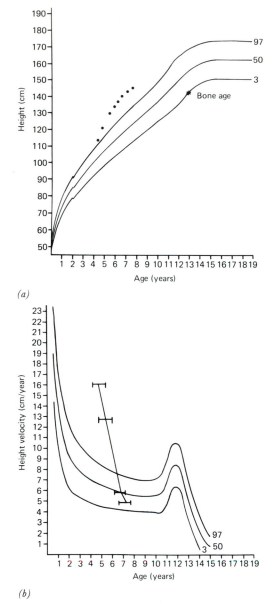

(a)

(b)

Figure 43.4. Serial measurements in a girl with precocious puberty. *(a)* Height chart. The patient's height is above the 97th centile between 4½–8 years of age. Her bone age is 13 years at the chronological age of 8. *(b)* Height velocity chart illustrating an abnormally fast rate of growth per year. The later deceleration in growth rate is related to premature closure of the epiphyses.

maturation at the left wrist and hand assessed from the Greulich and Pyle atlas (Greulich and Pyle, 1959) or by the radius-ulna score (Tanner *et al.*, 1975) is well advanced over the chronological age. If serial measurements are available, a greatly accelerated height velocity can be shown (*Figure 43.4*). Ultimately the rapidly advancing

bone age which is presumably due to the gonadal steroids leads to chronologically premature cessation of growth. The bone age can be so advanced and lead to such early epiphyseal fusion that the erstwhile oversized child is destined to become a growth-restricted adult (*Figure 43.5*).

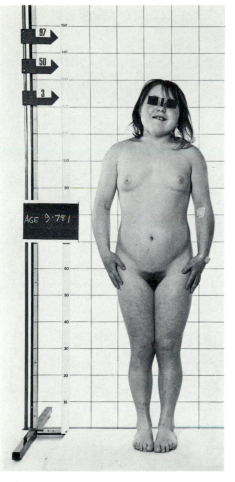

Figure 43.5. A 9-year-old girl with complete fusion of the epiphyses and an estimated bone age of 16 years. She has achieved her final adult height at the age of 9 years. The condition followed irradiation for medulloblastoma.

Neurogenic precocious puberty

These young children have a structural abnormality in the brain that is causally associated with precocious puberty and they should have as complete as possible an assessment of hypothalamic-pituitary function. The intracerebral lesion may lead to other endocrine dysfunction in addition to its effect on gonadotrophin secretion. In this group the difference in sex incidence is much less marked than with idiopathic precocious puberty although more girls than boys appear to develop isosexual precocity following hydrocephalus.

It is likely that structural lesions such as tuberous sclerosis and postirradiation damage disturb the intrahypothalamic function and the balance between RH and release-inhibiting hormone, or disrupt neurotransmitter elaboration in extrahypothalamic neurones that modulate the release of hypothalamic hormones into the portal hypophyseal circulation (Collu, 1977). Hypothalamic hamartomas may present a special situation where the tumour actually produces LH-RH and thus causes precocious puberty (Judge *et al.*, 1977). Since some of the intracerebral structural lesions leading to precocious puberty are small and not accompanied by neurological signs full use should be made of cranial computed tomography in children with precocious puberty (Hung *et al.*, 1980).

A striking clinical syndrome of neurogenic precocious puberty occurs with gelastic epilepsy (laughing seizures) often with a demonstrable lesion in the hypothalamus (Penfold, Manson and Caldicott, 1978). Management is directed to control of epilepsy and sexual precocity and, where feasible, tumour excision.

Untreated hypothyroidism

Hypothyroidism in childhood is a well documented but very unusual association with precocious puberty (Costin *et al.*, 1972). The patients have obvious symptoms and signs of juvenile hypothyroidism in addition to evidence of isosexual precocity. Recent studies have demonstrated that there are not only elevated plasma LH and FSH levels but also hyperprolactinaemia. There is an overlap between TSH and prolactin in response to TRH. In the presence of a low plasma thyroxine level the elevated TRH concentration results in hyperprolactinaemia which itself may mediate the release of FSH and LH (Barnes, Hayles and Ryan, 1973; Hemady, Siler-Khodr and Najjar, 1978). The clinical signs of sexual precocity largely resolve after the institution of treatment with thyroxine.

Russell-Silver syndrome (Silver syndrome)

This disorder includes a spectrum of congenital malformations (Silver, 1964; Smith, 1976). A number of affected children have variations in the pattern of sexual development including isosexual precocity with elevated urinary gonadotrophin concentrations. These patients therefore belong under the heading of precocious puberty. The accompanying major malformations include short stature of prenatal onset, skeletal asymmetry and clinodactyly. The aetiology of this syndrome is unknown and the incidence of precocious puberty is low.

Treated congenital adrenal hyperplasia

It is now apparent that boys with adequately treated congenital adrenal hyperplasia may develop precocious puberty. Their prolonged albeit intermittent exposure to elevated levels of sex steroids may lead to a premature reduction in hypothalamic sensitivity to sex steroids and consequently induce premature onset of hypothalamic-pituitary maturation (Penny, Olambiwonnu and Frasier, 1973). While the onset of puberty may be very early, in practice the affected boys only seem to present with testicular enlargement at or around the age of 9–10 years. Apart from counselling (see below) no treatment is necessary.

Investigations

In neurogenic precocious puberty due to various types of intracerebral pathology there may be additional clinical signs. These may be very obvious such as those in hydrocephalus or rapidly expanding tumours with neurological signs. On the other hand the symptom-free and sign-free child may have a very small neoplasm that is exerting its effects because of its site rather than its size. Consequently a complete history and clinical examination followed by a rational programme of investigation are always necessary in any child presenting with signs of isosexual precocity (*Table 43.7*).

The FSH/LH-RH test is done easily and without significant hazard. The synthetic form of hypothalamic RH, which is a decapeptide, is used. Following intravenous bolus administration of FSH/LH-RH 100 μg, blood should be

Table 43.7   Investigation of the child with clinically suspected precocious puberty

---

Measurement of height and weight
Examination of skeletal maturation at left hand and wrist
Skull X-ray
EEG
CT scan
FSH/LH-RH test
Examination under anaesthesia*

---

*Only where there is doubt concerning the presence of pelvic abnormality with or without precocious puberty. This opportunity should then be taken for obtaining a vaginal smear for evidence of oestrogenization.

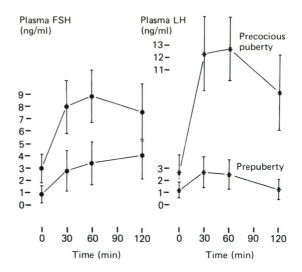

Figure 43.6. Comparisons of the response of plasma FSH and LH in 43 prepubertal patients and 10 patients with precocious puberty following intravenous FSH/LH-RH 100 μg.

taken at 15, 30, 45 and 60 minutes. In prepubertal subjects the response of plasma FSH and particularly plasma LH is significantly less than in the pubertal subject (*Figure 43.6*). Consequently a positive response differentiates precocious puberty from nonpubertal isosexual precocity. The author has demonstrated no difference between the response to FSH/LH-RH in patients with constitutional as opposed to neurogenic precocious puberty. A further blood sample can be taken at 240 minutes and measured for either plasma testosterone or beta oestradiol. In children with precocious puberty there may be a substantial increment at this time over the basal value.

Electroencephalographic changes are known to occur in constitutional precocious puberty where there is no detectable structural abnormality (Liu *et al.*, 1965). There may be a slow wave pattern in the absence of a recognizable neurogenic cause for precocious puberty.

Nonpubertal isosexual precocity (Table 43.4)

Tumours secreting gonadotrophin-like polypeptides

Nonpubertal isosexual precocity has been recognized accompanying embryonal tumours (teratomas) in children of either sex. These tumours are usually highly malignant and occur in the ovary and the brain (chorionepithelioma), the pelvis (presacral teratoma) and the liver (primary hepatoblastoma). Case reports have described the presence of gonadotrophins and sex steroids produced by the tumour (Seckel, 1946; Levine *et al.*, 1956; Bruton, Martz and Gerard, 1961; Hung *et al.*, 1963; Hutchinson *et al.*, 1969; Braunstein *et al.*, 1972). If these tumours secrete sex steroids then the clinical presentation may be with heterosexual precocity depending on the nature of tumour steroidogenesis.

Anabolic steroids and exogenous oestrogens

There have been instances of isosexual precocity developing after administration of anabolic (androgenic) steroids to young boys and inadvertent oestrogen administration to prepubertal girls. Androgenic steroids have been used in the treatment of hypoplastic anaemia in childhood and an inevitable unwanted side effect is the development of pubic hair and an increase in penile and scrotal size. Similar effects are encountered when anabolic steroids are used less discriminately in very young males ostensibly to promote growth. Oestrogens applied topically have led to isosexual precocity (Whittle and Lyell, 1948). Contamination of tablets and vitamin capsules by oestrogen has led to a number of girls and boys developing respectively isosexual and heterosexual precocity (Hertz, 1958; Weber *et al.*, 1963).

Premature thelarche

A relatively common form of isosexual precocity in young girls is premature isolated development of the breasts. In thelarche there are no other signs of sexual precocity and the girl does not show evidence of accelerated growth. However, some studies have demonstrated histological evidence of oestrogen effects on cells in urine sediment (Collet-Solberg and Grumbach, 1965). The natural history in the majority of patients is spontaneous resolution of the breast enlargement or no further progression after presentation. With further somatic growth the breast enlargement becomes increasingly less obvious. Puberty occurs at the normal time.

In males prepubertal gynaecomastia is a sign of heterosexual precocity. It is rare and may be idiopathic (August, Chandra and Hung, 1972) or due to an oestrogen-producing tumour.

Premature pubarche (adrenarche)

Pubic hair may develop as an isolated sign of sexual precocity and like thelarche may spontaneously remit. The isolated premature development of pubic hair has been attributed to the early attainment of adrenarche by the adrenal cortex and occurs much more frequently in girls (Silverman *et al.*, 1952; Warne *et al.*, 1978). Occasionally there may be accompanying axillary hair. In young girls the differential diagnosis includes congenital adrenal hyperplasia which may be excluded by the finding of normal levels of plasma 17-hydroxyprogesterone (August, Hung and Mayes, 1975) and urinary pregnanetriol. Adrenocortical tumours produce excess urinary dehydroepiandrosterone and oxosteroids and the raised levels are not suppressed by dexamethasone.

McCune-Albright syndrome

The association of polyostotic fibrous dysplasia and skin pigmentation with isosexual precocity is a readily recognizable but rare syndrome occurring in girls and in a very few boys (Albright *et al.*, 1937; Jolly, 1955; Benedict, 1962). Vaginal bleeding not uncommonly precedes the development of breasts and pubic hair. Luteinized follicular cysts are a recognized finding. Hyperthyroidism, Cushing's syndrome and acromegaly have been reported in association with McCune-Albright syndrome and this has led to the hypothesis that it is due to a congenital hypothalamic disorder (Hall and Warrick, 1972). Results of FSH/LH-RH tests on four occasions in three young female patients have not shown evidence of hypothalamic-pituitary maturation and so the author favours the concept of a peripheral endocrinopathy causing the sexual precocity (Danon and Crawford, 1974). Therefore McCune-Albright syndrome is considered in this chapter as a cause of nonpubertal isosexual precocity.

Heterosexual precocity

The major causes of heterosexual precocity are outlined in *Table 43.8*. They are discussed further in Chapters 44 and 47. It should be restated that heterosexual precocity is not a presentation of precocious puberty as defined in this chapter.

Table 43.8   Heterosexual precocity

Females	Congenital adrenal hyperplasia
	Androgen-producing adrenal carcinoma or adenoma
	Ovarian tumour (androgen producing)
	Anabolic steroids
Males	Adrenocortical adenoma or carcinoma (oestrogen producing)
	Testicular tumour (oestrogen producing)
	Exogenous oestrogens

Management

The specific treatment of children with sexual precocity depends on the underlying cause. All parents of affected young children together with older children themselves require counselling. In patients with nonpubertal isosexual precocity and heterosexual precocity specific treatment of the underlying cause is often available, for example in congenital adrenal hyperplasia (*see* Chapter 44), ovarian tumours (*see* Chapter 47) and testicular tumours (*see* Chapter 47). This present section is concerned with the treatment of the child with constitutional precocious puberty and neurogenic precocious puberty. The author's approach is based on the importance of counselling in addition to drug therapy for control of the secondary sexual development. In those cases of neurogenic precocious puberty where a structural lesion can be identified, treatment modalities such as surgery and irradiation would be considered.

Counselling

A major contribution to the understanding of the needs of children affected with precocious puberty and their parents has been made by Money (Hampson and Money, 1955; Money and Hampson, 1955). The child's psychological and psychosexual maturity is determined by life experience and is not an automatic product of somatic sexual maturation. The following are general guidelines to counselling (Wilkins, 1965):

1. Because children with sexual precocity are often physically robust and active they may appear hyperactive and clumsy. Parents and teachers require tolerance and discretion. The child's physical activity needs to be planned, taking into account physical robustness balanced against age.
2. Children capable of understanding benefit from being told in a simple way of the essential normality of their state.
3. Most parents require a lengthy explanation concerning the biology of sexual maturation.
4. Such information may not be sufficient to allay parental fears concerning promiscuity and perversion. These matters may have to be raised by the physician to reassure the parents about such taboo subjects which they are not likely to raise themselves.
5. Children with sexual precocity may or may not masturbate. It is unrealistic to forbid or punish them and they should be taught to use privacy and not to be ashamed.
6. Affected children may or may not be advanced in social maturity which is often outstripped by physical maturity. They should be treated in accordance with their level of social maturity.
7. If maladjustment does occur, it is more likely to be the result of life experience than to be related directly to the precocious puberty.
8. Parents, teachers and medical staff require to be reminded of the child's chronological age.
9. In the event of no treatment being administered to control secondary sexual maturation girls should be advised about the onset of menstruation.
10. Breast development and other evidence of secondary sexual maturity should be stressed as being early and normal.

Drug treatment

With support from their parents some girls cope with the onset of menstruation and secondary sexual development by the age of 6 years. There are other young children in whom drug control of secondary maturation is indicated because their parents have a high degree of anxiety and counselling alone does not provide sufficient support for them during the childhood years. Unfortunately the relative rarity of this group of disorders is such that very few clinics have had adequate experience of more than one drug. Currently there are three agents that have been used in the treatment of precocious puberty, namely danazol, medroxyprogesterone acetate and cyproterone acetate.

Danazol

This drug has been used by the author over the last 4 years in 11 children with precocious puberty, which was in eight of constitutional and in three of neurogenic origin (Smith and Harris, 1977, 1979). Danazol is an isoxasol derivative of 17-alpha-ethyltestosterone and is said to have only very weak androgenic properties. Evidence from studies in adult women demonstrates that the drug acts by interference with oestrogen receptors at all levels. From studies in children there is definite evidence of suppression of both LH and FSH in response to FSH/LH-RH (Smith and Harris, 1979). Danazol is given by mouth and is well tolerated. Good control of secondary sexual development is obtained with cessation of menstruation, reduction of breast size and no further increase in pubic hair. However, the drug does not reduce the acceleration of skeletal maturation and linear height and may enhance growth acceleration. Mild acne, some deepening of the voice and increase in body hair have occurred. Danazol may be administered once or twice daily by mouth in dosage of 5–10 mg/kg per 24 hours. Its availability only as 100 mg and 200 mg capsules is a constraint on dosage.

Medroxyprogesterone acetate

Medroxyprogesterone acetate is a 6-methyl derivative of 17-hydroxyprogesterone and has no androgenic or oestrogenic properties (Kupperman and Epstein, 1962). It has been used widely in the management of precocious puberty (Hahn, Hayles and Albert, 1964; Kaplan, Ling and Irani, 1968). Although there are variable responses in plasma gonadotrophin levels (Root *et al.*, 1970), the drug is effective in stopping menstruation and reducing breast size while there is no significant effect on pubic hair. Medroxyprogesterone acetate has no useful effect on the rate of skeletal maturation or the ultimate height attained by treated patients. It may be given orally as 10 mg daily or intramuscularly as 150 mg every 2 weeks. The drug has glucocorticoid-like properties which are dose dependent. Impairment of adrenocortical function in patients receiving it has been reported (Sadeghi-Nejad, Kaplan and Grumbach, 1971).

Cyproterone acetate

Cyproterone acetate is the most recent drug to be used in the management of precocious puberty. The author has had no experience with it. Cyproterone acetate is a 1,2-alpha methylene-substituted steroid with marked antiandrogenic effects (Werder *et al.*, 1974; Bierich, 1975). It is given orally as 70 mg/m² per day. While it is successful in suppressing menstruation and breast development there is no beneficial effect on growth and skeletal maturation. Recent reports indicate that cyproterone acetate decreases secretion of CRF and ACTH during stress. Appropriate care needs to be taken in patients on this drug who undergo surgery or suffer other stress.

References

Albright, F., Butler, A.M., Hampton, A.O. and Smith, P. (1937) Syndrome characterized by osteitis fibrosa discriminata, areas of pigmentation and endocrine dysfunction, with precocious puberty in females: report of five cases. *New England Journal of Medicine*, **216**, 727

August, G.P., Chandra, R. and Hung, W. (1972) Prepubertal gynaecomastia. *Journal of Pediatrics*, **80**, 259

August, G.P., Hung, W. and Mayes, D.M. (1975) Plasma androgens in premature pubarche: value of 17α hydroxyprogesterone in differentiation from congenital adrenal hyperplasia. *Journal of Pediatrics*, **87**, 246

Barnes, N.D., Hayles, A.B. and Ryan, R.J. (1973) Sexual maturation in juvenile hypothyroidism. *Mayo Clinic Proceedings*, **48**, 849

Benedict, P.H. (1962) Endocrine features in Albright's syndrome (fibrous dysplasia of bone). *Metabolism*, **11**, 30

Bierich, J.R. (1975) Sexual precocity. *In* Clinics in Endocrinology and Metabolism, Vol. 4 (edited by Bierich, J.R.). Saunders, Philadelphia. p.30

Braunstein, G.D., Bridson, W.E., Glass, A., Hull, E.W. and McIntire, K.R. (1972) In vivo and in vitro production of human chorionic gonadotrophin and alpha-feto-protein by a virilizing hepatoblastoma. *Journal of Clinical Endocrinology and Metabolism*, **35**, 857

Bruton, O.C., Martz, D.C. and Gerard, E.S. (1961) Precocious puberty due to secreting chorionepithelioma (teratoma) of the brain. *Journal of Pediatrics*, **59**, 719

Cloutier, M.D. and Hayles, A.B. (1970) Precocious puberty. *In* Advances in Pediatrics (edited by Schulman, I.). Year Book Medical Publishers, Chicago. p.125

Collett-Solberg, P.R. and Grumbach, M.M. (1965) A simplified procedure for evaluating estrogenic effects and the sex chromatin pattern in exfoliated cells in urine: studies in premature thelarche and gynaecomastia of adolescence. *Journal of Pediatrics*, **66**, 883

Collu, R. (1977) Role of Central Cholinergic and Aminergic Neurotransmitters in the Control of Anterior Pituitary Hormone Secretion in Clinical Neuroendocrinology (edited by Martini, L. and Besser, G.M.). Academic Press, London

Costin, G., Keishnar, A.K., Kogut, M.D. and Turkington, R.W. (1972) Prolactin activity in juvenile hypothyroidism and precocious puberty. *Pediatrics*, **50**, 881

Danon, M. and Crawford, J.D. (1974) Peripheral endocrinopathy causing sexual precocity in Albright syndrome. *Pediatric Research*, **8**, 368

Greulich, W.W. and Pyle, S.I. (1959) Radiographic Atlas of Skeletal Development of Hand and Wrist. Stanford University Press, Stanford, California

Hahn, H.B., Hayles, A.B. and Albert, A. (1964) Medroxyprogesterone and constitutional precocious puberty. *Mayo Clinic Proceedings*, **39**, 182

Hall, R. and Warrick, C. (1972) Hypersecretion of hypothalamic releasing hormones: a possible explanation of the endocrine manifestations of polyostatic fibrous dysplasia (Albright's syndrome). *Lancet*, i, 1313

Hampson, J.G. and Money, J. (1955) Idiopathic sexual precocity in the female. *Psychosomatic Medicine*, **17**, 16

Hemady, Z.S., Siler-Khodr, T.M. and Najjar, S. (1978) Precocious puberty in juvenile hypothyroidism. *Journal of Pediatrics*, **92**, 55

Hertz, R. (1958) Accidental ingestion of estrogens by children. *Pediatrics*, **21**, 203

Hung, W., Blizzard, R.M., Migeon, C.J., Camacho, A.M. and Nyhan, W.L. (1963) Precocious puberty in a boy with hepatoma and circulating gonadotrophin. *Journal of Pediatrics*, **63**, 895

Hung, W., August, G.P., Braillier, D.R. and Milhorat, T. (1980) Computerized tomography in the evaluation of isosexual precocity. *American Journal of Diseases of Children*, **134**, 25

Hutchinson, J.S.M., Brooks, R.V., Barratt, T.M., Newman, C.G.H. and Prunty, T.F.G. (1969) Sexual precocity due to an intracranial tumour causing unusual testicular secretion of testosterone. *Archives of Disease in Childhood*, **44**, 732

Jolly, H. (1955) Sexual Precocity. Blackwell, Oxford

Judge, D.M., Kulin, H.E., Page, R., Santen, R. and Trapukdi, S. (1977) Hypothalamic hamartoma: a source of luteinizing-hormone-releasing factor in precocious puberty. *New England Journal of Medicine*, **296**, 7

Kaplan, S.A., Ling, S.M. and Irani, N.G. (1968). Idiopathic sexual precocity: therapy with medroxyprogesterone. *American Journal of Diseases of Children*, **116**, 591

Kupperman, H.S. and Epstein, J.A. (1962) Medroxyprogesterone acetate in the treatment of constitutional sexual precocity. *Journal of Clinical Endocrinology and Metabolism*, **22**, 456

Levine, S.Z., Barnett, H.L., Shibuya, M. and Barker, J.K. (1956) Isosexual precocity in boys including a case of a gonadotrophin-producing teratoma. *In* Advances in Pediatrics, Vol.8 (edited by Levine, S.Z.). Year Book Medical Publishers, Chicago. pp. 58, 62

Liu, N., Grumbach, M.M., De Napoli, R.A. and Marishima, A. (1965) Prevalence of electroencephalographic abnormalities in idiopathic precocious puberty and premature pubarche. *Journal of Clinical Endocrinology and Metabolism*, **25**, 1296

Money, J. and Hampson, J.G. (1955) Idiopathic sexual precocity in the male. *Psychosomatic Medicine*, **17**, 1

Penfold, J.L., Manson, J.I. and Caldicott, W.M. (1978) Laughing seizures and precocious puberty. *Australian Paediatric Journal*, **14**, 185

Penny, R., Olambiwonnu, N.O. and Frasier, S.D. (1973) Precocious puberty following treatment in a six-year-old male with congenital adrenal hyperplasia: studies of

serum luteinizing hormone (LH), serum follicle-stimulating hormone (FSH) and plasma testosterone. *Journal of Clinical Endocrinology and Metabolism*, **36**, 920

Reiter, E.O. and Kulin, H.E. (1972) Sexual maturation in the female: normal development and precocious puberty. *Pediatric Clinics of North America*, **19**, 581

Rezek, P. and Hardin, H.C. (1955) Bilateral interstitial cell tumour of the testicle: report of one case observed fourteen years. *Journal of Urology*, **74**, 628

Root, A.W., Moshang, T., Bongiovanni, A.M. and Eberlein, W.R. (1970) Concentrations of plasma luteinizing hormone in infants, children and adolescents with normal and abnormal gonadal function. *Pediatric Research*, **4**, 175

Sadeghi-Nejad, A. Kaplan, S.L. and Grumbach, M.M. (1971) The effect of medroxyprogesterone acetate on adrenocortical function in children with precocious puberty. *Journal of Pediatrics*, **78**, 616

Schoen, E.J., Di Raimondo, V. and Dominguez, O.U. (1961) Bilateral testicular tumours complicating adrenal hyperplasia. *Journal of Clinical Endocrinology and Metabolism*, **21**, 518

Seckel, H.P.E. (1946) Precocious sexual development in children. *Medical Clinics of North America*, **30**, 183

Sigurjonsdottir, T.J. and Hayles, A.B. (1968) Precocious puberty. *American Journal of Diseases of Children*, **115**, 309

Silver, H.K. (1964) Asymmetry, short stature and variations in sexual development. *American Journal of Diseases of Children*, **107**, 495

Silverman, S.H., Migeon, C., Rosenberg, E. and Wilkins, L. (1952) Precocious growth of sexual hair without other secondary development; "premature pubarche" a constitutional variation of adolescence. *Pediatrics*, **10**, 426

Smith, C.S. and Harris, F. (1977) Preliminary experience with danazol in children with precocious puberty. *Journal of International Medical Research*, **5**, Suppl.3, p.109

Smith, C.S. and Harris, F. (1979) The role of danazol in the management of precocious puberty. *Postgraduate Medical Journal*, **55**, Suppl.5,p.81

Smith, D.W. (1976) Recognizable patterns of human malformation. *In* Major Problems in Clinical Paediatrics, 2nd edn. Saunders, Philadelphia. p.60

Tanner, J.S. (1962) Growth at Adolescence, 2nd edn. Blackwell, Oxford

Tanner, J.M. Whitehouse, R.H., Marshall, W.A., Healey, M.J.R. and Goldstein, H. (1975) Assessment of skeletal maturity and prediction of adult height. Academic Press, London

Warne, G.L., Carter, J.N. Faiman, C., Reyes, F.I. and Winter, J.S.D. (1978) Hormonal changes in girls with precocious adrenarche: a possible role for estradiol or prolactin. *Journal of Pediatrics*, **92**, 743

Weber, W.W., Grossman, M., Thom, J.V., Sax, J., Chan, J.J. and Duffy, M.P. (1963) Drug contamination with diethylstilbestrol. *New England Journal of Medicine*, **268**, 411

Werder, E.A., Murset, G., Zachman, M. and Brook, C.G.D. (1974) Treatment of precocious puberty with cyproterone acetate. *Pediatric Research*, **8**, 248

Whittle, C.H. and Lyell, A. (1948) Precocity in a girl aged 5: due to stilboestrol inunction. *Proceedings of the Royal Society of Medicine*, **41**, 760

Wilkins, L. (1965) The Diagnosis and Treatment of Endocrine Disorders in Childhood and Adolescence, 3rd edn. Thomas, Springfield, Illinois

44 Congenital Adrenal Hyperplasia and Female Pseudohermaphroditism

David B. Grant and J.H. Johnston

Female pseudohermaphroditism arises as a result of abnormal masculinization of the female external genitalia before birth. The degree of virilization can range from enlargement of the clitoris or fusion of the posterior parts of the labia to a completely male appearance (*Figure 44.1*). Such patients have normal female 46 XX karyotypes with normal differentiation and development of the ovaries and the müllerian derivatives.

Table 44.1 Classification of female pseudohermaphroditism

Congenital adrenal hyperplasia	21-Hydroxylase deficiency
	11-Hydroxylase deficiency
	3β-Hydroxysteroid-dehydrogenase deficiency
Virilization by a maternal tumour	
Iatrogenic	Progestin treatment in pregnancy
Pseudohermaphroditism associated with dysmorphic syndromes	
Pseudohermaphroditism associated with hindgut anomalies	
Unexplained pseudohermaphroditism	
Local lesions of the clitoris	

The commonest and most important cause of female pseudohermaphroditism is congenital adrenal hyperplasia with 21-hydroxylase deficiency but other conditions can also give rise to female intersex (*Table 44.1*). In a very small number of cases the aetiology remains uncertain even after extensive investigations.

Congenital adrenal hyperplasia

The association of female pseudohermaphroditism with bilateral hyperplasia of the adrenal glands (adrenogenital syndrome) has long been known. Nevertheless, the true nature of the

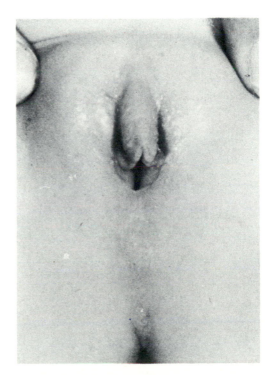

(a)

525

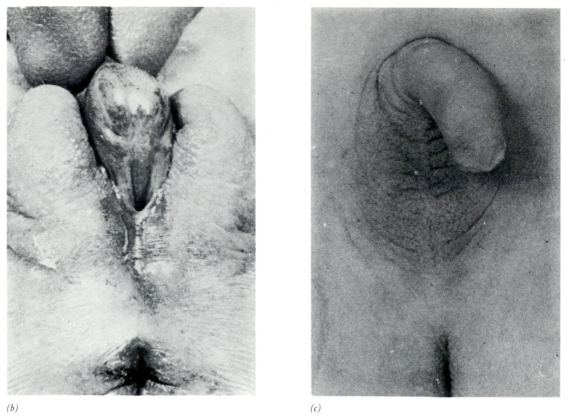

(b)   *(c)*

Figure 44.1. Genital appearance in female pseudohermaphroditism ranging from enlargement of the clitoris with slight labial fusion through an intermediate picture with a single opening into a urogenital sinus to a completely male appearance with a 'penile' urethra.

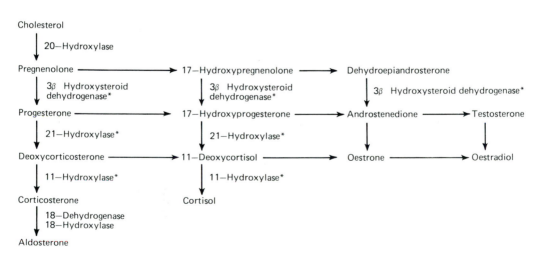

Figure 44.2. Enzyme defects of aldosterone and cortisol biosynthesis. *Defects of these enzymes cause female pseudohermaphroditism.

disorder was not appreciated until Wilkins *et al.* (1950) and Bartter, Forbes and Leaf (1950) independently showed that the elevated 17-oxosteroid excretion can be reversed by treatment with cortisone, thus indicating that the disorder is caused by a defect in cortisol biosynthesis.

It is now known that three different enzyme defects can lead to adrenal hyperplasia associated with female virilization. These are 21-hydroxylase, 11-hydroxylase and 3-beta-hydroxysteroid-dehydrogenase deficiencies (*Figure 44.2*). Further adrenal enzyme defects associated with incomplete male masculinization have been recognized, that is lipid adrenal hyperplasia and 17-hydroxylase deficiency, and these are discussed further under Male intersexual disorders in Chapter 39. Enzyme defects that selectively interfere with aldosterone biosynthesis have also been described, namely 18-oxidase and 18-hydroxylase deficiencies. While these conditions cause salt loss they are not associated with abnormal genital development and are not considered in this chapter.

Deficiency of 21-hydroxylase

This is the commonest cause of female pseudohermaphroditism and is inherited as a recessive disorder. Although both sexes are affected genital development is normal in males. The frequency of the condition varies in different populations, for example in Yupik Eskimos in Alaska the incidence is about one in every 500 births (Hirschfeld and Fleshman, 1969) while in Switzerland the frequency is about one in 5000 (Prader, 1958). It is now known that the gene or genes responsible for the enzyme defect are located on the short arm of chromosome pair no.6 where they are closely associated with the genes controlling HLA status (Levine *et al.*, 1978).

As a result of the enzyme defect the biosynthesis of cortisol and aldosterone is probably impaired to a greater or lesser extent in all patients (*Figure 44.2*) but there is wide variation in the severity of the disorder and clinical evidence of salt loss occurs in roughly half the cases (Marks and Fink, 1969). This variation does not occur within individual families and if one child suffers from severe salt loss then subsequent affected siblings are also likely to do so. Impaired aldo-

sterone secretion (New and Seaman, 1970) is thought to be the major factor behind this salt loss, which may be exaggerated by the natriuretic effect of other steroids such as 17-alpha-hydroxyprogesterone (Jacobs *et al.*, 1961) and progesterone (Landau and Lugibihl, 1958). These antialdosterone effects probably account for the apparently paradoxical finding of a normal aldosterone secretion rate in a child with early salt loss who was described by Visser and Degenhart (1967).

Deficiency of 21-hydroxylase coupled with excessive adrenal stimulation by ACTH following defective cortisol biosynthesis leads to overproduction of intermediate steroids. In particular this affects 17-alpha-hydroxyprogesterone (*Figure 44.2*) which can be metabolized to testosterone and in turn converted to dihydrotestosterone by the enzyme 5-alpha-reductase in the perineal tissues, thus causing virilization.

Excessive adrenal androgen production may start early in fetal life leading to complete masculinization of the external genitalia (*Figure 44.1*). On the other hand it may have a less marked effect producing enlargement of the clitoris, which is usually associated with posterior labial fusion and formation of a urogenital sinus. The openings of the urethra and the vagina into the urogenital sinus may be separate, although in very virilized patients the hypoplastic lower vagina opens into the posterior urethra as a result of androgen-induced inhibition of growth of the sinovaginal bulbs in early fetal life.

Testosterone secreted by the adrenal glands does not maintain the wolffian structures, and the male accessory ducts are absent. Ovarian differentiation and development are normal and the upper vagina, the cervix, the uterus and the fallopian tubes also develop normally since anti-müllerian hormone is not produced.

Deficiency of 11-hydroxylase

This is less common than 21-hydroxylase deficiency. It too results in female pseudohermaphroditism and can lead to marked virilization of the external genitalia in newborn girls. As in 21-hydroxylase deficiency ovarian and müllerian development are normal. In addition to causing excess testosterone production this enzyme defect leads to increased secretion of deoxycorticosterone and deoxycortisol or compound S (*Figure 44.2*) which are potent mineralocorticoids and compensate for the deficient aldosterone production, thereby preventing salt loss. These intermediate steroids account for the hypertension that often develops in later childhood in untreated cases (Bongiovanni and Eberlein, 1955). Glucocorticoid treatment in this condition can sometimes lead to salt loss by suppressing production of deoxycorticosterone and deoxycortisol and thus unmasking the deficiency of aldosterone production. With the exceptions of the development of hypertension and the absence of salt loss the clinical features of 11-hydroxylase and 21-hydroxylase deficiencies are the same.

Deficiency of 3-beta-hydroxysteroid-dehydrogenase

This uncommon enzyme defect has already been discussed under the causes of male pseudohermaphroditism due to defective testosterone biosynthesis. Paradoxically it is a well recognized cause of female pseudohermaphroditism as well. It is believed that the prenatal virilization of the female external genitalia is due to excess secretion of dehydroepiandrosterone which is a weak androgen. In addition to causing abnormal external genital development in both sexes deficiency of 3-beta-hydroxysteroid-dehydrogenase leads to defective aldosterone synthesis, and severe salt loss usually develops in early infancy (Bongiovanni and Kellenbenz, 1962). A few examples without salt loss have been described and presumably they result from incomplete enzyme deficiency (Kenny, Reynolds and Green, 1971).

Clinical features

Females

Girls with the three types of congenital adrenal hyperplasia described above can usually be recognized at birth by their abnormal external genitalia. Babies that are completely virilized may be mistaken for cryptorchid males and the true state of affairs may only become apparent when a salt-losing crisis develops or further virilization occurs in early childhood. In a small proportion of cases the genital anomaly is absent at birth or is so mild that it is overlooked. Such patients usually have a relatively mild biochemical disorder and rarely possess salt-losing symptoms. If the condition is not treated, 21-hydroxylase and 11-hydroxylase deficiencies cause further masculinization in early childhood with enlargement of the clitoris, growth of pubic hair, accelerated statural growth with rapid bone maturation and development of a muscular male habitus. When these are the presenting symptoms the condition must be differentiated from an adrenal tumour. Introduction of treatment in these late-diagnosed subjects, who usually have a very advanced bone age, may be followed by the rapid onset of puberty with breast development and menstruation (Wilkins, 1952).

Males

Boys with 21-hydroxylase or 11-hydroxylase deficiency have normal genital development, although excessive pigmentation of the penis and the scrotum is seen at birth in some cases. Unless a previous sibling has been affected or symptoms of salt loss evolve in the neonatal period the condition is likely to be overlooked until rapid growth occurs with development of the penis and appearance of pubic hair, which is usually between the ages of 3–5 years. Again an adrenal tumour must be considered in the differential diagnosis. Precocious puberty can generally be excluded by the absence of testicular development. However, as in girls, late-diagnosed cases with a very advanced bone age often show evidence of puberty with testicular enlargement soon after treatment is started. As noted above, males with deficiency of 3-beta-hydroxysteroid-dehydrogenase usually have poorly virilized external genitalia and commonly show severe salt loss.

Salt-losing crises

Failure to thrive, poor feeding and intermittent vomiting are the characteristic early symptoms of salt loss in congenital adrenal hyperplasia. They generally begin 6–10 days after birth but are occasionally delayed for several weeks. Rapid deterioration often occurs with dehydration and collapse if treatment is delayed. Laboratory investigation is usually straightforward since hyponatraemia with hyperkalaemia is present together with metabolic acidosis and a moderately elevated blood urea level.

As a rule congenital adrenal hyperplasia causing salt loss can be recognized with little difficulty in girls because of the genital anomaly. In boys conditions such as familial adrenal hypoplasia, aldosterone biosynthetic defects, pseudohypoaldosteronism and renal salt-wasting due to obstructive nephropathy must be considered in the differential diagnosis.

Diagnosis

Congenital adrenal hyperplasia is the most likely diagnosis in any child born with genital ambiguity and impalpable gonads, and should also be suspected in apparent males born with bilateral undescended testes. If symptoms of salt loss develop, the diagnosis of congenital adrenal hyperplasia is virtually certain. Demonstration of nuclear chromatin by the rapid and inexpensive buccal smear technique is normally adequate to indicate the true sex of the child. Investigation of either urinary or plasma steroids is required to confirm the diagnosis.

Until recently urinary steroid analysis provided the mainstay in the diagnosis of congenital adrenal hyperplasia, particularly since a raised 17-oxosteroid excretion rate occurs in all three types. Characterization of the exact type of enzyme defect requires more detailed steroid investigation. In 21-hydroxylase deficiency pregnanetriol (the main metabolite of 17-alpha-hydroxyprogesterone) and pregnanetriolone excretion rates are raised, while in 11-hydroxylase deficiency tetrahydrodeoxycortisol (tetrahydro-S) is the main metabolite. (Bongiovanni and Eberlein, 1955). In deficiency of 3-beta-hydroxysteroid-dehydrogenase there is increased excretion of Δ^5-pregnenetriol and Δ^5-pregnenediol (Bongiovanni and Kellenbenz, 1962). The excretion rate of pregnanetriol is also elevated, probably as a result of hepatic 3-beta-hydroxysteroid activity.

Estimation of urinary steroid excretion rates requires carefully timed urine collections which may not be possible if urgent treatment is indicated. Determination of the 11-oxygenation index on a random sample of urine may offset this difficulty since values raised above 0.6 are obtained in untreated congenital adrenal hyperplasia (Clayton, Edwards and Makin, 1971). While these diagnostic tests have served well false-positive and false-negative results have been reported in the neonatal period (Shackleton, Mitchell and Farquhar, 1972) and estimation of plasma steroid levels, particularly that of 17-alpha-hydroxyprogesterone, is becoming more widely used in the diagnosis of congenital adrenal hyperplasia (Atherden, Edmunds and Grant, 1974). These methods are not reliable immediately after birth because of placental steroid secretion but are usually accurate from the second day of life onwards (Hughes, Riad-Fahmy and Griffiths, 1979). In general the plasma concentration of 17-alpha-hydroxyprogesterone is related to the severity of the biochemical defect, and in mild cases the level may be only modestly elevated during the first 7–14 days after birth.

Treatment

In congenital adrenal hyperplasia the aims of treatment are to correct salt loss when this is present and to suppress adrenal androgen production thereby preventing progressive virilization with rapid bone maturation.

Salt loss

In young infants with severe salt loss emergency therapy with intravenous saline may be life-saving and is always the first line of treatment. Although mineralocorticoids prevent further urinary salt loss they cannot make good the existing sodium deficit and should never be used alone in the management of a salt-losing crisis. When the sodium balance has been re-established maintenance treatment with either intramuscular deoxycorticosterone trimethylacetate (Percorten) 12.5–25.0 mg every 3–4 weeks or oral fluorohydrocortisone acetate 0.05–0.10 mg/day should be given together with modest sodium supplements of 3–5 mmol/kg per day. The blood pressure must be checked regularly since overtreatment with mineralocorticoids can produce marked hypertension.

There has been debate regarding whether mineralocorticoid treatment is required on an indefinite basis. While significant salt loss seems to be a transient phenomenon in some cases in the majority it persists into adult life and withdrawal of mineralocorticoids is associated with a marked appetite for salt. If this cannot be met because of intercurrent illness a salt-losing crisis can rapidly develop (Loras, Haour and Bertrand, 1970). In addition growth may be impaired if mineralocorticoids are stopped in cases with persistent salt loss, and excess production of renin may itself lead to adrenal stimulation that cannot be completely suppressed with glucocorticoids (Rosler *et al.*, 1977). It thus appears that salt-retaining hormones should be continued indefinitely in patients with persistent salt loss as judged by a high urinary sodium excretion rate and markedly elevated plasma renin activity (Grant *et al.*, 1977).

Glucocorticoid therapy

Suppression of adrenal androgen secretion is achieved by giving glucocorticoids to inhibit ACTH production and thereby reduce adrenal activity. The synthetic preparations that are available have no obvious advantages over cortisol or cortisone in young children, and because of their potency they carry the risk of growth suppression due to overdosage. This can be a particular problem during the first year of life when growth is normally very rapid. The correct dosage of cortisol must be adjusted on an individual basis but a daily dose of around 25 mg/m^2 is likely to be satisfactory in most cases for maintenance therapy (Brook *et al.*, 1974). The parents should be told to double this dosage to cover intercurrent infections. There is still no consensus on the most effective timing of treatment. At present the authors favour giving two thirds of the daily dose as early as possible in the morning to try to mimic the normal pattern of cortisol secretion rather than giving equally divided doses throughout the day or a large evening dose to inhibit the early morning surge of ACTH.

Inadequate glucocorticoid treatment leads to rapid growth with even faster bone maturation and loss of long-term growth potential. Overtreatment may also compromise final height by inhibiting growth. Careful measurement of stature is thus a very valuable method of monitoring treatment which can be supplemented by bone age estimations and urinary steroid analyses at appropriate intervals. Plasma steroid estimations, particularly of 17-alpha-hydroxyprogesterone, are used in some units to evaluate treatment. However, because the levels show rapid changes both as a result of treatment and as part of a circadian cycle the results may be difficult to interpret.

While there is still debate about the need for long-term treatment in males without salt loss

glucocorticoid therapy must be continued indefinitely in females to prevent virilization. When growth is complete the steroid dose becomes less critical and better adrenal suppression may be obtained with prednisone or dexamethasone, possibly given as a single late-evening dose (Hayek, Crawford and Bode, 1971).

In adequately treated cases breast development usually occurs at an appropriate age although menstruation is often delayed. This has been attributed to inadequate suppression of adrenal androgens (Klingensmith *et al.*, 1977) but in the authors' experience this does not always seem to be the case. While one can speculate that amenorrhoea is due to earlier hypothalamic imprinting by adrenal androgens, there is no good evidence to support this view. Absent menstruation is sometimes due to vaginal obstruction but this is relatively uncommon. In a small proportion of cases primary ovarian failure probably accounts for the amenorrhoea (Levine *et al.*, 1977). Such patients have enlarged smooth ovaries that show fibrosis and few primary follicles on histological examination. The explanation for these changes is not known. Most subjects have normal ovarian function and a number of pregnancies have been reported in women with treated congenital adrenal hyperplasia.

Many girls with congenital adrenal hyperplasia are extrovert children who enjoy games and activities normally reserved for boys. There is still speculation as to the cause of this behaviour which is not related to inadequate treatment and may be due to the effects of androgens on fetal brain development. These children usually have no doubt that they are female, although they may become rather isolated adolescents when social pressures exclude them from their earlier tomboy interests and activities (Ehrhardt, Epstein and Money, 1968). Money and Daléry (1977) suggested that patients with complete masculinization of the external genitalia may fare better if raised as males but this view is by no means universally accepted.

Virilization by maternal androgens

Masculinization of the external genitalia by an androgen-secreting maternal tumour is an uncommon yet well recognized cause of female pseudohermaphroditism. The reported cases include virilization by both ovarian and adrenal tumours. In most of these babies the clitoris is enlarged and marked labial fusion is absent (Verhoeven *et al.*, 1973). However, in the case described by Mürset *et al.* (1970), which was caused by a maternal adrenal tumour, the infant had a male appearance at birth and was raised as a boy.

Iatrogenic fetal virilization

It has long been known that testosterone can produce fetal virilization when given to pregnant animals, for example rats (Greene, Burrill and Ivy, 1938) and rabbits (Jost, 1953). The clinical significance of these earlier observations became apparent in the late 1950s when synthetic progestin derivatives of testosterone became widely used in the management of threatened abortion, particularly in the USA. In 1958 Wilkins *et al.* described fetal virilization in a number of girls born to progestin-treated mothers, and 2 years later Wilkins (1960) reviewed no less than 70 cases.

Grumbach, Ducharme and Moloshok (1959) described 18 cases in detail. Nine were due to 19-nor-17-alpha-ethinyltestosterone (norethindrone) and eight to 17-alpha-ethynyltestosterone (ethisterone). These authors were able to show that the type of genital anomaly depended on the timing of maternal treatment, for instance fusion of the labia was only seen in cases treated before the 13th week of pregnancy. Similar findings were reported by Jacobson (1962) in 182 women treated with norethindrone for threatened abortion. Of the 82 female babies 15 showed some clitoral enlargement and labial fusion was present in two who had been exposed to the drug during the first trimester. Now that the virilizing effect of these progestins is widely known and their use in the management of threatened abortion has been largely abandoned iatrogenic female pseudohermaphroditism has become very uncommon in Europe and the USA.

Fetal virilization has been described following maternal treatment with testosterone (Grumbach and Ducharme, 1960) and aminoglutethimide (Le Maire *et al.*, 1972) and was probably a result of inhibition of 3-beta-hydroxysteroid-dehydrogenase in the fetal adrenals. Although it

has also been reported after therapy with progesterone, 17-alpha-hydroxyprogesterone, medroxyprogesterone and stilboestrol, the teratogenic effect of these preparations is still uncertain because other hormones were also given in most of the published cases. However, there is evidence to suggest that stilboestrol causes minor urethral anomalies in males (Henderson *et al.*, 1976) as well as predisposing female infants to later adenocarcinoma of the vagina (Herbst, Ulfelder and Pozkanzer, 1971).

Other causes of pseudohermaphroditism

Female pseudohermaphroditism associated with dysmorphic syndromes

Marked masculinization of the female genitalia is not a feature of most dysmorphic syndromes. Enlargement of the clitoris has been recorded in several conditions, for example Seckel's syndrome of bird-headed dwarfism, the Donohue syndrome of leprechaunism, the Fraser syndrome of cryptophthalmos, the Zellweger hepatorenal syndrome and the Beckwith-Wiedemann syndrome of macroglossia and exomphalos. In addition it is a fairly consistent feature of the Berardinelli syndrome of lipodystrophy and the Meldenhall syndrome of acanthosis, insulin resistance and pineal hyperplasia. Further details of these conditions are given by Rimoin and Schimke (1971) and Holmes *et al.* (1972). Familial clitoral enlargement associated with skeletal anomalies has also been described (Park, Jones and Melhem, 1972). The cause of clitoral enlargement in these conditions is not known.

Female pseudohermaphroditism with renal and anal anomalies

A number of authors have described congenital enlargement of the clitoris in girls with other developmental anomalies of the kidneys and hindgut (Sieber and Klein, 1958; Dubowitz, 1962). In some cases müllerian development was abnormal too and presumably these examples represent the result of a nonendocrine disturbance of renal and cloacal development.

Unexplained female pseudohermaphroditism

In rare cases the cause of female pseudohermaphroditism cannot be established. For example Wilkins *et al.* (1958) were not able to account for virilization in three of their patients. While some of these examples may be due to unrecorded progestin treatment during pregnancy Gordon *et al.* (1971) reported a girl with unexplained progressive enlargement of the clitoris. Increased tissue sensitivity to androgen was proposed as a possible explanation in this case.

Local lesions simulating female pseudohermaphroditism

Occasionally enlargement of the clitoris is due to a local lesion, and genital ambiguity in neurofibromatosis has been described (Kenny, Fetterman and Preeyasombat, 1966). Clitoral enlargement may also be caused by a haemangioma or a lipoma (Haddad and Jones, 1960). In premature infants the clitoris may appear abnormally prominent largely due to underdevelopment of the labia. Similarly the clitoris is prominent in the pterygium or webbing syndrome because of labial hypoplasia. Labial adhesions in older children are rarely confused with pseudohermaphroditism since their diaphanous appearance is quite characteristic. These adhesions are seldom seen in the newborn.

Surgical treatment

Rarely, but especially when the vagina and the urethra join at a high level, inadequate vaginal drainage results in the development of prenatal hydrocolpos so that surgical intervention is required urgently in the neonatal period. Ordinarily the timing of operative correction of the genital anomalies is a matter of choice. In the

commonest situation, namely the girl with 21-hydroxylase deficiency who is diagnosed and treated soon after birth, surgery can generally be carried out during the second 6 months of life, assuming that hormonal control and electrolyte balance are satisfactory. Such early correction is appreciated by the parents, who are always keen to have their baby girl looking feminine as soon as possible, and is important in avoiding psychological problems which may arise in the patient if intervention is delayed.

Surgery in subjects with congenital adrenal hyperplasia carries no extra risks if careful attention is paid to sodium balance and glucocorticoid therapy. Liberal doses of parenteral hydrocortisone 25–50 mg 8-hourly should be given in the immediate postoperative period and intravenous saline infusion 5–8 mmol/kg per day is required to offset urinary sodium losses.

In the feminization of the genitalia two aspects need to be considered. First, the laying open of the urogenital sinus so as to separate fused labia and provide separate urethral and vaginal openings on the vulva and, secondly, the management of the enlarged clitoris.

Vulvovaginoplasty

The technique required to exteriorize the vaginal and urethral orifices depends upon the degree of masculinization that exists. This is evident on clinical examination but preoperative determination of the length of the urogenital sinus is valuable in deciding the optimum method of management. The level of union between the vagina and the urethra can usually be demonstrated radiologically by retrograde injection of contrast medium into the sinus orifice. In some instances the vagina does not fill from the urogenital sinus and endoscopy is needed to determine its position.

With mildly masculinized patients in whom the urethra and the vagina join at a low level and there is a short urogenital sinus formed essentially by fusion of the posterior portions of the labia (*Figure 44.3a*) a simple cut-back procedure is all that is necessary. In the completely virilized girl (*Figures 44.3b and 44.4*) the urogenital sinus opens at the tip of the 'phallus', the labia are fused, the urethra and the vagina unite high up and the vagina is short. Following the laying open of the sinus to expose the separate

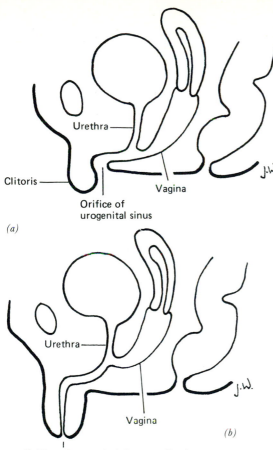

(a)

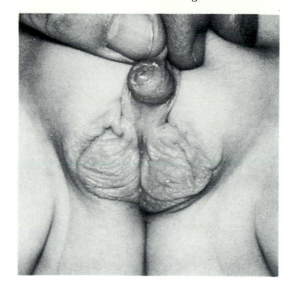

(a)

(b)

Orifice of urogenital sinus on clitoris

Figure 44.3. Sagittal sections through female genitalia in adrenogenital syndrome. *(a)* Mild masculinization. The vagina and the urethra unite near the surface and the urogenital sinus is short, opening proximal to the clitoris. *(b)* Complete masculinization. The vagina and the urethra unite high up and the long urogenital sinus opens at the tip of the phallus.

urethral and vaginal orifices the vagina can be freed posteriorly and laterally to permit it to descend nearer the surface. However, it is rarely possible for it to descend completely and at the beginning of the operation the problem is anticipated by raising an inverted-U skin flap on the perineum which is later swung inwards to be sutured to the posterior and lateral margins of the vaginal wall.

Hendren and Crawford (1969) described an alternative technique for subjects with high urethrovaginal union. The vagina is divided at its entrance into the urogenital sinus and the lumen exteriorized with the intervention of a skin flap as already mentioned. Following closure of the vaginal opening a portion of the urogenital sinus below that level is preserved to

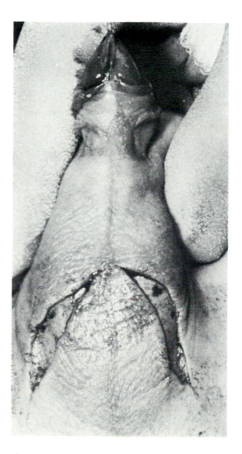

(b)

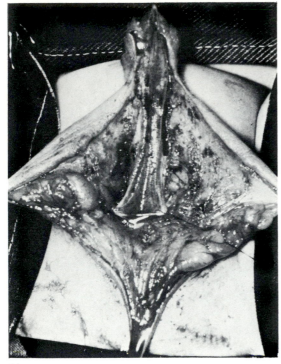

(c)

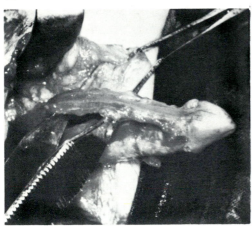

(d)

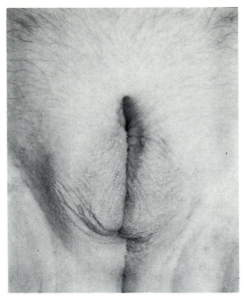

(e)

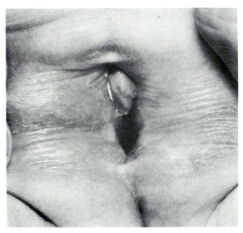

(f)

form the urethra. This method ensures that the urethral orifice is at a distance from the vaginal one, but the above authors considered its main advantage is that it avoids division of the external urethral sphincter which they believed often surrounds the urogenital sinus rather than the urethra. Such a position of the external sphincter has not been encountered in the present authors' experience and no patients treated along the lines shown in *Figure 44.4* have suffered any degree of postoperative urinary incontinence.

Figure 44.4. Girl with adrenogenital syndrome causing complete masculinization. *(a)* Aged 6 months showing clitoromegaly. The urogenital sinus opens at the tip of the clitoris and there is total labial fusion. *(b)* At operation an inverted-U flap is outlined on the perineum. *(c)* The urogenital sinus is laid open to expose the urethral and vaginal orifices. Dissection posterior to the vagina allows it to descend nearer the surface. The inverted-U flap is sutured to the posterior free margin of the vagina. *(d)* The clitoris is denuded by resection of dorsal skin and mobilization of a ventral mucosal strip. The dorsal neurovascular bundle with surrounding tissue is dissected from the corpora cavernosa. The body of the clitoris is excised, preserving the glans with its dorsal neurovascular and ventral mucosal pedicles. The glans is sutured to the pubic periosteum. *(e)* Aged 7 years showing the normal vulval appearance. *(f)* Aged 7 years showing the normal clitoral position.

Treatment of clitoromegaly

Infrequently with very mildly masculinized girls the clitoris shrinks sufficiently with medical treatment alone. Usually surgical correction is needed. Although Money, Hampson and Hampson (1955) reported that women could achieve a normal sexual orgasm following clitoridectomy it is nowadays fashionable to preserve the organ, or at least the glans, and to reduce it to more normal dimensions. Excision of the clitoris is therefore reserved for those cases, usually late-diagnosed non-salt-losing patients, in which the organ is excessively large.

Several techniques of clitoroplasty have been described. A reliable one is shown in *Figure 44.4*. The clitoral shaft is exposed by excising the redundant skin on the dorsum and dissecting free and preserving the mucosal strip on the ventrum. The dorsal neurovascular bundle passing from beneath the pubic symphysis to the glans is mobilized with a generous collar of surrounding tissue from the corpora cavernosa. The body of the clitoris between the glans and the crura is resected and the glans, which is attached dorsally to its neurovascular pedicle and ventrally to the mucosal strip, is sutured to the periosteum over the inferior aspect of the symphysis. A very large glans can be trimmed to a normal size by excision with resuture of a dorsal or ventral wedge.

Certain methods of clitoroplasty have been reported to lead to painful clitoral erections in adult life. Sotiropoulos *et al.* (1976) reported that 15 of 16 women treated by repositioning the mobilized and preserved clitoris were free of this complication. The possibility of its occurrence appears to be entirely avoided by the technique described above in which only the glans is retained.

Some authors have recommended that in severely masculinized girls vaginoplasty should be deferred until the child is prepubertal and that early intervention should be confined to dealing with the clitoral enlargement. However, an effective clitoroplasty virtually necessitates complete laying open of the urogenital sinus and there is in the authors' experience no disadvantage in carrying out full genital correction at one operation. The parents should be advised to ensure that the patient has a genital examination, if necessary under anaesthesia, at the age of 11–12 years to detect any introital narrowing that might need dilatation or operative treatment.

References

Atherden, S.M., Edmunds, A.T. and Grant, D.B. (1974) Plasma 17-hydroxyprogesterone in newborn infants with congenital adrenal hyperplasia and in infants with normal adrenal function. *Archives of Disease in Childhood*, **49**, 192

Bartter, F.C., Forbes, A.P. and Leaf, A. (1950) Congenital adrenal hyperplasia: attempts to correct disordered pattern. *Journal of Clinical Investigation*, **29**, 797

Bongiovanni, A.M. and Eberlein, W.R. (1955) Clinical and metabolic variations in the adrenogenital syndrome. *Pediatrics*, **16**, 628

Bongiovanni, A. and Kellenbenz, G. (1962) The adrenogenital syndrome deficiency of 3β-hydroxysteroid dehydrogenase. *Journal of Clinical Investigation*, **41**, 2086

Brook, C.G.D., Zachmann, M., Prader, A. and Mürset, G. (1974) Long-term therapy in congenital adrenal hyperplasia. *Journal of Pediatrics*, **85**, 12

Clayton, B.E., Edwards, R.W.H. and Makin, H.L.J. (1971) Congenital adrenal hyperplasia and other conditions associated with a raised urinary steroid 11-oxygenation index. *Journal of Endocrinology*, **50**, 251

Dubowitz, V. (1962) Virilization and malfunction of a female infant. *Lancet*, ii, 405

Ehrhardt, A.A., Epstein, R. and Money J. (1968) Gender identity in treated congenital adrenal hyperplasia. *Johns Hopkins Medical Journal*, **122**, 160

Gordon, L.S., Morillo-Gucci, G., Mulholland, G., Simpson, J.L. and German, J. (1971) Progressive idiopathic clitoral hypertrophy in a child. *In Birth Defects Original Article Series*, Vol.7, No. 6 (edited by Bergsma, D.).Liss, New York. p.201

Grant, D.B., Dillon, M.J., Atherden, S.M. and Levinsky, R.J. (1977) Congenital adrenal hyperplasia–renin and steroid values during treatment. *European Journal of Pediatrics*, **126**, 89

Greene, R.R., Burrill, M.W. and Ivy, A.C. (1938) Experimental production of intersexuality in the rat. *American Journal of Obstetrics and Gynecology*, **98**, 151

Grumbach, M.M. and Ducharme, J.R. (1960) The effects of androgens on fetal sexual development. *Fertility and Sterility*, **11**, 157

Grumbach, M.M., Ducharme, J.R. and Moloshok, R.E. (1959) On the fetal masculinizing action of certain oral progestins. *Journal of Clinical Endocrinology and Metabolism*, **19**, 1369

Haddad, H.M. and Jones, H.W. (1960) Clitoral enlargement simulating pseudohermaphroditism. *American Journal of Diseases of Children*, **99**, 282

Hayek, A., Crawford, J.D. and Bode, H.H. (1971) Single dose dexamethasone in the treatment of congenital adrenocortical hyperplasia. *Metabolism*, **20**, 897

Henderson, B.E., Benton, B., Cosgrove, M., Baptista, J., Aldrich, J., Townsend, D., Hart, W. and Mack, T.M. (1976) Urogenital tract anomalies in sons of women treated with diethylstilboestrol. *Pediatrics*, **58**, 505

Hendren, W.H. and Crawford, J.D. (1969) Adrenogenital syndrome: the anatomy of the anomaly and its repair – some new concepts. *Journal of Pediatric Surgery*, **4**, 49

Herbst, A.L., Ulfelder, H. and Pozkanzer, D.C. (1971) Adenocarcinoma of the vagina and maternal stilboestrol therapy: association of maternal stilboestrol with tumour in young women. *New England Journal of Medicine*, **284**, 878

Hirschfeld, A.J. and Fleshman, J.K. (1969) High incidence of salt-losing congenital adrenal hyperplasia in Alaska Eskimos. *Journal of Pediatrics*, **75**, 492

Holmes, L.B., Moser, H.W., Halldorsson, S., Mack, C., Pant, S.S. and Matzilevich, B. (1972) Mental retardation: an atlas of disorders with associated physical abnormalities. Macmillan, New York

Hughes, I.A., Riad-Fahmy, D. and Griffiths, K. (1979) Plasma 17-hydroxyprogesterone excretion in newborn infants. *Archives of Disease in Childhood*, **54**, 347

Jacobs, D.R., van der Poll, J., Gabrilove, J.L. and Soffer, L.J. (1961) 17α-hydroxyprogesterone – a salt-losing steroid: relation to congenital adrenal hyperplasia. *Journal of Clinical Endocrinology and Metabolism*, **21**, 909

Jacobson, B.D. (1962) Hazards of norethindrone therapy during pregnancy. *American Journal of Obstetrics and Gynecology*, **84**, 962

Jost, A. (1953) Problems of fetal endocrinology: the gonadal and hypophyseal hormones. *In* Recent Progress in Hormone Research, Vol. 8 (edited by Pincuss, G.). Academic Press, New York. p.379

Kenny, F.M., Fetterman, G.M. and Preeyasombat, C. (1966) Neurofibromata simulating a penis and gonads in a girl. *Pediatrics*, **37**, 456

Kenny, F.M., Reynolds, J.W. and Green, O.C. (1971) Partial 3β-hydroxysteroid dehydrogenase deficiency in a family with congenital adrenal hyperplasia: evidence for increasing 3β-HSD activity with age. *Pediatrics*, **48**, 756

Klingensmith, G.J., Garcia, S.C., Jones, H.W., Migeon, C.J. and Blizzard, R.M. (1977) Glucocorticoid treatment of girls with congenital adrenal hyperplasia: effects on weight, sexual maturation and fertility. *Journal of Pediatrics*, **90**, 996

Landau, R.L. and Lugibihl, K. (1958) Inhibition of sodium-retaining influence of aldosterone by progesterone. *Journal of Clinical Endocrinology and Metabolism*, **18**, 1237

Le Maire, W.J., Cleveland, W.W., Bejar, R.L., Marsh, J.M. and Fishman, L. (1972) Amino glutethimide: a possible cause of pseudohermaphroditism in females. *American Journal of Diseases of Children*, **124**, 421

Levine, L.S., Korth-Schutz, S., Saenger, P., Sweeney, W.J., Beling, C.G. and New, M.I. (1977) Disordered puberty in treated congenital adrenal hyperplasia. *In* Congenital Adrenal Hyperplasia (edited by Lee, P.A., Plotnick, L.P., Kowarski, A.A. and Migeon, C.J.). University Park Press, Baltimore. p.361

Levine, L.S., Zachmann, M., New, M.I., Prader, A., Pollack, M.S., O'Neill, G.J., Yang, S.Y., Oberfield, S.E. and Dupont, B. (1978) Genetic mapping; 21-hydroxylase-deficiency gene within the HLA linkage group. *New England Journal of Medicine*, **299**, 911

Loras, B., Haour, F. and Bertrand, J. (1970) Exchangeable sodium and aldosterone secretion in children with congenital adrenal hyperplasia due to 21-hydroxylase deficiency. *Pediatric Research*, **4**, 145

Marks, J.F. and Fink, C.W. (1969) Incidence of salt-losing congenital adrenal hyperplasia. *Pediatrics*, **43**, 636

Money, J. and Daléry, J. (1977) Hyperadrenocortical 46XX hermaphroditism with penile urethra. *In* Congenital Adrenal Hyperplasia (edited by Lee, P.A., Plotnick, L.P., Kawarski, A.A. and Migeon, C.J.). University Park Press, Baltimore. p.433

Money, J., Hampson, J.G. and Hampson, J.L. (1955) Hermaphroditism: recommendations concerning assignment of sex, change of sex and psychologic management. *Bulletin of the Johns Hopkins Hospital*, **97**, 284

Murset, G., Zachmann, M., Prader, A., Fischer, J. and Labhart, A. (1970) Male external genitalia of a girl caused by a virilizing adrenal tumour in the mother. *Acta Endocrinologica*, **65**, 627

New, M.I. and Seaman, M.P. (1970) Secretion rates of cortisol and aldosterone precursors in various forms of congenital adrenal hyperplasia. *Journal of Clinical Endocrinology and Metabolism*, **30**, 361

Park, I.J., Jones, H.W. and Melhem, R.E. (1972) Non-adrenal familial female pseudohermaphroditism. *American Journal of Obstetrics and Gynecology*, **112**, 930

Prader, A. (1958) Die häufigkeit des kongenitalen adrenogenitalen syndroms. *Helvetica Paediatrica Acta*, **13**, 426

Rimoin, D.A. and Schimke, R.N. (1971) Genetic disorders of the Endocrine Glands. Mosby, St Louis

Rosler, A., Levine, L.S., Schneider, B., Novogroder, M. and New, M.I. (1977) The interrelationship of sodium balance, plasma renin activity and ACTH in congenital adrenal hyperplasia. *Journal of Clinical Endocrinology and Metabolism*, **45**, 500

Shackleton, C.H., Mitchell, F.L. and Farquhar, J.W. (1972) Difficulties in the diagnosis of the adrenogenital syndrome in infancy. *Pediatrics*, **49**, 198

Sieber, W.K. and Klein, R. (1958) Cloaca with non-adrenal female pseudohermaphroditism. *Pediatrics*, **22**, 472

Sotiropoulos, A., Morishima, A., Homsy, Y. and Lattimer, J.K. (1976) Long-term assessment of genital reconstruction in female pseudohermaphrodites. *Journal of Urology*, **115**, 599

Verhoeven, A.T.M., Mostbloom, J.L., Van Lousden, H.A.I.M. and Van der Velden, W.H.M. (1973) Virilization in pregnancy co-existing with an ovarian mucinous cystadenoma: a case report and review of virilizing ovarian tumours in pregnancy. *Obstetrical and Gynecological Survey*, **28**, 597

Visser, H.K.A. and Degenhart, H.J. (1967) Salt-losing in an infant with congenital adrenal hyperplasia and normal aldosterone production. *Acta Paediatrica Scandinavica*, **56**, 216

Wilkins, L. (1952) Diagnosis of adrenogenital syndrome and its treatment with cortisone. *Journal of Pediatrics*, **41**, 860

Wilkins, L. (1960) Masculinisation of the female foetus due to the use of synthetic progestagens during pregnancy. *Acta Paediatrica Scandinavica*, Suppl.51, p.671

Wilkins, L., Lewis, R.A., Klein, R. and Rosemberg, E. (1950) Treatment of congenital adrenal hyperplasia with cortisone. *Bulletin of the Johns Hopkins Hospital*, **86**, 249

Wilkins, L., Jones, H., Holman, G.H. and Stempfel, R.S. (1958) Masculinization of the female fetus associated with administration of oral and intramuscular progestins during gestation: non-adrenal female pseudohermaphroditism. *Journal of Clinical Endocrinology and Metabolism*, **18**, 559

45 True Hermaphroditism and Mixed Gonadal Dysgenesis

David B. Grant and D. Innes Williams

Two different types of intersexual disorder each caused by abnormal gonadal differentiation are considered in this chapter. In true hermaphroditism histologically normal ovarian and testicular tissues are present in the same individual. In mixed gonadal dysgenesis abnormally differentiated testicular tissue is commonly associated with a contralateral streak gonad similar to the streak ovary found in Turner's syndrome.

While the aetiology and nature of these two disorders differ, both give rise to abnormal development of the external genitalia and both may be associated with persistence of müllerian and wolffian structures. The distinction between them sometimes depends only upon the histological interpretation of the biopsy of the gonad, namely whether it consists simply of ovarian stroma or whether follicles are also present. In general true hermaphroditism and mixed gonadal dysgenesis present similar problems in medical and surgical management and for this reason they are considered together here.

True hermaphroditism

Of all the different types of intersexual disorder true hermaphroditism has probably engendered most curiosity and speculation, and although it is an uncommon condition a relatively large number of case reports have been published (Van Niekerk, 1976). By definition both testicular tissue with well developed seminiferous tubules and ovarian tissue with follicles are present in hermaphrodites. Spermatogonia are usually only present in small numbers but Leydig cell are well represented in the testicular tissue.

Karyotype

No one chromosomal pattern characterizes true hermaphroditism and the relationship between sex chromosome content and gonadal development is largely unexplained. In a small proportion of cases there is an apparently satisfactory correlation in the findings of two populations of cells with respectively 46 XY and 46 XX karyotypes. It is easy to imagine that the XY cluster has given rise to a testicle and the XX cluster to an ovary, particularly when the type of gonad is different on either side. An XX/XY constitution cannot result from mosaicism (the presence in one individual of more than one cell population derived from a single zygote) although it may be due to chimerism in which there is fusion of two zygotes or double fertilization of one (*Figure 45.1*). With serological studies Josso, Crouchy and de Auvert (1965) recognized a double haptoglobulin phenotype in such a case and other authors have confirmed this finding. However, true mosaicism may be found in addition to hermaphroditism. Polani (1970) reviewed 108 cases and discovered 11 examples of chromosome constitution 45 X/46 XY, six of 46 XX/46 XY and five of 46 XX/47XXY, and six of other varieties.

In a small proportion of true hermaphrodites

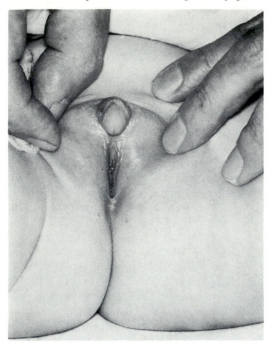

Figure 45.1. True hermaphroditism in an XX/XY chimera showing the external genitalia at 2 years of age. The child was raised as a girl and phallectomy and orchidectomy were performed.

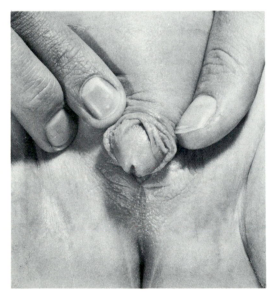

Figure 45.2. A hermaphrodite with bilateral ovotestes. The patient was initially considered a boy but was registered as female following demonstration of a 46 XX karyotype. Subsequent evaluation excluded congenital adrenal hyperplasia and showed a good testosterone response to gonadotrophin stimulation. Müllerian structures were absent and the child was reassigned as male with resection of the ovarian tissue and correction of chordee and hypospadias.

chromosome analysis shows a normal male karyotype, but it is possible that undetected mosaicism or chimerism may be present in some or all of these cases. The majority of true hermaphrodites have the karyotype 46 XX with no evidence of a Y cell line (*Figure 45.2*). In a few instances the condition appears to be familial, for instance XX hermaphroditism has occurred in several siblings (Rosenberg, Clayton and Hsu, 1963) and in one family an XX hermaphrodite had an XX male sibling (Kasdan *et al.*, 1973). There is no clear explanation of how a testicle comes to develop in an individual lacking a Y chromosome. Possible mechanisms are undetected mosaicism or chimerism, translocation of Y-located genes onto either an X chromosome or an autosome, and abnormal activation of a testis-regulating gene on an autosome. Although no Y fluorescence has so far been detected on any other chromosomes, Saenger (1976) demonstrated the presence of H-Y antigen in the testis of a 46 XX hermaphrodite.

Morphology of the gonads

The location and the distribution of the two types of gonadal tissue vary considerably between individual patients and in general three distinct morphological patterns can be distinguished. In the alternating form the testis and the ovary are on different sides, usually with the testis on the right. In the unilateral type testicular and ovarian tissues are present on the same side, sometimes separately but often in the form of an ovotestis, with a single gonad (either testis or ovary) on the opposite side. In the bilateral type ovarian and testicular tissues are present on both sides, as a rule in the form of ovotestes. Generally the location of the gonads corresponds with their histological characteristics, ovarian tissue lying within the abdomen and testes being situated in the inguinal canal or the labioscrotal folds. This also applies to ovotestes and the larger the testicular component the more likely they are to be located in the labioscrotal region. In the majority of ovotestes the ovarian and testicular components lie at opposite poles of the gonad. They are usually sharply demarcated from one another, a distinction that can sometimes be appreciated on clinical examination because the ovarian portion feels firmer and that is almost always evident when the gonad is exposed at operation. Less often the testicular tissue is located at the hilum of the gonad so that its true nature cannot be understood by examination with the the naked eye.

Genital ducts and external genitalia

A uterus is present in the majority of cases and almost invariably in those with an ovary on one side and an ovotestis on the other. Nevertheless, there is no relationship to a particular chromosome complement and absence of the uterus has been noted most often in the 46 XX group. Menstruation occurs after puberty in most individuals possessing a uterus, although it may be irregular and the flow scanty. Fallopian tube development is seen almost always in association with an ovary and sometimes with ovotestes, which is an interesting observation in relation to the expected production of anti-müllerian hormone by a testicular element. The epididymides and the vasa follow the testes and again are found with some ovotestes. In a few cases both müllerian and wolffian derivatives persist on the same side.

The external genitalia are most often ambiguous and the fact that over 80 per cent of true hermaphrodites are reared as males indicates moderate phallic development. Hypospadias is to be expected and in some cases the vaginal orifice is visible to clinical inspection. In others it opens into the urethra and can only be detected by radiological or endoscopic examination. The situation of the gonads relative to the scrotum has already been mentioned. These cases are unlikely to be mistaken for simple hypospadias if any careful palpation of the 'testicles' is undertaken. Some degree of hypogonadism is usual in true hermaphrodites reared as males, but a degree of penile enlargement and the appearance of pubic hair can be anticipated. Although sexual intercourse in the male role is possible for the majority of subjects, no case of paternity has yet been described.

Breast development occurs in almost all instances, sometimes late in development and occasionally even after removal of all recognizable ovarian tissue. The coincidence at puberty of both feminization and masculinization can be profoundly disturbing psychologically and the avoidance of this confusion is the best reason for early diagnosis and treatment.

Diagnosis

As has already been made evident the true hermaphrodite infant cannot be recognized on clinical grounds because the external appearances are in no way distinguishable from a variety of intersexual conditions. The karyotype alone can be equally unhelpful since even the 46 XY/46 XX pattern has been found in individuals without ovaries. While investigations using HCG and HMG stimulation may show the presence of both androgen-secreting and oestrogen-secreting tissues and may give some information on the likely pattern of adolescent development surgical exploration with gonadal biopsy remains the most important step in establishing the diagnosis of true hermaphroditism. This is not in itself an indication of the preferred sex of rearing and the decision must be made from an assessment of the size and the overall character of the phallus and the degree of development of the gonads.

If there is a well developed penis accompanied by one easily palpable scrotal testicle, and particularly if an HCG test shows a good testosterone response, the male role should be chosen whether the karyotype is 46 XX, 46 XY or some mosaic or chimera. Gonadal biopsy is required in all individuals other than 46 XY cases and if true hermaphroditism is diagnosed then appropriate surgery must be undertaken. When the phallus is small and resembles a large clitoris, the vaginal orifice is easily seen, and gonads if palpable are high in the groin the child is better off as a girl but the final diagnosis can be postponed. Thus the choice of sexual role is a decision for the neonatal period. A final diagnosis resulting from laparotomy may be immediately desirable when doubt exists but can in most instances be postponed for a year or two.

The exploratory operation should ordinarily be a laparotomy with exposure of both gonads either in the inguinal regions or in the abdomen. Biopsies should be taken from both sides, preferably by longitudinal strips including both poles of an ovotestis. Sometimes the gonad is embarrassingly small for biopsy and only a minute specimen can be removed. Frozen-section diagnosis is inadequate and following biopsy the gonad should be replaced either in the abdomen or within the hernial sac where it will not become too adherent to surrounding tissues and will therefore be available for a further surgical approach.

Surgical treatment

Definitive surgical treatment aims at removal of the gonad inappropriate to the chosen role together with correction of the external genitalia. In a 'boy' this implies hysterectomy and salpingectomy, orchidopexy if possible and repair of hypospadias. The vagina does not usually require removal but bilateral mastectomy may well be necessary at puberty. In a 'girl' orchidectomy and phallectomy are required. While the ovotestis can often be divided to remove the inappropriate half, where doubt exists it is better excised completely. Supplementary hormone treatment is likely to be required after puberty in a number of cases.

Mixed gonadal dysgenesis

The term mixed gonadal dysgenesis or asymmetric gonadal dysgenesis was introduced to describe the association of a dysplastic testis with a contralateral fibrous streak gonad (Sohval, 1964). This syndrome is usually the result of 45 X/46 XY chromosomal mosaicism probably following the loss of a Y chromosome from a cell line in early embryonic development as a result of mitotic nondysjunction or anaphase lag. Less often the disorder arises from more complex mosaic patterns such as 45 X/47 XYY or 45 X/46XY/47 XYY.

Morphology

In the classic form of mixed gonadal dysgenesis due to 45 X/46 XY mosaicism the external genitalia are abnormal with an enlarged phallus and a urogenital sinus. A dysgenetic testis which may be intra-abdominal or may lie in the labioscrotal fold is present on one side while the gonad on the opposite side is represented by fibrous tissue without any recognizable germinal cells lying in the position of an ovary. The histological appearance of this streak gonad is indistinguishable from that found in Turner's syndrome or pure XX or XY gonadal dysgenesis (*see* Chapter 42). A uterus which may be very hypoplastic is almost invariably present together with a fallopian tube on the side of the

fibrous streak. The dysgenetic testis is usually associated with a vas and an epididymis and the absence of a fallopian tube on this side indicates that antimüllerian hormone secretion by the dysplastic testis occurred normally during the early stages of genital differentiation.

While the combination of a dysgenetic testis and a streak gonad with abnormal genital differentiation is the most common expression of 45 X/46 XY mosaicism bilateral dysgenetic testes with apparently normal male external genitalia have been described, as have bilateral streak gonads with a completely female external genital pattern. It is clear that this chromosomal anomaly can have a wide phenotypic expression which is probably related to the distribution and the relative proportions of the two cell lines.

Clinical features

The appearance of the external genital anomaly in mixed gonadal dysgenesis is similar to that seen in other intersexual states and there is usually an enlarged phallus and a urogenital sinus. While there is considerable variation in the degree of masculinization of the genitalia many such children are raised as males. Patients with the disorder often show features of Turner's syndrome as a result of expression of the 45 X cell line (Davidoff and Federmann, 1973). In particular short stature is common and minor stigmata such as hypertelorism, a broad chest with hypoplastic nipples and webbing of the neck may be present (*Figure 45.3*). Breast development does not occur in the untreated case and uterine bleeding is not to be expected. Children raised as males usually show fairly good virilization at the time of adolescence with near normal circulating levels of testosterone. However, normal spermatogenesis does not occur and infertility is the rule.

There is an increased incidence of tumour formation in the intra-abdominal dysgenetic gonads. Benign gonadoblastoma is the most common neoplasm but it may be replaced by dysgerminoma or another malignant germ cell tumour. Such tumours arise during the first two decades and there is general agreement that the intra-abdominal dysgenetic gonads should be removed at an early age. The risk of malignancy in a normally descended gonad is less clear and there is debate as to whether extra-abdominal

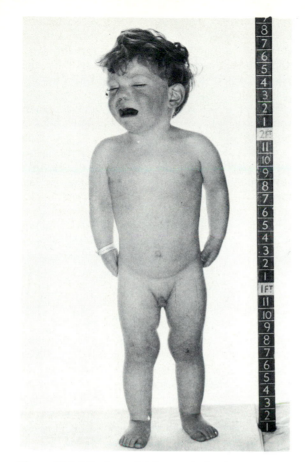

Figure 45.3. Mixed gonadal dysgenesis showing Turner's syndrome features in a boy with hypospadias, a unilateral streak gonad and a poorly developed testicle.

dysgenetic testes should be removed in children who have been brought up as males and can ordinarily be expected to show virilization at puberty.

Diagnosis

Although mixed gonadal dysgenesis can sometimes be recognized because of the somatic stigmata of Turner's syndrome or suspected because a single gonad is felt in a patient with anomalous genitalia, full chromosome analysis is required to demonstrate the presence of 45 X/46 XY mosaicism. Examination of a buccal smear is not sufficient because the chromatin-negative pattern is identical to that seen in normal males, and quinacrine staining shows Y-fluorescence in a proportion of the cell nuclei. In a small proportion of cases mosaicism is not detected since there is limited distribution of the 45 X cell line and then the karyotype appears to be a normal 46 XY. As in hermaphroditism laparotomy with gonadal biopsy is usually required to evaluate the morphology and the degree of development of the internal genital structures and thereby to obtain information that can be of value in deciding on the most appropriate gender. Further surgical management follows the lines suggested above for true hermaphroditism.

References

Davidoff, F. and Federmann, D.D. (1973) Mixed gonadal dysgenesis. *Pediatrics*, **52**, 725

Josso, N., Crouchy, J. and de Auvert, J. (1965) True hermaphroditism with XX–YY mosaicism, probably due to double fertilization of the ovum. *Journal of Clinical Endocrinology and Metabolism*, **25**, 114

Kasdan, R., Nankin, H.R., Troen, P., Wald, N., Pan, S. and Yanaihara, T. (1973) XX hermaphrodite and XX male siblings. *New England Journal of Medicine*, **288**, 539

Polani, P.E. (1970) Chromosome phenotypes – sex chromosomes in congenital malformations. Proceedings of the Third International Conference on Congenital Malformations (edited by Clarke Fraser, F. and McKusick, V.A.). International Congress Series, No. 204. Excerpta Medica, Amsterdam and New York. p.233

Rosenberg, H.S., Clayton, G.W. and Hsu, T.C. (1963) Familial XX hermaphroditism. *Journal of Clinical Endocrinology and Metabolism*, **23**, 203

Saenger, P. (1976) Presence of H-Y antigen and testis in 46 XX true hermaphrodite. *Journal of Clinical Endocrinology and Metabolism*, **43**, 1234

Sohval, A.R. (1964) Mixed gonadal dysgenesis, a variety of hermaphroditism. *American Journal of Medicine*, **36**, 281

Van Niekerk, W.A. (1976) True hermaphroditism, an analytic review. *American Journal of Obstetrics and Gynecology*, **126**, 890

46 Disorders of Sexual Development: Investigation and General Management

David B. Grant

The disorders of sexual development are discussed in detail in the previous chapters. This one aims to provide an outline guide to the assessment and the general management of these conditions.

The embryological and hormonal aspects of normal genital development are considered in Chapter 35. In particular the importance of the sex chromosomes in determining gonadal differentiation, the tendency of the internal and external genitalia to follow a female pattern in the absence of gonads, and the dual role of the testes in masculinizing the external genitalia and promoting involution of the müllerian ducts have been discussed.

Three rather broad groups of intersexual disorders can arise as a result of failure of normal development. They are the following:

1. Disorders due to abnormal gonadal differentiation and development
2. Imperfect masculinization in males with apparently normal testes (male pseudo-hermaphroditism)
3. Virilization of the external genitalia in females with normal ovaries and müllerian structures (female pseudohermaphroditism).

While a more detailed list of the causes of intersexual disorders is given in *Table 46.1* a completely satisfactory aetiological classification is not possible for several reasons. First, relatively little is known about the factors that regulate gonadal development and the initial differentiation of the internal ducts and the urogenital sinus. For example the presence of testes in XX males and the genital anomalies found in many dysmorphic syndromes cannot be entirely explained by current concepts of normal development. Secondly, although cytogenetic methods have clarified the nature of

Table 46.1 Aetiological classification of intersex disorders with their chromosome patterns

Abnormal gonadal differentiation and development

Turner's syndrome (45 X)
Pure gonadal dysgenesis (46 XX; 46 XY)
Agonadism or rudimentary testes (46 XY)
Mixed gonadal dysgenesis (45 X/46 XY)
True hermaphroditism (46 XX; 46 XY; 46 XX/46 XY; etc.)
XX males (46 XX)
Klinefelter's syndrome (47 XXY)
Various dysmorphic syndromes (46 XX; 46 XY)

Male pseudohermaphrodites (46 XY)

Impaired Leydig cell activity
    Enzyme defects in testosterone biosynthesis
    Leydig cell hypoplasia
    Fetal gonadotrophin deficiency
Impaired androgen metabolism by peripheral tissues
    5-alpha-reductase deficiency
    Partial androgen insensitivity
    Complete androgen insensitivity (testicular feminization)
Other forms
    Persistent müllerian structures (hernia uteri inguinale)
    ?Iatrogenic
    Various dysmorphic syndromes

Female pseudohermaphrodites (46 XX)

Congenital adrenal hyperplasia
Iatrogenic
Maternal virilizing tumour
Various dysmorphic syndromes
Local lesions

several intersexual disorders, classifications based on chromosome analyses are not satisfactory. For instance a 45 X/46 XY karyotype usually causes the syndrome of mixed gonadal dysgenesis but it has also been found in pure gonadal dysgenesis, Turner's syndrome and true hermaphroditism. Thirdly, a range of phenotypes have been described in male pseudohermaphroditism and it is not clear whether these represent separate entities or are different expressions of a single biochemical abnormality. Finally, a variety of phenotypic anomalies have been described in cases with abnormal differentiation and development of the testes, depending on the stage of development at which primary testicular failure occurred.

Clinical diagnosis

The author believes that it is useful to consider these disorders under the following clinical headings:

1. Patients in whom abnormal external genitalia are noted at or soon after birth
2. Children in whom an unexpected genital anomaly comes to light at examination or at laparotomy
3. Older children who show inappropriate secondary sexual development.

Abnormal genital appearance noted at birth

Generally two different types of genital anomaly are found at birth. In the first the appearance lies between the normal male and female patterns and ranges from a largely female picture with some enlargement of the clitoris to an almost completely male one with chordee and perineal hypospadias (*Figure 46.1*). Intermediate abnormalities with partial fusion of the labial folds and either a single urethral opening or separate urethral and vaginal orifices form a spectrum between the two extremes. In the second type there is no hypospadias but the penis and the scrotum are very underdeveloped and the testes usually impalpable. Alternatively

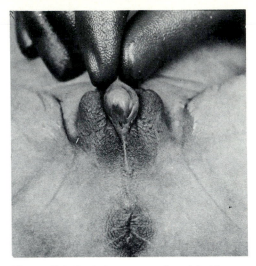

Figure 46.1. Genital appearance in a girl with congenital adrenal hyperplasia showing a single opening at the base of the phallus which is surrounded by rugose labioscrotal folds.

bilateral cryptorchidism may be associated with a relatively normal penis and scrotum.

The causes of these two types of genital anomaly differ and they are considered separately. Penile hypospadias is a relatively common malformation and is infrequently associated with other genital anomalies. Thus it is not discussed here.

Ambiguous genital appearance

It must be emphasized that the general appearance of the external genitalia is of very little help in defining the aetiology of the disorder, which is an essential step in planning long-term management. In the initial clinical assessment a history of a similar condition in other family members or of hormone treatment during pregnancy may shed light on the likely diagnosis. Careful examination for other anomalies may identify one of the dysmorphic syndromes known to be associated with abnormal genital development. However, the most important aspect of the examination is careful palpation to locate the gonads, and the choice of initial investigations is determined by these findings (*Figure 46.2*).

If *no gonads are palpable* the most likely diagnosis is female pseudohermaphroditism due to congenital adrenal hyperplasia, and this is virtually certain if symptoms of salt loss develop.

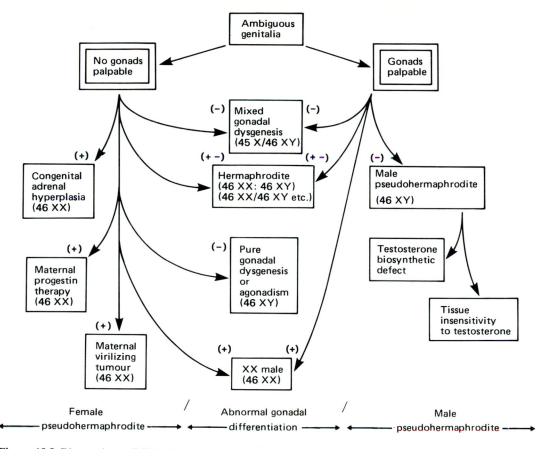

Figure 46.2. Diagnostic possibilities in abnormal external genital development. The nuclear chromatin pattern (+ or −) and the karyotypes are also shown.

An elevated urinary 17-oxosteroid excretion rate is the biochemical hallmark of the three types of virilizing adrenal hyperplasia, the commonest being caused by 21-hydroxylase deficiency. The next most frequent variety is due to 11-hydroxylase deficiency which is not associated with salt loss and the rarest results from 3-beta-hydroxysteroid-dehydrogenase deficiency which almost invariably causes severe salt loss. Initial investigation of either urinary steroid excretion or plasma 17-alpha-hydroxyprogesterone is indicated together with a buccal smear to confirm that the patient is chromatin positive. In relatively mild cases the results of steroid excretion tests may not be unequivocally abnormal in very early infancy and repeated investigations, possibly with adrenal stimulation, may be needed to establish the diagnosis.

If the steroid excretion rates do not confirm the presence of congenital adrenal hyperplasia and there is no history of hormone treatment during pregnancy or evidence of maternal virilization, more detailed investigation is necessary. Full chromosome studies and laparotomy with gonadal biopsy may be required to identify mixed gonadal dysgenesis, hermaphroditism, or the relatively unusual situation of cryptorchidism in a male pseudohermaphrodite. Patients with XY-gonadal dysgenesis or agonadism occasionally show some clitoral enlargement and again laparotomy with gonadal biopsy is required with chromosome analysis to establish the diagnosis.

When *both gonads are palpable* in the scrotum or the labial folds the most likely diagnosis is male pseudohermaphroditism due either to a defect in testosterone biosynthesis or more likely to tissue insensitivity to androgen. Full chromosome analysis is usually indicated to exclude a 46 XX or mosaic karyotype, and if a 46 XY pattern is found gonadal biopsy is rarely required. Estimation of plasma testosterone and related androgen levels, if necessary using stimulation with HCG, may provide evidence of a defect in testosterone or dihydrotestosterone synthesis. However, most male pseudohermaphrodites show normal testosterone production after HCG stimulation and further investigation to define the nature of the disorder is difficult, particularly as methods for studying the binding and metabolic effects of androgens *in vitro* are not yet available for routine clinical use.

In rare cases with bilateral palpable gonads the karyotype is 46 XX and surgical exploration is indicated to determine whether the patient is an XX male with hypospadias or a hermaphrodite with bilateral ovotestes. Very rarely a 45 X/46 XY karyotype is found and again laparotomy and gonadal biopsy are probably indicated.

The presence of only *one palpable gonad* raises the possibility of either mixed gonadal dysgenesis with a 45 X/46 XY karyotype or hermaphroditism with a separate testis and ovary on different sides. Chromosome analysis, laparotomy and gonadal biopsy are usually required.

Additional investigations such as genitography with contrast medium or pelvic ultrasound may be useful in some patients, especially those with mixed gonadal dysgenesis or true hermaphroditism. The presence of a well formed vagina with or without a uterus may influence the decision on the most suitable gender.

Underdeveloped male genitalia

In newborn infants without hypospadias but with a very small penis and scrotum (*Figure 46.3*) the differential diagnosis usually lies between rudimentary testes and gonadotrophin deficiency either as an isolated defect or in association with other anterior pituitary disorders. Neonatal hypoglycaemia strongly suggests the last. Marked hypotonia and severe feeding difficulties point to the Prader-Willi syndrome. Other congenital anomalies may indicate one of the many conditions associated with male hypogonadism such as the Laurence-Moon-Biedl syndrome. A chromatin-positive buccal smear is found in patients with Klinefelter's syndrome and in XX males and chromosome analysis differentiates these disorders.

Estimation of gonadotrophin levels after stimulation with LH-RH, and of testosterone concentrations following HCG administration is

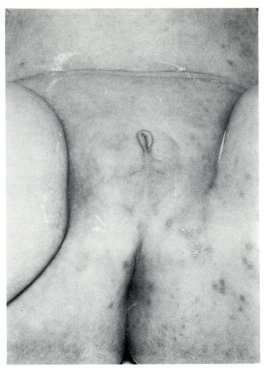

Figure 46.3. Severe micropenis in an infant with a 46 XY karyotype and rudimentary testes.

usually helpful in this group of patients during the first weeks of life when there is commonly increased gonadotrophin and testosterone secretion. An exaggerated response to LH-RH, especially of FSH, together with a poor rise in the plasma testosterone level after HCG clearly indicates the presence of rudimentary or vanishing testes. An absent or trivial response to LH-RH strongly suggests gonadotrophin deficiency. In the latter situation the testosterone response to HCG is often also severely impaired.

Incidental finding of abnormal genital development

The discovery of testes in an apparently normal girl at herniorrhaphy or laparotomy is the commonest of these situations. Most such children have male pseudohermaphroditism due to complete tissue insensitivity to androgen (testicular feminization syndrome) and it is best to preserve the testes to allow spontaneous feminization at adolescence. In some cases previously unrecognized enlargement of the clitoris indicates that tissue insensitivity is not complete and raises the possibility that virilization will occur at puberty. In these patients there is probably a strong case for early gonadectomy. Rarely laparotomy for another condition reveals a normal uterus and fallopian tubes with fibrous streak gonads in an apparently normal girl. This condition of pure gonadal dysgenesis, which can be associated with either a 46 XX or a 46 XY karyotype, usually presents due to lack of secondary sexual development at the time of puberty (see below).

Very infrequently herniorrhaphy or laparotomy demonstrates the presence of a uterus and fallopian tubes in a male with normal testes and accessory structures. This disorder of hernia uteri inguinale results from failure of the testes to induce müllerian regression and is inherited as a recessive condition.

Inappropriate sexual development in later childhood

In girls relatively mild congenital adrenal hyperplasia occasionally presents with virilization of the external genitalia in later childhood. Similarly in some male pseudohermaphrodites the genitalia may be considered entirely female at birth and the condition only becomes evident when virilization takes place at puberty. Identification of gonads in the labia virtually confirms the latter diagnosis. Very rarely adolescent virilization brings to light unsuspected mixed gonadal dysgenesis of 45 X/46 XY karyotype or true hermaphroditism. In all these situations virilization by an androgen-secreting adrenal or ovarian tumour is the most important differential diagnosis.

In boys gynaecomastia at adolescence is common and is rarely due to any obvious disorder. Sometimes it is a presenting feature of Klinefelter's syndrome, true hermaphroditism or some types of male pseudohermaphroditism. Again the most important differential diagnosis is an adrenal or testicular tumour.

Absence of female secondary development is a feature of Turner's syndrome and pure gonadal dysgenesis. Primary amenorrhoea and scant growth of body hair with normal breast development are the commonest presenting features of complete androgen insensitivity (testicular feminization).

Lack of normal male secondary sexual development is usually due to genetically determined delayed puberty but can be caused by many general medical disorders. In a small proportion of cases it results from gonadotrophin deficiency or the condition of vanishing testes. In most disorders causing delayed puberty the diagnosis can be established by endocrine and chromosomal investigation and surgical exploration is not commonly called for.

General management and choice of gender

Most parents are very distressed when they learn that there is uncertainty about the sex of their child and they often press for an early answer as they fear that it may grow up to be neither male nor female. The temptation to give a provisional assignment of gender must be avoided until the nature of the condition is known and an informed answer can be given.

In the newborn the decision on the most appropriate gender is mainly based on the appearance of the external genitalia, particularly the amount of erectile tissue in the phallus, and on the likely pattern of secondary sexual development at puberty. While it is relatively easy to predict the pattern of adolescent development in many intersexual disorders this aspect can be very difficult in some male pseudohermaphrodites with genital tissues that respond poorly to androgens. It is probably safe to conclude that patients with disorders caused by defective testosterone biosynthesis will show an adequate response to androgen therapy at the time of puberty. In doubtful cases early treatment with a short course of three injections of depot testosterone 50 mg at monthly intervals may clarify whether the phallus is likely to respond to androgens in later life.

The karyotype has virtually no direct bearing on the choice of gender. However, it often has indirect importance in elucidating the nature of the disorder and allowing prediction of the likely pattern of adolescent development.

In some cases detailed knowledge of the histological features of the gonads is valuable in deciding on future gender. For example in patients with bilateral ovotestes it is important to assess whether the ovarian or testicular components predominate. Investigation of potential gonadal endocrine function with stimulation tests may be helpful in some of these subjects. The question of future fertility is not relevant in deciding on gender in most male pseudohermaphrodites and patients with abnormal gonadal differentiation because few of them escape germ cell failure. This is not the case in the majority of female pseudohermaphrodites, who have essentially normal potential for childbearing, and there is usually little doubt that these patients should be raised as girls.

Although in the neonatal period psychological and social considerations are relatively unimportant in Western cultures, in some societies the advantages of being male far outweigh all other factors in the parents' view of their child's future. Psychological and social factors become much more important, and are often decisive, when a change of sex assignment is considered in older children. Examples are a child with micropenis who has been brought up as a boy

because of the chromosomal findings but has no prospect of functional genitalia in later life, and a female with congenital adrenal hyperplasia who has been mistakenly raised as a male and could have normal reproductive function if the sex were reassigned. In many cultures it may be impossible for the family to accept a change of gender after early infancy even if the child has not yet established his own gender identity.

Management of male pseudohermaphrodites who have been raised as girls and show pubertal virilization and some potential for male sexual function can also be extremely difficult. Change of gender is unacceptable to most families but the author is aware of a few patients who decided for themselves that they wish to be male. Adolescents faced with this problem should be aware that they have the alternative choices of further virilization and its implications or gonadectomy to prevent it. While this can usually be explained to the patient and family in terms of the bisexual potential present in every individual it is important to have experienced psychological assistance in such cases.

47 Gonadal Tumours

D. Innes Williams

Gonadal tumours, although rare, have features that give them scientific interest beyond the immediate clinical problem. For instance advances in the knowledge of teratoma have resulted from the study of ovarian tumours in the embryonic stage (Stevens, 1976) while the biochemical activity of tumour cells evidenced by the excretion of tumour markers has provided an important instrument for assessing the progress of disease. From the pathological viewpoint testicular and ovarian tumours have much in common despite the differences of anatomy in presentation and it is therefore convenient to consider them together.

Testicular tumours

Testicular tumours are much less commonly encountered than malignancies of the kidney or the lower urinary tract. Marsden and Steward (1968) estimated that when considering only fatal cases of solid tumour in children under 15 years less than 0.5 per cent arise in the testicle. Other assessments give higher figures, perhaps due to the fact that a fatal outcome is rare in some forms of neoplasm. The British Testicular Tumour Panel (Brown, 1976) derived 4.4 per cent of its specimens from children and of these some 40 per cent were yolk-sac tumours. Next in order of frequency were paratesticular rhabdomyosarcomas and differentiated teratomas, and other forms were represented by only a few examples. The peaks of age incidence were in the first 3 years and later around puberty.

Most testicular tumours present with symptomless enlargement, of insidious onset, of the testicle. Pain is uncommon in the early stages and older boys often conceal their knowledge of the swelling for some time before seeking medical advice. A more abrupt presentation with pain and slight pyrexia occurs in malignant teratomas of prepubertal boys. Clinical examination usually leaves little doubt as to the diagnosis since the mass is hard, irregular and opaque on transillumination. Hydrocele may accompany the tumour and in the common hydrocele of infancy the possibility of a tumour must be eliminated by careful transillumination and, if necessary, palpation after the aspiration of fluid. Torsion may be a differential diagnosis in the case of acute onset and it, too, requires surgery. Tumour in an undescended testis may be of any histology (Batata and Whitmore, 1980).

Full investigation of suspected testicular tumour requires thorough clinical examination of the abdomen, the breasts and the genital tract, and a search for enlarged lymph nodes at distant sites and particularly in the left scalene area. Intravenous urograms may give an important indication of the presence of enlarged abdominal nodes from the position of the ureters. Chest X-rays are obligatory. Although lymphography has been regarded as a useful investigation in some centres, cannulation of the pedal lymphatics in infants presents considerable difficulty and the procedure is very time consuming. Moreover, involved nodes often fail to opacify.

For these reasons lymphography has largely given way to ultrasound and CT scanning. The choice between these two methods depends upon local availability of equipment and expertise. Most paediatric centres now have well staffed ultrasound units capable of achieving excellent delineation of posterior abdominal wall structures and therefore of enlarged lymph nodes. Full blood counts are required in all these children and biochemical estimations should include plasma testosterone, alpha-fetoprotein (AFP) and beta-HCG levels.

As with testicular tumours in adults some cases are finally diagnosed only at operation. Exploration should be undertaken through an inguinal incision. The cord is isolated and a soft clamp applied. The testicle is then mobilized and the tunica vaginalis opened to inspect the organ. At this stage the diagnosis is usually obvious and the surgeon can proceed to orchidectomy without removing the clamp, tying the vessels as high up as possible. In a few cases a biopsy with frozen-section histology is required.

The investigations and the operative findings should enable satisfactory staging on the following scheme:

1. Stage I. No evidence of spread beyond the testicle.
2. Stage II. Lymph-node involvement in the iliac or para-aortic region but confined to areas below the diaphragm.
3. Stage III. Lymph-node involvement of mediastinal and scalene nodes.
4. Stage IV. Generalized metastases in lung, bone, liver, and so on.

The pathological classification of testicular tumours in children, as in adults, is an area of vigorous debate and some terminological confusion. The scheme adopted here is that put forward by the British Testicular Tumour Panel and fully described by Pugh (1976). The classification used in most American works is set out by Mostofi and Price (1973). The reader is referred to these works for full discussions of the origin, the pathogenesis and the histological characteristics of testicular tumours. Overall results with the various categories were reported by Exelby (1980).

Yolk-sac tumour

This rapid-growing malignant tumour is variously known as endodermal sinus tumour, orchidoblastoma, embryonal carcinoma and adenocarcinoma of the infant testicle. Following the work of Teilum (1959, 1965, 1971) it is now usually believed to be derived from extra-embryonic yolk-sac tissues because of the resemblance of the cellular pattern to that seen in human yolk-sac endoderm and in the endodermal sinus of the rat (a structure not found in the human). Similar cellular elements are occasionally found in teratomas and seminomas and some pathologists regard the tumour as teratomatous in origin. Yolk-sac tumours are also found, though less often, in the ovary and rarely in the sacrococcygeal region.

In the testicle most cases present during the first 3 years of life with painless enlargement and are not clinically distinguishable from teratomas. However, characteristically there is an associated considerable rise in the serum AFP level, which falls to normal after complete extirpation of the tumour. The marker may thus indicate the nature of the pathological cells and the presence of metastases. Interestingly alpha-fetoprotein values may be slightly raised in malignant teratomas and this may correlate with the inclusion of yolk-sac cellular elements.

The primary treatment is radical orchidectomy and the histological diagnosis can be made only after this operation. Subsequent management depends upon the age of the child and the evidence of spread of the disease. Overall mortality figures of 60 per cent were quoted by Woodtli and Hedinger (1974) but younger children usually do well. Those with a short history and no evidence of lymph-node involvement are almost always cured by orchidectomy alone. Thus in the boy of 2 years or less when radiological films and ultrasound scans are negative for enlarged nodes it is advisable to follow the progress of the AFP concentration. If it falls to normal within 3 months no further treatment needs to be administered, although supervision by chest X-ray and AFP estimation should continue at 3-month intervals for 3 years. When the abdominal nodes are enlarged or high AFP levels persist yet there is no evidence of mediastinal or generalized metastases radical nodal dissection or radiotherapy should be considered.

The surgical approach is seldom adopted in British practice, although it has enthusiastic protagonists in North America. Young, Mount and Foote (1970) regarded the case in favour of radical surgery to be unproven since those series with higher survival rates after dissection include many children with negative nodal histology. Radiotherapy is employed in the author's cases but is of doubtful benefit. The place of chemotherapy is also debatable and insufficient evidence is available to indicate any specific regimen. In the very young boy suffering from stage I disease it can scarcely be justified as a postoperative routine. However, in children over 2 years or with a long history of tumour it might perhaps be so employed. In cases of stage II tumours chemotherapy can be used as an adjuvant to radiotherapy, and in disseminated disease it is the treatment of choice. Until some clearer guidance emerges a regimen similar to that for rhabdomyosarcoma using vincristine, actinomycin and cyclophosphamide should be employed.

Teratoma

The fully differentiated teratoma is sometimes erroneously described as a dermoid and is a characteristic tumour of young boys, although it is perhaps no more than half as common as the yolk-sac tumour. Again boys in the first 3 years of life are chiefly affected and the presentation is unremarkable. On section and histological examination the tumour shows cysts and solid masses of squamous epithelium, bone, cartilage, fibrous and adipose tissue, and sometimes neural elements. In adults with superficially similar tumours it is not uncommon to find malignant areas but this is very rare in children. The disease is essentially benign and no dissemination is found. Levels of tumour marker substances are not elevated and simple orchidectomy suffices for cure.

At the other end of the scale of differentiation the malignant anaplastic teratomas (teratocarcinomas) scarcely ever occur in the prepubertal male and need not be considered here. The 'malignant teratoma intermediate' of the British Testicular Tumour Panel classification is encountered in older children from 8 years upwards and follows the same pattern as in adult life. Gynaecomastia is an occasional feature and the beta-HCG level may be raised. If so it provides a useful marker for assessing progress because the AFP concentration is less often affected. For the malignant teratoma postoperative chemotherapy and irradiation of the lymph nodes should be routine even if there is no evidence of metastasis. Where bulky nodes are present surgical excision of residual masses followed by further chemotherapy may be required (Peckham, 1976). The therapeutic regimen devised by Einhorn and Donoghue (1977) has been successful in adult cases and will probably be adopted for children.

Rhabdomyosarcoma

This tumour characteristically arises in the paratesticular tissue of the cord structures rather than in the epididymis. While the lesion is small the testicle may be palpable as a separate mass so that a clinical diagnosis of rhabdomyosarcoma may be made. There are no hormonal effects and no nodal tumour markers. The age incidence ranges from infancy through childhood to adolescence and early adult life.

The prognosis is best in early childhood and when the diagnosis is made before metastasis has occurred. Once the para-aortic nodes are involved the outcome is likely to be fatal even when radical nodal dissection is undertaken. Recent experience of aggressive chemotherapy for rhabdomyosarcoma in other sites suggests that it should be possible in future to save some of these children.

Seminoma

This characteristic tumour of young adults is very rarely seen in childhood and then only in the later years. There are no features peculiar to early presentation and the reader is therefore referred to the adult literature.

Sertoli cell and mesenchymal tumours

In this group are a variety of tumours that Mostofi (1959) regarded as derived from the specialized gonadal stroma on the principle that Sertoli cells, Leydig cells and interstitial fibroblasts have a common origin. Granulosa cell tumours of the ovary may have a similar histological appearance. The term androblastoma was used by Teilum (1958) but the word suggests a malignant tumour with marked androgenic effects, which is not the case.

These tumours can occur at any age and the British Testicular Tumour Panel found they comprised 1.2 per cent of a whole series, seven out of 32 occurring during the first decade of life. They are relatively small tumours often with cystic change and well demarcated from the testicle. Histologically epithelial and stromal elements are found and the former are often arranged in columns or tubules. While Mostofi indicated that 10 per cent only are malignant metastasis can occur in children as well as in adults. Isosexual precocity has been recorded, as has gynaecomastia in postpubertal cases (Gabrilove *et al.*, 1980). Insufficient information is available with regard to tumour markers. The need for postorchidectomy treatment by radical nodal dissection, radiotherapy or chemotherapy must be determined by the degree of malignancy as judged histologically and the evidence of spread from radiological or ultrasound data.

Leydig cell tumour

The Leydig cell tumour is often discussed because of its remarkable endocrine effects, although it is very rare. It can occur at any age and many childhood examples are recorded. This tumour is ordinarily unilateral and the bilateral cases described may be in fact examples of adrenocortical hyperplasia. Leydig cell tumours are relatively small and slow-growing, often appearing at around 4–5 years of age. Attention is frequently directed towards the testicle only after signs of isosexual precocity are noticed. There is acceleration of growth and muscular development and pubic hair appears together with facial hair and acne. The penis enlarges and erections occur. The opposite testicle remains infantile in size. Surprisingly in adolescent boys gynaecomastia may be a feature. Pathologically the Leydig cell tumour is a well defined lobulated growth which is yellowish-brown in colour. It contains histologically compact masses of strongly eosinophilic cells with granular and sometimes vacuolated cytoplasm. Crystalloids of Reinke are an occasional feature but are not necessary for diagnosis. Approximately 10 per cent of such tumours overall are malignant but no prepubertal fatal case has been described.

Endocrinologically the cells produce testosterone, 4-androstenedione and dehydroepiandrosterone. Clinically the plasma testosterone level is raised, as is the urinary excretion rate of 17-oxosteroids. Some excess oestrogen is also produced.

Orchidectomy should suffice for treatment, although evidence of malignancy must be sought. After operation signs of precocity regress but the temporary acceleration of the growth processes results in premature fusion of bony epiphyses and ultimately the child's full stature is not reached (Turner, 1976).

Lymphoma and leukaemia

Although lymphoblastoma may on rare occasions affect the child's testicle and Burkitt's syndrome does so more often, the common problem is in leukaemia. A child with acute lymphoblastic leukaemia in remission due to chemotherapy may develop a unilateral or bilateral testicular swelling. A study by Pincott and Ransley (1979) demonstrated the frequency with which leukaemia cells can be found histologically in the testicles in these circumstances. There is an immediate response to chemotherapy, which is the treatment of choice for the testicle.

Gonadoblastoma

Tumours of the dysgenetic gonad were fully reviewed by Scully (1953, 1970) and named by him gonadoblastoma, and they occur chiefly in intersexual states. The gonad may be identifiable as an underdeveloped and undescended testis in a phenotypic male or may be represented only by a fibrous streak found in the anatomical position of an ovary. Eighty per cent of cases occur in phenotypic females with or without virilization, but when the karyotype is determined a Y chromosome is almost always present. The lesion may be unilateral or bilateral. While such tumours are seldom large they may completely replace the gonad so that its original nature is obscured. Histologically the cells are of two types. Some are large with rounded vesicular nuclei and vacuolated cytoplasm and are probably of germinal origin. Others resemble Leydig cells and are smaller and often arranged around the margin of laminated Call-Exner-like bodies. Hormonal effects may be evident clinically, as a rule in the shape of virilization, although the initial intersexual state may cause confusion. Mackay (1974) showed that the gonadoblastoma was capable of secreting both androgens and oestrogens.

Gonadoblastomas must be considered benign tumours but seminoma-like areas can be seen and on very rare occasions metastasis occurs. Other types of tumour may be found in association in the same or the opposite gonad.

Miscellaneous tumours

In the epididymis the adenomatoid tumour believed to be of müllerian-remnant origin seldom occurs in childhood. It is benign. Cystadenoma of the epididymis is associated with Lindau's disease. Fibroma and fibrosarcoma are recorded occasionally. Haemangiomas affect the external genitalia often and the testicle exceptionally. Secondary tumours are rare while spread of nephroblastoma down the spermatic cord is widely recognized.

Ovarian tumours

Tumours of the ovary may seem to be of less immediate concern to the urologist, but because of both their presentation as pelvic masses and their endocrine effects a familiarity with their general characteristics is essential. A high proportion of these tumours are cystic and, although many cysts are not true tumours, for the clinician's convenience they are all described together here. In the past almost all ovarian tumours were suspected on clinical examination and diagnosed at laparotomy. This is particularly true of the common case where torsion occurs and the child presents with an acute abdomen.

However, it is desirable to go through a series of investigations before operation—not only to establish the diagnosis beyond doubt but also to determine whether local removal of the cyst, complete salpingo-ovariectomy or wider excision should be undertaken. Intravenous urograms not infrequently show outward displacement of the ureters and pressure upon the bladder. Ultrasound demonstrates a simple or loculated cystic swelling, or in the case of malignant disease a solid mass with possible extensions. In such cases a search must be made for distant metastases. With solid tumours the AFP level should be estimated since in the case of a yolk-sac tumour it is helpful to follow serum levels postoperatively. Cases with endocrine effects require appropriate hormone assays in addition.

Follicular cysts

Minute pinhead cysts are commonly observed on the surface or deep within the normal ovary in the child. They represent atretic follicles after the disappearance of the oocytes and usually involute spontaneously. Some continue to enlarge and present as an abdominal swelling or with an acute episode of torsion. Many authors group them together with lutein cysts. They are not neoplastic. Huffman (1968) found 19 per cent of children's ovarian tumours to be of this type.

Follicular cysts do not usually enlarge beyond 12 cm in diameter and they are unilocular, smooth-walled and lined by a thin layer of granulosa cells. Haemorrhage sometimes fills them with bloody fluid. They can present in the neonate or later in childhood as pelvic masses or can be found during laparotomy, for instance at the time of appendicectomy. At operation it is usually possible to distinguish the healthy ovarian tissue and therefore to excise only the cyst. They have a tendency to undergo torsion, in which case total ovariectomy may be required.

Some girls with precocious puberty are found to have solitary or multiple follicular cysts, although it is by no means always certain that they are the causative lesion. Where possible they should be excised and this operation is followed by a regression of precocious signs (Monteleone, 1973) but it is not justifiable to perform bilateral ovariectomy.

Cystadenoma

Serous and pseudomucinous cystadenomas are among the commonest ovarian tumours and occur at all ages. The simple variety is benign while the papillary forms may be malignant. All are slow-growing and usually painless, and are discovered as a result of abdominal enlargement, torsion or necrosis. Serous cystadenomas are seldom very large. They are translucent and ovarian cystectomy is an acceptable treatment. Papillary tumours are frequently bilateral and are multilocular with doughy areas containing papillomatous masses. Papillary formations may occur on the outer surface in which case the cystadenoma spreads to other pelvic organs even though histologically it appears benign. Necrosis and rupture may also disseminate the papillary tumour. The cysts should never be opened or drained within the abdomen and should be removed complete and examined outside the body. Pseudomucinous cystadenomas contain jelly-like fluid and may reach an enormous size but do so more commonly in adolescence or adult life. Externally they are smooth, shiny and lobulated, and they seem to contain solid areas. Salpingo-ovariectomy is the treatment of choice.

The frankly malignant forms are cystic or semisolid serous cystadenocarcinomas with papillary outgrowths and are associated with ascites and involvement of adjacent organs.

Teratoma

Benign cystic teratomas or dermoids are common. They are composed of well differentiated tissues which are sometimes epidermal in nature such as skin, hair and teeth and also of derivatives of all three tissue layers. While the dermoids have a soft cystic consistency in the body the contents when cooled outside form a sticky putty-like substance. Some solid areas are always present.

Dermoids present with abdominal swelling or torsion. Occasionally their presence causes local irritation and chronic pain or frequency. Radiologically they may be diagnosed by the presence of teeth. They are benign and can be treated by simple ovariectomy or even cystectomy.

Malignant teratomas are relatively uncommon in childhood. They are small solid tumours that invade adjacent organs at an early stage. Welch (1979) reviewed the relevant literature and recognized four types: immature, a tumour of intermediate malignancy with a 56 per cent survival rate; embryonal, corresponding to teratocarcinoma of the testis with a 30 per cent

survival rate; chorionic, which is exceptionally rare in childhood; and neurectodermal. The last named has a tendency to diffuse abdominal metastatic spread, and later to spontaneous involution and a benign course. Salpingo-ovariectomy is appropriate for the malignant teratoma and should be followed by chemotherapy and radiotherapy.

Yolk-sac tumour

This tumour, the embryonal carcinoma, has already been described in its testicular form. In the ovary it has a later onset and is more apt to follow a malignant course. It is symptomless in the early stages and therefore likely to have involved the pelvic wall before being diagnosed. AFP estimations may be helpful for diagnosis and monitoring progress. Ovariectomy or biopsy should be followed by radiotherapy and chemotherapy.

Dysgerminoma

The dysgerminoma is the counterpart of the seminoma of the testis and may be histologically indistinguishable. However, a greater proportion of cases present in the early years of life. The tumour spreads to local lymph nodes and invades adjacent organs relatively early on. It therefore presents as a painful swelling in the pelvis. The right side is more commonly involved. Local excision of the tumour is undertaken at the time of laparotomy. The opposite ovary and the uterus should be preserved if possible. As with seminoma, radiotherapy has a dramatic effect and is routine whatever stage has been reached. Cure rates are encouraging and figures such as 95 per cent survival for localized disease and 78 per cent after spread are quoted. Nevertheless, mixed tumours containing malignant teratoma as well as dysgerminoma elements have a poor prognosis. Hormonal effects described with dysgerminoma are probably due to the inclusion of other elements.

Granulosa cell tumour

This is the commonest hormone-producing neoplasm and like the Leydig cell tumour of the testis the precocity it causes has given it greater notoriety than its numbers justify. These tumours may be unilateral or bilateral. They are relatively small and solid with small areas of cystic degeneration and necrosis. Histologically the cells resemble the granulosa cells of the normal follicle and are arranged in an alveolar pattern. The degree of differentiation varies and some lesions are frankly malignant.

Characteristically the presentation is of isosexual precocity. There is an acceleration of growth, breast development, pubic hair and pubertal changes in the external genitalia. Although uterine bleeding occurs it does not show any periodicity, a fact that on the history may distinguish it from the very much commoner precocious puberty. On examination a mass is palpable, while it may not be large and may require bimanual palpation under anaesthesia to detect it. Hormone studies reveal raised oestrogen and progestin levels. For the usual benign tumour ovariectomy suffices and careful follow-up is required.

Other tumours

Involvement of the ovary is seen during the course of prolonged treatment of leukaemia in childhood and the clinical situation closely parallels that seen in testicular involvement. Sarcomas are recorded and very rarely masculinizing arrhenoblastomas. Yolk-sac tumours and mesenchymal tumours occur as in the male. Rhabdomyosarcomas may arise in the broad ligament region. Secondary tumours are very unusual in childhood.

References

Batata, M.A. and Whitmore, W.P. (1980) Cryptorchidism and testicular cancer. *Journal of Urology*, **124**, 382

Brown, N.J. (1976) Testicular tumours in children. *In* Pathology of the Testis (edited by Pugh, R.C.B.). Blackwell, Oxford. p.79

Einhorn, L.H. and Donoghue, J.P. (1977) Improved chemotherapy in disseminated testicular cancer. *Journal of Urology*, **117**, 65

Exelby, P.R. (1980) Testicular cancer in children. *Cancer*, **45**, 1803

Gabrilove, J.L., Freiberg, E.K., Leiter, G. and Nicolis, G.L. (1980) Feminizing and non-feminizing Sertoli cell tumours. *Journal of Urology*, **124**, 757

Huffman, J. (1968) The Gynaecology of Childhood and Adolescence. Saunders, Philadelphia

Mackay, A.M. (1974) Tumours of dysgenetic gonads (gonadoblastomas): ultrastructural and steroidogenic aspects. *Cancer*, **34**, 1108

Marsden, H.G. and Steward, J.K. (1968) Recent results in cancer research. *In* Tumours in Children. Springer, Berlin. p.1

Monteleone, J.A. (1973) Pseudoprecocious puberty associated with isolated follicular cyst of the ovary. *Journal of Pediatric Surgery*, **8**, 949

Mostofi, F.K. (1952) Infantile testicular tumours. *Bulletin of the New York Academy of Medicine*, **28**, 684

Mostofi, F.K. (1959) Tumors of specialized gonadal stroma in human male patients. *Cancer*, **12**, 944

Mostofi, F.K. and Price, E.B. (1973) Tumors of the male genital system. *In* Atlas of Tumor Pathology, Second Series. AFIP, Washington, DC

Peckham, M.J. (1976) *In* Scientific Foundations of Urology, Vol. 2 (edited by Williams, D.I. and Chisholm, G.D.). Heinemann, London. p.400

Pincott, J.R. and Ransley, P.G. (1979) Personal communication

Pugh, R.C.B. (1976) Pathology of the Testis. Blackwell, Oxford

Scully, R.E. (1953) Gonadoblastoma: a gonadal tumor related to the dysgerminoma (seminoma) and capable of sex-hormone production. *Cancer*, **6**, 455

Scully, R.E. (1970) Gonadoblastoma: a review of 74 cases. *Cancer*, **25**, 1340

Stevens, L.C. (1976) *In* Scientific Foundations of Urology (edited by Williams, D.I. and Chisholm, G.D.). Heinemann, London.

Teilum, G. (1958) Classification of testicular and ovarian androblastoma and Sertoli cell tumors: a survey of comparative studies with consideration of histogenesis, endocrinology and embryological theories. *Cancer*, **11**, 769

Teilum, G. (1959) Endodermal sinus tumors of the ovary and testis: comparative morphogenesis of the so-called mesonephroma ovarii (Schiller) and extraembryonic (yolk-sac-allantoic) structures of the rat's placenta. *Cancer*, **12**, 1092

Teilum, G. (1965) Classification of endodermal sinus tumour (mesoblastoma vitellinum) and so-called "embryonal carcinoma" of the ovary. *Acta Pathologica et Microbiologica Scandinavica*, **64**, 407

Teilum, G. (1971) Special Tumors of Ovary and Testis. Munksgaard, Copenhagen

Turner, W.R. (1976) Leydig cell tumour in identical twins. *Urology*, **7**, 194

Welch, K.J. (1979) Ovarian Tumours. *In* Pediatric Surgery, 3rd edn (edited by Ravitch, M.M., Welch, K.J., Benson, C.D., Aberdeen, E. and Randolph, J.G.). Yearbook Medical Publishers, Chicago. p.1437

Woodtli, W. and Hedinger, C. (1974) Endodermal sinus tumor or orchioblastoma in children and adults. *Virchows Archiv. A. Pathological Anatomy and Histology*, **364**, 93

Young, P.G., Mount, B.M. and Foote, F.W. (1970) Embryonal adenocarcinoma in the prepubertal testis. *Cancer*, **26**, 1065

48 Adrenocortical Tumours and Cushing's Syndrome

David B. Grant and D. Innes Williams

The great majority of adrenocortical tumours occurring during childhood are endocrinologically active and present as a result of excessive steroid secretion, usually with either virilization or Cushing's syndrome or a combination of these two clinical patterns. Feminizing tumours and aldosterone-secreting tumours are very uncommon, as are hormonally inactive neoplasms. The main clinical importance of tumours of the adrenal cortex lies in the facts that they may mimic other virilizing disorders such as congenital adrenal hyperplasia which require medical as opposed to surgical treatment and that relatively early diagnosis is often possible because of the endocrine manifestations. In addition cortisol-secreting tumours may lead to serious hazards in the postoperative period.

Pathological features

Tumours of the adrenal cortex are most common in early childhood, often presenting between the ages of 2–4 years but sometimes becoming manifest during the first year or in later childhood. These lesions are about twice as common in girls and are sometimes related to other congenital disorders such as hemihypertrophy (Fraumeni and Miller, 1967). They may also be associated with nonadrenal malignant tumours: for example two of the authors' patients died as a result of second tumours (these were an osteogenic sarcoma and a medulloblastoma) following successful removal of an adrenal one. Similar cases were described by Levine (1978).

In the literature carcinomas appear to be commoner than adenomas (Gilbert and Cleveland, 1970) but it is often difficult to distinguish between the two on histological examination

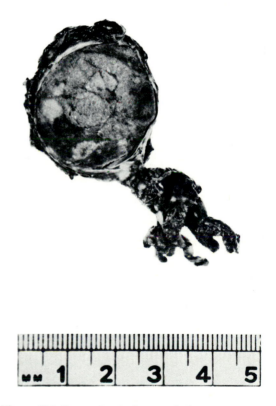

Figure 48.1. Encapsulated adrenocortical tumour removed at operation from the patient illustrated in *Figure 48.4.*

557

because frequent mitoses and cellular pleomorphism can occur in both types. The macroscopic appearance probably gives a better guide to the prognosis. Adenomas are usually relatively small, that is 1–5 cm in diameter, with a smooth well defined capsule (*Figure 48.1*) and a yellowish colour on cut section. Small areas of haemorrhagic necrosis or calcification may be present. Carcinomas are generally larger with more marked areas of necrosis. The capsule is poorly defined or incomplete and the tumour is adherent to adjacent structures. Histological examination shows breaching of the capsule by tumour cells with invasion of blood vessels in the surrounding tissues (special staining may be required to detect the latter). Metastases, as a rule in the liver or the lung, may be present at the time of diagnosis.

There is usually no obvious correlation between the histological appearance of the tumour and the pattern of steroid synthesis. However, the authors anticipate that cell culture studies will reveal selective enzyme defects. While some tumours have the potential to synthesize cortisol or testosterone others can only produce intermediate compounds such as dehydroepiandrosterone.

Most adrenocortical tumours are probably largely autonomous with regard to steroid production. A few cases have been reported in which the tumour was stimulated by ACTH (Korth-Schutz *et al.*, 1977).

There have been a number of reports of Cushing's syndrome due to tumours arising outside the adrenal cortex, for example neuroblastomas and ganglioneuromas. It is still uncertain whether this is due to ectopic ACTH production or to steroid secretion by the tumour itself.

Atrophy of the contralateral gland is almost invariable in cortisol-secreting adrenal tumours and occurs as a result of suppression of pituitary ACTH secretion. The zona glomerulosa which secretes aldosterone and is largely controlled by the renin-angiotensin system is usually normal in the contralateral gland. This adrenal atrophy, which does not occur with pure virilizing tumours, can lead to adrenal insufficiency in the postoperative period (see below).

Clinical and endocrinological features

Virilizing tumours

The classic features of virilizing tumours are growth of pubic hair and enlargement of the penis or clitoris. Acne and greasiness of the hair with an adult body odour are common, as are

(b)

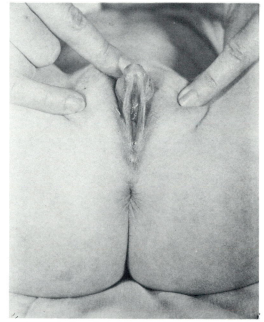

(a)

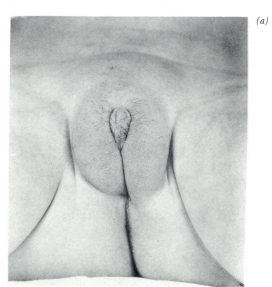

Figure 48.2. Adrenocortical adenoma. The external genitalia of this 2-year-old girl show enlargement of the clitoris, rugosity of the labia and development of pubic hair.

acceleration of growth and bone maturation. Although examination may reveal an abdominal mass this is relatively uncommon.

In boys the main differential diagnoses are non-salt-losing congenital adrenal hyperplasia and true precocious puberty. The latter can usually be excluded on clinical examination because the testes are infantile. In girls the differential diagnoses are very mild virilizing congenital adrenal hyperplasia and premature pubarche, that is premature growth of pubic hair as a result of androgen secretion by normal adrenal glands (*Figure 48.2*). The presence of clitoral enlargement and the absence of breast development exclude true precocious puberty.

Laboratory investigation may show grossly elevated urinary 17-oxosteroid excretion rates which are largely due to excess secretion of the weakly androgenic steroid dehydroepiandosterone which can also be estimated in plasma. In some cases urinary 17-oxosteroid levels are only moderately elevated and raised plasma testosterone concentrations account for the virilization. As a rule dexamethasone suppression tests clearly indicate the presence of a tumour as opposed to congenital adrenal hyperplasia and premature pubarche. In the latter condition the urinary and plasma steroids are suppressed completely after 3 days administration of dexamethasone 4–8 mg/day, and this does not happen if a tumour is present. As noted above a few tumours are ACTH-dependent and in these cases dexamethasone leads to incomplete suppression.

Tumours causing Cushing's syndrome

The clinical features of Cushing's syndrome, namely a round plethoric face, obesity (particularly of the trunk) and striae are well known. However, recognition of the disorder is often

Figure 48.3. Cushing's syndrome due to bilateral adrenal hyperplasia. *(a)* Pretreatment. *(b)* Two years after bilateral adrenalectomy.

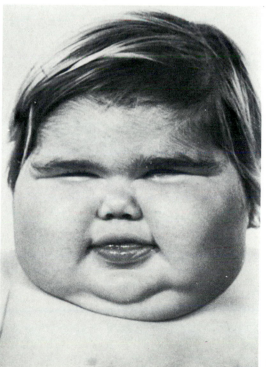

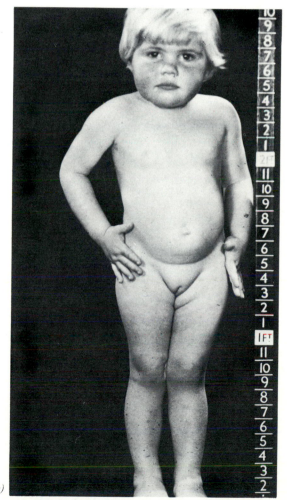

(a) *(b)*

delayed in young children since their rosy cheeks and generous build are popularly considered signs of vigorous good health. The authors have seen patients in whom the diagnosis was not considered for many months because of this. In extreme cases there is stunting of growth with osteoporosis, myopathy, hypertension and glycosuria.

The main differential diagnosis is excessive cortisol secretion as a result of bilateral adrenal hyperplasia (*Figure 48.3*). This is usually due to excess stimulation by pituitary ACTH (Cushing's disease) and occasionally to ectopic ACTH secretion by a neuroblastoma or other tumour. In general the younger the patient the more likely is the diagnosis of an adrenal tumour, although in some cases presenting soon after birth bilateral nodular adrenal hyperplasia is present (Klevit *et al.*, 1966). The nature of the latter condition is largely unknown and it does not seem to be caused by excessive production of pituitary ACTH.

Cushing's syndrome is sometimes suspected in cases of simple obesity, particularly if striae are present, but can normally be readily excluded by laboratory investigation. Probably the most useful test is estimation of morning and late evening plasma cortisol concentrations. In Cushing's syndrome the two values are very similar because of loss of the normal circadian pattern which by contrast is preserved in simple obesity. Urinary steroid studies are often less helpful since 17-hydroxysteroid levels are increased in obesity. However, in this case they are suppressed by low doses of dexamethasone 0.5–2.0 mg/day and this test has its advocates. More complicated techniques such as estimation of the cortisol production rate by isotopic dilution are occasionally required in difficult cases.

Having established the presence of excess cortisol secretion a suppression test with high doses of dexamethasone is generally indicated to differentiate an adrenal tumour from bilateral hyperplasia. Marked reductions in plasma and urinary steroid concentrations occur in bilateral hyperplasia due to pituitary overactivity and there is little change when a tumour is present. In adults estimation of plasma ACTH by radioimmunoassay has been helpful in distinguishing between an adrenal tumour, ectopic ACTH secretion and pituitary-dependent disease. The respective findings are undetectable, markedly elevated and high normal ACTH levels. While this may also be the case in children the authors' experience with the method has been disappointing because some patients with bilateral hyperplasia show very low ACTH values erroneously suggesting the presence of a tumour.

Tumours causing both virilization and Cushing's syndrome

A combination of some virilization with features of Cushing's syndrome is relatively common. The exact clinical manifestations depend on the relationship between androgen and cortisol secretion. If the latter predominates then growth and bone age may be retarded and vice versa.

Whereas the clinical features of Cushing's syndrome serve to distinguish the condition from congenital adrenal hyperplasia or premature pubarche it must be noted that hirsutism with growth of pubic hair is common in patients with pituitary-dependent Cushing's disease. Nevertheless, the presence of penile or clitoral enlargement virtually excludes the latter diagnosis.

Feminizing tumours

Tumours that produce gynaecomastia with no evidence of virilization are very uncommon in children and Bhettay and Bonnici (1977) were able to find only eight cases of feminizing tumours in the paediatric age range. Most of these tumours are adenomas in contrast to the high proportion of carcinomas reported in adults. In prepubertal boys the most important differential diagnosis is a testicular tumour. In girls the clinical features may closely mimic true precocious puberty but menstruation is unusual (*Figure 48.4*). Urinary 17-oxosteroid excretion was raised in all but one of the reported cases and usually provides an important clue to the diagnosis (Bhettay and Bonnici, 1977).

While gynaecomastia is not a feature of congenital adrenal hyperplasia it has been recorded in 11-hydroxylase deficiency. At adolescence gynaecomastia is common and is rarely due to a serious endocrine disorder.

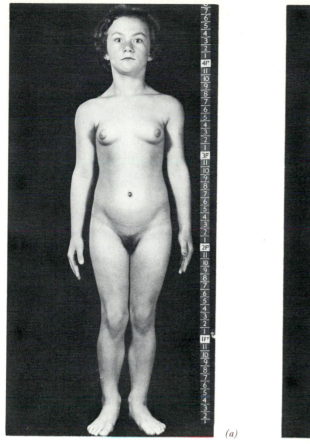

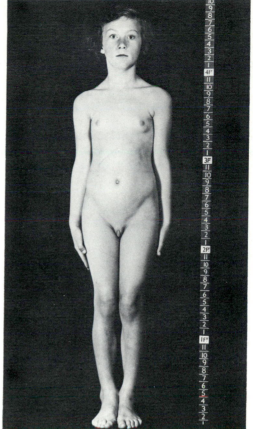

(a)

(b)

Figure 48.4. Feminizing adrenocortical tumour in an 8-year-old girl. *(a)* Pretreatment. *(b)* One year after adrenalectomy.

Aldosterone-secreting tumours

Aldosterone-secreting tumours are very uncommon in children and Kafrouni *et al.* (1975) found just six cases below the age of 16 in their survey of the literature. The clinical features are similar to those described in adults, with hypertension, polyuria and hypokalaemia as the salient features. Plasma renin activity is suppressed, thus differentiating the condition from Bartter's syndrome in which hypokalaemia is associated with elevated plasma renin activity (Dillon, Shah and Mitchell, 1979). Removal of the adrenal tumour resulted in full clinical and biochemical cure in all the reported cases.

As in adults excess aldosterone secretion is occasionally due to bilateral adrenal hyperplasia but this is very uncommon (Grim *et al.*, 1967). Bilateral adrenalectomy may be necessary in these cases.

Localization of adrenal tumours

While the presence of an adrenal tumour can be strongly suspected from the clinical and endocrinological findings its localization is necessary for correct surgical management. When a large tumour is present it may be detected on clinical examination and its presence confirmed by a plain abdominal X-ray which shows displacement of the renal shadow and calcification within the tumour. Further investigation is then probably unnecessary. However, in the majority of cases, especially when a small adenoma is present, detailed investigation is called for. The classic methods of intravenous urography and tomography are being supplanted by newer techniques, in particular abdominal ultrasound.

Perirenal insufflation is now rarely performed and has been largely replaced by selective arteriography in difficult cases. Computed tomography of the abdomen or adrenal scanning with isotopically labelled iodocholesterol may also be helpful, although the authors' limited experience with these methods has been rather disappointing.

If the tumour is very small, exact localization is not always possible. In such cases surgical exploration by the anterior approach may be needed to inspect both adrenal glands.

Operative treatment

In young infants large tumours can be satisfactorily approached from the front through a long transverse incision. In older children a thoracoabdominal incision may be better but for a small adenoma the simple loin approach through the bed of the 12th rib is adequate.

When using the laparotomy incision the left adrenal gland is best demonstrated by drawing the spleen forward and incising the lienorenal fold of the peritoneum. Continued gentle traction on the spleen is helpful while the vessels are identified and ligated. On the right the colon and, if necessary, the duodenum are mobilized by an incision along their lateral borders exposing the kidney, which is gently pushed downwards, together with the adrenal above it. The gland itself must be cautiously freed from the surrounding areolar tissue and the veins ligated in continuity before they are cut. On the right a short straight vein enters the vena cava directly and must be carefully sought if troublesome haemorrhage is to be avoided.

With large tumours there may be a few remnants of normal adrenal tissue on the surface which are inevitably removed with the growth. Small adenomas are apt to shell out during mobilization but it is probably wise to remove the gland intact because of the risk of malignancy.

Postoperative management

Very careful medical supervision is required following removal of a tumour associated with features of Cushing's syndrome. The contralateral gland is likely to be atrophic and severe shock and hypotension occur unless generous amounts of cortisol are given in the postoperative period (Raiti *et al.*, 1972). This is not a risk with tumours causing pure virilization although it can occur in the mixed form with cushingoid features. Some information on the state of the contralateral gland can be obtained by preoperative measurement of plasma cortisol levels. If the late evening values are low then adrenal suppression is unlikely. In doubtful cases it is probably wise to assume that adrenal atrophy has occurred and large doses of parenteral hydrocortisone 100–150 mg/m^2 per day should be given. Salt-retaining hormone is not usually required since aldosterone secretion is not suppressed. The dose of hydrocortisone should be reduced progressively to reach physiological replacement levels of 20–30 mg/m^2 per day 8–12 days after surgery, and then slowly phased out over the next 2–3 months. By this time ACTH secretion is likely to be normal and the remaining gland should have recovered full function. During this phase steroid therapy should be doubled or tripled if there is severe stress or infection. After about 3 months steroid cover should no longer be necessary.

Postoperative follow-up

After removal of the tumour the signs of virilization or Cushing's syndrome usually regress almost completely unless there is residual or metastatic tumour tissue. During follow-up plasma or urinary steroid determinations can be used to detect tumour recurrence before clinical signs become manifest. Metastatic disease or local recurrence of the tumour can occur several years after surgery but generally declares itself within a few months. Further surgical treatment is rarely possible and the prognosis is poor. While most tumours respond unsatisfactorily to radiotherapy the drug mitotane (o,p'DDD) may be of some help in arresting tumour growth because it causes necrosis of adrenal cells. This agent has been used extensively in adults with adrenal carcinoma (Lubitz, Freeman and Okun, 1973) but there is relatively little information on its place in the management of children with disseminated adrenal carcinoma.

Cushing's disease due to bilateral adrenal hyperplasia

During the past decade it has become apparent that pituitary-dependent Cushing's disease is not as uncommon in childhood as was once supposed. There are a number of well documented reports of its occurrence, usually after the age of 10 years. In some of these cases the disorder was relatively mild and arrest of growth with slight obesity was the only clinical manifestation (Grant and Atherden, 1979). While the clinical aspects and laboratory investigation of pituitary-dependent Cushing's disease have been outlined above, management differs to some extent from that of adrenal tumours and must be considered further.

There is still no consensus on the most appropriate treatment for pituitary-dependent Cushing's syndrome in childhood. Bilateral adrenalectomy has been the most widely used procedure and total adrenalectomy is recommended as there is no merit in subtotal resection which carries the risk of regrowth of the adrenal remnant with recurrence of symptoms. The early results of bilateral adrenalectomy are generally good with complete regression of the clinical manifestations and good catch-up growth. As with adrenal tumours generous hydrocortisone cover is indicated immediately after surgery and treatment with salt-retaining hormone is also necessary. Steroid replacement therapy is required on a life-long basis. The long-term results of bilateral adrenalectomy are less satisfactory because pituitary adenomas with excessive pigmentation (Nelson, Sprunt and Mims, 1966) are common and further treatment with pituitary surgery or radiotherapy is needed (McArthur, Hayles and Salassa, 1979).

A number of children with pituitary-dependent Cushing's disease have been treated with external irradiation (Jennings, Liddle and Orth, 1977). While this has been successful in a fairly high proportion of cases the response to treatment is relatively slow and the clinical features may not begin to resolve for many months. Pituitary function is usually normal after treatment but catch-up growth is often poor (Fontanellaz, 1971). Internal irradiation of the pituitary has also been used and Cassar *et al.* (1979) reported good results in nine patients aged 10–18 years after ^{198}Au or ^{90}Y implantation. Although this technique seems to produce a much more rapid clinical remission than external irradiation it calls for considerable technical expertise.

Corticotrophin-secreting pituitary microadenomas are probably present in a high proportion of children with pituitary-dependent Cushing's syndrome. Trans-sphenoidal exploration with removal of the microadenoma may be the treatment of choice if experienced neurosurgical assistance is easily available (Tyrrell *et al.*, 1978).

In some patients there may be a case for a trial of medical therapy, particularly since spontaneous remission has been recorded in mild cases. The serotonin antagonist cyproheptadine, which suppresses ACTH secretion in normal subjects, was used with some success by Krieger, Amorosa and Linick (1975) in a small number of adult patients. However, general experience with this drug has been disappointing. Aminoglutethimide, which is a drug that blocks early steroid biosynthesis, has been used with some success in a few patients. Metyrapone inhibits 11-hydroxylation and has also been used to block cortisol biosynthesis. It is probably most useful in preparing severely ill patients for surgery or reducing the symptoms while waiting for external irradiation of the pituitary to take effect.

References

Bhettay, E. and Bonnici, F. (1977) Pure oestrogen-secreting feminizing adrenocortical adenoma. *Archives of Disease in Childhood*, **52**, 241

Cassar, J., Doyle, F.M., Mashiter, K. and Joplin, G.F. (1979) Treatment of Cushing's disease in juveniles with interstitial pituitary irradiation. *Clinical Endocrinology*, **11**, 313

Dillon, M.J., Shah, V. and Mitchell, M.D. (1979) Bartter's syndrome: 10 cases in childhood. Results of long-term Indomethacin therapy. *Quarterly Journal of Medicine*, **48**, 429

Fontanellaz, H-P. (1971) Das Cushing-syndrom im kindesalter. *Helvetica Paediatrica Acta*, **26**, 28

Fraumeni, J.F. and Miller, R.W. (1967) Adrenocortical neoplasms with hemihypertrophy, brain tumours and other disorders. *Journal of Pediatrics*, **70**, 129

Gilbert, M.G. and Cleveland, W.W. (1970) Cushing's syndrome in infancy. *Pediatrics*, **46**, 217

Grant, D.B. and Atherden, S.M. (1979) Case report: Cushing's syndrome presenting with growth failure. Clinical remission during cyproheptadine therapy. *Archives of Disease in Childhood*, **54**, 466

Grim, C.E., McBryde, A.C., Glenn, J.F. and Gunnells, J.C. (1967) Childhood primary hyperaldosteronism with bilateral adrenocortical hyperplasia: plasma renin activity as an aid to diagnosis. *Journal of Pediatrics*, **71**, 377

Jennings, A.S., Liddle, G.W. and Orth, D.N. (1977) Results of treating childhood Cushing's disease with pituitary irradiation. *New England Journal of Medicine*, **297**, 957

Kafrouni, G., Oakes, M.D., Lurvey, A.N. and de Quattro, V. (1975) Aldosteronism in a child with localization by adrenal vein aldosterone: review of literature. *Journal of Pediatric Surgery*, **10**, 917

Klevit, H.D., Campbell, R.A., Blair, H.R. and Bongiovanni, A.M. (1966) Cushing's syndrome with nodular adrenal hyperplasia in infancy. *Journal of Pediatrics*, **68**, 912

Korth-Schutz, S., Levine, L.S., Roth, J.A., Saenger, P. and New, M.I. (1977) Virilizing adrenal tumour in a child suppressed with dexamethasone for three years: effect of o,p'-DDD on serum and urinary androgens. *Journal of Endocrinology and Metabolism*, **44**, 433

Krieger, D.T., Amorosa, L. and Linick, F. (1975) Cyproheptadine-induced remission of Cushing's disease. *New England Journal of Medicine*, **293**, 893

Levine, G.W. (1978) Adrenocortical carcinoma in two children with subsequent primary tumours. *American Journal of Diseases of Children*, **132**, 238

Lubitz, J.A., Freeman, L. and Okun, R. (1973) Mitotane use in inoperable adrenal cortical carcinoma. *Journal of the American Medical Association*, **223**, 1109

McArthur, R.G., Hayles, A.B. and Salassa, R.M. (1979) Childhood Cushing's disease: results of bilateral adrenalectomy. *Journal of Pediatrics*, **95**, 214

Nelson, D.H., Sprunt, J.G. and Mims, R.B. (1966) Plasma ACTH in 58 patients before or after adrenalectomy for Cushing's syndrome. *Journal of Clinical Endocrinology and Metabolism*, **26**, 722

Raiti, S., Grant, D.B., Williams, D.I. and Newns, G.H. (1972) Cushing's syndrome in childhood: post-operative management. *Archives of Disease in Childhood*, **47**, 597

Tyrrell, J.B., Brooks, R.M., Fitzgerald, P.A., Cofoid, P.B., Forsham, P.H. and Wilson, C.B. (1978) Cushing's disease: selective trans-sphenoidal resection of pituitary micro-adenomas. *New England Journal of Medicine*, **298**, 753

Index